NAD	nicotinamide adenine dinucleotide
NMS	neuromuscular spindle
P	pressure
P_B	barometric pressure
P_A	pressure in the alveoli
P_G	pressure of a gas
PaO_2	partial pressure of oxygen in arterial blood
P_AO_2	partial pressure of oxygen in the alveoli
$PaCO_2$	partial pressure of carbon dioxide in arterial blood
P_ACO_2	partial pressure of carbon dioxide in the alveoli
PvO_2	partial pressure of oxygen in venous blood
$PvCO_2$	partial pressure of carbon dioxide in venous blood
PO_2	partial pressure of oxygen
PCO_2	partial pressure of carbon dioxide
PN_2	partial pressure of nitrogen
P_i	inorganic phosphate
PC	phosphocreatine
pH	hydrogen ion concentration
PNF	proprioceptive neuromuscular facilitation
$\dot{Q}$	cardiac output
R_a	rate of appearance
R_d	rate of disappearance
R	resistance
RER	respiratory exchange ratio
RH	relative humidity
RHR	resting heart rate
RM	repetition maximum
ROM	range of motion
RPP	rate pressure product
RQ	respiratory quotient
RV	residual volume
$SaO_2\%$	percent saturation of arterial blood with oxygen

$SbO_2\%$	percent saturation of blood with oxygen
$SvO_2\%$	percent saturation of venous blood with oxygen
SBP	systolic blood pressure
SSC	stretch shortening cycle
SO	slow, oxidative muscle fibers
SR	sarcoplasmic reticulum
ST	slow-twitch muscle fibers
STPD	standard temperature and pressure, dry air
SV	stroke volume
T	temperature
Tamb	ambient temperature
Tco	core temperature
Tre	rectal temperature
Tsk	skin temperature
Ttym	tympanic temperature
TC	total cholesterol
TPR	total peripheral resistance
URTI	upper respiratory tract infection
V	volume
V_D	volume of dead space
V_E	volume of expired air
V_G	volume of a gas
V_I	volume of inspired air
V_T	tidal volume
$\dot{V}O_2cons$	volume of oxygen consumed
$\dot{V}O_2max$	maximal volume of oxygen consumed
$\dot{V}O_2peak$	peak volume of oxygen consumed
$\dot{V}CO_2prod$	volume of carbon dioxide produced
$v\dot{V}O_2max$	velocity at maximal oxygen consumption
VC	vital capacity
VEP	ventricular ejection period
VFP	ventricular filling period
WT	weight

EXERCISE PHYSIOLOGY

for Health, Fitness, and Performance

EXERCISE PHYSIOLOGY

for Health, Fitness, and Performance

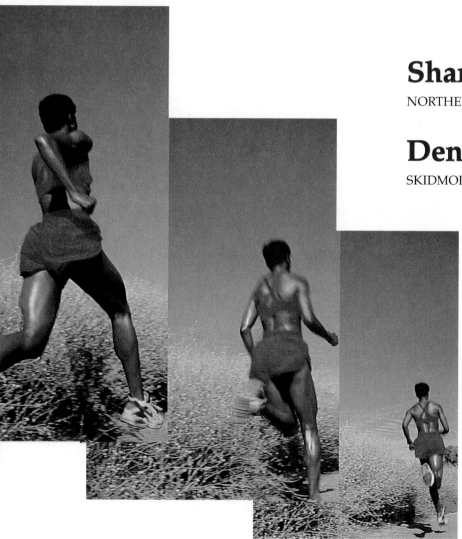

Sharon A. Plowman
NORTHERN ILLINOIS UNIVERSITY

Denise L. Smith
SKIDMORE COLLEGE

Allyn and Bacon   BOSTON   LONDON   TORONTO   SYDNEY   TOKYO   SINGAPORE

Senior Editor: Suzy Spivey
Editorial Assistant: Lisa Davidson
Marketing Manager: Quinn Perkson
Production Administrator: Deborah Brown
Editorial Production Service: Woodstock Publishers' Services
Text Designer: Deborah Schneck
Photo Director: Susan Duane
Composition and Prepress Buyer: Linda Cox
Cover Administrator: Linda Knowles
Cover Designer: Studio Nine
Manufacturing Buyer: Megan Cochran

Copyright © 1997 by Allyn and Bacon
A Viacom Company
160 Gould Street
Needham Heights, MA 02194

Internet: www.abacon.com
America Online: keyword: College Online

Library of Congress Cataloging-in-Publication Data

Plowman, Sharon A.
    Exercise physiology for health, fitness, and performance / Sharon
A. Plowman, Denise L. Smith
        p. cm.
    Includes bibliographical references and index.
    ISBN 0–205–16202–9 (casebound)
    1. Exercise—Physiological aspects.   I. Smith, Denise L.
    II. Title
QP301.P585   1996
612'.044—dc20   96–38343
                                                       CIP

Printed in the United States of America

10 9 8 7 6 5 4 3 2 1   01 00 99 98 97 96

The credits appear on page 557 following the index. They should be considered an extension of the copyright page.

To our teachers and students, past, present, and future:
sometimes one and the same.

Brief Contents

Contents

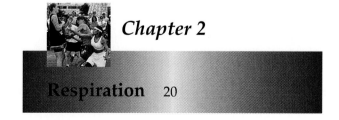

Chapter 3

Respiratory Exercise Response, Training Adaptations, and Special Considerations   47

Chapter 4

The Cardiovascular System

Chapter 5

Cardiovascular Responses to Exercise   111

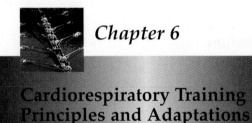

Chapter 6

Cardiorespiratory Training Principles and Adaptations

Chapter 7

Thermoregulation   172

Chapter 8

Cardiorespiratory System in Health and Disease   189

Unit

Metabolic System   211

Chapter 9

Energy Production   212

Chapter 10

Anaerobic Metabolism During Exercise   243

Chapter 11

Aerobic Metabolism During Exercise 274

Chapter 15

Body Composition and Weight Control   375

Chapter 14

Body Composition: Determination and Importance   351

Chapter 18

Muscular Contraction and Human Movement   445

Chapter 19

Muscular Principles and Adaptations   471

Chapter 20

Neuromuscular Aspects of Movement   485

List of Figures

List of Tables

Preface

The purpose of *Exercise Physiology for Health, Fitness, and Performance* is to present concepts in a clear and comprehensive way that will allow students to apply the principles of exercise physiology in the widest variety of possible work situations. The primary audience is kinesiology and physical education majors and minors, including students in traditional teaching preparation programs (with or without a coaching emphasis) and students in exercise and sport science tracts where the goal is to prepare for careers in fitness, rehabilitation, athletic training, or physical therapy.

As with other textbooks in the field, a great deal of information is presented. Most of the information has been summarized and conceptualized based on research. However, we have occasionally included specific research studies to illustrate certain points, believing that students need to develop an appreciation for research and the constancy of change that research precipitates. The chapters are thoroughly referenced and a complete list of references, in scientific format, is provided at the end of each chapter. These references should prove to be a useful resource for students to explore topics in more detail for laboratory reports or term projects.

The body of knowledge in exercise physiology is extensive and growing every day. Each individual faculty member must determine what is essential for his or her students. To this end, we have tried to allow for choice and flexibility, particularly in the organization and content of the book.

A Unique Integrative Approach

The intent of this textbook is to present the body of knowledge based on the traditions of exercise physiology but in a way that is not bound by those traditions. Instead of proceeding from a unit of basic science, through one or more units of applied science, to a final unit of special populations or situations (which can lead to the false sense that scientific theories and applications can and should be separated), we have chosen a completely integrative approach to make the link between basic theories and applied concepts both strong and logical.

Flexible Organization

The introductory chapter explains the text organization, provides an overview of exercise physiology, and establishes the basic concepts that will be covered in each unit. Three major units follow the introduction: cardiovascular-respiratory system, metabolic system, and neuromuscular-skeletal system. Although the units are presented in this order, each unit is intended to stand alone and has been written in such a way that it may be taught before or after each of the other two.

Consistent Sequence of Presentation

The chapters in each unit follow a consistent sequence of presentation: basic anatomy and physiology (including neuro-hormonal regulation), the measurement and meaning of variables important to understanding exercise physiology, exercise responses, training principles and adaptations, and special applications, problems, and considerations.

Basic Sciences It is assumed that the students using this text will have had a basic course in anatomy, physiology, chemistry, and math. However, it is also acknowledged that reviewing specific aspects of these courses is essential for many students. Some students do not need this review and for them the basic chapters can be de-emphasized.

Measurement Inclusion of the measurement sections serves two purposes. The first purpose is to identify how the variables most frequently used in exercise physiology are obtained. The second purpose is to contrast criterion or laboratory test results, essential for accurate determination and understanding of the exercise responses and training adaptations, with field test results, often the only items available to the professional in school or health club settings.

Exercise Responses and Training Adaptations The chapters or sections on exercise responses and training adaptations present the definitive and core information for exercise physiology. The exercise response chapters are organized by exercise modality and intensity. Specifically, physiological responses to the following five categories of exercise (based on the duration, intensity, and type of muscle contraction) are presented: (1) short-term, light to moderate dynamic aerobic submaximal exercise; (2) long-term, moderate to heavy dynamic submaximal aerobic exercise; (3) incremental aerobic exercise to maximum; (4) static exercise; and (5) dynamic resistance exercise. Training principles specific to each unit are provided prior to the discussion of adaptations so that the student can see the connection between what must be done from an exercise prescription standpoint and what will be achieved.

Special Applications The special applications chapters always relate the unit topic to health-related fitness and then deal with such diverse topics as altitude, thermoregulation and immunology (cardiovascular-respiratory units); making weight and eating disorders (metabolic unit); and anabolic steroids (neuromuscular-skeletal unit).

Complete Integration of Age Groups and Sexes

A major departure from tradition in the organization of this text is the complete integration of information relevant to all age groups and both sexes. In the past, there was good reason to describe evidence and derive concepts based on information from male college students and elite male athletes. These were the populations most involved in physical activity and sport and they were the groups most frequently studied. As more women, children, and elderly began participating in sport and fitness programs, information became available on these groups. Chapters on females, children, and the elderly were added to the back of exercise physiology texts as supplemental material. However, most physical education and exercise professionals will be dealing with both males and females, children and adolescents in school settings, average middle-aged adults in health clubs or fitness centers, and the elderly in special programs. Very few will be dealing strictly with college-age students, and fewer still will work with elite athletes. This does not mean that information based on the young adult male populations has been excluded or even de-emphasized. However, it does mean that it is time to remove the individuals who make up most of the population from the back of the book. Therefore, we have integrated information about males and females at various ages throughout the text.

Pedagogical Considerations

Most of the pedagogical techniques used in this textbook are straightforward. These techniques include a list of learning objectives at the beginning of each chapter as well as a chapter summary, review questions, and references at the end of each chapter. Another pedagogical aid is the use of margin definitions. Terms are boldfaced and defined in the text where they first appear as well as in the margin to emphasize the context in which the terms are used. A glossary is also included.

To aid the student, a complete list of commonly used symbols and abbreviations with their meanings is printed on the front and back endpapers of the text. Each chapter contains a multitude of tables, graphs, charts, diagrams, and photographs to underscore the pedagogy and enhance the visual appeal of the text.

Unique Color Coding

A unique aspect of the graphs is color-coding for quick recognition of the condition each represents. For the exercise responses, each exercise type has its own shaded background color. Similarly, training adaptations are presented on a specific tinted background. General information graphs are coded generically. Finally, the most frequent comparisons (training status, sex, and age) have consistent line or bar profile colors. The selected colors are shown in the accompanying table.

Table of Color Coding

Unit Colors

Cardiovascular-Respiratory System

Metabolic System

Neuromuscular-Skeletal System

Background Tints

Basic or generic

Short-term, light to moderate, dynamic aerobic submaximal exercise

Long-term, moderate to heavy, dynamic aerobic submaximal exercise

Incremental aerobic exercise to maximum

Static exercise

Dynamic resistance exercise

Training adaptations

Lines or Bar Profiles

Young (<20 years)

Adult (20–50 years)

Elderly (50+ years)

Male

Female

Untrained

Trained

Active Learning

An attempt has been made to engage the student in active learning beyond just reading. In some instances, students are referred to highlighted boxes to work through problems that address their understanding of the material. Answers to these questions of understanding are presented at the end of the chapter in which they appear. In other instances, students are also asked to interpret a set of circumstances or deduce an answer based on previously presented information before continuing to read. Where appropriate, equations are highlighted and examples worked out in the text. Each chapter ends with a set of essay review questions.

Appendixes

Appendix A provides information on the metric system, units, symbols, and conversions both within the metric system and English system and between the metric and English systems. Appendix B is intended to be supplementary material. It consists of three parts, all dealing with aspects of oxygen consumption calculation.

Supplements

A comprehensive set of ancillary materials designed to facilitate classroom preparation and ease the transition into a new text is available to adopters of *Exercise Physiology*.

- **Instructor's Manual and Test Bank** prepared by the authors and Pat Fehling at Skidmore College. This comprehensive teaching tool provides chapter-by-chapter outlines with comparisons to corresponding chapters in the leading competing texts, suggested laboratory activities, answers to the review questions at the end of each chapter, and multiple-choice test questions. In addition, an appendix on incorporating the Internet into the classroom with many useful World Wide Web addresses is included as well as transparency masters.

- **Computerized Test Bank.** ESATest III, the best selling, state-of-the-art test generation software package, is available free to adopters of *Exercise Physiology*. Designed to operate on IBM (DOS and Windows) and Macintosh computers, this program allows you to create and print tests quickly, add your own questions, edit questions, scramble questions, create multiple versions of tests, and much more. In addition, ESATEST III offers many unique features, including pop-up help screens, a toll-free number for technical support, on-line testing, and a comprehensive grading system.

- **Transparency Set.** A set of 100 full-color transparency acetates representing illustrations, charts, and graphs from the text are available to adopters.

- **Presentation Package.** A presentation package with art from the text is available to qualified adopters. Ask your local Allyn & Bacon sales representative for more information.

Acknowledgments

The completion of this textbook required the help of many people. A complete list of individuals is impossible, but four groups to which we are indebted must be recognized for their meritorious assistance. The first group is our families and friends who saw less of us than either we or they desired due to the constant time demands. Their support, patience, and understanding were much appreciated. The second group contains our many professional colleagues, known and unknown, who critically reviewed the manuscript at several stages and provided valuable suggestions for revisions along with a steady supply of encouragement. This kept us going. The third group is our students who provided much of the initial motivation for undertaking the task. Some went far beyond that and pro-

vided meaningful feedback by using the text in manuscript form. The final group is the editors and staff at Allyn and Bacon whose faith in the project and commitment to excellence in its production are responsible for the finished product you now see. We thank you all.

Acknowledgment of Reviewers

The following publisher's reviewers provided excellent feedback and criticism throughout the development of the text. To the following, a grateful acknowledgment of their expertise and thorough review:

Jerry Brandon
Georgia State University

Ronnie Carda
University of Wisconsin

Jan Claiborne
Gettysburg College

James H. Johnson
Smith College

Frank A. Kulling
Oklahoma State University

Barry McKewen
University of Texas

Russel Pate
University of South Carolina

Wendy E. S. Repovich
Eastern Washington University

J. Frank Smith
St. Edward's University

Joseph F. Smith
University of Alabama

Pat Vehrs
University of Houston

Philip B. Watts
Northern Michigan University

Michael J. Webster
Western Illinois University

About the Authors

SHARON A. PLOWMAN is a Professor in the Department of Physical Education at Northern Illinois University and Director of the Exercise Physiology Laboratory. She has taught for 29 years including classes in Exercise Physiology, Stress Testing, and Exercise Bioenergetics. She has published over sixty scientific and research articles in the field with emphasis on females and children in such journals as *Annals of Nutrition and Metabolism; Medicine and Science in Sports and Exercise; Research Quarterly for Exercise and Sport;* and *Human Biology.* She is a co-author with M. H. Anshel (ed.) et al. of the *Dictionary of the Sport and Exercises Sciences* (1991).

Dr. Plowman is a Fellow in the American College of Sports Medicine and served on the Board of Trustees of that organization from 1980–1983. In 1992 she was elected an Active Fellow by the American Academy of Kinesiology and Physical Education. The American Alliance for Health, Physical Education, Recreation and Dance (AAHPERD) recognized her with the Mable Lee Award in 1976 and the Physical Fitness Council Award in 1994. Dr. Plowman received the Excellence in Teaching Award at Northern Illinois University at the department level in 1974 and 1975 and at the university level in 1975.

DENISE L. SMITH is an Associate Professor in the Department of Physical Education and Dance at Skidmore College. She has taught classes in Anatomy and Physiology, Exercise Physiology, and Cardiorespiratory Aspects of Human Performance for six years and is the Director of the Human Performance Laboratory at that institution. She has published fourteen scientific articles in such journals as *Ergonomics; European Journal of Applied Physiology; Journal of Cardiopulmonary Rehabilitation;* and *Aviation, Space and Environmental Medicine.*

Dr. Smith has served on the Executive Board and as an officer for the MidAtlantic Regional Chapter of the American College of Sports Medicine. She regularly presents her research on both the national and international levels. One of her specialties is research concerning the physiological effects of fire-fighting, and since 1994 she has been a visiting professor at the University of Illinois Fire Service Institute in Urbana–Champaign.

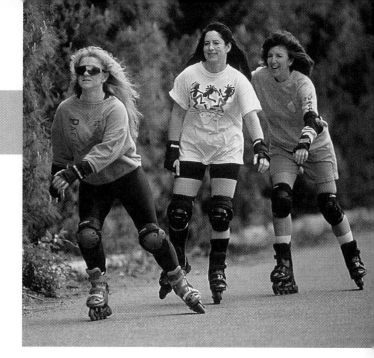

Introduction:
The Warm-Up

After studying this chapter, you should be able to:

- Describe what exercise physiology is and discuss why you need to study it.

- Identify the organizational structure of this text.

- Differentiate between exercise responses and training adaptations.

- Explain the baselines against which exercise responses and training adaptations are compared.

- List and explain the factors that must be considered in a description of the exercise response.

- Compare the levels of training adaptation.

- List and explain the training principles.

- Describe the differences and similarities between health-related and sport-specific physical fitness.

- Define and explain periodization.

- Discuss the physiological basis of exercise and exercise training as stressors.

- Identify performance, physiological and behavioral signs, and symptoms of overtraining.

What Is Exercise Physiology and Why Study It?

In a 1966 science fiction movie called *Fantastic Voyage* (CBS/Fox), a military medical team is miniaturized in a nuclear-powered submarine and injected through a hypodermic needle into the carotid artery. Anticipating an easy float into the brain, where they plan to remove a blood clot by laser beam, they are both awed and imperiled by what they see and what befalls them. They see erythrocytes turning from an iridescent blue to vivid red as oxygen bubbles replace carbon dioxide; nerve impulses appear as bright flashes of light; and when air pressure is lost, all they need to do is tap into an alveoli. All of their encounters are not so benign, however: They are sucked into a whirlpool caused by an abnormal fistula between the carotid artery and jugular vein. They have to get the outside team to stop the heart so that they will not be crushed by its contraction. They are jostled about by the conduction of sound waves in the inner ear. They are attacked by antibodies. And finally, their submarine is destroyed by a white blood cell—they are, after all, foreign bodies to the natural defense system. Of course, in the end, the "good guys" on the team escape through a tear duct and all is well.

Although the journey you are about to take through the human body will not be quite so literal, nor anywhere near as dangerous, it should be just as incredible and probably more fascinating, for it goes beyond the basics of anatomy and physiology into the realm of the moving human. The body is capable of great feats, whose limits and full benefits in terms of exercise and sport are still unknown.

Consider these events and changes, all of which have probably taken place within the life span of your parents.

- President Dwight D. Eisenhower suffered a heart attack on September 23, 1955.[11] At that time six weeks of bed rest and a lifetime of curtailed activity was normal medical treatment and advice.[6] Eisenhower's rehabilitation, including a return to golf, was, if not revolutionary, certainly progressive. Today, cardiac patients are mobilized within days and frequently train for and safely run marathons.

- The 4-min mile was considered an unbreakable limit until May 6, 1954, when Roger Bannister ran the mile in 3:59.4. Hundreds of runners (including some high school boys) have since accomplished that feat. The 1995 men's world record for the mile, which was set in 1993, is 3:44.39.

- The 800-m run was banned from the Olympics from 1928 to 1964 for women because females were "too weak and delicate" to run such a "long" distance. In the 1950s when the 800-m run was reintroduced for women in Europe, ambulances were stationed at the finish line, motors running, to carry off the casualties.[13] In 1963 the women's world marathon record (then not an Olympic sport for women) was 3:37.07, a time now commonly achieved by females not considered to be elite athletes. In 1995 the women's world record (set in 1985) was 2:21.06, an improvement of 1:16:01 (35%).

- In 1954 Kraus and Hirschland published a report indicating that American children were less fit than European children.[8] At that time being *fit* was defined as being able to pass the Kraus-Weber test of minimal muscular fitness, which consisted of one each of the following: bent-leg sit-up; straight-leg sit-up; standing toe touch; double-leg lift, prone; double-leg lift, supine; and trunk extension, prone. Today, physical fitness is more broadly defined in terms of both physiology and age span and is even more sought after.

These changes and a multitude of others that we readily accept as a normal part of our daily lives have come about as a combined result of formal medical and scientific research and informal experimentation by individuals with the curiosity and courage to try new things.

These events and changes also typify the concerns with which the broad area of exercise physiology deals—that is, athletic performance, physical fitness, and rehabilitation. **Exercise physiology** can be defined as both a basic and an applied science that describes, explains, and uses the body's re-

Exercise Physiology A basic and an applied science that describes, explains, and uses the body's response to exercise and adaptation to exercise training to maximize human physical potential.

sponse to exercise and adaptation to exercise training to maximize human physical potential.

Any single course or textbook cannot, of course, provide all the information a prospective professional in one of these related areas will need. However, a knowledge of exercise physiology and an appreciation for basing practice on research findings goes a long way in setting professionals in the field apart from mere practitioners. It is one thing to be able to lead aerobic dances. It is another to be able to design routines based on predictable short- and long-term responses of given class members, to be able to evaluate those responses, and then to be able to modify the sessions as needed. Thus, it is deemed important for the exercise science students intent on becoming respected professionals in any of the related fields to learn exercise physiology in order to:

1. Understand how the basic physiological functioning of the human body is modified by short- and long-term exercise and the mechanisms that bring about these changes. Unless one knows what responses are normal, it is not possible to recognize an abnormal response or adjust to it.

2. Be able to apply the results of scientific research to maximize health, rehabilitation, and/or athletic performance in a variety of subpopulations.

3. Be able to respond accurately to questions and to recognize and react to myths and misconceptions that appear in relation to exercise. Good advice should be based on scientifically determined evidence.

Overview of the Text

So that students can accomplish the goals just outlined, this text has been divided into three units: cardiovascular-respiratory system, metabolic system, and neuromuscular-skeletal system. Within each unit the following format is followed.

1. basic information
   a. anatomical structures
   b. physiological function, including regulatory mechanisms
   c. laboratory techniques and variables typically measured.

2. exercise responses

3. training
   a. application of the training principles
   b. adaptations to training

4. special applications, problems, and considerations

The first part of each unit deals with the basic anatomical and physiological structures and functions necessary to understand the material that follows. The next part of each unit deals with the acute responses to exercise. This is followed by a specific application of the training principles and the adaptations that typically occur if the training principles are applied correctly. Finally, each unit ends with one or more special application topics, such as thermal concerns, weight control/body composition, and osteoporosis.

This integrated approach is intended to provide fairly immediate relevancy of application of the basic information. More information continues to be available on college-age males or elite male athletes than for any other portion of the population. Wherever possible, though, we have attempted to expand beyond this base and to compare both sexes, not only as young or middle-aged adults but also as children and adolescents at one end of the age spectrum and as the elderly at the other.

Each unit is intended to be independent of the other two, although the body obviously functions as a whole. The separation is designed to provide each individual faculty member flexibility in determining the sequence of his or her course. It is possible to start with any unit and proceed in any order through the other two. This concept is represented by the circle in Figure 1.1.

The neuromuscular-skeletal unit is presented last in our sequencing (see Figure 1.1) because movement (locomotion or exercise) is the ultimate goal. For the body to perform movement, energy must be available. Hence, the metabolism unit, which deals with how fuels or substrates are used to produce the needed energy, is presented prior to the neuromuscular-skeletal unit. Most of the energy that supports muscle activity is produced through the use of oxygen. Providing that oxygen requires the combined efforts of respiration and circulation. Thus, we start with the cardiovascular-respiratory unit as the first link in the chain that proceeds through metabolism and ends with muscle action.

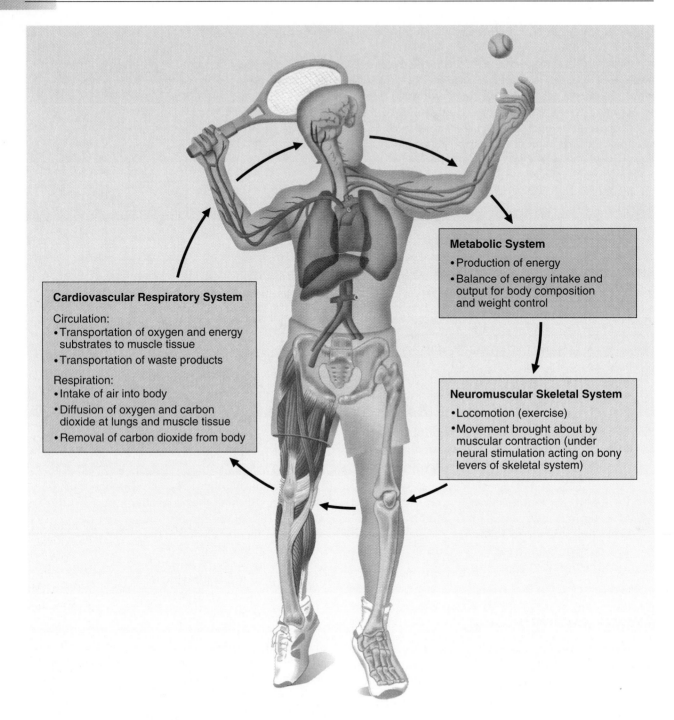

Metabolic System
- Production of energy
- Balance of energy intake and output for body composition and weight control

Cardiovascular Respiratory System

Circulation:
- Transportation of oxygen and energy substrates to muscle tissue
- Transportation of waste products

Respiration:
- Intake of air into body
- Diffusion of oxygen and carbon dioxide at lungs and muscle tissue
- Removal of carbon dioxide from body

Neuromuscular Skeletal System
- Locomotion (exercise)
- Movement brought about by muscular contraction (under neural stimulation acting on bony levers of skeletal system)

FIGURE 1.1 Schematic Representation of Text Organization

Each unit is divided into chapters as the length and depth of the material dictates. Each chapter begins with a list of learning objectives. The objectives will help you get an overall picture of what is to be presented and to understand what you should be learning in the chapter. Definitions are highlighted in the margins as they are introduced. Each chapter ends with a summary and review questions. Scattered throughout the text, primarily in separate boxes, are problems for you to complete; answers to these will also be presented at the end of each chapter. When appropriate, worked-out calculations are presented in examples. The appendices and endpapers provide supplemental information. For example, Appendix A contains a listing of the basic physical quantities, units of measurement, and conversions within the Systeme International d'Unités (SI or metric system of measurement commonly used in scientific work) and between the metric and English measurement systems. You will find on the endpapers a list of symbols and abbreviations and their meanings used throughout the book. You may need to refer to these appendices frequently since many of these symbols and measurement units may be new to you.

The field of exercise physiology is a dynamic area of study with many practical implications. At the very least over the next few months you should gain an appreciation for the tremendous range over which the human body can function. At the very best you will become better prepared as a professional for the safe and effective execution of the responsibilities of your chosen field. Somewhere along the way, you will probably also learn something about yourself. Enjoy the voyage.

*T*he Exercise Response

Let's begin with some definitions and concepts that are basic to all of the units and thus need to be established right away. **Exercise** is a single acute bout of bodily exertion or muscular activity that requires an expenditure of energy above resting level and generally results in voluntary movement. The term *physical activity,* while not completely synonymous, will be used interchangeably with exercise in this text. Where the amount of exercise can actually be measured, the term *work* or *workload* may be used as well.

Exercise disrupts the homeostatic state of the body. These disruptions or changes represent the body's response to exercise. An example with which you are undoubtedly already familiar is the elevation in heart rate that occurs with exercise. However, although all exercises require the expenditure of energy and a rise in heart rate, and most involve

the voluntary movement of muscles, not all bring about the same acute responses. Four factors need to be considered in order to determine or describe the acute response to exercise:

1.   the exercise modality
2.   the exercise intensity
3.   characteristics of the exerciser
4.   the exercise task (or test) used.

Exercise Modalities

Exercise modality (or **mode**) means the type of activity or the particular sport. For example, rowing has a very different effect on the cardiovascular-respiratory system than does football. Modalities are often classified by the type of energy demand (aerobic or anaerobic) or the major muscle action (continuous and rhythmical, resistance, or static). Walking, cycling, and swimming are examples of continuous, rhythmical aerobic activities; jumping, sprinting, and weight lifting are anaerobic and/or resistance activities. Thus, when you are trying to determine the effects of exercise on a particular system, you must first know what type of exercise is being performed.

Exercise Intensities

Exercise intensity is most easily described as maximal or submaximal. Of these, **maximal (max) exercise** is the most straightforward; it simply refers to the highest intensity, greatest load, or longest duration an individual is capable of doing. Motivation plays a large part in the achievement of maximal

---

Exercise A single acute bout of bodily exertion or muscular activity that requires an expenditure of energy above resting level and that in most, but not all, cases results in voluntary movement.

Exercise Modality or Mode The type of activity or sport; usually classified by energy demand or type of muscle action.

Maximal Exercise The highest intensity, greatest load, or longest duration exercise of which an individual is capable.

levels of exercise. Most maximal values are reached at the endpoint of an incremental work task. That is, the exercise task begins at a level the individual is comfortable with and gradually increases until he or she can do no more. The values for the physiological variables measured at this time are labeled as max; for example, maximum heart rate is symbolized as HR max.

Submaximal exercise may be described in one of two ways. The first involves a *set load*, which is a load that is known or is assumed to be below an individual's maximum. This load may be established by some physiological variable, such as working at a specific heart rate (perhaps $150 \text{ b} \cdot \text{min}^{-1}$); at a specific workload (for example, $600 \text{ kgm} \cdot \text{min}^{-1}$ on a cycle ergometer), or for a given distance (perhaps a 1-mi run). Such a load is called an **absolute workload.** If an absolute workload is used, and the individuals being tested vary in their fitness level, then some individuals will be challenged more than others. Generally, those who are more fit in terms of the component being tested will be less challenged and so will score better than those who are less fit and more challenged. For example, suppose the exercise task is to lift 80 lb in a bench press as many times as possible. If each of four individuals tested were able to lift a maximum of 160, 100, 80, and 60 lb once, respectively, it would be anticipated that the first individual could do more repetitions than anyone else. Similarly, it would be expected that the second individual could do more repetitions than the third and fourth, that the third individual could do only 1 repetition, and the fourth individual could not do any. The assumption that the load was submaximal for all individuals would not be upheld. However, the use of an absolute load does allow for a ranking among individuals in a single exercise bout and is most often the type of task used in physical fitness screenings or tests.

Absolute Submaximal Workload A set exercise load performed at any intensity from just above resting to just below maximum.

Relative Submaximal Workload A workload above resting but below maximum that is prorated to each individual; typically set as some percentage of maximum.

The second way to describe submaximal exercise is as a percentage of the maximum. Thus, a load may be set at a percentage of maximal heart rate, a percentage of the maximal ability to use oxygen, or a percentage of a maximal workload. This value is called a **relative workload** because it is prorated or relative to each individual. It is both the intent and expectation that all individuals will then be equally challenged by the task and that the same amount of time or number of repetitions can be completed by most, if not all, individuals. For example, for the individuals described in the previous paragraph, suppose that the task now is to lift 75% of the maximal load each individual could lift once as many times as possible. Now the individuals will be lifting 120, 75, 60, and 45 lb, respectively. If each person is equally motivated, there should be no meaningful difference in the total number of repetitions each can perform. Relative workloads are occasionally used in physical fitness testing. They are more frequently used to describe exercises that are light, moderate, or heavy in intensity or to give guidelines for exercise prescription.

Characteristics of the Exerciser

Certain characteristics of the exerciser can make a difference in the magnitude of the exercise response. The basic pattern of the response will be similar, but the magnitude of the response can vary with the sex, age (child/adolescent, adult, elderly) and/or physiological status such as health and training level of the individual. Where possible, we will point out these differences in response. They are important in interpreting any given individual's results.

Exercise Task (or Test) Used

The test utilized to evoke the exercise response needs to be taken into account when interpreting the results. One concern is that the mode of the test should match the system you are most interested in evaluating or have predominantly trained. For example, you cannot determine cardiovascular condition utilizing weight-lifting tests, although you may want to know how the cardiovascular system responds to such a task.

Another concern is the degree of accuracy of the test. The most accurate tests are called **criterion**

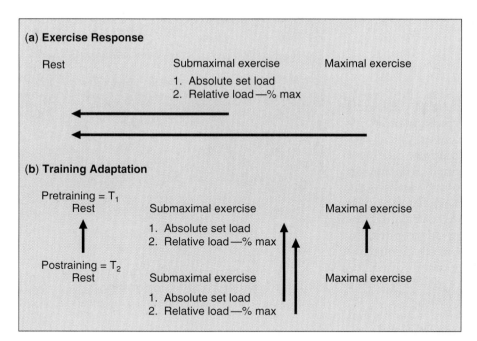

(a) Exercise Response

(b) Training Adaptation

FIGURE **1.2**

The Comparative Basis for Exercise Responses and Training Adaptations
The arrows indicate the direction of the comparisons. The baseline is at the point of the arrow.

tests; they represent a standard against which other tests are evaluated. Most criterion tests are **laboratory tests**—precise, direct measurements of physiological function that usually involve monitoring, collection, and analysis of expired air, blood, or electrical signals—and require expensive equipment and trained technicians. All laboratory tests, however, are not criterion tests.

Field tests are tests that can be conducted almost anywhere, such as school gymnasia, playing fields, or health clubs. Field tests are often performance-based and estimate the values measured by the criterion test. The mile run is a field test used to assess cardiovascular-respiratory fitness, which is more directly and accurately measured by maximal oxygen consumption ($\dot{V}O_2$max). Both laboratory and field tests will be discussed in this text.

Exercise Response Comparisons

Figure 1.2a diagrammatically depicts the comparisons that are made in describing the exercise response. Note that the baseline for the comparisons is always the resting value. That is, submaximal exercise values will be either higher, lower, or unchanged in relation to the resting value. In general, most physiological variables that are measured will be higher during submaximal exercise than at rest. The higher the exercise intensity, the greater the change from rest is. Maximal values (100% intensity) represent the greatest possible change from rest. For example, suppose that an individual has a resting heart rate of 60 b·min^{-1}, a light submaximal exercise heart rate of 110 b·min^{-1}, and a maximal heart rate of 180 b·min^{-1}. The submaximal heart rate is an increase of 50 b·min^{-1} over rest, and the maximal heart rate is a 120 b·min^{-1} increase above rest. Exercise responses also can and will be described as graphic patterns in relation to time and intensity.

Criterion Test The standard against which other tests are judged.

Laboratory Test Precise, direct measurement of physiological functions for the assessment of exercise responses or training adaptations; usually involves monitoring, collection, and analysis of expired air, blood, or electrical signals.

Field Test A test that can be conducted anywhere; is performance-based and estimates the values measured by the criterion test.

*T*raining

Training Adaptations

Training is a consistent or chronic progression of exercise sessions designed to improve physiological function for better health or sport performance (Figure 1.3). Training brings about changes typically labeled *adaptations*. **Training adaptations** represent adjustments that promote optimal functioning. Whereas exercise responses use resting values as the baseline, training adaptations are evaluated against the same condition after as opposed to before training. Figure 1.2b depicts training adaptations. At pretraining (Time$_1$, T$_1$) there are three baseline conditions: rest, submaximal exercise, and maximal exercise. After a training program of generally 8 to 20 weeks (labeled posttraining or Time$_2$, T$_2$), an individual is tested under these same conditions and the values compared with the pretraining, T$_1$, responses. For instance, the posttraining heart rate at rest is compared with the pretraining heart rate at rest; the posttraining heart rate at a selected absolute or relative submaximal heart rate is compared to the pretraining heart rate at the same selected absolute or relative submaximal heart rate; and, the posttraining maximal heart rate is compared with the pretraining maximal heart rate. Thus, the following information might result.

Response	T$_1$	T$_2$
Resting heart rate (b·min^{-1})	66	56
Heart rate at 600 kgm·min^{-1} (b·min^{-1})	140	128
Heart rate at maximum (b·min^{-1})	190	190

We can conclude that the resting heart rate decreased 10 b·min^{-1}, the submaximal exercise heart rate decreased 12 b·min^{-1}, and the maximal exercise heart rate did not change. Any measured physio-

> **Training** A consistent or chronic progression of exercise sessions designed to improve physiological function for better health or sport performance.
>
> **Training Adaptations** Physiological changes or adjustments resulting from an exercise training program that promote optimal functioning.

FIGURE 1.3

Training to Improve Physiological Function and Skill for Improved Sport Performance
Photo courtesy of Northern Illinois University Media Services.

logical variable can be substituted for heart rate, although the conclusions may differ.

Training adaptations at rest show more variation than either submaximal or maximal changes; increases, decreases, and no change are all common. In general, if the exercise test is an absolute submaximal test, the physiological responses will probably be decreased after training. If the exercise test is a relative submaximal test, the physiological responses will probably show no change after training. And if the comparison is made at maximal effort, most physiological responses will be increased. These results do not hold for all variables that are measured but are general patterns.

The predominant way of looking at training adaptations is that not only do they result from the chronic application of exercise but also that they themselves represent *chronic changes*. Such adaptations become greater with harder training, are thought to exist as long as the training continues, and gradually return to baseline values when training stops (detraining). In point of fact, not all training adaptations follow this standard pattern. Some benefits occur only immediately after the exercise session. These effects are called *last-bout effects* and should not be confused with the exercise response. For example, a last-bout effect occurs with blood pressure levels. The acute response of blood pressure to continuous aerobic endurance exercise is an increase in systolic blood pressure but no change in diastolic blood pressure. The last-bout effect in individuals with high blood pressure is a decrease below their resting level for up to 3 hr after exercise. Then the high resting values return. In some cases the last-bout effect can be augmented. That is, for a period of one to several weeks the positive change occurring after the exercise bout can be increased. In the example just referred to, the decrease in systolic blood pressure after several weeks would be more than the initial decrease. However, the adjustments that can occur are finite. Once the level of the *augmented last-bout effect* is reached, no further increase in training will bring about additional benefit.[5] This may be the reason why reductions in high blood pressure that occur with training rarely result in normal resting values.

Thus, the adaptations that result from training can occur on three levels: (1) a chronic change, (2) a last-bout effect, and (3) an augmented last-bout effect. The majority of the training adaptations will be dealt with in this text as if they are chronic changes.

Training Principles

While there is much we do not know about training, and new techniques of training are always appearing, there are eight well-established fundamental guidelines that should form the basis for the development of any training program. These **training principles** are defined and briefly discussed here. The specific details for applying each principle, as well as the anticipated results or adaptations, will be discussed in connection with each physiological system in the units that follow.

1. *Specificity.* This principle is sometimes called the SAID principle, which stands for specific adaptations to imposed demands . . . that is, what you do is what you get.

Thus, when you develop a training program, you must first determine what the goal is. Fitness programs for children and adolescents will differ from those for the elderly. Physical fitness programs for nonathletes will vary from fitness programs for athletes. Athletic training programs will vary by sport, by event, or even by position within the same sport.

Second, you must be able to analyze the goal in terms of its physiological requirements. What system is being stressed, the cardiovascular-respiratory,

the metabolic, or the neuromuscular-skeletal? What is the major energy system involved? What motor fitness attributes (agility, balance, flexibility, strength, power, muscular endurance) need to be developed? The closer the training program matches the answers to these questions, the greater the chance for success.

2. *Overload.* To overload is to place a demand on the body greater than that to which it is accustomed. To determine what an overload might be, you must first evaluate each individual on the critical physiological variables discussed under specificity. Then, three factors must be considered: frequency—the number of training sessions on a daily or weekly basis; intensity—the level of work, energy expenditure, or physiological response in relation to the maximum; and duration—the amount of time spent training per session or per day.

3. *Adaptation.* Adaptation is the change in physiological function that occurs in response to training. Adaptation allows the individual to either do more work or do the same work with a smaller disruption of baseline values. Keeping records and retesting individuals are generally necessary to determine the degree of adaptation.

4. *Progression.* Progression is the change in overload in response to adaptation. Progression implies that the increments in training load are small, controlled, and flexible.

5. *Retrogression/Plateau/Reversibility.* Progress is rarely linear, predictable, or consistent. When an individual's adaptation or performance levels off or gets worse, a plateau has been reached or retrogression has occurred. Retrogression may signal overtraining. The ultimate retrogression is the reversal of achieved physiological adaptations that occurs when training stops (detraining).

6. *Maintenance.* Maintenance refers to sustaining the achieved adaptation with the most efficient use of time and effort. At this point the individuals have reached an acceptable level of

Training Principles Fundamental guidelines that form the basis for the development of an exercise training program.

physical fitness or training. The amount of time and effort required to maintain their adaptation depends on the systems involved; it is higher, for example, in the cardiovascular system than in the neuromuscular system.

7. *Individualization.* Individuals require both personalized exercise prescriptions based on their fitness levels and goals and adapt differently to the same training program. A major reason for these differences is lifestyle, particularly nutritional and sleep habits and substance use (such as tobacco or alcohol). Finally age, sex, genetics, and disease conditions all affect individual exercise prescriptions and adaptations.

8. *Warm-Up/Cool-Down.* A warm-up prepares the body for activity by elevating the body temperature. Conversely, a cool-down allows for a gradual return to normal body temperature. The best type of warm-up is specific to the activity that will follow and individualized so as not to produce fatigue.

A nonphysiological consideration is needed at this point. Except at a military boot camp, it is very difficult to force anyone to train. Therefore, some motivation is needed. Thus, it is important that there be an element of fun in any training program.

Health-Related Physical Fitness That portion of physical fitness directed toward the prevention of or rehabilitation from disease as well as the development of a high level of functional capacity for the necessary and discretionary tasks of life.

Hypokinetic Diseases Diseases caused by and/or associated with lack of physical activity.

Sport-Specific Physical Fitness That portion of physical fitness which is directed toward optimizing athletic performance.

Physical Fitness A physiological state of well-being that provides the foundation for the tasks of daily living, a degree of protection against hypokinetic disease, and a basis for participation in sport.

Periodization Plans for training based on a manipulation of the fitness components with the intent of peaking the athlete for the competitive season or varying health-related fitness training in cycles of harder or easier training.

Intersperse games, variations, and special events, and make normal training sessions as enjoyable as possible.

Health-Related Versus Sport-Specific Physical Fitness

As alluded to in the description of specificity, there are two main goals for exercise training: (1) health-related physical fitness and (2) sport-specific physical fitness, sometimes called athletic fitness.

In this text the concept of **health-related physical fitness** means that portion of physical fitness which is directed toward the prevention of or rehabilitation from disease as well as the development of a high level of functional capacity for the necessary and discretionary tasks of life. Thus, the goal may be to participate minimally in an activity to achieve some health benefit before a disease state occurs. The goal may be to participate in a substantial amount of activity to improve or maintain a high level of physical fitness. Or the goal may be to participate in an activity that allows a disabled individual to recover and/or attain the maximal function possible. All goals should be attained while avoiding injury.

Three components of health-related physical fitness are generally recognized: cardiovascular-respiratory endurance, body composition, muscular fitness (strength, muscular endurance, and flexibility). Figure 1.4 shows that the components of health-related physical fitness form the core of physical fitness. The relationship between each of these fitness components and hypokinetic disease will be described in the appropriate units of the text. For now it is sufficient to know that **hypokinetic diseases** are diseases which are caused by and/or associated with a lack of physical activity. Health-related physical fitness is important for everyone.

Sport-specific physical fitness has a more narrow focus; it is that portion of physical fitness directed toward optimizing athletic performance. To develop this type of fitness program, you must first analyze the physiological demands of the sport. Second, you must evaluate where the athlete is in terms of these requirements. Once you know both of these elements, you can develop a specifically designed individualized program. This program should work the specific musculature involved while achieving a proper balance between agonistic and antagonistic muscle groups; use the muscles in the biomechanical patterns of the sport; match the metabolic requirements; and incorporate any motor fitness attributes that are needed at a starting level that is appropriate for the athlete. The demands of the sport will not change to accommodate the athlete. The athlete must be the one to meet the demands of the sport if reasonable success is desired. Figure 1.4 shows that sport-specific athletic fitness builds on the core of health-related physical fitness and expands from there.

Putting all of these elements together, **physical fitness** may be defined as a physiological state of well-being that provides the foundation for the tasks of daily living, a degree of protection against hypokinetic disease, and a basis for participation in sport.[1]

Periodization

Once a training program is designed, it should be applied in a pattern that will be most beneficial. Such a pattern is called the *training cycle* or **periodization.** Periodization plans for training based on a manipulation of the fitness components and training principles with the intent of peaking the athlete for the competitive season or some part of it. An individual training for any level of health-related physical fitness should also utilize periodization to build in cycles of harder or easier training. In this latter case, however, the variation will be neither as great as nor as rigidly tied to a specific event as the athlete is tied to the competitive season.

Figure 1.5 shows how periodization might be arranged for an athlete. In the figure, the time

FIGURE 1.4

Physical Fitness

Cardiovascular-respiratory endurance; Aerobic power and capacity

Anaerobic power and capacity

Cardiovascular-respiratory endurance; Aerobic power

Muscular strength

Power

Muscular strength

Muscular endurance

Body composition values associated with low risk of hypokinetic disease

Muscular endurance

Flexibility

Balance

Body composition values that will optimize performance

Flexibility

Agility

☐ Sport-specific physical fitness   ☐ Health-related physical fitness frame, most likely a year, has been divided into four phases or cycles. These are active rest, off-season, preseason, and in-season. Each main cycle or macrocycle in turn is usually divided into 4-week mezocycles and 1-week microcycles. Each type of cycle aims for an optimal mixture of work and rest.[3,7]

The active rest phase begins immediately after the last competition of the previous year. The athlete should take a couple days of complete rest at this point and then participate in noncompetitive physical activities that are not his or her primary sport. This type of activity is called cross training.[7]

The off-season phase should be preceded by a sport-specific fitness evaluation to provide guidance for both the off-season and the preseason training programs. Another evaluation might be conducted prior to the preseason if desired, or evaluations might be systematically done throughout the year to determine how the individual is re-

sponding to the training and to make any necessary adjustments. The off-season is a time of general preparation when the health-related physical fitness components are emphasized to develop a basis of cardiovascular-respiratory endurance (an *aerobic base*), flexibility, and heavy resistance training. Any needed changes in body composition should be addressed here.[7]

During the preseason phase a shift is made to specific preparation for the intended sport in all components. The training program at this time is very heavy and generally occupies the 6–8 weeks prior to the first competition.[7]

Once the athlete begins the in-season phase, the early emphasis shifts to maintaining the sport-specific fitness that was developed during the preseason. What heavy work is done should immediately follow a competition instead of directly preceding one. During the late season, when the most important competitions are held (such as conference

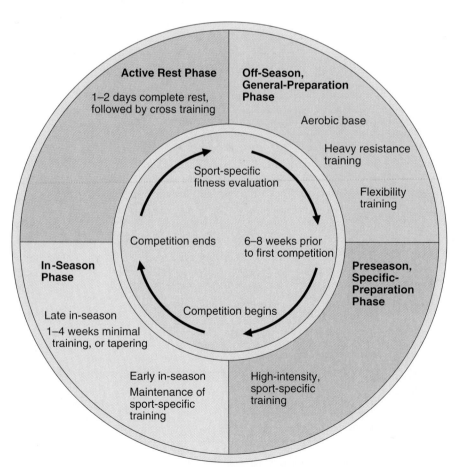

FIGURE 1.5

Periodization for Training Athletes

championships or bowl games), the athlete should do only a minimum of training or taper gradually by decreasing training frequency and duration but maintaining intensity so that he or she is rested without being detrained.[7]

Where possible throughout this text, periodization will be considered in the application of the training principles.

Exercise and Training as Stressors

Individuals in the professional fields that depend on exercise and training typically think of these activities as universally positive factors. However, both acute exercise and chronic training are stressors.

Selye's Theory of Stress

A *stressor* is any activity, event, or impingement which causes stress. **Stress** is most simply defined as a disruption in body homeostasis and all attempts by the body to regain homeostasis. Selye, however, defines stress more completely as the state manifested by a specific syndrome that consists of all the nonspecifically induced changes within a biological system. The biological system here is the human body. The specific syndrome is the *general adaptation syndrome* (GAS), a step-by-step description of the bodily reactions to a stressor. It consists of three major stages:

1. the alarm reaction, shock and countershock
2. the stage of resistance
3. the stage of exhaustion[12]

In the alarm reaction stage the body responds to a stressor with a disruption of homeostasis (shock). It immediately attempts to regain homeostasis (countershock). If the body is able to adjust, the response is mild and advantageous to the organism; the stage of resistance or adaptation ensues. If the stress becomes chronic or the acquired adaptation is lost, the stage of exhaustion is entered. At this point the nonspecifically induced changes, which are apparent during the alarm reaction but disappear during the stage of resistance, become paramount. These changes are labeled the *triad of symptoms* and include adrenal enlargement, thymus and lym-

phatic shrinkage, and bleeding ulcers of the digestive tract. Specifically induced changes directly related to the stressor may also occur. An example of a specifically induced change might be shivering if the stressor is cold. Ultimate exhaustion is death.[12]

Physiological Basis of Stress: Neurohormonal Control

There are two complementary, and often overlapping, physiological pathways through which the body responds to all stressors: the nervous system and the hormonal system. Because these two systems function so closely together, they are often referred to as the *neurohormonal system.*

The *nervous system* is the fast-acting regulatory center of the body. It communicates by nerve fibers that release chemical neurotransmitters at the target locations. The portion of the nervous system that predominates in stress responses is the *sympathetic nervous system.* The sympathetic nervous system is a division of the *autonomic nervous system,* which controls involuntary bodily functions by regulating cardiac muscle, smooth muscle, and glands. The sympathetic nervous system is sympathetic to or supportive of physiological changes that enable the individual to increase movement—to fight or to flee. Such changes are often labeled *fight or flight responses.*

The *endocrine system* is the slower of the two regulatory systems. It relies on chemical signals, by way of hormones, that are transported in the blood to communicate with target organs and cells at specific receptor sites.

Both the neural and the hormonal regulatory systems are involved in the stress response system. A schematic outline of the two regulatory pathways is presented in Figure 1.6. The primarily neural component is called the brain stem (locus ceruleus)–sympathetic nervous system pathway; it is shown on the left in Figure 1.6. The primarily hormonal component is called the hypothalamus-

Stress The state manifested by the specific syndrome that consists of all the nonspecifically induced changes within a biological system; a disruption in body homeostasis and all attempts by the body to regain homeostasis.

pituitary-adrenal axis and is the pathway on the right in Figure 1.6.[2]

When the individual is presented with a stressor, the hypothalamus coordinates the response. The hypothalamus is both a neural structure and an endocrine gland. Thus, it can orchestrate the body's response by stimulation of both the sympathetic nervous system and the endocrine glands.

The sympathetic nerve fibers originate in the brain stem and travel throughout the body to a variety of target sites. The sympathetic nerve fibers also go to and control the adrenal medulla. Norepinephrine (NE) is released by sympathetic nerve fibers and both norepinephrine and epinephrine (E) are secreted by the adrenal medulla. The NE released from the sympathetic nerve endings and from the adrenal medulla is the same chemical. However, when NE is released by the nerves, it is considered to be a neurotransmitter; when it is released by the adrenal medulla, it is considered to be a hormone. The NE and E secreted by the adrenal medulla circulate in the bloodstream to the target sites, where they mimic and reinforce the actions of the sympathetic nerve fibers that innervate these same target sites. This response pattern is often referred to as symptho-adrenal activation. Both NE and E may also influence other endocrine glands, as indicated by the connecting line to the anterior pituitary gland in (Figure 1.6).

The hypothalamus directly regulates endocrine glands both neurally and through a series of releasing factors, sometimes called releasing hormones. In the generic stress response corticotrophic-releasing hormone (CRH) is released by the hypothalamus and stimulates the anterior pituitary to secrete adrenocorticotrophic hormone (ACTH). ACTH in turn stimulates the adrenal cortex to release cortisol, which acts on specific target sites.

Both neural and hormonal regulation of the body's exercise response and training adaptations go beyond this basic stress response. For example, hormones are involved in metabolic processes, bone remodeling, and maintenance of fluid balance. Thus, one key to understanding the body's response to exercise and adaptation to training is understanding the coordinated functioning of the neuro-

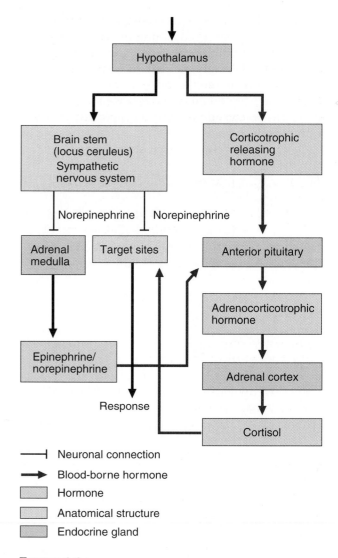

FIGURE 1.6

Pathways of Neurohormonal Regulation of the Exercise Stress Response

hormonal system. Throughout this text these functions will be dealt with specifically as they are related to the material in each unit.

Overtraining

Although there are historical examples of the ultimate stage-of-exhaustion response—that is, death caused by unrelenting exercise under inadequate nutritional conditions—such an occurrence is a very

Overtraining   A state of overstress or failure to adapt to an exercise training load.

extreme and statistically unlikely possibility. A more realistic everyday concern for individuals involved in a fitness program or athletic training program is that overstress can result in temporary exhaustion known as staleness, burnout, or **overtraining.** This condition is of special concern since stress is additive. That is, environmental, psychological, and social factors such as weather extremes, exercise physiology examinations, competitive pressures, and interpersonal relationships can also cause stress; and the effects do not act independently but are cumulative.

Overtraining can range from mild to severe. It is most likely to occur in individuals who are highly motivated, in instances where large increases in training occur abruptly, and in situations where in-

sufficient rest and recovery are included in the periodization training program. The sooner overtraining is recognized and dealt with, the faster recovery can be expected. The recognition of overtraining necessitates a familiarity with its signs and symptoms. A list of such signs and symptoms is given in Table 1.1. These are outward manifestations of neuroendocrine imbalances, immune system suppression, or a reversal of normal physiological training adaptations.[3,9,10] This list is by no means all-inclusive, and no single indicator other than a decrement in performance is likely to be common to all individuals who are overtrained. Only those signs and symptoms that require minimal testing or that can be detected by astute observation have been included. Above all, this list should point to the

TABLE 1.1 ▪ Signs and Symptoms of Overtraining

PERFORMANCE-RELATED

Consistent decrement in performance

Persistent fatigue and sluggishness that leads to several days of poor training

Prolonged recovery from training sessions or competitive events

Reappearance of already corrected errors

PHYSIOLOGICAL

Decreased maximal work capacities

Increased disruption of homeostasis at submaximal workloads

Headaches or stomachaches out of proportion to life events

Insomnia

Persistent low-grade stiffness and soreness of the muscles and joints

Frequent sore throats, colds, and/or cold sores

Constipation or diarrhea

Loss of appetite; loss of body weight and/or muscle mass when no conscious attempt is being made to diet or when weight loss is undesirable

An elevation of approximately 10% in the morning heart rate taken immediately upon awakening

Amenorrhea

PSYCHOLOGICAL/BEHAVIORAL

Feelings of depression

General apathy, especially toward previously enjoyable activities

Decreased self-esteem

Emotional instability or mood changes

Difficulty concentrating

Loss of competitive drive or desire

importance of monitoring and interacting with those entrusted to your guidance. One of the most helpful things that the exerciser can do is to keep a training log including heart rates, body weight, other physical or mental feelings, and planned versus achieved workouts. With this information and periodic testing in all cycles of the training program, adjustments can be made to reverse or, even better, prevent overtraining. Improving performance and avoiding overtraining are the intended results of a careful application of the training principles described throughout this text.

From the standpoint of stress theory, *physical fitness* may be defined as achieved adaptation to the stress imposed by muscular exercise. Physical fitness results from a properly applied training program, is usually exhibited in response to an acute exercise task, and implies avoidance of overtraining.

SUMMARY

1. The purpose of this chapter has been both to acquaint you with the general organization of the text and to provide background information that will help you interpret and understand the information that will subsequently be presented.

2. The response to exercise, which is always a disruption in homeostasis, depends upon the exercise modality, the exercise intensity, the characteristics of the exerciser, and whether the test is a criterion- or field-based task.

3. The baselines against which the exercise-caused disruptions of homeostasis are compared are normal resting values of the measured variables.

4. Exercise training brings about adaptations in physiological function. The baselines against which training adaptations are compared are the corresponding pre-training conditions.

5. Training adaptations may occur on at least three levels: a last-bout effect, an augmented last-bout effect, or a chronic change.

6. Eight general training principles provide guidance for establishing and applying training programs: specificity, overload, adaptation, progression, retrogression-plateau-reversibility, maintenance, individualization, warm-up and cool-down.

7. Health-related physical fitness is composed of components representing cardiovascular-respiratory en-

durance, metabolism, muscular fitness (strength, muscular endurance, and flexibility).

8. Sport-specific physical fitness should build on health-related physical fitness, adding motor fitness attributes (such as agility, balance, and power) and anaerobic power and capacity, as needed.

9. Periodization provides a timeline for the planning of training programs that cycles through four phases: active rest, off-season, preseason, and in-season.

10. Both a single acute bout of exercise and chronic exercise training are stressors.

11. To prescribe a training program:
- Analyze the physiological demands of the physical fitness program, rehabilitation, or sport goal;
- Evaluate the individual relative to the established physiological demands;
- Apply the training principles relative to the established physiological demands in periodization cycles that allow for a pattern of varying levels of exercise and rest or recovery.

12. The physiological responses to stress are mediated through the hypothalamus by way of the hypothalamic-pituitary-adrenal axis and the brain stem (locus ceruleus)–sympathetic nervous system pathway.

13. Overtraining is an indication that the individual is not physiologically adapting to the stress of exercise training, probably because large increases in training have occurred abruptly or insufficient attention has been paid to rest and recovery.

REVIEW QUESTIONS

1. Define *exercise physiology, exercise,* and *exercise training*.

2. Explain the comparisons used to describe the exercise response and training adaptations.

3. Differentiate between an absolute and relative submaximal workload, and give an example using a situation other than weight lifting.

4. Fully describe an exercise situation, including all elements that are needed to accurately evaluate the exercise response.

5. Differentiate between the three levels of training adaptation, and state which level of adaptation is most common.

6. List and explain the training principles.

7. Compare the components of health-related physical fitness with those of sport-specific physical fitness.

8. Diagram and give an example of periodization for a sport of your choice.

9. Prepare a line chart of the neurohormonal physiological basis of the exercise and exercise training stress response.

10. Identify the performance-related, physiological, and behavioral signs and symptoms of overtraining that can be evaluated with little if any laboratory testing.

REFERENCES

1. American Alliance for Health, Physical Education, Recreation and Dance: Physical Best: *A Physical Fitness Education and Assessment Program.* Reston, VA: Author (1988).

2. Chrousos, G. P., & P. W. Gold: The concepts of stress and stress system disorders. *Journal of the American Medical Association.* 267(4):1244–1252 (1992).

3. Fry, R. W., A. R. Morton, & D. Keast: Overtraining in athletes. *Sports Medicine.* 12(1):32–65 (1991).

4. Halpern, A. A., & E. E. Bleck: Sit-up exercises: An electromyographic study. *Clinical Orthopaedics and Related Research.* 145:172–178 (1979).

5. Haskell, W. L.: Health consequences of physical activity: Understanding and challenges regarding dose response. *Medicine and Science in Sports and Exercise.* 26 (6):649–660 (1994).

6. Hellerstein, H. K.: Cardiac rehabilitation: A retrospective view. In M. L. Pollock & D. H. Schmidt (eds.), *Heart Disease and Rehabilitation.* Boston: Houghton Mifflin, 511–514 (1979).

7. Kibler, W. B., & T. J. Chandler: Sport-specific conditioning. *American Journal of Sports Medicine.* 22(3):424–432 (1994).

8. Kraus, H., & R. Hirschland: Minimum muscular fitness tests in school. *Research Quarterly.* 25:178–188 (1954).

9. Kuipers, H., & H. A. Keizer: Overtraining in elite athletes: Review and directions for the future. *Sports Medicine.* 6:79–92 (1988).

10. Morris, A. F.: *Sports Medicine: Prevention of Athletic Injuries.* Dubuque, IA: Brown (1984).

11. Raab, W.: Heart attack—Number one killer of Americans. In *The Healthy Life: How Diet and Exercise Affect Your Heart and Vigor.* New York: Time Incorporated (1966).

12. Selye, H.: *The Stress of Life.* New York: McGraw-Hill (1956).

13. Ullyot, J.: *Women's Running.* Mountain View, CA: World Publications (1976).

Cardiovascular-Respiratory System

2

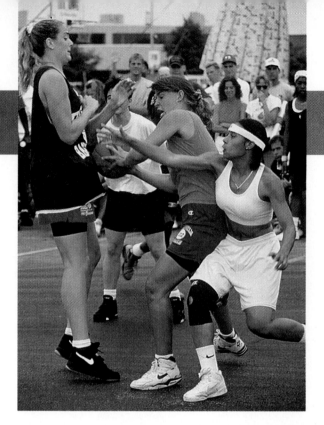

Respiration

After studying the chapter, you should be able to:

- Distinguish between and explain the component variables of pulmonary ventilation, external respiration, and internal respiration.

- Identify the conductive and respiratory zones of the respiratory system and compare the functions of the two zones.

- Explain the mechanics of breathing.

- Differentiate between pulmonary circulation and bronchial circulation.

- Describe static and dynamic lung volumes.

- Distinguish between the conditions under which respiratory measures are collected and reported.

- Calculate minute and alveolar ventilation, the partial pressure of a gas in a mixture, the amount of oxygen carried per deciliter of blood; and the arteriovenous oxygen difference.

- Explain how respiration is regulated at rest and during exercise.

- Explain how oxygen and carbon dioxide are transported in the circulatory system and how oxygen is released to the tissues.

- Explain the role of respiration in acid-base balance.

Introduction

The common denominator for all sports and physical fitness is muscle action. For muscles to be able to act, energy must be provided. The first link in the chain of supplying a large portion of this energy is respiration, for it is respiration that provides oxygen to and removes carbon dioxide from the body.

Although it is typical to think of respiration as being synonymous with breathing and/or ventilation, technically it is not. Figure 2.1 presents an overview of respiration. As the figure shows, the volume of air flowing into the lungs from the external environment through either the nose or mouth is called **pulmonary ventilation.** Ventilation is accomplished by breathing, the alternation of inspiration and expiration that causes the air to move. The actual exchange of the gases oxygen (O_2) and carbon dioxide (CO_2) between the lungs and the blood is known as **external respiration.** At the cellular level oxygen and carbon dioxide gases are again exchanged; this exchange is called **internal respiration. Cellular respiration** is the utilization of oxygen by the cells to produce energy with carbon dioxide as a by-product. Cellular respiration includes both aerobic (with O_2) and anaerobic (with-

out O_2) energy production and will be discussed in Chapter 9. This chapter concentrates on pulmonary ventilation, external respiration, and internal respiration.

Structure of the Pulmonary System

The respiratory system consists of two major portions: (1) the conductive zone, which transports the air to the lungs; and (2) the respiratory zone, where gas exchange takes place.

The Conductive Zone

The basic structure of the conductive zone is shown in Figure 2.2. Everything from the nose, or mouth,

---

Pulmonary Ventilation   The process by which air is moved into the lungs.

External Respiration   The exchange of gases between the lungs and the blood.

Internal Respiration   The exchange of gases at the cellular level.

Cellular Respiration   The utilization of oxygen by the cells to produce energy.

FIGURE 2.1

Overview of Respiration

Respiration consists of four separate parts. The first is pulmonary ventilation in which air is moved into and out of the body. The second, external respiration, involves the exchange of oxygen and carbon dioxide between the lungs and the blood. The third is internal respiration, which involves the exchange of oxygen and carbon dioxide at the cellular or tissue level. Finally, cellular respiration is the utilization of oxygen to produce energy, which also produces carbon dioxide as a by-product.

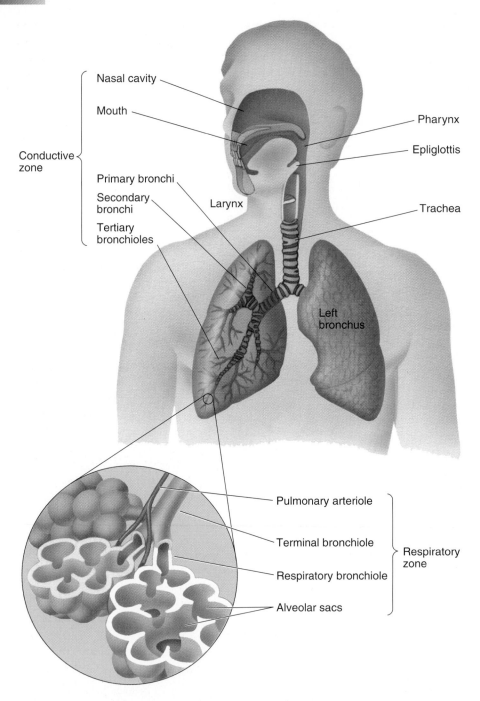

FIGURE 2.2

Anatomy of the Pulmonary System

The pulmonary system is divided into two zones— the conductive zone transports air to the lungs, and the respiratory zone is where gas exchange takes place.

Nasal cavity

Mouth

Conductive zone

Primary bronchi

Secondary bronchi

Tertiary bronchioles

Larynx

Pharynx

Epiglottis

Trachea

Left bronchus

Pulmonary arteriole

Terminal bronchiole

Respiratory zone

Respiratory bronchiole

Alveolar sacs

to the terminal bronchioles comprises the *conductive zone*.[8] The primary role of the conductive zone is to transport air. Because no exchange of gases takes place, this zone is also called *anatomical dead space*. As a general guideline, the amount of anatomical dead space can be estimated as 1 mL for each 1 lb of "ideal" body weight.[11] Hence, a 130-lb female who is at her ideal weight has an estimated 130 mL of anatomical dead space. However, if this individual were to gain 20 lb, she would not then also gain anatomical dead space; that estimate would remain at 130 mL. Anatomical dead space is important in determining alveolar ventilation, as discussed later in the chapter.

A second important role of the conductive zone is to warm and humidify the air. By the time the air reaches the lungs, it has been warmed to body temperature (normally ~37°C) and has been 99.5% saturated with water vapor. This protective mechanism maintains core body temperature and protects the lungs from injury.[11] The warming and humidifying of air is easily accomplished over a wide range of environmental temperatures under resting conditions when the volume of air transported is small and the air is inhaled through the nose. During heavy exercise, however, large volumes of air are inhaled primarily through the mouth, thus bypassing the warming and moisturizing sites of the nose and nasal cavity. As a result, the mouth and throat may feel dry. If heavy exercise takes place in cold weather (especially at subzero temperatures), dryness increases and actual throat pain may be felt. These uncomfortable feelings are not a symptom of freezing of the lungs; rather they are the result of the drying and cooling of the upper airway. The lower portions of the conductive zone still moisturize and warm the air sufficiently before it reaches the lungs. A scarf worn across the mouth will trap both the moisture and the heat from the exhaled air and decrease or eliminate the uncomfortable sensations.

A third role of the conductive zone is to filter incoming air. The nasal cavity, pharynx, larynx, trachea and bronchial system are all lined with ciliated mucous membranes (Figure 2.2). These membranes trap impurities and foreign particles (particulates) that are inhaled. Both smoke and environmental air pollutants diminish ciliary activity and can ultimately destroy the cilia.

The Respiratory Zone

The *respiratory zone* consists of the respiratory bronchioles, the alveolar ducts, alveolar sacs (or grapelike clusters), and the alveoli (see Figure 2.2). The *alveoli* are the actual site of gas exchange between the pulmonary system and cardiovascular system. At birth humans possess approximately 24 million alveoli. This number increases to about 300 million by the age of 8 yr and remains constant until 30 yr of age, when it begins a gradual decline. Although each individual alveolus is small, only about 0.2 mm in diameter, collectively the alveoli in a young adult

have a total surface area of 70 to 80 m².[11] This area would cover a badminton court or even a tennis court if flattened out. Despite this large surface area, the lungs weigh only about 2.2 lb (1 kg). The membrane between the alveoli and capillaries is actually composed of five very thin layers, two of which are the endothelial cells which comprise the alveoli and capillaries themselves. Despite the number of layers, the thickness is less than the paper this book is printed on, and gas exchange takes place easily.[8]

Some alveoli have no capillary blood supply and can therefore not participate in gas exchange; these alveoli make up a *physiological dead space*. The amount of physiological dead space is minimal in healthy individuals; thus, the total dead space is only slightly larger than the anatomical dead space.[11]

Mechanics of Breathing

The movement of air into the lungs from the atmosphere depends upon two factors—pressure gradient (ΔP) and resistance (R). The relationship between these factors is expressed by the equation for *airflow* ($\dot{V}$):

(2.1)

$$\text{airflow (L} \cdot \text{min}^{-1}) = \frac{\text{pressure gradient (mm Hg)}}{\text{resistance (R unit)}}$$

or

$$\dot{V} = \frac{\Delta P}{R}$$

A *pressure gradient* is simply the difference (difference is represented by the Greek capital letter Δ, delta) between two pressures. The larger the differences in pressure, the larger the pressure gradient is. Gases—in this case air, which is a mixture of gases—move from areas of high pressure to areas of low pressure.

Resistance is the sum of the forces opposing the flow of the gases. About 20% of the resistance to airflow is caused by tissue friction as the lungs move during inspiration and expiration. The remaining 80% is due to the friction between the gas molecules and the walls of the airway (airway resistance) and the internal friction between the gas molecules themselves (viscosity). Airway resistance is determined by the size of the airway and the smoothness or turbulence of the airflow.

Equation 2.1 indicates that in order for air to flow, the pressure gradient must be greater than the resistance to the flow. Thus, for inspiration to take place, pressure must be higher in the atmosphere than in the lungs; for expiration, pressure in the alveoli of the lungs must be higher than in the atmosphere. Figure 2.3 shows how the inspiratory pressure gradient is created.

A key to understanding Figure 2.3 is Boyle's law. *Boyle's law* states that the pressure of a gas is inversely related to its volume (or vice versa) under conditions of constant temperature: Low pressure is associated with large volume, and high pressure is associated with small volume.

For pulmonary ventilation, an increase in chest cavity volume is accomplished by muscle contraction for inspiration. This increase in volume leads to an internal lung pressure decrease, according to Boyle's law. As a result, the chest cavity exhibits a negative pressure relative to the atmosphere. Thus, a pressure gradient has been created. Air flows into the chest cavity in an attempt to equalize this pressure difference.

The main inspiratory muscle is the dome-shaped diaphragm. Upon neural stimulation the di-

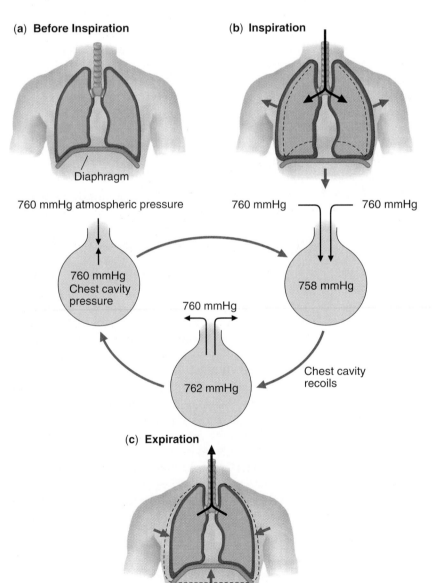

(a) Before Inspiration

Diaphragm

760 mmHg atmospheric pressure

760 mmHg
Chest cavity
pressure

(b) Inspiration

760 mmHg — 760 mmHg

758 mmHg

760 mmHg

762 mmHg

Chest cavity
recoils

(c) Expiration

FIGURE 2.3

Inspiratory and Expiratory Pressure Gradients

Inspiration and expiration are accomplished by the creation of pressure gradients. (a) The respiratory musculature is relaxed, atmospheric pressure equals chest cavity pressure, and so no air movement occurs. (b) The external intercostals and diaphragm contract, moving the ribs up and out and the diaphragm down, respectively. This muscle action enlarges the chest cavity laterally, anterioposterially, and downward, increasing the volume. As a result chest cavity pressure is lower than atmospheric pressure and air flows in. (c) The inspiratory muscles relax, and the chest cavity recoils, creating a pressure higher than atmospheric pressure. Air flows out. The respiratory cycle then begins again.

aphragm contracts and moves downward, elongating the chest cavity (see Figure 2.3b). Further enlargement of the chest cavity can come from the action of the external intercostal muscles as well as others (known collectively as the accessory muscles), which elevate the rib cage and bring about expansion both laterally (side to side) and anteroposteriorly (front to back). The extent of accessory muscle activity and the resultant drop in pressure depends on the depth of the inspiration.

The changes in chest cavity volume are transferred to the lungs themselves owing to the presence and function of pleura. *Pleura* is a thin, double-layered membrane that lines both the chest cavity (the inner surfaces of the thorax, sternum, ribs, vertebrae, and diaphragm) and the external lung surfaces. The portion covering the chest cavity is called *parietal pleura*; the portion covering the external lung surfaces is called the *visceral* or *pulmonary pleura*. A fluid secreted by the pleura fills the space between the pleura (the intrapleural space) and allows the lungs to glide smoothly over the chest cavity walls. It also causes the parietal and pulmonary pleura to adhere to each other in the same way that two pieces of glass are held together by a thin film of water. Because of this adhesion, the lungs themselves move when muscle action causes movement of the chest cavity.[6,8]

During normal resting conditions expiration occurs simply because the diaphragm and other inspiratory muscles relax. When the muscles are relaxed, both the lungs and the muscles, which are highly elastic, recoil to their original positions. This elastic recoil decreases lung volume, and thus creates a pressure inside the chest cavity that is higher than the atmospheric pressure. As the chest cavity decreases in volume, the intrathoracic pressure increases slightly above that of the atmosphere. The result is that air moves out of the lungs into the atmosphere. The pressures equalize again and the cycle repeats itself with the next inspiration. A complete respiratory cycle includes both inspiration and expiration.

During heavy breathing, as in exercise, expiration is an active process. The primary expiratory muscles are the abdominals and the internal intercostals. The abdominals (rectus abdominus, the obliques, and the transverse abdominus) push the abdominal organs—and hence the diaphragm—upward; the internal intercostals pull the ribs inward

and down. This decrease in chest volume increases intrathoracic pressure quicker than passive elastic recoil does, and the air is forced out of the lungs faster.

The pleura also serve a purpose during expiration. Pressure in the intrapleural space fluctuates with breathing in a way that parallels pressure within the lungs. However, the intrapleural pressure is always negative (-4 to -8 mmHg) relative to the intrapulmonary (lung) pressure. This negative pressure protects the lungs from collapsing. If the intrapleural pressure were equal to the atmospheric pressure, the lungs would collapse at the end of expiration because of the elastic recoil.

Because muscle activity is involved during the respiratory cycle of inhalation and exhalation, energy is consumed. During rest, however, this energy consumption (restricted to inspiratory muscles) amounts to only 1–2% of the total energy expenditure in nonsmokers.[10]

Respiratory Circulation

The lung has two different circulatory systems: pulmonary circulation, which serves the external respiratory function, and bronchial circulation, which supplies the internal respiration needs of the lung tissue itself.

Pulmonary circulation parallels the divisions of the structures in the conductive zone, branching in a treelike manner called arborization. Arborization ends in a dense alveolar capillary network, blanketing most but not all alveoli. **Perfusion of the lung** is the phrase used to describe the capillary blood flow through this network.[6,8]

The pulmonary artery exits from the right ventricle of the heart and gives rise to the capillary network in the lungs. The pulmonary vein arises from this capillary network and enters the heart at the left atrium. As with pulmonary airflow and the rest of the circulatory system, blood flows through this circuit owing to differences in pressure—that is, a pressure gradient that can overcome resistance to the flow. Normal pulmonary artery blood pressure

Perfusion of the Lung   Pulmonary circulation, especially capillary blood flow.

is low, only 25/10 mmHg; but venous pulmonary blood pressure is even lower, only 7 mmHg. Although this pressure gradient between the pulmonary artery and vein is not large, it is sufficient to bring about the blood flow. However, because of these low pressures, gravity affects pulmonary circulation more than the systemic or total body circulation. Thus, whatever portion of the lungs is lowest is perfused best. Whichever portion of the lungs is better perfused with blood is also better ventilated.[6,7,8]

Bronchial circulation consists of relatively small systemic arteries that originate from the aorta, travel through the lungs, and return as veins that empty into the pulmonary venous system. Thus, not all of the pulmonary venous blood is oxygenated.[11]

Minute Ventilation

Measurement of pulmonary ventilation as either the amount of air inspired or the amount of air expired in 1 min is known as **minute ventilation** or **minute volume.** The most common units of measurement are liters per minute ($L \cdot min^{-1}$) and milliliters per minute ($mL \cdot min^{-1}$). Inspired minute ventilation is symbolized as $\dot{V}_I$, where V is volume, the "dot" indicates per unit of time, and the subscript I stands for inspired. The symbol for expired ventilation $\dot{V}_E$ merely substitutes a subscripted E, meaning expired, for the I.

Minute ventilation is dependent upon **tidal volume** (V_T), the amount of air inhaled or exhaled per breath and the frequency (f) of breaths per minute. The equation is

> **(2.2)**   minute ventilation ($mL \cdot min^{-1}$)
> = tidal volume ($mL \cdot br^{-1}$) × frequency ($br \cdot min^{-1}$)
>
> or $\dot{V} = V_T \times f$

> **Minute Ventilation (Minute Volume) ($\dot{V}_I$ or $\dot{V}_E$)**
> The amount of air inspired or expired each minute; the pulmonary ventilation rate per minute; calculated as tidal volume times frequency of breathing.
>
> **Tidal Volume (V_T)**   The amount of air that is inspired or expired in a normal breath.
>
> **Alveolar Ventilation ($\dot{V}_A$)**   The volume of air available for gas exchange; calculated as tidal volume minus dead space volume times frequency.

Milliliters per minute are then commonly converted to liters per minute by dividing by 1000.

At rest a normal young adult will ventilate at a frequency of 12–15 times per minute and have a tidal volume of 400–600 mL. Children ventilate at a much faster rate but with a smaller tidal volume.

■ EXAMPLE

Compute $\dot{V}_E$ when f = 15 $br \cdot min^{-1}$ and V_T = 400 mL. You should have set up and solved the equation as follows:

$$\dot{V}_E = (400 \text{ mL} \cdot br^{-1}) \times (15 \text{ br} \cdot min^{-1}) = 6000 \text{ mL} \cdot min^{-1}$$
$$6000 \text{ mL} \cdot min^{-1} \div 1000 \text{ mL} \cdot L^{-1} = 6.0 \text{ L} \cdot min^{-1} \quad ■$$

Since minute ventilation represents the total amount of air moved into or out of the lungs per minute, it includes the portion of air that fills the conduction zone. Thus, this is not the amount of air that is available for gas exchange. The amount of air that is available for gas exchange is termed **alveolar ventilation** (or anatomical effective ventilation). Alveolar ventilation ($\dot{V}_A$) takes into account tidal volume ($\dot{V}_T$), dead space ($\dot{V}_D$), and the frequency (f) of breathing. The equation for calculating $\dot{V}_A$ is

> **(2.3)**   alveolar ventilation ($mL \cdot min^{-1}$)
> = [tidal volume ($mL \cdot br^{-1}$) – dead space ($mL \cdot br^{-1}$)] × frequency ($br \cdot min^{-1}$)
>
> or $\dot{V}_A = (V_T - V_D) \times f$

■ EXAMPLE

Calculate alveolar ventilation using the values of f and V_T given in the previous example, for a female who is at her ideal weight of 130 lb. This problem becomes

$$\dot{V}_A = [(400 \text{ mL} \cdot br^{-1}) - (130 \text{ mL} \cdot br^{-1})]$$
$$\times (15 \text{ br} \cdot min^{-1})$$
$$= 4050 \text{ mL} \cdot min^{-1} \div 1000 \text{ mL} \cdot L^{-1}$$
$$= 4.05 \text{ L} \cdot min^{-1}$$

Typically, approximately 70% of $\dot{V}_I$ reaches the alveoli for gas exchange. In this example, the percentage is 67.5% [(4050 $mL \cdot min^{-1}$) ÷ (6000 $mL \cdot min^{-1}$)].   ■

As with minute ventilation, alveolar ventilation can be calculated from either $\dot{V}_E$ or $\dot{V}_I$. The physiological dead space is so negligible in normal healthy individuals that it does not need to be taken into account in these calculations. To be sure you understand the implications of this concept, complete the problems in Box 2.1.

Measurement of Lung Volumes

Lung volumes can be measured either statically or dynamically. Static lung volumes are anatomical measures; since they are independent of time, they do not measure flow. Dynamic lung volumes depend on time and hence measure airflow in addition to air volume.

Static Lung Volumes

Take as deep a breath as you can. At this point your lungs contain the maximum amount of air they can hold. This amount of air is called **total lung capac-**ity (TLC). Figure 2.4 shows that TLC can be divided into four volumes and three other capacities. The definition of each volume and capacity are included on the table. Note that the four capacities are combinations of two or more volumes. All of these volumes and capacities have clinical significance, but only those important in the study of exercise physiology will be discussed briefly here.

As mentioned previously, tidal volume (V_T) represents the amount of air either inhaled or exhaled in a single breath. A normal V_T inflates the lungs to about half of the TLC in the erect sitting or standing position and only about a third in the supine position.[11] When the demand for energy increases during exercise, V_T increases by expanding into both the inspiratory reserve volume (IRV) and expiratory reserve volume (ERV). Thus, the limits of the vital capacity (VC = IRV + V_T + ERV) represent the absolute limits of tidal volume increase during exercise.

Residual volume (RV) is the amount of air left in the lungs following a maximal exhalation. This leftover air is important because it allows for a continuous gas exchange between the alveoli and the capillaries between breaths. If all of the air were forced out, no gas would be available for exchange. During exercise, when V_T expands, the functional residual capacity (FRC) assists in maintaining a smooth exchange, in the following way. The V_T can and does expand into both the IRV and the ERV, but it expands more into the IRV than the ERV, leaving a relatively large FRC intact. This large FRC dilutes the gas changes (the decrease in oxygen and increase in carbon dioxide) caused by the increased energy production and expenditure of exercise. By reducing fluctuation, the FRC stabilizes and smooths the gas exchange.

Despite its beneficial physiological aspects, residual volume also presents a measurement difficulty. When body composition is determined by hydrostatic (underwater) weighing (see Chapter 14), residual volume must be measured. Residual air makes the body buoyant; if it is not accounted for, it reduces the underwater weight. The less an

---

Box 2.1 A Question of Understanding

1. Given two breathing patterns, A and B, in the accompanying table, calculate the alveolar ventilation.

	Breathing Pattern	
	A	**B**
$\dot{V}_E$ (L·min^{-1})	6	6
V_T (mL·br^{-1})	600	200
f (br·min^{-1})	10	30
V_D (mL·br^{-1})	150	150
$\dot{V}_A$ (mL·min^{-1})	?	?

On the basis of your calculations, is it better to breathe fast and shallowly or slowly and deeply?

2. Individuals learning the front-crawl swimming stroke are often reluctant to exhale air while their faces are in the water. They then try to inhale more air when their faces are turned to the side or to both exhale and inhale in the short time available during the head turn. Why is this not an effective breathing technique?

3. What is the effect of a snorkel on the dead space? What implication does this effect have for breathing with a snorkel?

Total Lung Capacity (TLC)   The greatest amount of air that the lungs can contain.

Residual Volume (RV)   The amount of air left in the lungs following a maximal exhalation.

Inspiratory reserve volume IRV:
  The greatest amount of air that
  can be inspired at the end of
  a normal inspiration

Tidal volume V_T:
  The amount of air that is inspired
  or expired in a normal breath

Expiratory reserve volume ERV:
  The greatest amount of air that
  can be expired at the end of a
  normal expiration

Residual volume RV:
  The amount of air that is left in
  the lungs following a maximal
  exhalation

Inspiratory capacity IC:
  The greatest amount of air that can
  be inspired from a resting expiratory
  level
  $IC = IRV + V_T$

Vital capacity VC:
  The greatest amount of air that can
  be exhaled following a maximal
  inhalation
  $VC = IRV + V_T + ERV$

Functional residual capacity FRC:
  The amount of air left in the lungs
  at the end of a normal expiration
  $FRC = ERV + RV$

Total lung capacity TLC:
  The greatest amount of air that can
  be contained in the lungs
  $TLC = VC + RV$
      $= IC + FRC$
      $= IRV + V_T + ERV + RV$

FIGURE 2.4

Static Lung Volumes

Total lung capacity (TLC) can be subdivided several ways into four volumes (IRV, V_T, ERV, and RV) and into three other capacities (IC, FRC, and VC). From the normal resting depth of inspiration and expiration (indicated by the wavy line moving up and down, respectively, in the box labeled V_T), both inspiration and expiration can be expanded into the IRV and ERV until all possible air is inhaled and exhaled (VC). The RV remain in the lungs at all times.

individual weighs underwater, the higher the measured percentage of body fat is. Thus if residual volume is not accounted for, it will be measured as fat. This is the most common reason for determining residual volume in exercise physiology. Sometimes residual volume is estimated from vital capacity.[13] When it is, residual volume is calculated as 24% of vital capacity for males and 28% of vital capacity for females.

Vital capacity (VC) itself is simply the largest amount of air that can be exhaled following a maximal inhalation. The common way of testing vital capacity is to ask the individual to inhale maximally

---

Vital Capacity (VC) The greatest amount of air that can be exhaled following a maximal inhalation.

---

and then forcefully exhale all of the air as quickly as possible. Because the exhalation is forced, the designation *forced vital capacity*, FVC, is used.

Dynamic Lung Volumes

If volumes are measured at specified time intervals (usually 1 and 3 sec) during a forced vital capacity test, the name is changed to *forced expiratory volume*, specifically, FEV_1 and FEV_3. This provides information not only on the total volume of air moved but also on the rate of flow of that movement. Normal healthy individuals should be able to exhale at least 80% of their FVC in 1 sec. Because time is now a factor, this measurement is labeled FEV_1. FEV_1 values below 65–70% are indicative of moderate to severe restriction to airflow.[1]

The second commonly measured dynamic lung volume is a test of ventilatory capacity called *maxi-*

mal voluntary ventilation (MVV). In this test a timed maximal ventilation of either 12 or 15 sec is recorded and then multiplied by 5 (if 12 sec) or 4 (if 15 sec) to extrapolate to the volume that could be ventilated in 1 min. This value is usually higher than what can actually be achieved during exercise in untrained individuals, but it does give a rough estimation of exercise ventilation potential. Low values can reflect not only airway resistance but also poorly conditioned or poorly functioning ventilatory muscles.

Both forced expiratory volume and maximal voluntary ventilation tests are often used as screening tests prior to maximal exercise tests of oxygen consumption.

Spirometry

All of the lung volumes and capacities described in the preceding paragraphs—except for total lung capacity, functional residual capacity, and residual volume—can be measured using a spirometer. *Spirometers* typically consist of an inverted container called a bell that fits inside another container usually filled with water. An air tube reaches from the subject's mouth to about the water line. When air is exhaled into the tube, the bell is pushed up; inhalation moves the bell down. A pen connected to the pulley system follows the movements of the bell. In this way, the volumes of air inspired and expired can be measured, and the various volumes, capacities, and flow rates can be calculated. A spirometer that measures air volumes over water is called a

wet spirometer. Some newer spirometers do not use water and therefore are called *dry spirometers* (Figure 2.5).

Gas Dilution

Total lung capacity, functional residual capacity, and residual volume cannot be measured by simple spirometry because each one includes air that cannot be exhaled voluntarily from the lungs. Thus, it is necessary to determine the volume of air that remains in the lungs. The most common technique for this measurement is gas dilution. One technique involves the dilution of an inert, insoluble, foreign gas such as helium (He). A second technique involves the dilution of medical grade oxygen and the measurement of nitrogen (N_2) and is called the nitrogen washout technique.

Standardization

The respiratory measures detailed above are collected under ambient, or atmospheric, conditions. That is, the temperature measured is the temperature of the room or in the spirometer; the pressure is the barometric pressure of the room; and because the air is exhaled from inside the human body, which is a wet environment, the air is saturated with water vapor. The designation is thus ATPS: ambient (A) temperature (T) and pressure (P), saturated (S). Because ATPS volumes vary from situation to situation, they must be converted to standardized conditions on the basis of the effects of pressure, temperature, and water vapor on gas volumes. Figure 2.6 illustrates these three effects, which are described in the following paragraphs.

1. The volume of a given quantity of gas is inversely related to the pressure exerted on it when the temperature remains constant. This effect is Boyle's law and was discussed previously in the explanation of the mechanics of breathing. As shown in Figure 2.6a, when pressure is reduced from 760 to 600 mmHg, 5 L of air expands to 6.3 L. The reverse is also true. If the pressure increases from 600 to 760 mmHg, the volume is reduced, from 6.3 to 5.0 L.[11]

2. The volume of a given quantity of gas is directly related to the temperature of the gas when the pressure remains constant. This effect is described by *Charles's law*. As shown in Figure 2.6b,

FIGURE 2.5

A Spirometer

(a)   Effect of Pressure on Volume

(b)   Effect of Temperature on Volume

(c)   Effect of Water Vapor on Volume

FIGURE 2.6

Effects of Pressure, Temperature, and Water Vapor on Air Volume

(a) The volume of a given quantity of a gas is inversely related to the pressure exerted on it, if the temperature remains constant (Boyle's law). (b) The volume of a give quantity of gas is directly related to the temperature of the gas if the pressure remains constant (Charles's law). (c) The volume of a gas increases as the content of water vapor increases.

if the temperature is reduced from 37°C to 0°C, the volume of the gas is also reduced, from 5 to 4.4 L. The reverse is also true. If the temperature rises from 0°C to 37°C, the volume also rises, from 4.4 to 5.0 L.

3.   Water molecules evaporate into a gas such as air and are responsible for part of the pressure of that gas. The amount of pressure accounted for by the water vapor is related exponentially to

temperature. As shown in Figure 2.6c, when a volume of air is converted from saturated to dry air at a constant temperature, the volume is reduced, from 5.0 to 4.7 L. Once again, the reverse is also true. If a gas volume goes from dry to wet at a given temperature, the volume increases.[11]

The numbers representing temperature and pressure in Figure 2.6 were not chosen arbitrarily. They are involved in the two standardized conditions to which ATPS lung volumes are converted: BTPS and STPD. The abbreviation BTPS means body temperature (37°C), ambient pressure, and fully saturated with water vapor. Remember that in its passage through the conduction zone the air was both warmed and humidified to achieve these values. When converting from ATPS to BTPS, the temperature increases; and the pressure, adjusted for the effects of temperature on water vapor pressure, decreases. From Charles's law (an increase in temperature causes an increase in volume) and Boyle's law (a decrease in pressure causes an increase in volume), the BTPS volume is larger than the originally measured ATPS volume. BTPS is typically used when the anatomical space from which the volume of gas originated is of primary importance. Hence, most lung volumes and capacities are conventionally expressed as BTPS.

STPD means standard temperature (0°C) and pressure (760 mmHg), dry.

■ EXAMPLE

Based on the previous discussion, decide whether you think STPD volumes will be greater or smaller than ATPS volumes. Explain your decision. Your reasoning should be as follows. Under typical testing conditions temperature decreases from ATPS (≈20°C) to STPD (0°C), and by Charles's law, so does volume. Unless the testing is done at sea level, pressure increases from ATPS (variable, but around 735–745 mmHg before considering the influence of water vapor) to STPD (760 mmHg), and according to Boyle's law, volume decreases. Going from wet to dry conditions also decreases the volume. Therefore, the STPD volume is smaller than the originally measured ATPS volume.   ■

STPD volumes are used when it is necessary to know the amount of gas molecules present. Minute ventilation, whether measured as inspired or ex-

TABLE 2.1 ■ **Approximate Gas Partial Pressures in Ambient Air and Selected Ventilatory and Respiratory Sites**

Gases	(a) Dry Atmospheric Air, Sea Level			(b) Dry Atmospheric Air, Altitude = 14,000 ft (4268 m) (Pike's Peak)			(c) Alveolar Air, Sea Level		
	%	P_B (mmHg)	P (mmHg)	%	P_B (mmHg)	P (mmHg)	%	P_B (mmHg)	P (mmHg)
O_2	20.93	760	159	20.93	440	92	13.7–14.6	760	104–98*
CO_2	0.03	760	0.3	0.03	440	0.1	5.3	760	40
N_2	79.04	760	600.7	79.4	440	348	73.9–74.8	760	561–569
H_2O	0.00	760	0.0	0.00	440	0.0	6.2	760	47†
						440			760

*Owing to minor variations in percentage, the PO_2 in alveolar air is often rounded to 100 mmHg.

†Assumes a body temperature of 37°C.

pired, is typically converted and reported in STPD conditions, although sometimes it may be expressed as BTPS.

*P*artial Pressure of a Gas: Dalton's Law

Dry, unpolluted atmospheric air is a mixture of gases including oxygen, carbon dioxide, nitrogen, argon, and krypton. Since the latter three are considered to be inert in humans, they are generally linked together and labeled simply as nitrogen, because nitrogen comprises by far the largest amount. Thus, air is said to be composed of 79.04% nitrogen, 20.93% oxygen, and 0.03% carbon dioxide. These percentages are also referred to as fractions of each gas and are then given in a decimal form 0.7904 nitrogen, 0.2093 oxygen, and 0.0003 carbon dioxide. Another way to describe the composition of a gas mixture such as air is by the partial pressures exerted by each gas.[7]

All gases exert pressure. In a mixture of gases the total pressure exerted by the gases is the sum of the pressure of individual gases making up the mixture. Total pressure is standardized to the sea-level barometric pressure of 760 mmHg, but at altitudes above sea level the actual barometric pressure, P_B, must be used. The **partial pressure of a gas (P_G)** is that portion of the total pressure exerted by any single gas within the mixture. The partial pressure of any gas is proportional to its percentage in the total

gas mixture. These relationships are known as *Dalton's law of partial pressures.*

The partial pressure of any gas is the product of the total pressure and the fraction of the gas (as a decimal).

(2.4)   partial pressure of a gas (mmHg)
= total pressure (mmHg) × fraction of the gas
or
$$P_G = P_B \times F_G$$

For example, the standardized partial pressure of nitrogen, PN_2, is 760 mmHg × 0.7904 = 600.7 mmHg.

Substituting the appropriate fractions, calculate the PO_2 and PCO_2 of dry atmospheric air. Table 2.1, column a, shows the answers. For extra practice also calculate the partial pressure of dry atmospheric air at altitude and of alveolar air. Look first at Table 2.1, columns a and b. Notice that the gas percentages are the same at sea level and at altitude, in this case 14,000 ft (4268 m). These percentages would be true no matter what the selected altitude. Conversely, the barometric pressure (P_B) is lower at both the selected altitude and any other altitude in comparison with sea level. Exactly how much lower than sea

Partial Pressure of a Gas (P_G) The pressure exerted by an individual gas in a mixture; determined by multiplying the fraction of the gas by the total barometric pressure.

level the P_B is depends on how high the altitude is. At 14,000 ft P_B is 440 mmHg. As the altitude increases, the barometric pressure decreases. Now compare Table 2.1, columns a and c. Notice that now the barometric pressure values are the same, that is, they are both standardized to 760 mmHg. However, the fractions of the gases are different. This variation in alveolar air from atmospheric air occurs as the percentage of oxygen is diminished by diffusion into the capillary blood and the percentage of carbon dioxide is enlarged by diffusion out of the capillary blood. In addition, water vapor now occupies a percentage of the total air mixture.

Knowledge of the partial pressure of gases is important for at least two reasons. The first is that the partial pressures of oxygen and more definitively carbon dioxide serve to regulate pulmonary ventilation to bring air into the lungs. The second reason is that both external and internal respiration depend on pressure gradients.

Regulation of Pulmonary Ventilation

Breathing, or pulmonary ventilation, is the result of inspiratory and expiratory muscle contraction and relaxation. The muscle action—and hence the rate, depth, and rhythm of breathing—is controlled by the brain and nervous system and is tightly coupled to the body's overall need for oxygen and the subsequent production of energy and carbon dioxide. The coordinated control of the respiratory muscles is a very complex process that is not yet fully understood.[7,8]

The Respiratory Centers

Two respiratory centers, composed of anatomically distinct neural networks, are located within the medulla oblongata of the brain stem. These two centers are schematically diagramed in Figure 2.7. The more important of the two is the *inspiratory center* (I),

> **Respiratory Cycle**   Inspiration and expiration.
>
> **Eupnea**   Normal respiration rate and rhythm.

also called the *dorsal respiratory group* (DRG). The other center is the *expiratory center* (E), sometimes called the *ventral respiratory group* (VRG). The nerves that make up the inspiratory center depolarize spontaneously in a cyclic, rhythmical on-off pattern. During the "on" portion of the cycle nerve impulses traveling via motor neurons in the phrenic nerve stimulate the diaphragm and external intercostal inspiratory muscles to contract. Inhalation occurs when the thoracic cavity is enlarged and intrathoracic pressure decreases. During the "off" portion of the cycle the nerve impulses are interrupted, the inspiratory muscles relax, and exhalation occurs. Without outside influence and at rest, the inspiratory center brings about a **respiratory cycle** of approximately 2 sec for inspiration and 3 sec for exhalation (for a rate of 12–15 br$\cdot$min^{-1}). This normal respiratory rate and oscillating rhythm is known as **eupnea.**[7]

The expiratory center appears to have two functions. The first is to maintain inspiratory muscle tone or low-level contraction such that the inspiratory muscles never completely relax. The second is to bring about active contraction of the expiratory muscles (internal intercostals and abdominals) when forceful breathing is required, such as during moderate to heavy exercise. This latter action is instigated by the inspiratory center, which recruits additional accessory muscles at the same time.[7,8]

Two neural centers in the pons area of the brain stem also act as respiratory centers and seem to be important for ensuring that the transitions between inhalation and exhalation are smooth. The *pneumotaxic center* constantly transmits inhibitory (indicated on the diagram by a minus sign, –) neural impulses directly to the inspiratory center and situationally to the apneustic center. This limits or, in some cases, shortens inspiration and promotes expiration—thus fine tuning the breathing pattern and preventing lung overinflation. The *apneustic center* continually stimulates (indicated on the diagram by a plus sign, +) the inspiratory center unless inhibited situationally by the pneumotaxic center.[7,8]

Anatomical Sensors and Factors Affecting Control of Pulmonary Ventilation

The inspiratory, expiratory, pneumotaxic, and apneustic centers are influenced by a number of fac-

FIGURE 2.7

Brain Stem Control of Pulmonary Ventilation

Schematic representation of the respiratory centers that control ventilation.

tors through a variety of anatomical sensors that are important during exercise. Figure 2.8 schematically presents the major factors and where each factor operates. Without outside influences the rate (frequency) of breathing and tidal volume (depth of breathing) exhibit the greatest changes. A disruption in rhythm rarely occurs except under voluntary control.[6,7,8,12]

Higher Brain Centers   Both the hypothalamus and the cerebral cortex can influence breathing. The first operates involuntarily and the second voluntarily.

Hypothalamus.   The sympathetic nervous system centers in the hypothalamus are activated by pain or strong emotions. They, in turn, send neural messages to the respiratory centers. The reaction can be either stimulatory or inhibitory to breathing.

Hyperventilation by an individual who is emotionally upset is an example of hypothalamic stimulation and having your breath taken away when you jump into very cold water exemplifies hypothalamic inhibition. This hypothalamic control mechanism is also very important in bringing about the increase in respiration upon initiation of movement and sustaining the increase throughout the duration of an activity.[4]

Cerebral Cortex.   Cerebral control of breathing originates in the motor cortex. Such control is important to musicians, singers, and athletes such as swimmers, weight lifters, archers, and shooters, to name just a few. The motor cortex may also operate such that the conscious anticipation of exercise unconsciously increases ventilation. Neural impulses from the motor cortex pass directly to the respiratory muscles, bypassing the control centers in the

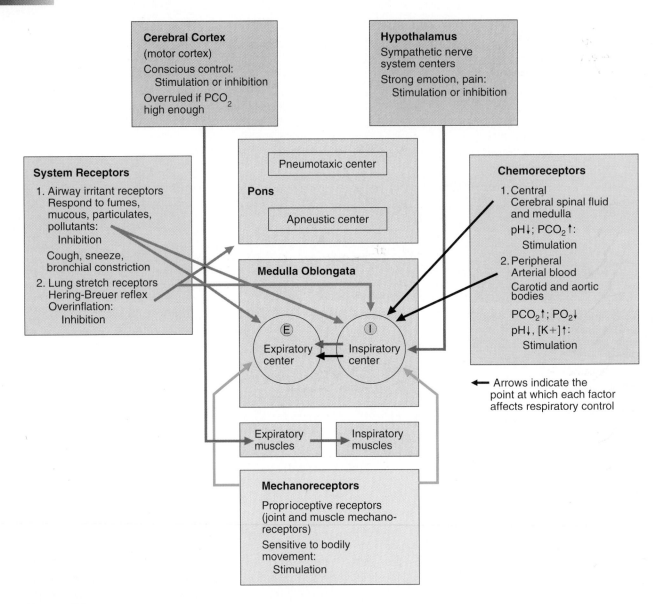

FIGURE 2.8

Anatomical Sensors and Factors That Influence the Control of Pulmonary Ventilation

Schematic representation of the pathways of action of the factors that influence the brain stem control of ventilation.

medulla. Voluntary control is limited, however.[7,8] If you doubt this, take a reading break now and jog in place at a fast pace for 3 min. Sit down immediately upon stopping, and try holding your breath for 1 min. If you can do that, great; but even if you can, you will probably feel a desire to breathe. More than

likely, the automatic drive to breathe will overrule your conscious signal not to; and at some point before the end of the minute, you will gasp for air.

Systemic Receptors   The lungs themselves contain several types of receptors that provide sensory information to the respiratory control centers and result in reflex action. Chief among them are irritant receptors and stretch receptors.[7,8] Both of these receptors are more important as protective devices than as regulators of normal resting or exercise ventilation.

Irritant Receptors. *Irritant receptors* within the conduction zone respond to foreign substances such as chemicals, noxious gases, cold air, mucus, and   dust other pollutant particulates and bring about a reflex response. Depending on the irritating substance and the anatomical location, the response may be a cough, a sneeze, or a bronchial constriction, all of which disrupt the normal breathing pattern.[7,8]

Stretch Receptors. *Stretch receptors* in the lung respond to deep, fast inflation. Increases in lung volume stimulate the stretch receptors, which send inhibitory impulses to both the apneustic center and the inspiratory center. As a result, inspiration ceases. This reflex is called the *Hering-Breuer reflex*. The threshold for this reflex is quite high. It does not appear to function at rest and plays a minor role in exercise.

Mechanoreceptors   Specific *mechanoreceptors* called proprioceptors exist in skeletal muscles (including respiratory muscles) and joint capsules. These receptors provide information to a variety of sites in the brain about movement and body position in space. Input from these receptors probably plays some minor role in the stimulation of respiration during exercise but are not involved in respiration during rest.[7]

Chemoreceptors   *Chemoreceptor sensors* that respond to fluctuations in chemical substances important to respiration are found in two major anatomical locations. *Central chemoreceptors* are located in the medulla oblongata (but not in the respiratory control centers) and are sensitive to an increased carbon dioxide partial pressure ($PCO_2\uparrow$) and an increased acidity ($pH\downarrow$). *Peripheral chemoreceptors* are located in large arteries, specifically, at the aortic body and the carotid body. In addition to being sensitive to $\uparrow PCO_2$ and $\downarrow pH$, these receptors are also sensitive to a decrease in the partial pressure of oxygen ($\downarrow PO_2$) and an increase in the con-

centration of potassium ions ($[K^+]\uparrow$). Each of these factors is explained in the following subsections.

Influence of PO_2.   The peripheral carotid body chemoreceptors are the main oxygen sensors. Under normal circumstances decline in PO_2 has very little impact on minute ventilation other than enhancing sensitivity to $PCO_2\uparrow$.[7]

Figure 2.9 shows that from the normal arterial PO_2 of 95 mmHg (Table 2.1) to a value of about 60 mmHg, minute ventilation does not change if the arterial PCO_2 remains normal (approximately 36–42 mmHg). However, if the arterial PO_2 decreases below 60 mmHg, minute ventilation is stimulated to rise exponentially. This decrease is not a normal physiological event at sea level, even at very heavy levels of exercise, because the arterial PO_2 mmHg is maintained within narrow limits. However, arterial PO_2 may fall below 60 mmHg at altitudes at or above 14,000 ft (4268 m), triggering the graphically depicted increase in minute ventilation.[7,8]

FIGURE 2.9

The Effect of Arterial PO_2 (PaO_2) on Minute Ventilation

At a normal $PaCO_2$ of 36–42 mmHg, reduced PaO_2 does not stimulate ventilation until the value of PaO_2 is less than 60 mmHg.

Source: A. R. Leff & P. T. Schumacker. *Respiratory Physiology: Basics and Applications.* Philadelphia: W. B. Saunders Company (1993). Reprinted by permission.

Influence of PCO₂. Both the central and the peripheral chemoreceptors are sensitive to an increase in arterial PCO_2. However, the peripheral chemoreceptors respond more directly to PCO_2 than the central chemoreceptors do. The central chemoreceptors respond initially to rising PCO_2 levels but thereafter primarily to the effect these rising PCO_2 levels have on pH. The ventilatory response to PCO_2 is split 40–60% between peripheral and central chemoreceptors, respectively. At rest, the regulation of pH in the cerebrospinal fluid is the primary control mechanism of ventilation.

Figure 2.10 shows the influence of increasing arterial PCO_2 values on minute ventilation. Even a small deviation from the normal value of PCO_2 of approximately 40 mmHg (Table 2.1) causes a large rectilinear increase in minute ventilation when arterial PO_2 is maintained at approximately normal levels (≈95 mmHg). The steepness and the immediacy of this rectilinear increase indicates that the ventilation is much more sensitive to an increase in PCO_2

FIGURE 2.10

The Ventilatory Response to Carbon Dioxide

At a normal P_AO_2 of approximately 100 mmHg, a rise in $PaCO_2$ from the normal value of 40 mmHg to just 45 mmHg almost doubles pulmonary ventilation (from approximately 17 L·min⁻¹ to 27 L·min⁻¹, as indicated by the dashed lines intersecting the Y-axis) showing how sensitive ventilation is to $PaCO_2$.

Source: Modified from M. Nielsen & H. Smith. Studies on the regulation of respiration in acute hypoxia. *Acta Physiologica Scandinavica* 24:293–313 (1951). Reprinted by permission.

than to a decrease in PO_2. Hence, PCO_2 is the stronger regulating factor. An increase as small as 5 mmHg in PCO_2 will almost double ventilation.[7]

Holding your breath will cause an increase in arterial PCO_2. This buildup of CO_2 is the reason your conscious control of respiration was overruled when you tried not to breathe after doing the 3-min jog in place. On the other hand, hyperventilation—whether caused by an altitude response to a decreased PO_2, an involuntary response during an anxiety attack, or a conscious attempt to extend breath-holding time—will decrease PCO_2 and the drive to breathe.

The decrement in PCO_2 with hyperventilation can have serious consequences. Most people know that hyperventilating will extend breath-holding time, but many erroneously believe it does so because more oxygen is taken in. They are unaware that it is CO_2 that is changing (being blown off) and that respiration is more sensitive to PCO_2 changes than to PO_2 changes. Craig[2] presented a summary of 58 cases of loss of consciousness during underwater swimming and diving following hyperventilation. Of these cases, 40% (23 cases) ended as fatalities, and most of these cases occurred in guarded pools. Because an individual continues patterned motor activity (swimming) after loss of consciousness caused by a lack of oxygen to the brain, these life-threatening cases are difficult for a lifeguard to detect quickly. The beginning swimmer who is frustrated at trying to coordinate arms, legs, and breathing and simply puts his or her head in the water and tries to go as far as possible without breathing is also vulnerable. It is recommended that underwater swimming be limited to one length of a standard 25-yd or 25-m pool.

Influence of pH. As with an increase in arterial PCO_2 both the peripheral and central chemoreceptors are sensitive to decreases in pH. The pH level is partially related to CO_2 level. When CO_2 is hydrated, it forms carbonic acid (H_2CO_3) and degrades readily into hydrogen ions (H^+) and bicarbonate (HCO_3^-) according to the following reactions:

$$CO_2 + H_2O \leftrightarrow H_2CO_3 \leftrightarrow H^+ + HCO_3^-$$

$$\underset{\text{dioxide}}{\text{carbon}} + \text{water} \leftrightarrow \underset{\text{acid}}{\text{carbonic}} \leftrightarrow \underset{\text{ions}}{\text{hydrogen}} + \text{bicarbonate}$$

In blood the H^+ can be buffered; but if that capacity is exceeded, any change in arterial pH is detected by the aortic and carotid bodies. The brain and spinal cord are bathed by a protein-free solution known as *cerebrospinal fluid* (CSF). CO_2 easily diffuses across the blood-brain barrier and into the CSF. Because brain cells also produce CO_2 and because CSF has no protein buffers, the pH of CSF is slightly more acidic than that of blood. An excess of H^+ in CSF acts directly on the central chemoreceptors to increase respiration; a decrease in H^+ suppresses respiration.

All changes in pH are, of course, not related to CO_2. For example, during high-intensity exercise large quantities of lactic acid accumulate. If the blood's ability to buffer the resultant H^+ is exceeded, pH will decrease and respiration will increase.

Influence of [K^+]. Of the chemical factors mentioned so far ($\downarrow PO_2$, $\uparrow PCO_2$, $\downarrow pH$), only $\downarrow pH$ changes enough during exercise to cause the needed increase in ventilation known as *hyperpnea*. An increase in [K^+] may be another factor that changes sufficiently in exercise to increase ventilation. Potassium moves from the working muscles to blood during all intensities of exercise as a result of the establishment of neural impulses. This increased [K^+], called *hyperkalemia*, directly stimulates the carotid bodies. At rest [K^+] is not a factor.[4,5,9]

Figure 2.8 presented earlier schematically depicts the factors that control the rate and depth of ventilation. It would be logical to assume that changes in arterial PO_2 and PCO_2 occur during exercise and have the primary role in control. However, this is not what happens. Neither PO_2 nor PCO_2 change enough, especially early in exercise or at low to moderate to heavy intensities in untrained individuals to play a major role in ventilatory control during exercise. Exactly which factor is most important is not known precisely, and changes may take place in the sensitivity of the medullary respiratory control centers themselves during exercise. Neural messages from the motor cortex, muscle proprioceptors, and hypothalamic sympathetic nervous system activity as well as increases in the hydrogen ion and potassium ion concentrations all appear to have a role during exercise.[4,8]

Gas Exchange and Transport

Gas Exchange: Henry's Law

As mentioned previously, knowledge of the partial pressure of gases is important for two reasons. One is that the partial pressures of gases control pul-

monary ventilation. The second reason is that the movement of O_2 and CO_2 between the alveoli and capillaries (defined as external respiration) and between the capillaries and tissues (defined as internal respiration) occurs by the process of diffusion. **Diffusion** is defined as the tendency of gaseous, liquid, or solid molecules to move from areas of high concentration to areas of low concentration by constant random action. Diffusion can only occur if there is a pressure gradient (a difference in the partial pressures of the gas) between the capillary and the tissue. Gases diffuse down a pressure gradient from areas of high pressure to areas of low pressure. The rate of diffusion depends on the magnitude of the pressure gradient (millimeters of mercury at the high end minus millimeters of mercury at the low end), the surface area available for diffusion, the thickness of the barrier between the two locations, and the solubility (ability to be dissolved) of the gas in the barrier liquid. *Henry's law* states that when a mixture of gases is in contact with a liquid, each gas dissolves in the liquid in proportion to its partial pressure and solubility until equilibrium is achieved and the gas partial pressures are equal in both locations.[7,8]

External Respiration

External respiration is the movement of gases at the alveolar–pulmonary capillary level. Specifically oxygen diffuses from the alveoli into the pulmonary capillaries, and carbon dioxide diffuses from the pulmonary capillary to the alveoli. This exchange is diagramed in Figures 2.11a and 2.11d.

Remember that pulmonary circulation originates from the right ventricle of the heart. By definition, an artery is a vessel carrying blood away from the heart. Unlike systemic arteries, the pulmonary artery carries partially deoxygenated blood. The pulmonary arteries quickly branch into capillaries that parallel the alveoli. While they are small, the capillaries do have a definable length.

When the capillary and alveoli first make contact at the arterial end of the capillary, PO_2 in the

Diffusion The tendency of gaseous, liquid, or solid molecules to move from areas of high concentration to areas of low concentration by constant random action.

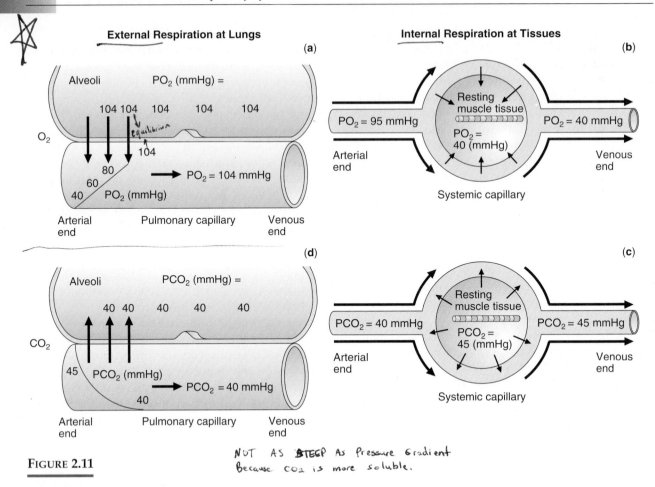

External Respiration at Lungs (a)

Internal Respiration at Tissues (b)

(d)

(c)

NOT AS STEEP As Pressure Gradient
Because CO_2 is more soluble.

FIGURE 2.11

Oxygen and Carbon Dioxide Exchange

Gas exchange takes place at two anatomical locations: the alveoli-pulmonary capillary interface (called external respiration) and the systemic capillary tissue interface (called internal respiration). (a) External respiration for oxygen, (b) internal respiration for oxygen, (c) internal respiration for carbon dioxide, and (d) external respiration of carbon dioxide.

alveoli (P_AO_2) is high (98–104 mmHg) (see Table 2.1) and PO_2 in the capillary (PaO_2) is low (40 mmHg). The net diffusion of oxygen is from high to low down the pressure gradient until an equilibrium is reached. Note in Figure 2.11a that this equalization of pressure occurs within the first third of the capillary length. Refer again to Table 2.1 and Figures 2.11a and 2.11b. In Figure 2.11b, notice that PaO_2 is listed as 95 mmHg, not as 98–104 mmHg as given in Table 2.1 and Figure 2.11a. The lower value results because the fully oxygenated blood in the pulmonary vein is diluted with partially oxygenated venous blood (PvO_2 = 40 mmHg) from bronchial vein as blood from both veins flows into

the left atrium. Remember that the bronchial artery, the capillaries, and the vein provide blood to and return it from the lungs as part of the systemic circulation and so have the normal systemic gas contents and pressures. Although blood from the bronchial vein amounts to only about 2% of the total blood returning to the left atrium, it is sufficient to bring the PaO_2 of systemic arterial blood down to approximately 95 mmHg.[6]

At the same time that oxygen is diffusing from the alveoli to the pulmonary capillaries, carbon dioxide is diffusing from the pulmonary capillaries to the alveoli. When any given capillary and alveoli first make contact at the arterial end of the capillary,

PCO_2 in the capillary is high (about 45 mmHg) and PCO_2 in the alveoli is low (40 mmHg) (see Table 2.1). The net diffusion of carbon dioxide is also from high to low pressure down the gradient until an equilibrium is reached. Note in Figure 2.11d that this equalization of pressure occurs within the first third of the capillary length. Note also that the pressure gradient for CO_2 is not nearly as steep (5 mmHg) as it is for O_2 (64 mmHg). Carbon dioxide simply does not need as great a pressure gradient because it is more soluble. Again, remember that each gas moves down its own concentration gradient irrespective of the concentration of any other gas.

Internal Respiration

Internal respiration is the movement of gases at the capillary-tissue level. Although the tissue can be any tissue, it is particularly relevant for exercise physiology students to think of the tissue as skeletal muscle tissue. Internal respiration is diagramed in Figures 2.11b and 2.11c. Skeletal muscle fibers are well supplied with capillaries. When blood enters the arterial end of any capillary, PaO_2 is high (95 mmHg). Within the tissue PO_2 at rest is low (40 mmHg). The net diffusion of oxygen is once again from high to low pressure until an equilibrium is reached. Blood exiting into the venous system thus has a PvO_2 of 40 mmHg, which is maintained until oxygenation occurs again at the alveoli.

Carbon dioxide is produced at the tissue level as a direct result of cellular respiration. Thus, PCO_2 levels are higher (about 45 mmHg) in the tissues than elsewhere in the system. Diffusion occurs as always from the area of high pressure (45 mmHg in the tissue) to the area of low pressure (40 mmHg in the systemic capillary), once again achieving equilibrium. The venous level of PCO_2 is also maintained until it reaches the alveoli, where the carbon dioxide diffuses out of the bloodstream and is exhaled. To make sure that you understand what is happening here, complete the question in Box 2.2.

Oxygen Transport

Oxygen is carried two ways in the blood. The first way oxygen is transported is in a dissolved form in the liquid portion of the blood. The amount of oxygen transported in this fashion is only about 1.5–3% of the total oxygen transported. However, it is this

---

Box 2.2 A Question of Understanding

Follow oxygen around the body from the alveoli to the pulmonary capillaries, through the left side of the heart, the systemic arteries, the tissue, the systemic capillaries, the systemic veins, the right side of the heart, and back to the alveoli. Give the PO_2 at each site and any net movement of oxygen. Do the same thing for carbon dioxide, giving PCO_2, but start at the tissue level where carbon dioxide is produced and follow it through the systemic capillaries and veins, the right side of the heart, the pulmonary capillaries and alveoli, the pulmonary vein, the left side of the heart, the systemic arterial system, and back to the systemic capillaries at the tissue level. Check your answer with the one provided in the answer section.

---

dissolved component that is responsible for the partial pressure of oxygen in the blood (see Figure 2.11). The dissolved oxygen content is determined by the PO_2 and the solubility of oxygen, which is a constant of 0.00304 mL $\cdot$ dL^{-1} $\cdot$ mmHg at 37°C. The formula is[6,7,8]

(2.5)   dissolved O_2 content (mL $\cdot$ dL^{-1}) = PO_2 (mmHg) $\times$ solubility (mL $\cdot$ dL^{-1} $\cdot$ mmHg^{-1})

■ EXAMPLE

In normal arterial blood with a PaO_2 of 95 mmHg the calculation becomes

dissolved O_2 content = (95 mmHg) $\times$
(0.00304 mL $\cdot$ dL^{-1} $\cdot$ mmHg^{-1})
= 0.29 mL $\cdot$ dL^{-1}

Thus, only 0.29 mL of oxygen is dissolved in a deciliter of arterial blood. You may also see this result expressed in units of milliliters per 100 milliliters (mL $\cdot$ 100 mL^{-1}) of blood or as milliliters percent (mL%). All are comparable.   ■

The second way oxygen is transported in the blood is bound to hemoglobin. The vast majority, 97–98.5%, of the oxygen is transported in the bloodstream bound to hemoglobin.

Red Blood Cells and Hemoglobin   Red blood cells (RBC), or erythrocytes, are small, flexible cells shaped like biconcave disks, or miniature doughnuts, with the hole squished in but not pushed out (Figure 2.12). Females typically have a RBC count of 4.3–5.2 million per cubic milliliter of blood; the male count is generally between 5.1 and 5.8 million per cubic milliliter of blood. The total number for the average person is about 35 trillion, with a total surface area of about 2000 times the total body surface area. **Hemoglobin,** which is the protein portion of the RBC that binds with oxygen, constitutes about one third of a RBC by weight if water is included, but 97% if water is excluded. Normal values for hemoglobin for adult females are 12–16 g · 100 mL^{-1} blood, with a mean of 14 g · 100 mL^{-1} blood. For adult males the values are 14–18 g · 100 mL^{-1} blood, with a mean of 16 g · 100 mL^{-1} blood. Children have slightly lower values.[8]

Hemoglobin consists of four iron-containing pigments called *hemes* and a protein called *globin.* Each iron atom can combine reversibly with one molecule of oxygen. Therefore, each hemoglobin molecule can transport four molecules of oxygen. The chemical symbol for hemoglobin not bound to oxygen, sometimes called deoxyhemoglobin or reduced hemoglobin, is Hb. Hemoglobin bound to oxygen is symbolized HbO$_2$ and is termed oxyhemoglobin. None of the oxygen bound to hemoglobin is used by the RBC.

The Binding of Oxygen with Hb: The Oxygen Dissociation Curve

All four oxygen molecules do not bind with the four heme atoms at the same time. Binding of one oxygen molecule onto a fully deoxygenated hemoglobin molecule changes the shape and increases the binding affinity for the next oxygen molecule. Thus, each succeeding oxygen molecule binds more easily than the preceding one. The result, when graphed, gives the characteris-

FIGURE 2.12

Red Blood Cells

An electron micrograph of erythrocytes or red blood cells (RBC) dyed red and showing the biconcave disk shape.

tic sigmoid-shaped curve of oxyhemoglobin shown in Figure 2.13. This curve is called the *oxygen dissociation curve,* for reasons that will become clear later.

When all four of its heme groups are bound to oxygen, the hemoglobin molecule is said to be fully saturated. All hemoglobin may not be fully saturated, though. The amount of the oxygen-carrying capacity that is utilized is referred to as **percent saturation of hemoglobin** and is designated as SbO$_2$%. Percent saturation is calculated as

$$(2.6) \qquad SbO_2\% = \frac{O_2 \text{ combined with Hb}}{O_2 \text{ capacity for combining with Hb}} \times 100$$

The symbols SaO$_2$% and SvO$_2$% may be used to distinguish percent saturation of blood in the arteries and veins, respectively, whereas Sb refers nonspecifically to blood.

Percent saturation depends primarily on the partial pressure of oxygen. In arterial blood at a PO$_2$ of 95 mmHg the percent saturation is 97%. Find this value on Figure 2.13 where PO$_2$ is on the X-axis and SbO$_2$% is on the left Y-axis. On the same figure determine the SbO$_2$% in normal venous blood. Since the PO$_2$ in normal venous blood is 40 mmHg, you should have determined that the SbO$_2$% was 75%. This value is also shown in Figure 2.13.

The oxygen content of hemoglobin depends upon the hemoglobin level and the physiological

---

Hemoglobin (Hb)   The protein portion of the red blood cell that binds with oxygen, consisting of four iron-containing pigments called hemes and a protein called globin.

Percent Saturation of Hemoglobin (SbO$_2$%)   The ratio of the amount of oxygen combined with hemoglobin to the total oxygen capacity for combining with hemoglobin, expressed as a percentage; indicated generally as SbO$_2$% or specifically as SaO$_2$% for arterial blood or as SvO$_2$% for venous blood.

Assumes Hb = 15g·dL⁻¹ blood; Body temperature = 37°C
a = arterial blood; $PaCO_2$ = 40 mmHg; pH = 7.4
v = venous blood; $PvCO_2$ = 45 mmHg; pH = 7.38

FIGURE 2.13

Oxygen Dissociation Curve
Under normal resting conditions approximately 25% of the oxygen being transported in arterial blood is dissociated (released or exchanged by internal respiration) for use by body tissues. The shaded area at the top of the diagram represents this in percentage on the left Y-axis and as an absolute amount on the right Y-axis. See text for full explanation and calculations.

oxygen-binding capacity according to the following formula

> **(2.7)**   oxygen content of hemoglobin (mL · dL⁻¹)
> = hemoglobin level (gm · dL⁻¹) × oxygen-binding capacity (mLO₂· gm Hb⁻¹) × percent saturation (expressed as a decimal fraction)
>
> or $HbO_2 = Hb \times 1.34 \times SbO_2\%$

In this equation the hemoglobin level will, of course, vary from individual to individual. The physiological oxygen-binding capacity is a constant 1.34 mLO₂· gmHb⁻¹, and the percent saturation of hemoglobin will vary between arterial and venous blood and resting and exercise conditions.

■ EXAMPLE

Using an average hemoglobin level of 15 gm · dL⁻¹, calculate the oxygen content for arterial blood where the percent saturation is 97%.

$$HbO_2 \text{ mL} \cdot \text{dL}^{-1} = 15 \text{ gm} \cdot \text{dL}^{-1}$$
$$\times 1.34 \text{ mLO}_2 \cdot \text{gmHb}^{-1} \times .97$$
$$= 19.5 \text{ mL} \cdot \text{dL}^{-1}$$

Check Figure 2.11 and look at the right side Y-axis. This axis is of O_2 content in mL · dL⁻¹ rounded to the nearest whole number. The value for normal arterial blood at 97% saturation is the value just calculated.   ■

Arteriovenous Oxygen Difference   The amount of oxygen released (dissociated) from the blood during one circuit through the systemic system is called the **arteriovenous oxygen difference (a-vO₂ diff)**. That is, the a-vO₂ diff is the difference between the amount of oxygen returned in venous blood and the amount originally carried in arterial blood. Before we can subtract to obtain the a-vO₂ diff, we must calculate the total oxygen in both the arteries and the veins. The amount normally carried in arterial blood has already been determined. It is

$$\text{dissolved } O_2 = \quad 0.29 \text{ mL} \cdot \text{dL}^{-1}$$
$$HbO_2 = \quad \underline{19.50 \text{ mL} \cdot \text{dL}^{-1}}$$
$$19.79 \text{ mL} \cdot \text{dL}^{-1} = \text{total } O_2 \text{ content in arterial blood (aO}_2)$$

■ EXAMPLE

Calculate the dissolved O_2 and HbO_2 in venous blood.

The calculations are as follows:

$$\text{dissolved } O_2 \text{ (venous)} = 40 \text{ mmHg}$$
$$\times 0.00304 \text{ mLO}_2 \cdot \text{dL}^{-1} \cdot \text{mmHg}$$
$$= 0.12 \text{ mL} \cdot \text{dL}^{-1}$$
$$HbO_2 \text{ (venous)} = 15 \text{ g} \cdot \text{dL}^{-1} \times 1.34 \text{ mL} \cdot \text{g}^{-1}$$
$$\times 0.75 = 15.08 \text{ mL} \cdot \text{dL}^{-1}$$

Now, add these values.

$$\text{dissolved } O_2 = 0.12 \text{ mL} \cdot \text{dL}^{-1}$$
$$HbO_2 = \underline{15.08 \text{ mL} \cdot \text{dL}^{-1}}$$
$$15.20 \text{ mL} \cdot \text{dL}^{-1} = \text{total } O_2 \text{ content in venous blood (vO}_2) \quad ■$$

Arteriovenous Oxygen Difference (a-vO₂ diff)
The difference between the amount of oxygen returned in venous blood and the amount originally carried in arterial blood.

The a-vO_2 diff is calculated by the formula

(2.8)	a-vO_2 diff = O_2 in arterial blood (mL · dL^{-1}) – O_2 in venous blood (mL · dL^{-1})
	or a-vO_2 diff = aO_2 – vO_2

Hence, the difference, using the values already calculated, is

$$\text{a-v}O_2 \text{ diff} = 19.79 \text{ mL} \cdot \text{dL}^{-1} – 15.20 \text{ mL} \cdot \text{dL}^{-1}$$
$$= 4.59 \text{ mL} \cdot \text{dL}^{-1}$$

Therefore, approximately 5 mL $O_2 \cdot$ dL^{-1} are transported to and used by the tissue to support cellular metabolism under normal resting conditions. This means that approximately 25% (4.59 ÷ 19.79 = 0.23 × 100 = 23%) of the oxygen is actually released from the hemoglobin to the tissues and used during rest. And thus, approximately 75% of the oxygen is held in reserve for use during such events as physical exercise. The actual amount of oxygen used, measured as the a-vO_2 diff, is called the *coefficient of oxygen utilization*. The normal resting coefficient of oxygen utilization is 4.59 mL · dL^{-1}.

Note that the 75% is also the SbO_2% value for venous blood. Refer to Figure 2.13 again. The shaded area at the top—between the SbO_2% values of 97 and 75% on the left axis and between the values 19.79 and 15.20 mL · dL^{-1} on the right axis—represents these relative and absolute amounts of O_2 that have been released or dissociated primarily from the RBC cells. On this basis, the curve is called the oxygen dissociation curve. The separation or release of oxygen from the red blood cells to the tissues is called **oxygen dissociation.**

Carbon Dioxide Transport

Carbon dioxide is carried three ways in the blood from muscle or other tissue where it is produced to the lungs where it is eliminated from the body. As with O_2, the first way it is transported is dissolved in blood plasma. The amount of CO_2 transported in this fashion is only about 5–10% of the total CO_2 transported. However, as with dissolved O_2, it is

> **Oxygen Dissociation** The separation or release of oxygen from the red blood cells to the tissues.

this dissolved CO_2 component that determines the partial pressure of CO_2 in the blood. Since the exchange of CO_2 in internal and external respiration depends largely upon the PCO_2, this is a critical role for dissolved CO_2. The remaining 90–95% of the CO_2 diffuses into the RBCs.

As CO_2 enters the RBC, about 20% combines chemically with the globin portion of the Hb molecule to produce the second form of CO_2 transport—namely, as *carbamino hemoglobin* (HbCO_2). Some small quantity may combine with proteins in the plasma as well. Note that when CO_2 combines with Hb, the CO_2 is not competing with oxygen for space on the heme units, since it combines with the globin portion. However, more CO_2 can combine with Hb if it is deoxygenated. That is, the lower the PO_2 and SbO_2%, the greater is the amount of CO_2 that can be carried in the blood. This reaction is known as the *Haldane effect*.[7]

At the lung the situation is reversed: As O_2 saturates the Hb, less CO_2 can be combined; so the release of CO_2 is stimulated. Thus, Hb is really a transport vehicle carrying O_2 from the alveoli to the cells and CO_2 from the cells to the alveoli. This task is made easier by the fact that the dissociation (dropping off) of one molecule facilitates the binding (picking up) of the other at both sites.

The third way that CO_2 can be transported is as bicarbonate ions. Approximately 70–75% of the CO_2 is transported in this way. When CO_2 diffuses into the RBCs, it combines with water under the influence of the enzyme carbonic anhydrase and forms carbonic acid (H_2CO_3). Carbonic acid is both weak and unstable and quickly dissociates into hydrogen ions (H^+) and bicarbonate ions (HCO_3^-). The chemical reaction is depicted as

$$\overset{\text{carbonic}}{\underset{}{\text{anhydrase}}}$$
$$CO_2 + H_2O \leftrightarrow H_2CO_3 \leftrightarrow H^+ + HCO_3^-$$

The H^+ binds to Hb (H^+ + Hb → HHb), thus preventing much change in pH; and the HCO_3^- diffuses into plasma. To counteract this loss of negative charges, chloride ions (Cl$^-$) move from plasma to the RBC. This ion exchange is called the *chloride shift*. At the lungs, where PCO_2 is relatively low, the reactions are all reversed. The chemical reactions are

$$O_2 + \text{HHb} \rightarrow \text{Hb}O_2 + H^+$$
$$H^+ + HCO_3^- \rightarrow H_2CO_3 \rightarrow CO_2 + H_2O$$

Once back in the form of CO_2, the CO_2 diffuses along its partial pressure gradient from the blood to the alveoli and is exhaled.[6,7,8]

Figure 2.14 summarizes the transport of both oxygen and carbon dioxide in arterial and venous blood. Take time to study that and relate it to the textual information.

The Respiratory System and Acid-Base Balance

The ability of hemoglobin to bind the hydrogen ions (H^+) produced during the transport of carbon dioxide and the ability of pulmonary ventilation to both respond to (Figures 2.8 and 2.10) and eliminate carbon dioxide are very important in the maintenance of acid-base balance. These reactions exemplify two of the three lines of defense for regulating acid-base balance, namely, the chemical buffer system and the respiratory system. Furthermore, the partial pressure of carbon dioxide is also directly involved in the third line of defense, renal regulation by the kidneys.

Acid-base balance is defined as a series of mechanisms that attempt to regulate the concentration of hydrogen ions in body fluids. It is vitally important, since virtually all biochemical reactions in the human body require the pH to be maintained within very narrow limits for proper functioning.[8,11] Hydrogen ions originate from a number of sources in the human body, but the majority appear as a result of the production of energy when oxygen is used and carbon dioxide is generated or when lactic acid is accumulated without the use of oxygen.

Chemical buffers are either weak acids or weak bases that respectively release or bind hydrogen ions. They respond instantaneously. Hemoglobin is not the only chemical buffer, but in terms of capacity it is the most important buffer in the blood. Bicarbonate (HCO_3^-) is another important base.[11]

The carbonic acid–bicarbonate system (H_2CO_3/HCO_3^-) not only allows for the temporary buffering of hydrogen ions as they travel through the circulatory system but also provides for the removal from the body of the carbon dioxide formed in the buffering process. The sensitivity of pulmonary ventilation to PCO_2 and pH enables varying amounts of acid production to be dealt with, since increased levels of carbon dioxide can be exhaled as necessary. This respiratory compensation reacts within a matter of 1–3 min.[8,11]

The kidney's role in acid-base balance is twofold: (1) to conserve or eliminate bicarbonate ions, hence stabilizing the amount in the body, and (2) to excrete hydrogen ions. Renal bicarbonate retention or excretion depends upon the PCO_2 in arterial blood. The kidneys are the most potent of the acid-base mechanisms. However, they require hours or even days to effectively change pH.[8,11]

In the normal resting condition venous pH is slightly lower than arterial pH (venous = 7.35, arterial = 7.4), but this difference has very little affect on most physiological functions. The key is maintaining arterial pH levels. Thus, not only does the respiratory system deliver oxygen for the production of energy, but it also contributes to the effective functioning of all biochemical reactions through its role in maintaining acid-base balance.

SUMMARY

1. Respiration consists of pulmonary ventilation and oxygen and carbon dioxide gas exchange at the alveolar (external) and tissue (internal) levels.

2. Structurally, the pulmonary system can be divided into the conductive and respiratory zones. The conductive zone serves to transport air, warm and humidify air, and filter the air. Gas exchange takes place in the respiratory zone.

3. At rest inspiration is an active process brought about by a pressure gradient that exceeds resistance to the flow of air. Resting expiration is a passive process accomplished primarily by elastic recoil.

4. The conductive zone makes up the anatomical dead space. A physiological dead space occurs when functional alveoli are not supplied with capillaries.

5. Minute ventilation ($\dot{V}_E$ or $\dot{V}_I$) is the respiratory variable most commonly measured in exercise situations. However, alveolar ventilation is the best measure of air available for gas exchange.

6. Residual volume, the amount of air remaining in the lungs after a maximal expiration, must be accounted for when one determines body composition by underwater weighing.

7. Respiratory measures are collected under ambient conditions (ATPS). Most lung volumes and capacities are then converted to body temperature values (BTPS). Minute ventilation may also be converted to standard temperature and pressure, dry (STPD) conditions.

8. Primary control of respiration resides in the medulla oblongata (inspiratory and expiratory centers),

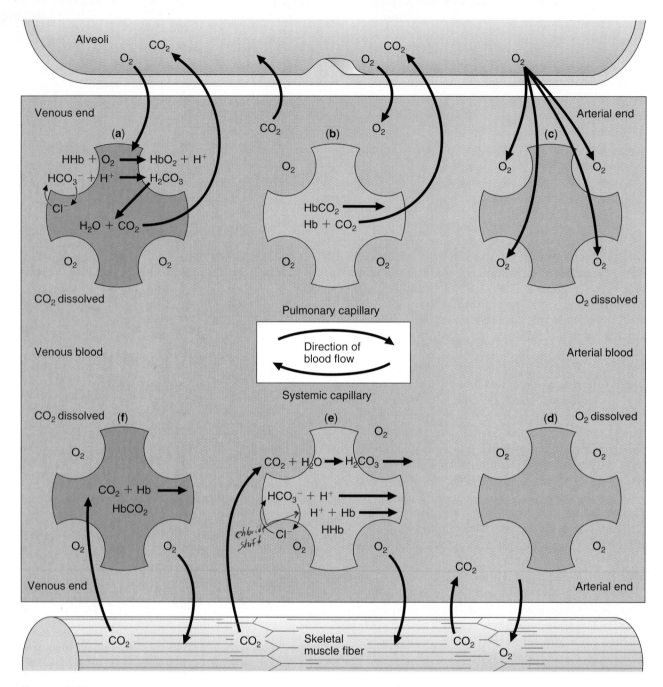

FIGURE 2.14

Summary of Oxygen and Carbon Dioxide Transport

Oxygen is transported two ways in the circulatory system—dissolved and bound to the heme units of hemoglobin (RBC). Carbon dioxide is transported three ways in the circulatory system—dissolved, bound to the globin portion of hemoglobin, and as bicarbonate. (a) The oxygenation of hemoglobin and diffusion of carbon dioxide from bicarbonate, (b) the diffusion of carbon dioxide from the globin portion of hemoglobin, (c) transport of oxygen on heme portions of hemoglobin, (d) diffusion of oxygen from heme portion of hemoglobin, (e) transport of carbon dioxide as bicarbonate, (f) transport of carbon dioxide on globin portion of hemoglobin.

with fine tuning provided by the pneumotaxic and apneustic centers in the pons. Factors affecting these centers include:

    (a) Conscious thought through the cerebral cortex.
    (b) Sympathetic nerve reactions through the hypothalamus.
    (c) Irritants or lung inflammation through systemic receptors in the airways and lungs.
    (d) PO_2, PCO_2, pH, and K^+ through central and peripheral chemoreceptors.
    (e) Movement via proprioceptive stimulation from mechanoreceptors and muscles and joints.

    9. Gases flow from areas of high pressure to areas of low pressure—that is, always down a pressure gradient. Each gas moves independently. Oxygen moves from the alveoli into arterial blood and red blood cells and then from the red blood cells and capillary blood into the muscle tissues. Carbon dioxide moves from the muscle tissues into capillary blood and red blood cells and then from the venous blood and red blood cells into the alveoli. The P values driving these exchanges are given in the answer section that follows this summary for Box 2.2.

    10. Hemoglobin is composed of four iron heme units and one globin (a protein). When fully saturated, each hemoglobin molecule will have oxygen bound to each of its four heme structures. Normal arterial saturation ($SaO_2\%$) is 97%; normal resting venous saturation ($SvO_2\%$) is 75%.

    11. Oxygen that is released from the red blood cells at the tissue level is said to have been dissociated. At rest the primary drive for this dissociation is the pressure gradient for oxygen.

    12. At rest only about 25% of circulated oxygen is used; 75% remains saturated in venous blood. These percentages translate into an arteriovenous oxygen difference of approximately 4.6 $mL \cdot dL^{-1}$.

    13. Carbon dioxide is transported from the tissue to the lungs in three ways: dissolved, as carbamino hemoglobin, and as bicarbonate ions. The chemical buffering and removal of carbon dioxide from the body are important in maintaining acid-base balance.

At identical minute ventilations alveolar ventilation is greatly reduced as the depth (tidal volume) of the ventilation decreases. Increasing the frequency of breathing does not compensate for a small tidal volume at the alveolar level. Shallow, frequent breathing is not as effective as deep, infrequent breathing.

2. Both situations decrease alveolar ventilation. When tidal volume is low, as in trying to inhale without exhaling first or in taking short, quick gulps of air, the volume of the dead space has a negative impact on the amount of air available for exchange (the alveolar ventilation). This result is exemplified by the calculations in problem 1. Inadequate alveolar ventilation can lead to dizziness or unconsciousness, which are dangerous situations, especially in water.

3. A snorkel extends the dead space. Thus, the tidal volume must be increased sufficiently to compensate for that volume as well as the anatomical dead space to maintain an effective alveolar ventilation.

Box 2.1 Answers

1. Pattern A:
$$[(600 \text{ mL} \cdot br^{-1}) - (150 \text{ mL} \cdot br^{-1})] \times$$
$$(10 \text{ br} \cdot min^{-1}) = (450 \text{ mL} \cdot br^{-1}) \times$$
$$(10 \text{ br} \cdot min^{-1}) = 4500 \text{ mL} \cdot min^{-1}$$

Pattern B:
$$[(200 \text{ mL} \cdot br^{-1}) - (150 \text{ mL} \cdot br^{-1})] \times$$
$$(30 \text{ br} \cdot min^{-1}) = (50 \text{ mL} \cdot br^{-1}) \times$$
$$(30 \text{ br} \cdot min^{-1}) = 1500 \text{ mL} \cdot min^{-1}$$

Box 2.2 Answers

Site	PO_2	PCO_2
Alveoli	104 mmHg	
Pulmonary capillary	40 mmHg, arterial end; 104 mmHg, venous end	
Left side of heart	95 mmHg	
Systemic arteries	95 mmHg	40 mmHg
Tissue (resting)	40 mmHg	45 mmHg
Systemic capillary	95 mmHg, arterial end; 40 mmHg venous end	40 mmHg, arterial end; 45 mmHg, venous end
Systemic veins	40 mmHg	45 mmHg
Right side of heart	40 mmHg	45 mmHg
Pulmonary artery	40 mmHg	45 mmHg
Alveoli		40 mmHg
Pulmonary capillary		45 mmHg, arterial end; 40 mmHg, venous end
Left side of heart		40 mmHg

REVIEW QUESTIONS

1. Define *pulmonary ventilation, external respiration,* and *internal respiration.* Define the following variables and classify each as involved in pulmonary ventilation, external respiration, or internal respiration. Some may be classified in more than one way.

(A-a)PO$_2$ diff

a-vO$_2$ diff

V_D

f

$\dot{V}_E$ and $\dot{V}_I$

V_T

PaO$_2$

P$_A$O$_2$

PaCO$_2$

PvCO$_2$

PvO$_2$

SaO$_2$%

SbO$_2$%

SvO$_2$%

2. Diagram the conductive and respiratory zones of the respiratory system. Compare the function of the two zones.

3. Why does air flow into and out of the lungs?

4. What is the functional difference between pulmonary circulation and bronchial circulation? How does bronchial circulation affect the PaO$_2$?

5. Identify the three capacities and four volumes into which total lung capacity can be divided. Which of them is most responsive during exercise? Which must be accounted for when one determines body composition by hydrostatic (underwater) weighing?

6. Explain the conditions represented by the volume designations ATPS, BTPS, and STPD. Where is each condition most appropriately used? Which volume is typically the largest? Which is the smallest? Name and explain the gas laws that cause these differences.

7. Discuss the primary control of respiration and the factors that affect such control.

8. Describe how oxygen and carbon dioxide are transported in the circulatory system. Note in particular the importance of each transport form and any interaction between the movements of the individual gases.

9. Explain how the transport and removal of carbon dioxide relate to acid-base balance. Why is the maintenance of acid-base balance important?

10. Graph a normal resting oxygen dissociation curve. What percentage of the available oxygen is normally dissociated at rest?

REFERENCES

1. Adams, G. M.: *Exercise Physiology Laboratory Manual* (2nd edition). Dubuque, IA: Brown (1994).
2. Craig, A. B.: Summary of 58 cases of loss of consciousness during underwater swimming and diving. *Medicine and Science in Sports.* 8(3):171–175 (1976).
3. Dempsey, J. A., E. H. Vidruk, & G. S. Mitchell: Pulmonary control systems in exercise: Update. *Federation Proceedings.* 44:2260–2270 (1985).
4. Eldridge, F. L.: Central integration of mechanisms in exercise hyperpnea. *Medicine and Science in Sports and Exercise.* 26(3):319–327 (1994).
5. Forster, H. V., & L. G. Pau: The role of the carotid chemoreceptors in the control of breathing during exercise. *Medicine and Science in Sports and Exercise.* 26(3):328–336 (1994).
6. Guyton, A. C.: *Textbook of Medical Physiology* (7th edition). Philadelphia: Saunders (1986).
7. Leff, A. R., & P. T. Schumacker: *Respiratory Physiology: Basics and Applications.* Philadelphia: Saunders Company (1993).
8. Martin, B. J., K. E. Sparks, C. W. Zwillich, & J. V. Weil: Low exercise ventilation in endurance athletes. *Medicine and Science in Sports.* 11(2):181–185 (1979).
9. Nye, P. C. G.: Identification of peripheral chemoreceptor stimuli. *Medicine and Science in Sports and Exercise.* 26(3):311–318 (1994).
10. Pardy, R. L., S. N. A. Hussain, & P. T. Macklein: The ventilatory pump in exercise. *Clinics in Chest Medicine.* 5(1):35–49 (1984).
11. Slonim, N. B., & L. H. Hamilton: *Respiratory Physiology* (3rd edition). St. Louis: Mosby (1976).
12. Whipp, B. J., S. A. Ward, N. Lamarra, J. A. Davis, & K. Wasserman: Parameters of ventilatory and gas exchange dynamics during exercise. *Journal of Applied Physiology: Respiratory, Environmental and Exercise Physiology.* 52(6):1506–1513 (1982).
13. Wilmore, J. H.: The use of actual, predicted, and constant residual volumes in the assessment of body composition by underwater weighing. *Medicine and Science in Sports.* 1:87–90 (1969).

3

Respiratory Exercise Response, Training Adaptations, and Special Considerations

After studying the chapter, you should be able to:

- Graph and explain the pattern of response for the major respiratory variables during short-term, light to moderate submaximal dynamic aerobic exercise.

- Graph and explain the pattern of response for the major respiratory variables during prolonged, heavy submaximal dynamic aerobic exercise.

- Graph and explain the pattern of response for the major respiratory variables during dynamic, incremental exercise to maximum.

- Graph and explain the pattern of response for the major respiratory variables during static exercise.

- Compare and contrast the pulmonary ventilation, external respiration, and

internal respiration responses to short-term, light to moderate submaximal dynamic aerobic exercise; prolonged, heavy submaximal dynamic aerobic exercise; dynamic aerobic incremental exercise to maximum, and static exercise.

- List the adaptations that consistently occur in the respiratory system as a result of exercise training.

- Identify variations in resting volumes, exercise responses, and training adaption among young adults, children and adolescents, and the elderly and between males and females.

- Determine the value of altitude training, hypoxic swim training, and training in polluted conditions.

Response of the Respiratory System to Exercise

During exercise the demand for energy increases, varying, of course, with the type, intensity, and duration of the exercise. In most exercise situations much of the body's ability to respond to the demand for more energy depends upon the availability of oxygen. To provide the needed oxygen for aerobic energy production the respiratory system—including pulmonary ventilation, external respiration, and internal respiration—must respond. Pulmonary ventilation increases to enhance alveolar ventilation; external respiration adjusts in such a way as to maintain the relationship between ventilation and perfusion in most cases; internal respiration responds with the increased extraction of oxygen by the muscles. These changes in respiration not only provide adequate oxygenation for the muscles but also play a major role in the maintenance of acid-base balance, which is, in turn, closely related to carbon dioxide levels.

In general, all levels of respiratory activity are precisely matched to the rate of work being done. Furthermore, because of this precise control and the large reserve built into the system, respiration in normal, healthy, sedentary or moderately fit individuals is generally not a limiting factor in activity. This is true despite the perception of feeling out of breath during exercise. Only in the rare situation of some highly trained, elite, male endurance athletes do the capacities of the cardiovascular and metabolic systems exceed that of the respiratory system such that respiration can be considered a limitation to maximal work.

Of course, changes in pulmonary ventilation would be of little benefit if parallel changes in pulmonary blood volume and flow and total body circulation did not also occur. The specific details of the accompanying cardiovascular responses will be discussed later in this unit.

This section will concentrate on pulmonary ventilation, external respiration, and internal respiration responses to dynamic aerobic activity, including short- and long-term, constant-load submaximal activity and incremental work to maximum. The most prominent changes in the respiratory system occur within these classifications of activity. A few comments will also be made concerning static exercise responses. However, the response to dynamic resistance activity has not been specifically documented and therefore will not be discussed. When reading this discussion and studying the accompanying graphs, you may wish to refer to the glossary of respiratory symbols summarized in Table 3.1.

TABLE 3.1 ■ Respiratory Symbols

Pulmonary Ventilation	External Respiration	Internal Respiration
$\dot{V}_E$ = minute ventilation	$\dot{V}_A$ = alveolar ventilation	a-vO_2 diff = amount of oxygen carried in the arteries minus the amount carried in the veins
V_D = dead space	P_AO_2 = partial pressure of oxygen at the alveoli	
V_T = tidal volume	PaO_2 = partial pressure of oxygen in arterial blood	$PaCO_2$ = partial pressure of carbon dioxide in arterial blood
f = frequency of breathing		$PvCO_2$ = partial pressure of carbon dioxide in venous blood
V_D/V_T = ratio of dead space to tidal volume	(A-a)PO_2 diff = oxygen or PO_2 pressure gradient between the alveoli and arteries	SvO_2% = percent saturation of venous blood with oxygen
	SaO_2% = percent saturation of arterial blood with oxygen	PvO_2 = partial pressure of oxygen in venous blood
	P_ACO_2 = partial pressure of carbon dioxide at the alveoli	

Short-Term, Submaximal, Light-to Moderate-Intensity Dynamic Aerobic Exercise

The responses to short-term (meaning 5–10 min), light- to moderate-intensity (defined as 30–74% of maximal work capacity), dynamic aerobic exercise are diagramed in Figures 3.1, 3.2, and 3.5. These responses are discussed in detail in the subsections that follow.

Pulmonary Ventilation   The most obvious response to an increased metabolic demand, such as exercise, is an increase in pulmonary ventilation ($\dot{V}_E$ L·min^{-1}), which is called **hyperpnea.** What is perhaps a little surprising is the initial immediate reaction. In Figure 3.1a, note that between the onset of exercise at 0 min and 2 min into the exercise, a triphasic response in $\dot{V}_E$ has occurred. Within the first respiratory cycle at the onset of exercise, there is an initial abrupt increase in $\dot{V}_E$, which is phase 1. It is maintained for approximately 10–20 sec. Phase 2 is the slower exponential rise from the initial elevation to the steady-state leveling off. At the low to moderate workload depicted here, this exponential rise should be completed in 2–3 min. At this point phase 3, or the new steady state, is achieved. The actual level of the achieved exercise steady state depends upon a number of factors, including the workload, the fitness of the individual, and the environmental conditions. In the time span depicted the steady-state level is maintained. The three-phase response at the onset of activity is typically not seen when $\dot{V}_E$ is reported or graphed minute by minute, but it has occurred.[76, 113, 114, 115]

The initial rise in ventilation occurs primarily because of an increase in tidal volume.[66] Theoretically, the potential range of tidal volume is from the resting level to the limits of vital capacity. In reality, rarely is more than 50–65% of vital capacity reached before a plateau occurs. Furthermore, although tidal volume encroaches into both the inspiratory reserve capacity (IRC) and the expiratory reserve capacity (ERC), it encroaches much more into IRC than ERC.[63,78,105,117]

At light to moderate workloads the contribution of increases in breathing frequency to minute ventilation is minimal and gradual. Both tidal volume and frequency level off at a steady state that satisfies the requirements of the short submaximal activity (Figures 3.1b and 3.1c).

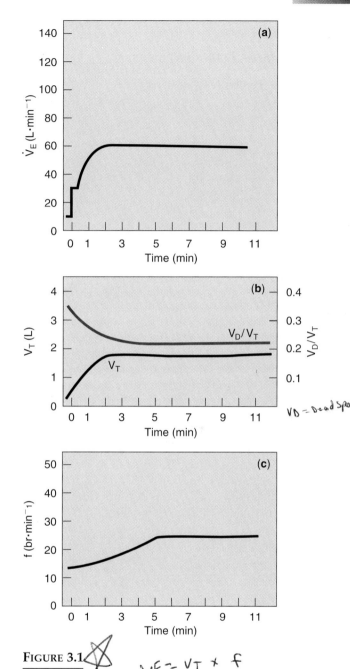

FIGURE 3.1

$$V_E \sim V_T \times f$$

Responses of Pulmonary Ventilation Variables to Constant (5–10 min), Submaximal (light to moderate) Dynamic Exercise

---

Hyperpnea Increased pulmonary ventilation that matches an increased metabolic demand, as in an exercise situation.

FIGURE 3.2

Responses of External Respiration Variables to Constant (5–10 min), Submaximal (light to moderate) Dynamic Exercise

Airway resistance decreases owing to bronchodilation as soon as any intensity of exercise begins. Likewise, the ratio of dead space (V_D) to tidal volume (V_T) decreases, and in this case the largest changes are evident at the lowest work rate.[111, 114] This result is shown in Figure 3.1b. The depth of the drop in V_D/V_T is moderate at low to moderate exercise intensities. The V_D itself changes minimally with bronchodilation, but with the proportionally larger increase in V_T the ratio declines.[44] This result is important because alveolar ventilation ($\dot{V}_A$) thus increases from about 70% of the total pulmonary ventilation at rest to a higher percentage during exercise. Since $\dot{V}_A$ is the critical ventilation, this reduction in the V_D/V_T ratio means that the appropriate level of $\dot{V}_A$ can be achieved with a smaller rise in $\dot{V}_E$ than would be needed if the ratio did not change.[112]

External Respiration   The $\dot{V}_A$ response to low to moderate exercise is depicted in Figure 3.2a. This curve parallels the change in $\dot{V}_E$, except that the initial adjustments seen in $\dot{V}_E$ are not depicted for $\dot{V}_A$. The rise in $\dot{V}_A$ is sufficient to maintain PO_2 at the alveolar level (P_AO_2) during short-term submaximal exercise (Figure 3.2b). Maintenance of P_AO_2 is important because it represents the driving force for oxygen transfer across the alveolar-capillary interface.[81,110]

As explained earlier, under resting conditions there is an inequity in PO_2 between the alveoli (P_AO_2) and arterial blood (PaO_2) owing to the dilution of the systemic arterial blood with the bronchial venous blood. During short-term, low-intensity submaximal exercise PaO_2 is maintained and the *alveolar–to–arterial oxygen partial pressure difference,* depicted as (A-a)PO_2 diff in Figure 3.2c, either does not change or decreases slightly.[58, 66, 112] At moderate workloads a slight increase may be seen. The (A-a)PO_2 diff reflects the efficiency and/or adequacy of oxygen transfer in the lungs during exercise. At the steady-state submaximal levels described here, there is, in essence, no noticeable change in this efficiency.

Gas exchange and blood perfusion in the lungs during low to moderate exercise is sufficient to maintain the saturation of red blood cells with oxygen (SaO_2%) within a narrow range approximating resting levels (Figure 3.2d).[46]

Internal Respiration   Recall that internal respiration involves the dissociation of oxygen from the red blood cells so that it may diffuse down the pressure gradient into the muscles and other tissues.

Refer to Figure 3.3 and re-familiarize yourself with the resting relationships described in Chapter 2 and labeled again in this figure. The line for resting arterial blood at 95 mmHg on the X-axis represents the PaO_2. It intersects with the middle curve and indicates a percent saturation of hemoglobin (SbO_2%) of approximately 97% on the left Y-axis. The line for resting venous blood at 40 mmHg on the X-axis represents the PvO_2. This line also inter-

sects with the middle curve and indicates a SbO_2 of 75%. That is, at rest 75% of the oxygen remains associated with the red blood cells in venous blood. Thus, a great deal more oxygen could be extracted at the tissue capillary level than normally is.

Four factors are involved in accomplishing the increased oxygen extraction during exercise: (1) an increased PO_2 gradient; (2) an increased PCO_2; (3) a decreased pH; and (4) an increased temperature. Each is depicted in the oxygen dissociation curve in Figure 3.3. The way each factor operates is described in the following list.

1. *Increased PO_2 gradient.*   Under resting conditions sufficient oxygen remains in the muscle tissue to maintain a PO_2 of 40 mmHg. When exercise increases the demand for energy, the oxygen already in the muscle tissue is used immediately. Since the oxygen is used, the muscle tissue partial pressure is reduced correspondingly. The PO_2 of arterial blood remains unchanged. Therefore, the pressure gradient can be widened from 55 mmHg

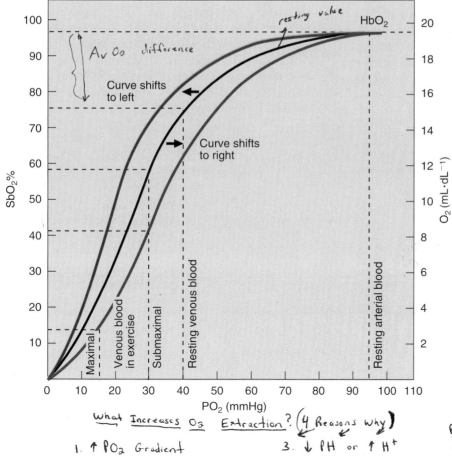

FIGURE 3.3

Oxygen Dissociation During Exercise (Internal Respiration)
The center curve represents normal resting values: $PaCO_2$ = 40 mmHg, pH = 7.4, body temperature = 37 degrees Celsius. During all intensities and types of exercise the $PaCO_2$ increases, pH decreases (becomes more acidic), and body temperature increases. Each of these conditions causes the curve to shift to the right with the result that more oxygen is dissociated from red blood cells to be used by the muscles. Consequently, both the oxygen content of the venous blood and the SbO_2% in venous blood is lower the higher the intensity of exercise to a minimum of approximately 15%.

(95 mmHg at the arterial end of the capillary minus 40 mmHg in the muscle tissue) to possibly 65 mmHg (95 mmHg at the arterial end of the capillary minus 30 mmHg in the muscle tissue) during light submaximal exercise.

Equilibrium is reached between the muscle tissue and the blood by the venous end of the capillary, so the returning venous blood also has the lower PO_2. Refer to Figure 3.3 and find the line labeled submaximal for venous blood in exercise above the X-axis value of 30 mmHg. Assume for the moment that this is the only change that occurs (a false assumption, as will be detailed later, but one which does no harm here). From the figure you can see the effect this increased pressure gradient has on the dissociation of oxygen. By following this submaximal exercise line to where it intersects the solid line middle curve and then to the left Y-axis, you can see that the corresponding $SbO_2\%$ (actually $SvO_2\%$ now) is 60%, not 75%. Thus, instead of 23% of the oxygen being dissociated as it was at rest (97% $SaO_2\%$ − 75% $SvO_2\%$ = 22%; 22% ÷ 97% = 23%) now 38% (97% $SaO_2\%$ − 60 $SvO_2\%$ = 37%; 37% ÷ 97% = 38%) has been released from the red blood cells just by changing the pressure gradient. Hence, an additional 15% of the available oxygen (38% − 23% = 15%) has been dissociated and is used for energy production. Not all submaximal exercise requires the same amount of oxygen, so these numbers are simply illustrative of the effect of a widening pressure gradient.

2. Increased PCO_2. When oxygen is used to provide energy, carbon dioxide is produced as a by-product. Increasing levels of carbon dioxide mean that PCO_2 increases. An increase in PCO_2 shifts the oxygen dissociation curve to the right. This shift was seen in a minimal way even at rest in the venous curve depicted in Figure 2.13. However, during exercise the shift is further to the right. Exactly how far the curve shifts depends upon how hard the exercise is and how much carbon dioxide is produced. The shift in the curve to the right means that at any given PO_2 more dissociation occurs, as shown in Figure 3.3. Follow the line for venous blood in exercise from the value of 30 mmHg on the PO_2 X-axis until it intersects the right-hand curve. A horizontal line from this intersection to the left Y-axis yields a saturation value of about 41%. Thus, more oxygen is dissociated than would have been if the pressure gradient had been operating alone. Figure 3.4 emphasizes that the actual shift occurs during the red blood cell transit through the capillary before reaching the actual venous blood.

3. Decreased pH or increased hydrogen ion concentration. Hydrogen ions (H^+) come from two primary sources during exercise. First, carbon dioxide combines with water to form carbonic acid. The carbonic acid then breaks down into hydrogen ions and bicarbonate. Second, lactic acid breaks down into lactate and hydrogen ions. The presence of increased levels of hydrogen ions lowers the pH to a

Skeletal muscle fiber

Fuel + O_2 ⟶ CO_2 + heat + energy

Fuel without O_2 ⟶ lactic acid + energy
(⟶ H^+)

Arterial end   Systemic capillary   Venous end

FIGURE 3.4

Factors Influencing Oxygen Dissociation During Exercise

The by-products of the production of energy, namely carbon dioxide, heat, and hydrogen ions (H^+), in skeletal muscle fibers stimulate the dissociation of oxygen from red blood cells as they traverse systemic capillaries.

more acidic level. This more acidic pH shifts the oxygen dissociation curve to the right in the same way that an increased PCO_2 did and with the same results: a greater dissociation of oxygen from red blood cells. How far to the right the curve shifts depends on the amount of hydrogen ions released. As with carbon dioxide, this effect is taking place during the red blood cell's transit through the muscle capillaries. The interactive effect of carbon dioxide and pH on the affinity of hemoglobin for oxygen is known as the *Bohr effect*.[47,62]

4. Increased temperature. Another by-product of muscle energy production is heat. Heat is also transferred from the muscle tissue (high heat) to the capillary (low heat) (Figure 3.4). The resultant rise in temperature shifts the oxygen dissociation curve to the right. The action is precisely the same as that for the increase in PCO_2 and the decrease in pH, and so it is again depicted by the same shift in Figure 3.3.

Thus, the elevation in the use of oxygen to produce energy during exercise and the by-products of that energy production operate together to make the reserves of oxygen available.

The exercise responses for the variables from the oxygen dissociation curve are depicted in Figure 3.5. The best overall indicator of internal respiration is the arteriovenous oxygen difference (a-vO_2 diff).[46] Since PaO_2 (Figure 3.5a) and SaO_2% (Figure 3.2d) do not change with short-term, low-intensity exercise, the actual amount of oxygen being carried in the arteries (in milliliters per deciliter) also does not change.[111] However, since the production of energy uses more oxygen even at these low intensities, the venous oxygen value as well as the PvO_2 (Figure 3.5c) and SvO_2% (Figure 3.5f) will decrease. With an equal arterial oxygen and lower venous oxygen content, the a-vO_2 diff (Figure 3.5e) will increase. Since this is a steady-state submaximal situation, the a-vO_2 diff will level off when sufficient oxygen is being extracted to supply the needs of the cell.[27, 30, 59]

Because the production of energy not only uses oxygen but also produces carbon dioxide, it would be anticipated that the PvCO_2 value would increase. As shown in Figure 3.5d, this increase does occur, but it is not particularly large at these low to moderate workloads. The extra carbon dioxide is exhaled easily from the lungs and the hyperpnea of

exercise may even blow off a little extra carbon dioxide, resulting in a slight decrement in PaCO_2 (Figure 3.5b). Regulation of ventilation maintains PaCO_2 very close to resting values.[27,30,59,111,114]

These combined responses are well within the reserve capacity of the respiratory system for normal, healthy individuals.

Prolonged, Constant, Relatively Heavy, Submaximal Dynamic Aerobic Exercise

If submaximal aerobic exercise is increased in duration and maintained at high-moderate to heavy intensity (60–75% of maximal working capacity), respiratory responses vary primarily in magnitude when compared with the changes just discussed for low- to moderate-intensity, short-term exercise. In addition, several of the variables exhibit a drifting pattern.

Pulmonary Ventilation

Figure 3.6a shows that $\dot{V}_E$ increases to a higher level than during light- to moderate-intensity exercise before plateauing at a steady state. The achievement of the steady state may take somewhat longer than at lower work intensities and often is not held throughout the duration of the exercise. Note that after approximately 30 min a gradual rise in $\dot{V}_E$ occurs, despite an unchanging workload, an effect called *ventilatory drift*.[30,50,110] The precise reason for this drift is unknown,[96] although a rising body temperature is most often speculated as the reason. This drift is both inefficient and advantageous. It is inefficient because it is in excess of the workload demand. It is advantageous to gas exchange since alveolar ventilation parallels the drift and acid-base balance is maintained.[30,50]

As for lower-intensity submaximal exercise, the initial change in $\dot{V}_E$ is due primarily to an increase in V_T (Figure 3.6b). However, in the later stages of heavy submaximal work tidal volume may decrease slightly. The drift in $\dot{V}_E$ comes about primarily as a result of increased breathing frequency (Figure 3.6c). The V_D/V_T ratio (Figure 3.6b) still decreases primarily at the onset of activity, but it does so to a greater extent with the heavier workload than at lighter loads. After about an hour of heavy submaximal work the V_D/V_T ratio may increase very slightly.

FIGURE 3.5

Reponse of Internal Respiration Variables to Constant (5-10 min), Submaximal (light to moderate) Dynamic Exercise

* Best overall indicator of internal respiration.

External Respiration   As stated earlier, the drift in $\dot{V}_E$ is paralleled by a similar drift in $\dot{V}_A$ (Figure 3.7a). P_AO_2 remains constant (Figure 3.7b), as it did with lower-intensity submaximal work. How-ever, PaO_2 decreases slightly until about the time when ventilatory drift occurs.[30] It then returns to-ward baseline values. This variation in PaO_2 while P_AO_2 remains unchanged is reflected in a mirror

FIGURE 3.6   *1. Vary in Magnitude*   *2 differences*   *2. Drifting Patterns*   *than short*

Responses of Pulmonary Ventilation Variables to Prolonged (60 min), Constant, Submaximal (60–75% of maximum) Dynamic Exercise

Vent. Drift - Rising Body temp? - Inefficient by breathing hard. - Advantageous by gas exchange.

FIGURE 3.7

Responses of External Respiration Variables to Prolonged (60 min), Constant, Submaximal (60–75% of maximum) Dynamic Exercise

Drift

↑ at Drift.

image relationship in the (A-a)PO$_2$ diff (Figure 3.7c). The initial increase in the (A-a)PO$_2$ diff is not a desirable change. It indicates inefficiency in gas exchange. However, the small loss of efficiency seen here has very little practical meaning and does not limit the exercise.[50,111]

Internal Respiration Other than differences in magnitude, all of the internal respiration variables respond in the same way during prolonged, constant, relatively heavy submaximal dynamic exercise as during the shorter, lighter dynamic exercise previously described.

Despite the higher workload PaO$_2$ is maintained relatively constant (Figure 3.8a). Because of the heavier workload more oxygen is dissociated and used, and the PvO$_2$ (Figure 3.8c) and SvO$_2$% (Figure 3.8f) decrease to lower levels than in shorter, lighter workloads. The result is a widening of the a-vO$_2$ diff (Figure 3.8e). The factors responsible for the dissociation of oxygen are the same as those for lower-intensity exercise. PaCO$_2$ (Figure 3.8b) decreases slightly due to the increased volume of air being exhaled. PvCO$_2$ (Figure 3.8d) increases because the greater use of oxygen to produce energy also results in more carbon dioxide that must be carried in the venous system to the lungs to be exhaled.

Incremental Dynamic Aerobic Exercise to Maximum

An incremental aerobic exercise bout consists of a series of progressively increasing work intensities, which stop when the individual cannot do any more. The length of each work intensity, often called a *stage*, may vary from 1 to 3 min to allow for the achievement of a steady state, at least until the higher workloads, when a steady state cannot be maintained.

Pulmonary Ventilation It might be anticipated that since $\dot{V}_E$ rises and levels off at submaximal workloads, that this rise would be proportional,

direct, and rectilinear throughout the entire range, from rest to maximal exercise. However, as shown in Figure 3.9a, a smooth rise is not completely descriptive of the response. At light to moderate and even heavy intensities, up to approximately 50–75% of maximum workload, $\dot{V}_E$ does increase in a rectilinear fashion. At this point a break in the linearity occurs, and a second, steeper linear rise ensues. This proportional rise continues until approximately 85–95% of maximum workload, when a second break in linearity occurs. The slope of the third linear rise to maximum that follows is even steeper yet.[63,80,110] These points where the rectilinear rise in minute ventilation breaks from linearity during incremental exercise to maximum are called **ventilatory thresholds.** The first breakpoint is called the first ventilatory threshold (VT1), and the second breakpoint is called the second ventilatory threshold (VT2).

Precisely what causes these breakpoints is unknown. One theory has linked them with an excess of carbon dioxide resulting from the buffering of lactic acid, and this theory calls the breakpoints anaerobic thresholds. Although carbon dioxide is a known respiratory stimulator, this theory is probably not accurate (for reasons to be fully discussed in the unit on metabolism). Therefore, the term *ventilatory thresholds* is preferred. Other possible mechanisms—including catecholamine or potassium stimulation of the carotid bodies; limitations in changes in V_T, f, and V_D/V_T to maintain $\dot{V}_A$; increasing body temperatures; and feedback from the skeletal muscle proprioceptors—have been suggested as causes of the ventilatory thresholds, but their role remains unproven. It is likely that a combination of factors is responsible.[68,101,109]

Knowledge of the ventilatory thresholds, regardless of why they occur, has some practical benefit. The workloads at which the ventilatory thresholds occur are related to endurance exercise performance. That is, the higher the workload where the breaks occur, the greater the intensity of activity that can be sustained.[68,109]

Once again, the changes in minute ventilation ($\dot{V}_E$) during low to moderate workloads are achieved primarily by an increase in V_T (Figure 3.9b). At very heavy workloads, however, the depth of breathing not only may cease to increase but also may decrease.[28,117] When V_T reaches its highest point, any further increase in ventilation can only be

---

Ventilatory Thresholds Points where the rectilinear rise in minute ventilation breaks from linearity during an incremental exercise to maximum.

FIGURE 3.8

Responses of Internal Respiration Variables to Prolonged (60 min), Constant, Submaximal (60–75% of maximum) Dynamic Exercise

Same response

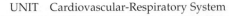

What's causing VE to go up, from beg. to end?
What's diff. bet. linear & Exponential?

Stages 1-3 For steady state

Practical Value (End Exercise)

★The higher the workload, where the break occurs, the greater the intensity of activity that can be sustained.

Vent. threshold ~excess CO₂ from buffering of LA?

↑ temp
Feedback from muscle
Limitations in changes in VT, f & VD/VT to maintain VA.

60% of max reduction
0.1 = 90% of VT Avail. for exchange

90% of VT is available for exchange.

Exponential at higher workloads.

FIGURE 3.9

Responses of Pulmonary Ventilation Variables to Incremental Dynamic Exercise to Maximum

Exercise-Induced Hypoxemia (EIH) A condition found in elite male endurance athletes in which the amount of oxygen carried in arterial blood is severely reduced.

the result of an increase in breathing frequency.[110] The rise in breathing frequency is exponential at the higher work levels (Figure 3.9c). As for submaximal workloads, the V_D/V_T ratio decreases the most in the initial light to moderate stages of the incremental work.[44] The maximal reduction is reached at about 60% of maximal work, and this value is maintained to maximum. Since the V_D/V_T ratio is reduced to 0.1 (or 10% of V_T), 90% of V_T is available for exchange at the alveoli ($\dot{V}_A$), providing a more efficient ventilation.[44,58,111,112]

External Respiration Changes in $\dot{V}_A$ parallel the changes in $\dot{V}_E$, including the slope of the rectilinear rises and the two breakpoints (Figure 3.10a). The breakpoints in $\dot{V}_A$, however, occur prior to the breakpoints in $\dot{V}_E$—that is, at slightly lower percentages of maximal work.[58,110]

The rise in $\dot{V}_A$ is sufficient to maintain P_AO_2 and subsequently PaO_2 through the light-to-moderate-intensity exercise stages (Figure 3.10b). As the workload becomes higher, P_AO_2 rises exponentially to maximum. This rise provides the driving force that hastens the rate of equilibrium of alveolar gas with mixed venous blood and in so doing maintains PaO_2 and SaO_2% within narrow limits in normal or moderately fit individuals (Figure 3.10d).[28, 44, 98, 111, 112] The (A-a)PO₂ diff follows the pattern of the exponential rise in P_AO_2 (Figure 3.10c). The increase of the (A-a)PO₂ diff to approximately 30 mmHg shown in Figure 3.10c is still considered to be a small increase.[58]

Refer again to the PaO_2 graph in Figure 3.10b. Note the dotted line, which shows a steep decrease in PaO_2. Such a decrease is called **exercise-induced hypoxemia (EIH)**; it is a condition in which the amount of oxygen carried in arterial blood is insufficient. Surprisingly, 40–50% of highly trained, healthy, elite, male cyclists and runners exhibit this response at work rates approaching maximum. Whether elite endurance athletes in other sports or female athletes in these or other sports show the same response is unknown. During EIH the individual's ability to process oxygen and, hence, to perform high-intensity activity is lower than normal, although both may be higher than those of untrained or moderately trained individuals. In other words, respiration—more specifically, external respiration—is a limitation to exercise in some highly trained athletes. Furthermore, athletes who exhibit EIH at sea level suffer

FIGURE 3.10

Responses of <u>External</u> Respiration Variables to Incremental Dynamic Exercise to Maximum

more severe gas exchange impairments during short-term exposure to higher altitudes than do athletes who do not exhibit EIH at sea level.[81]

As shown on the graph in Figures 3.10b and 3.11a, the decline in PaO_2 with EIH can be considerable, ranging from 18 to 38 mmHg below resting values (96 − 18 = 78 mmHg; 96 − 37 = 59 mmHg). At the same time, the SaO_2% (Figure 3.10d) will be reduced to possibly 84% instead of 97%.[16, 81]

What causes EIH? Both theoretical and experimental evidence support an inequality between ventilation and perfusion as one reason and a limitation in diffusion as another. In turn, the failure to achieve complete diffusion equilibrium may be related to the faster transit time of red blood cells through the capillary bed of athletes with a highly developed cardiovascular system.[81, 98] In normal sedentary or moderately trained individuals pulmonary capillary blood volume increases with exercise. This increases the surface area for diffusion and slows down the red blood cell transit time sufficiently to allow complete diffusion and equilibration of the gases. In highly trained athletes pulmonary capillary blood volume reaches its maximum at relatively low workloads.[98] Hence, when these elite athletes continue to increase their workloads and total body circulation, pulmonary capillary volume cannot expand anymore. Instead, blood flow velocity increases and red blood cell transit time decreases. As a result, the red blood cell transit time in elite endurance athletes is estimated to be considerably less than that required for gas equilibration.[108] Thus, EIH may be attributed in part to a diffusion limitation as a consequence of this reduced red blood cell transit time. Why EIH occurs in some athletes and not others has not been determined.

With EIH the (A-a)PO$_2$ diff curve would increase even more than shown in Figure 3.10c, and the SaO_2% curve would decline as shown in Figure 3.10d. The (A-a)PO$_2$ diff then becomes a definite indication of lack of efficiency in respiration.[89, 99]

Internal Respiration   The dissociation or release of oxygen reaches its limit during incremental

* Lowest Limit (Tot. Max Exercise)
95-15 ←
↳means alot O₂ being diffused.

FIGURE 3.11

Responses of Internal Respiration Variables to Incremental Dynamic Exercise to Maximum

exercise to maximum. At low and moderate workloads more and more oxygen is released according to the sigmoid-shaped curve in Figure 3.3. The factors that stimulate the dissociation of oxygen during incremental exercise to maximum are the same as always, but they typically are greater in magnitude. That is, the pressure gradient will be wider, PCO_2 will be higher, pH will be lower and temperature will be higher as the exercise load increases.[108] It is not possible to extract all the oxygen from the blood perfusing heavily or even maximally exercising muscles. Thus, a muscle PO_2 of 15 mmHg is considered a reasonable lower limit for heavy exercise, with a corresponding maximal pressure gradient of close to 80 mmHg (95 mmHg at the arterial end of the capillary minus 15 mmHg in the muscle tissue). Therefore, some oxygen is always returned in the venous blood. The result is a venous saturation (SvO_2%) of oxygen of approximately 15–35% (Figure 3.11f), which exerts a partial pressure of 15–25 mmHg (Figure 3.11c).

As more oxygen is used to produce more energy, more carbon dioxide is produced. This metabolic carbon dioxide—as well as nonmetabolic carbon dioxide produced in the effort to buffer the lactic acid that accumulates at the higher workloads—brings about the slightly curvilinear rise in $PvCO_2$ shown in Figure 3.11d. Conversely, $PaCO_2$ (Figure 3.11b) is maintained at first and then decreases. This fall in arterial carbon dioxide partial pressure reflects the excess removal of carbon dioxide brought about by alveolar hyperventilation.[30, 44, 58] The a-vO_2 diff (Figure 3.11e) parallels the changes in oxygen dissociation, gradually increasing with the incremental workloads until it can increase no more. It plateaus at approximately 50–60% of the maximal workload.[88, 93]

Thus, even maximal exercise is well within the respiratory reserves for most individuals. Only highly trained male endurance athletes whose metabolic and cardiovascular systems have increased greatly exceed their respiratory reserves.

Static Exercise

Static exercise involves the production of force or tension with no mechanical work being done. Therefore, gradations of static exercise are usually expressed relative to an individual's own ability to produce force, called the *maximal voluntary contrac-*

tion (MVC), for a given muscle group and held for a specified period of time. This activity is much the same as performing a dynamic exercise at a selected percentage of maximal work, except that in dynamic work the total musculature is generally greater.

In terms of actual energy cost, static exercise is very low in its requirements. However, when static and dynamic exercise require relatively equal amounts of energy, ventilation increases correspondingly. One major difference is apparent, though. At the onset of exercise the initial (0–2 min) three-phase response in $\dot{V}_E$ is absent in static activity. In addition, the a-vO_2 diff either remains the same or decreases slightly during static exercise in contrast to the consistent elevation during dynamic exercise. The maintenance or slight decrease in a-vO_2 diff is undoubtedly related to the occlusion of circulation to the statically contracting muscles. In all other aspects the respiratory responses are similar in static exercise and in low-intensity, dynamic endurance exercise. Static exercise does not push the reserve capacity of the respiratory system.[4]

Table 3.2 summarizes the respiratory responses to exercise that have been discussed in these sections.

Entrainment of Respiration During Exercise

In some, but not all, individuals the performance of rhythmical exercise (such as walking, running, cycling, and rowing) is accompanied by a synchronization of limb movement and breathing frequency called **entrainment**.[11,17,19,52,56,61,71] Entrainment means, for example, that an individual always inhales during the recovery phase of rowing and always exhales during the drive portion of the stroke. Or the walker, runner, or cyclist always exhales on the push-off phase of one leg or the other. Unlike swimming, where the coordination of breathing is a function of head placement during

---

Entrainment The synchronization of limb movement and breathing frequency that accompanies rhythmical exercise.

TABLE 3.2 ■ Respiratory Responses to Exercise*

	LIGHT- TO MODERATE-INTENSITY, SHORT-TERM SUBMAXIMAL EXERCISE†	HEAVY, LONG-DURATION† SUBMAXIMAL EXERCISE	INCREMENTAL-TO-MAXIMUM EXERCISE	STATIC EXERCISE
PULMONARY VENTILATION				All responses the same as for light-to moderate-intensity, short-term submaximal exercise
$\dot{V}_E$	Increases rapidly; levels off	Increases rapidly; levels off; drifts upward	Shows initial rectilinear rise; has two breakpoints	
V_D	Decreases	Decreases	Decreases	
V_T	Increases rapidly; levels off	Increases rapidly; levels off	Has truncated, inverted U-shaped curve; increases greatly; has incomplete reversal	
f	Slowly increases; levels off	Increases slowly; levels off; drifts upward	Has exponential curvilinear rise	
V_D/V_T	Decreases initially; levels off	Decreases rapidly initially; levels off	Decreases rapidly initially; levels off at 60% of maximum and is maintained	
EXTERNAL RESPIRATION				
$\dot{V}_A$	Increases rapidly; levels off	Increases rapidly; levels off; drifts upward	Shows initial rectilinear rise; has two breakpoints	
P_AO_2	Shows no change	Shows no change	Shows no change until approximately 75% of maximum; then has exponential rise	
PaO_2	Shows no change	Has small U-shaped curve	Shows no change until approximately 75% of maximum; then increases slightly	
$(A-a)PO_2$ diff	Decreases slightly or shows no change (light); increases slightly (moderate)	Has truncated, inverted U-shaped curve; increases rapidly initially; has incomplete reversal	Shows no change until approximately 75% of maximum; then has exponential rise‡	
$SaO_2\%$	Decreases less than 1%; has U-shaped curve	—	—	
INTERNAL RESPIRATION				
$PaCO_2$	Is level; then decreases slightly	Is level; the decreases slightly	Is level; then decreases	
$PvCO_2$	Shows slight linear rise	Shows linear rise; levels off	Has sharp rise; levels slightly	
PvO_2	Decreases rapidly; levels off	Decreases rapidly; levels off	Decreases sharply; levels off	
$SvO_2\%$	Decreases initially; levels off	Decreases initially; levels off	Decreases sharply; never reaches 0	
a-vO_2 diff	Increases rapidly; levels off	Increases rapidly; levels off	Shows rectilinear rise to highest possible value that is maintained to maximum	Shows no change or decreases slightly

*Resting values are taken as baseline.
†The difference between leveling during the light to moderate short-term and heavy long-duration submaximal exercise responses is one of magnitude; that is, leveling occurs at a higher value with higher intensities.
‡Hypoxemia may occur in higher altitudes.

any given stroke, and hence a learned response, entrainment occurs without conscious thought.

Subjects who entrain naturally have a lower energy cost during exercise when they entrain but not when they breathe randomly. However, subjects forced to breathe in specific entrainment patterns rather than being allowed to breathe spontaneously do not exhibit any reduction in energy cost nor perceive any decrement in breathing effort with entrained breathing.[69]

Beginning exercisers often ask how and when they should breathe. The best advice for land activity appears to be to just do whatever comes naturally, be it in a spontaneous or an entrainment pattern. The one exception is weight training. The static component of weight training can cause the **Valsalva maneuver**, a breath-holding action that involves closing of the glottis (which keeps air in the lungs) and contraction of the diaphragm and abdominal musculature. The result is an increase in intra-abdominal pressure and, concomitantly, an abnormal increase in blood pressure. Blood pressures are much lower if breathing is done during the contraction. For this reason it is generally recommended that inhalation occur during the lowering phase of a resistance exercise and exhalation occur during the lifting phase of each repetition.[41]

The Influence of Age and Sex on Respiration at Rest and During Exercise

Children and Adolescents

Lung Volumes and Capacities

In general, the total lung capacity and each of its subdivisions increase in a pattern that deviates only slightly from a straight rectilinear relationship for both males and females as they age from approximately 6 yr to the late teens or early twenties. The forced expiratory volume at one second and maximal voluntary ventilation follow essentially the same incremental pattern in children.[6,8,14,63,72] From birth to approximately age 10 these changes depend largely upon the growth and development of the respiratory system. After that, cell proliferation ceases and hypertrophy of existing structures occurs until maturity. Thus, these changes are primarily, but not ex-

clusively, the result of structural enlargement and are strongly related to body height.[14,57] When the subdivisions of total lung capacity are expressed as a percentage of the total volume, the proportions remain the same from about age 8 to age 20. The anatomical dead space increases in proportion to maturity.[3, 87]

Pulmonary Ventilation

The control of ventilation appears to be similar in children and adults. However, there are some minor differences in minute ventilation and its components across the age span.[119]

Rest. The $\dot{V}_E$ at rest is surprisingly consistent regardless of age.[87] Figure 3.12 shows that this value in males varies less than 2 L·min^{-1} from ages 6 to 76. Comparable data are not available for females. When $\dot{V}_E$ is related to body weight, younger boys have a higher $\dot{V}_E$ than older adolescents or adults; but from adolescence to old age there is basically no difference.

The remarkably consistent $\dot{V}_E$ is achieved differently by children than by older adolescents and adults. Figure 3.13a shows that breathing frequency is higher and tidal volume lower in youngsters than in older adolescents and adults. From approximately the midteen years until old age, the breathing frequency stabilizes at 10–15 br·min^{-1}, and tidal volume stabilizes at about 500 mL in males.[72, 87] Younger children use a higher portion of their vital capacity as a tidal volume than do older adolescents and young adults (Figure 3.13b).

Submaximal Exercise. Children's and adolescent's respiratory responses to exercise are quite similar to those of adults, with only some quantitative differences. Thus, $\dot{V}_E$ will rise in response to greater oxygen needs. However, the higher $\dot{V}_E$ in relation to body weight seen at rest is maintained, as is the variation in how $\dot{V}_E$ is obtained. That is, children exhibit a higher breathing frequency and lower tidal volume at any given submaximal load than adults. They also respond with a higher $\dot{V}_E$ in rela-

Valsalva Maneuver Breath-holding that involves closing of the glottis and contraction of the diaphragm and abdominal musculature.

FIGURE 3.12

Minute Ventilation at Rest and During Maximal Exercise for Males Age 6–76

Source: Based on data from Robinson.[87]

tion to body weight at an equal workload. These differences are considered negative, indicating a wasteful ventilation, and gradually disappear by late adolescence.[10, 87, 91, 92] The differences are exemplified for 11-yr-old girls and boys in comparison to 29-yr-old adults in Figures 3.14a and Figure 3.14b.[91,92] The speeds are different for the males and females, so direct comparison between the sexes cannot be made. In addition to the differences shown in Figure 3.14, younger children use a marginally lower proportion of their vital capacity during submaximal exercise than do adults.

FIGURE 3.13

Frequency of Breathing, Tidal Volume, and the Percentage of Vital Capacity Used as Tidal Volume at Rest and During Maximal Exercise for Males Age 6–76

Source: Based on data from Robinson.[87]

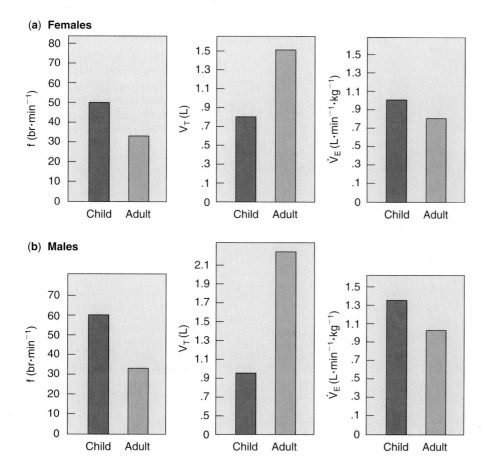

(a) Females

(b) Males

FIGURE 3.14

Pulmonary Ventilation Responses to Submaximal Exercise in Male and Female Children and Adults

Source: Based on data from (a) Rowland and Green [92] and (b) Rowland et al.[91]

Females: Mean age child = 11.3 yr; adult = 28.7 yr, treadmill speed = 7.3 kph (122 m · min⁻¹).
Males: Mean age child = 11.6 yr; adult = 29.2 yr, treadmill speed = 9.6 kph (160 m · min⁻¹).

During prolonged submaximal exercise children and adolescents exhibit the same ventilatory drift as adults. There is nothing in the respiratory response to prolonged exercise that would indicate that children are not suited for such activity.[72]

Maximal Exercise. In general, children's responses to maximal exercise parallel the differences seen at rest and during submaximal work. That is, the older the child, the higher the $\dot{V}_E$ that can be achieved in absolute terms. The $\dot{V}_E$ in relation to body weight gradually declines from about age 7 until adulthood is achieved at about 20 years of age, although in 4–6-yr-olds this value is comparable to that of young adults (Figure 3.15a).[6,8,39,64,87,90,92] Breathing frequency decreases consistently from the youngest children tested to approximately age 20 while tidal volume shows a steady rise over the same time span (Figure 3.15b). The percentage of vital capacity used as tidal volume rises slightly from childhood to young adulthood.

Children exhibit the ventilatory breakpoints during incremental exercise to maximum. However, the breakpoints appear earlier, at lower workloads, than they do for either adolescents or adults. The physiological mechanisms for the ventilatory breakpoints in children are as unclear as they are for adults.[10, 92]

External and Internal Respiration   Little is known about the changes in gas exchange and transport that occur during normal growth and maturation. The relatively higher breathing frequency and lower tidal volume of children in relation to adolescents and adults, at rest and during exercise, seem to be offset by their smaller anatomical dead space. Consequently, alveolar ventilation is more than adequate at all values of $\dot{V}_E$.[10, 72, 119]

Pulmonary diffusion during exercise does not appear to differ by age. Likewise, there does not appear to be any meaningful aging trends for P_AO_2, PaO_2, or $(A\text{-}a)PO_2$ diff at rest or during exercise.

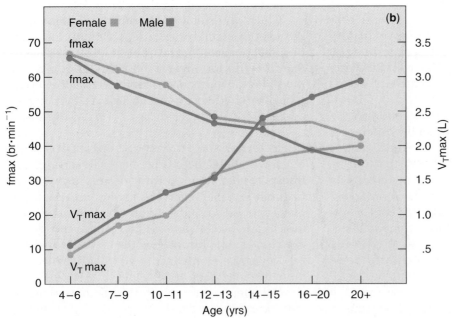

FIGURE 3.15

Pulmonary Ventilation Responses to Maximal Treadmill Exercise as Children Age to Adulthood for Males and Females

Source: Based on data from Åstrand.[6]

However, PaO_2 decreases slightly and the $(A-a)PO_2$ diff increases slightly as children mature to adulthood.[10,37,87] As a consequence, the percent saturation of arterial blood is also relatively constant across the age span.[87]

The arteriovenous oxygen differences are also very similar at both rest and maximal exercise levels from childhood to maturity. If anything, children may be able to extract about 5% more oxygen during maximal exercise than adults.[38] Alveolar and arterial oxygen partial pressure levels are slightly lower in young children than in adolescents or adults, possibly reflecting the child's relative hyperventilation.[119]

The Elderly

Lung Volumes and Capacities
The effect of aging on total lung capacity is controversial. There is evidence that total lung capacity both decreases and stays the same in individuals over the age of 50.[54,55,57,62,103,104] On the other hand, research has firmly established that vital capacity and inspiratory capacity decrease with age and that residual volume and functional residual capacity increase, thus changing the percentage of total volume that each occupy.[5,6,36,102,103,105] For example, the ratio of residual volume to total lung capacity doubles from about 15 to 30% in the elderly.[21, 57]

The forced expiratory volume in 1 second (FEV_1) and maximal voluntary ventilation decline steadily after approximately age 35 in both males and females.[3,36,100,102,103] These declines are brought about by a combination of structural and mechanical changes in the respiratory system. These changes include (1) a decrease in the elastic recoil of the lung tissue; (2) a stiffening of the thoracic cage, which decreases chest mobility, necessitating a greater reliance on the diaphragm; (3) a decrease in the intervertebral spaces, which in turn decreases height and changes the shape of the thoracic cavity; (4) losses in respiratory muscle force and velocity of contraction. Of all these changes, the loss of elastic recoil appears to be the most important.[57, 105]

Pulmonary Ventilation
Rest. Resting $\dot{V}_E$ (Figure 3.12) and its components V_T and f (Figure 3.13a) are remarkably consistent across the entire age span. However, at rest the percentage of vital capacity used as V_T does show a very slight U-shaped curve (Figure 3.13b). That is, both young children and the elderly use slightly more of their vital capacity for V_T at rest than do young adults.[87]

Submaximal Exercise. $\dot{V}_E$ rises in the elderly in response to increased energy needs. As for young adults, this increase is accomplished mainly by an increase in V_T at lighter workloads and then by an increased frequency of breathing, if needed. Like children, the elderly seem to have an exaggerated response in $\dot{V}_E$ when compared with younger adults. That is, the absolute $\dot{V}_E$ is higher at any given workload in the elderly than in young adults. Because the vital capacity decreases with age and V_T remains fairly stable, V_T represents a higher percentage of the elderly's vital capacity.[5, 6, 26, 31, 87, 100]

Maximal Exercise. With aging both the ability to exercise maximally and the ability to process air decline. The decrement in pulmonary function contributes to the decline in work capacity but probably simply parallels the changes in circulation, metabolism, and muscle function that are also occurring.

The highest $\dot{V}_E$ values are typically seen in young adults, and these may decline by almost half by the seventh decade of life (Figure 3.12). This decline is evident both in absolute values ($\dot{V}_E$ in liters per minute) and in values related to body weight ($\dot{V}_E$ in liters per kilogram per minute). Most of this decline is brought about by a reduction in tidal volume, although maximal breathing frequency does decrease slightly.

The percentage of vital capacity used during maximal work is relatively stable with age from young adulthood on. However, the dead space–to–tidal volume ratio is consistently 15–20% higher in older adults than in younger adults.[87] The ventilatory breakpoints occur at lower absolute and relative workloads in older adults than in younger adults.[100]

External Respiration
Rest. The loss of elastic recoil in the lungs not only affects the static and dynamic lung volumes but also influences the distribution of air in the lungs. Thus, ventilation may not be preferentially directed to the base of the lung in the upright

posture at rest, although the majority of blood flow is still directed there. Thus, there may be an imbalance between alveolar ventilation and pulmonary perfusion.[57]

In addition, structural changes in the aging lung lead to a decrease in alveolar capillary surface area, which in turn means a decrease in diffusion capacity.[33, 57] Furthermore, pulmonary capillary blood volume decreases owing to a stiffening of both pulmonary arteries and capillaries. The cumulative effects of these changes are a decrease in arterial oxygen partial pressure, but not alveolar, and a widening of the alveolar-to-arterial oxygen difference, although the changes are neither inevitable nor large. The saturation of hemoglobin with oxygen in arterial blood declines about 2–3% from age 10 to age 70.[87, 100]

Exercise.   During exercise the increased ventilation that is required results in a more homogeneous distribution of ventilation in the lungs. Although the decreases noted at rest in diffusion surface and pulmonary capillary blood volume remain, the matching of ventilation and perfusion improves during exercise as more of the lung is used. The available reserve is sufficient to meet the demands for oxygen transport even to maximal exercise levels.

Nevertheless, alveolar ventilation is a smaller portion of minute ventilation in older adults than in younger adults. This change does indicate a slightly decreased efficiency of respiration; but general arterial hypoxemia is prevented, and carbon dioxide elimination is adequate. That is, the arterial oxygen and carbon dioxide partial pressures are maintained within narrow limits and are similar to those for younger adults. The alveolar-to-arterial oxygen differences are more variable in the elderly than in younger adults but, on average, are only slightly wider than the usual mean values for younger individuals.[57, 87, 100]

Internal Respiration   At rest and at any given submaximal level of exercise the arteriovenous oxygen difference is greater in older adults than in younger adults. Thus, venous saturation of oxyhemoglobin is lower. Conversely, at maximal exercise the arteriovenous oxygen difference is lower in the elderly than in younger individuals. Maximal values average 14–15 mL · dL^{-1} in older adults but

average 15–20 mL · dL^{-1} in younger adults. Some of these changes in the arteriovenous oxygen difference can be attributed to a shift in the oxygen dissociation curve to the left, which makes the release of oxygen to the tissues more difficult.[62, 100] Refer to Figure 3.3 to see this effect.

Male-Female Respiratory Differences

Lung Volumes and Capacities   Values for total lung capacity and each of its subdivisions are lower for females than males across the entire age span, with the possible exception of around 12–13 yr, when girls have had their pubertal growth spurt and boys have not. These differences are carried over into the dynamic measurements of maximal voluntary ventilation and forced expiratory volume in 1 sec. Part of these differences can be attributed in general to the smaller size of the female. However, even prorating values according to height, weight, or surface area does not totally eliminate the difference.[69, 21, 40]

Pulmonary Ventilation   At rest there is no consistent difference in breathing frequency between males and females.[72] However, at the same submaximal ventilation females typically display a higher breathing frequency and a lower tidal volume than males. This pattern is maintained at maximal exercise.[95] Also, at maximal exercise males exhibit higher minute ventilation at all ages than females, although these differences are narrowed considerably when prorated by body weight.[5, 6] Figures 3.15a and 3.15b show these differences for children and young adults.

External and Internal Respiration   Data to compare males and females are unavailable for most of the external and internal respiratory measures. The arteriovenous oxygen difference has been measured at rest and during submaximal and maximal exercise, but the results show little consistency.[7, 12, 121]

Respiratory Training Adaptations

No training principles or guidelines are presented for the respiratory system because training specifically directed toward this system is very rare in nondiseased individuals. What few training adaptations occur do so as a by-product of training for cardiovascular and/or metabolic improvement. Applications of the training principles are presented for these systems in their respective units. The few training adaptations of the respiratory system follow.

Lung Volumes and Capacities

Whether the chronic but intermittent elevations in respiratory demand that occur with physical training actually change the lung itself is unknown. Studies in which the training modality is land-based (running, cycling, wrestling, and the like) have found no consistent significant changes in total lung capacity, vital capacity, residual volume, functional residual capacity, or inspiratory capacity in either males or females of any age; nor have they found any differences favoring athletes over nonathletes.[9,25,29,37,60,75,85,94] Studies where the activities are water-based (swimming and scuba diving), however, have shown that swimmers have higher volumes and capacities than both land-based athletes and nonathletes.[25,67] In addition, swim training studies have demonstrated increases in total lung capacity and vital capacity in both children and young adults. Similar generalizations can be made for the dynamic measures of forced expiratory volume in 1 sec and maximal voluntary ventilation.[2, 9, 18, 106, 109]

Precisely why swimmers, and not land-based athletes, show improvements in static and dynamic lung volumes is not known. However, swimmers in all but the backstroke are breathing against the resistance of water in a restricted breathing pattern with repeated expansion of the lungs to total lung capacity. Swimming also takes place with the body in a horizontal position, and this posture is optimal for perfusion of the lung and diffusion of respiratory gases.[24, 74]

Pulmonary Ventilation

Changes in $\dot{V}_E$ are the primary and most consistent adaptations seen in the respiratory system as a result of endurance training. While $\dot{V}_E$ itself does not change at rest, a shift occurs in its components: V_T increases, and f decreases. Not only is this shift maintained during submaximal work, but also the

$\dot{V}_E$ is lower as a result of the training. At maximal work $\dot{V}_E$ is higher after training than before, accompanying the ability to do more work. The major component change is an increase in f, but V_T will increase as well.[30,71,82,84,113,116] In addition, the capacity for sustaining high levels of voluntary ventilation is improved, reflecting an increase in both the strength and the endurance of the respiratory muscles.[64, 86]

These adaptations are seen within the first 6–10 weeks of a training program and reverse just as quickly upon detraining.[84] They occur as a result of both land- and water-based activities across the entire age span.[10, 42, 79, 97, 118, 119] The ventilatory thresholds shift to a higher workload as a result of training in children and in adults.[48, 77]

External and Internal Respiration

In a healthy individual of any age and either sex, gas exchange varies little as a result of training.[84] The diffusion capacity has been reported to be higher in elite swimmers[21, 70, 74, 107] and runners,[60] but it does not consistently increase either at submaximal or maximal work as a result of training.[94] This observed result may be an example of genetic selection for specific athletes.[21, 28, 30, 75, 85, 106, 108] Even in studies where diffusing capacity has shown an increase, it is most likely due to circulatory changes (an increase in pulmonary capillary volume) and not to any pulmonary membrane change per se.

Arterial values of pH and PCO_2 do not change with training, but venous pH levels increase (become less acidic) and PCO_2 values decrease[82] during the same submaximal exercise. The alveolar-to-arterial oxygen pressure difference decreases at submaximal workloads as a result of training, indicating greater efficiency.[94] Training may also cause the oxygen dissociation curve to shift to the right, facilitating the release of oxygen from the blood into the muscle tissue.[82]

In children neither the submaximal nor maximal arteriovenous oxygen difference adapts as a result of training.[10,38] In young adults the arteriovenous oxygen difference increases at rest[20, 94] and at maximal exercise as a result of training.[15, 23, 94] Both increases and decreases in the arteriovenous oxygen difference have been found during submaximal exercise as a result of endurance training.[20,34,35,94] Changes in middle-aged and elderly adults are less likely than in younger adults.[43, 93] None of the other partial pressure or saturation variables change significantly and/or consistently with training.

Table 3.3 summarizes the respiratory training adaptations discussed in this section.

Why Are There So Few Respiratory Adaptations to Exercise Training?

The most commonly accepted answer to the question of why there are so few respiratory adaptations to exercise training is that the pulmonary system is endowed with a tremendous reserve capacity that is more than sufficient to meet the demands of even very heavy physical exercise. Thus, when physical training is undertaken, the various components of the respiratory system are not stressed to any significant limits and so do not need to change. At the same time, the cardiovascular and metabolic capacities of muscle are being stressed and do respond by adapting. The adaptations in these systems may ultimately exceed the capability of the respiratory system, as seen in highly trained male athletes with exercise-induced hypoxemia. Otherwise, there is no need for great changes in the respiratory system in the normal healthy individual.[28, 30]

Special Considerations

The Impact of Altitude on Exercise and Training

The effects of altitude were alluded to several times in Chapter 2. It is time now to deal more directly with the effects of both acute and chronic exposure to altitude and with the issue of whether participation in altitude training can improve athletic performance. Referring back to Table 2.1 and Equation 2.4 may be helpful in comprehending the following discussion.

The percentage of oxygen in air remains constant at 20.93% no matter what the altitude. However, the barometric pressure (P_B) decreases exponentially with an increase in altitude. For instance, at Denver (5280 ft, or 1600 m) P_B is 630 mmHg, and at Colorado Springs (7590 ft, or 2300 m) P_B is 586 mmHg (Figure 3.16). Therefore, the oxygen partial pressure (PO_2) in atmospheric air is reduced. At Denver the PO_2 is 132 mmHg (630 mmHg × 0.2093), and at Colorado Springs it is 123 mmHg (586 mmHg × 0.2093); as compared to 159 mmHg at

TABLE 3.3 ■ Respiratory Training Adaptations

	REST	SUBMAXIMAL EXERCISE	MAXIMAL EXERCISE
Lung volumes and capacities	Show no changes from land-based activities; swimming and diving show increases, especially in total lung capacity and vital capacity	—	—
Pulmonary ventilation			
$\dot{V}_E$	Shows no change	Decreases	Increases
V_T	Increases	Increases	Increases
f	Decreases	Decreases	Increases
External respiration, (A-a)PO_2 diff	Shows no change	Decreases	Shows no change
Internal respiration, $PvCO_2$	—	Decreases	—
Oxygen dissociation curve	—	Curve shifts to the right	Curve shifts to the right
a-vO_2 diff	Shows no change in children; increases in young adults	Shows no change in children; inconsistent changes in adults	Shows no change in children, increases in young adults

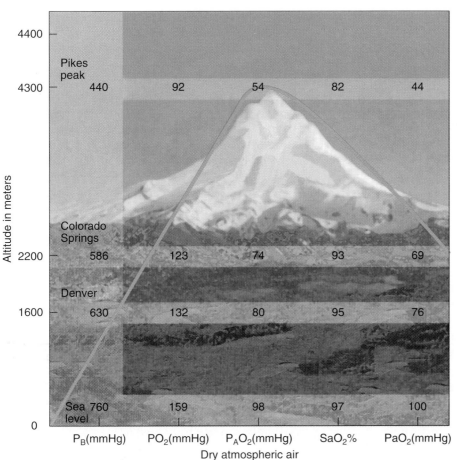

P_B(mmHg)	PO_2(mmHg)	P_AO_2(mmHg)	SaO_2%	PaO_2(mmHg)
Pikes peak 440	92	54	82	44
Colorado Springs 586	123	74	93	69
Denver 630	132	80	95	76
Sea level 760	159	98	97	100

Dry atmospheric air

FIGURE 3.16

The Impact of Altitude on External Respiration

*As altitude ↑ the PO_2 ↓.

sea level (760 mmHg × 0.2093). Because the partial pressure of the inspired oxygen decreases with altitude, the alveolar oxygen partial pressure P_AO_2 also decreases to 80 mmHg and 74 mmHg, respectively, at Denver and Colorado Springs:

[(630 mmHg) – (47 mmHg)] × (.137 O_2) = 80 mmHg;
[(586 mmHg) – (47 mmHg)] × (.137 O_2) = 74 mmHg

This decrease in P_AO_2 reduces the pressure gradient between the returning venous blood (PvO_2) and the alveoli, resulting in a lower percent saturation (SaO_2%) and arterial partial pressure (PaO_2):

80 mmHg × .95 = PaO_2 of 76 mmHg at Denver;
74 mmHg × .93 = PaO_2 of 69 mmHg at Colorado Springs

This decrement in PaO_2 stimulates an increase in $\dot{V}_E$ via the aortic and carotid body chemoreceptors, as compensation to provide more oxygen for alveolar ventilation. The initial increase in $\dot{V}_E$ is **hyperventi-**lation, defined as an increase in pulmonary ventilation that exceeds metabolic requirements, and is achieved primarily by an increase in respiratory frequency. Altitude-induced hyperventilation increases the amount of carbon dioxide exhaled. In turn, the increased exhalation of carbon dioxide decreases alveolar and arterial carbon dioxide partial pressure as well as pH. The decrease in percent saturation (SaO_2%) and the other resultant changes at Denver and Colorado Springs are minimal, perhaps 2–5% because of the flatness of the oxygen dissociation curve (Figure 2.13) in that range. However, at the top

Hyperventilation Increased pulmonary ventilation, especially ventilation that exceeds metabolic requirements; carbon dioxide is blown off, leading to a decrease in its partial pressure in arterial blood.

of Pikes Peak (14,100 ft, or 4300 m) SaO_2% is 82%, and the full effect of altitude is seen.[49,51,83] Table 2.1 and Figure 3.16 show the external respiration values. The SaO_2% is approximately 15% less at Pikes Peak than at sea level.

Within the red blood cells a chemical called 2,3-diphosphoglycerate (2,3-DPG) increases at altitude. The effect of the increase in 2,3-DPG is the same as an increase in carbon dioxide partial pressure, hydrogen ion concentration, and body temperature on the oxygen dissociation curve (Figure 3.3). That is, it causes a shift of the oxygen dissociation curve to the right, thus offsetting the shift to the left (and decreased release of oxygen) that would occur owing to the decrement in carbon dioxide partial pressure and pH.

Within two days of altitude exposure hemoglobin concentration increases, which in turn increases the amount of oxygen transported per deciliter of blood. Unfortunately, the hemoglobin concentration increases only because total blood volume initially decreases. That is, the same number of red blood cells are simply distributed in a smaller volume of blood, a process called *hemoconcentration*. The blood volume loss reflects a total body water loss through the kidneys and through increased respiratory evaporation owing to the compensatory hyperventilation. Such hemoconcentration increases the viscosity of the blood, which means increased resistance to blood flow. In an attempt to maintain blood flow, heart rate increases.[51,83]

These changes are compounded during exercise. The normal exercise increase in diffusion capacity does not exceed that at sea level, because arterial oxygen partial pressure is decreased and venous oxygen partial pressure remains the same. As a result, the normal exercise increase in arteriovenous oxygen difference is not as great at altitude as it is at sea level.

Although the individual probably does not perceive any of the aforementioned changes, except possibly hyperventilation, some unpleasant sensations may mark the onset of altitude sickness. These sensations include the loss of appetite, dizziness, fatigue, nausea, vomiting, dehydration, and weakness.[47, 51]

The acute effects of altitude are experienced most directly in terms of the intensity at which an aerobic endurance activity can be maintained. The higher the altitude, the greater the impact and the sooner fatigue is felt. Thus, the intensity at which any endurance event can be performed will be lower, as will the ability to sustain that activity at higher elevations. This result is true for all individuals at all age levels, although high-altitude mountain climbers are impacted the most. Sprints and other muscular strength, muscular endurance, and power events do not appear to be disadvantaged from a physiological standpoint and may even be enhanced because of a reduction in air resistance at higher elevations.[51, 83]

Teachers giving fitness tests to students can adjust the cardiovascular endurance items detailed in Chapter 4 as follows:

4000–7500 ft (1200–2270 m)	7.5%
7600–9000 ft (2300–2730 m)	10.0%
9100–12,000 ft (2750–3640 m)	15.0%

This adjustment would involve either adding time to do the 1-mi run or decreasing the number of laps needed to meet the criterion score for the PACER.[22,51] For example, the criterion-referenced standard (minimally acceptable score) for a 14-yr-old boy in the 1-mi run is 11:00. To increase this acceptable time to account for the altitude at Denver (5280 ft, or 1600 m), we can convert the target time to seconds and multiply by 0.075:

$$[(11 \text{ min}) \times (60 \text{ sec} \cdot \text{min}^{-1})] \times 0.075 = 660 \text{ sec} \times 0.075$$
$$= 49.5$$

Thus, an acceptable score might be 11:50 instead of 11:00. Similarly, for the PACER the criterion-referenced standard for a 16-yr-old girl is 28 laps. To account for altitude, we calculate $28 \times 0.075 = 2.1$. Therefore, the criterion target would be 26 laps, not 28 laps.

Athletes who wish to compete at altitude have two choices in attempting to minimize the adverse environmental effects. The first is to arrive at the altitude site no more than 12 hr prior to the activity. This is what many collegiate and some professional teams do, even at the moderate altitudes where they compete. Although this strategy does not prevent the effects of altitude, it does minimize the chances that acute altitude sickness will impair performance.[51, 83]

The second choice is to train at the same altitude as the eventual competition. During this time the athletes can acclimatize somewhat to the altitude. Full acclimatization can take at least a year, and even then the former sea-level resident will not be as physiologically adapted as the individual who was born and has always lived at altitude. In the initial days of such training a gradual change in altitude may be helpful, and the advice to "work high and sleep low" is often given, until the desired level of altitude can be somewhat tolerated.

Acclimatization involves subtle but important shifts in the initial attempts of adjusting to the lower oxygen partial pressure. That is, hemoconcentration continues, but the cause shifts from being a decrease in plasma volume with no change in red blood cell count to an increase in both red blood cells and blood volume.[47] Likewise, hyperventilation is maintained, but instead of an increased frequency of breathing, an increase in tidal volume occurs. Increased tidal volume allows a more effective pulmonary gas exchange. Arterial carbon dioxide partial pressure remains depressed, but arterial oxygen partial pressure increases somewhat as acclimation proceeds.[1,45,47,49,51,83] Females seem to acclimatize to altitude more readily than do males.[45]

Unfortunately, these processes of acclimatization do not completely counteract the fundamental hypoxic stress of altitude. Thus, individuals training at altitude cannot train at the same level of intensity for the same period of time as they could at sea level. Consequently, highly trained athletes (especially those prone to exercise-induced hypoxemia) are likely to benefit the least from altitude training. Untrained individuals may still be doing more than before, and reap the benefits of the training.

Despite the drawbacks, athletes who train at altitude usually see positive results from that training if the competition is at the same altitude and occurs directly following the training period. The effect of altitude training on later sea-level maximal performance is highly controversial, showing large individual variations. In general, there does not appear to be any advantage to altitude training over that gained from the exercise training itself. That is, the response to the two stressors is not additive.[1, 51]

If an individual chooses to train at moderate altitude, the following guidelines are suggested.

1. Spend a minimum of two to four weeks at altitude.

2. Maintain the same intensity of exertion that you would use at sea level, but decrease the duration and increase the frequency.

3. Lengthen rest periods.

4. Replace fluids even to the point of hyperhydration.[83]

Hypoxic Swim Training

Swimmers have tried their own version of altitude training, called *hypoxic training* or *controlled-frequency breathing*. The general assumption is that if a swimmer inhales once every third, fifth, or seventh arm stroke, instead of every other arm stroke, then the reduced volume of air taken in decreases oxygen partial pressure and creates hypoxia, a decrease in available oxygen. Hypoxia is supposed to bring about the same beneficial effects to the swimmer that running at altitude does for the track athlete.

There are several problems with this idea. First, as you have already learned, altitude training is probably beneficial only for competition at altitude, not at seal level. This restricted benefit is apparent despite the fact that the track athletes both train and live at altitude for 24 hr a day and do not just experience hypoxia for a few minutes a day. Second, controlled-frequency breathing does not produce hypoxia. What is produced instead is *hypercapnia*, an increase in the partial pressure of carbon dioxide. Third, hypercapnia often causes headaches that last for 30 min or more after the workout ceases. These headaches are painful and may interfere with training.

On the positive side, controlled-frequency breathing may increase buoyancy and improve body position, enabling the swimmer to concentrate on the biomechanics of the stroke. However, it is simply not an effective technique for the training of respiratory, circulatory, metabolic, or neuromuscular functions. At best, controlled-frequency breathing should be used very sparingly and be closely monitored.[32, 53, 65, 120]

Exercise Training and Pollution

The impairment of cilia function mentioned in Chapter 2 is not the only respiratory effect of inhaling cigarette smoke and other environmental pollutants. Inhalation of several pollutants (smog and its secondary product, ozone; sulfur dioxide from the burning of coal or oil; particulates such as dust or ashes) brings about a reflex bronchioconstriction in the upper airways. If inhalation of pollutants occurs while an individual is exercising, the problem is confounded. As the intensity of exercise increases, both the rate and the depth of breathing also increase. To accommodate this increase, the individual switches from nose to mouth breathing and hence bypasses the cleansing filtration of the nose. As a result, a greater percentage of inhaled pollutants penetrate deeper into the respiratory tract than would if the individual were at rest. Results may include chest pain (due to the airway constriction), difficulty in breathing, coughing, nose and throat irritation, and decreased performance.[51, 73]

If the pollutant is carbon monoxide (CO), it reduces both the ability to carry oxygen and the ability to release oxygen already bound to red blood cells. The affinity of hemoglobin for carbon monoxide is 210 times greater than its affinity for oxygen, and carbon monoxide binds at the same site where oxygen would. Thus, when carboxyhemoglobin (COHb) is formed, the arterial percent saturation of oxygen decreases. The release of oxygen from hemoglobin is impaired by a shift in the oxygen dissociation curve to the left (see Figure 3.3). A 4% carboxyhemoglobin level will have a detrimental effect on exercise time and intensity. This level may result if training is done near heavy traffic. Also, individuals smoking 10 or fewer cigarettes per day average approximately 4% carboxyhemoglobin, and a two-pack-a-day habit almost doubles this value. Nonsmokers riding in a car for 1 hr with a smoker can reach 3% carboxyhemoglobin.[51]

Athletes are often affected by pollution levels that do not bother spectators. Individuals with cardiovascular and respiratory diseases and children are also particularly vulnerable.[73] The following recommendations are suggested to minimize the impact of pollutants upon an exercise training session or competition.

1. Individuals with health problems making them particularly susceptible to the effects of pollution should not exercise outside when air quality warnings are in effect but, instead, should seek sites where the air is filtered.

2. Prolonged heavy exercise should be avoided by everyone when hazardous warnings are in effect. Individuals can adapt to breathing pollutants; however, in the long term adaptation is harmful, because it suppresses normal defense mechanisms. Therefore, adaptation should not be attempted.

3. Workouts should be scheduled in the early morning and the late evening to avoid the peak hours of pollution. Runners, cyclists, and in-line skaters should seek locations that are lightly traveled by vehicles. Locations upwind with at least 50 ft between motor vehicles and exercisers are best. Trailing close to a pace car or waiting at stoplights behind cars' exhaust pipes should be avoided.

4. At the very least, smoking should be banned from all indoor training and competition sites. Smoking should be discouraged at all times.[73]

SUMMARY

1. During short-term, light to moderate dynamic aerobic exercise, minute ventilation, alveolar ventilation, and the arteriovenous oxygen difference increase rapidly and reach a steady state within approximately 2–3 min. The partial pressure of oxygen at the alveolar and arterial levels does not change, and as a result the alveolar to arterial oxygen pressure gradient and percent saturation of arterial hemoglobin with oxygen are maintained. The ratio of dead space to tidal volume, percent saturation of oxygen in venous blood, and the partial pressure of oxygen in venous blood decrease rapidly and reach a steady state within approximately 2–3 min. The partial pressure of carbon dioxide increases in the venous blood as the result of the increased energy production, but the partial pressure of carbon dioxide decreases slightly due to the hyperpnea.

2. During the first 30 min of prolonged moderate to heavy dynamic aerobic exercise the only meaningful differences in respiratory responses from short-term light exercise are in magnitude and a slight drop in the arterial partial pressure of oxygen, which, in turn, widens the alveolar to arterial oxygen pressure gradient. After approximately 30 min, minute ventilation, alveolar ventilation, and the arteriovenous oxygen difference exhibit an upward drift. This respiratory drift is associated with a rising body temperature.

3. During incremental aerobic exercise to maximum both minute ventilation and alveolar ventilation exhibit a rectilinear rise interrupted by two breakpoints that change the slope upward. The arteriovenous oxygen difference rises rectilinearly until approximately 60% of maximal work, where it levels off. The partial pressure of both alveolar and arterial oxygen, and the resultant alveolar to arterial oxygen pressure gradient and percent sat-

uration of arterial blood, remain constant until approximately 75% of maximal work. At this point the first three exhibit a slight exponential rise and the arterial oxygen saturation percent decreases slightly as a result. The percent saturation of oxygen in venous blood and venous oxygen partial pressure both decrease rectilinearly until approximately 60% of maximal work, where they level off. As the oxygen is extracted and used, carbon dioxide is produced so that the partial pressure of carbon dioxide in venous blood rises sharply at first and then more slowly. The arterial partial pressure of carbon dioxide is maintained initially but then declines as additional carbon dioxide is blown off by the increasing hyperpnea.

4. All of the respiratory responses to static exercise are the same as for light- to moderate-intensity, short-term submaximal aerobic exercise except that oxygen extraction, as denoted by the arteriovenous oxygen difference, either shows no change or decreases slightly.

5. During exercise increased oxygen dissociation is accomplished by a widening of the O_2 pressure gradient, an increase in PCO_2, a decrease in pH, and an increase in body temperature. The changes in PCO_2, pH, and body temperature increase oxygen release by causing a shift to the right of the oxygen dissociation curve. At altitude the tendency for the decrease in PCO_2, caused by the compensatory hyperventilation, to shift the curve to the left and impair oxygen dissociation is counteracted by an increase in 2,3-DPG activity.

6. Individuals should select the breathing pattern, entrainment or spontaneous, that comes most naturally to them when exercising.

7. Many of the differences in respiratory measures when comparing children and adolescents with young adults or males with females are at least partially related to size. Smaller individuals have smaller values.

8. In general, exercise responses are in the same direction but may vary in magnitude across the age span for both males and females.

9. Respiratory training adaptations are minimal in land-based athletes or fitness participants. The most consistent change is in minute ventilation, which goes down during submaximal work and increases at maximum. Swimming and diving show increases in most static and dynamic lung volumes and capacities, particularly in total lung capacity and vital capacity.

10. The relative percentages of oxygen, carbon dioxide, and nitrogen remain the same regardless of the altitude. However, because the barometric pressure goes down exponentially as altitude increases, the partial pressures exerted by oxygen and carbon dioxide also decrease with altitude. The result is a decrease in percent saturation of oxygen and a decreased ability to maintain high-intensity aerobic exercise.

11. Individuals who must compete at altitude should arrive at the location either less than 12 hr or 2–4 weeks prior to the event. Acclimatization and training at altitude appear to be beneficial for competing at that same altitude but not for subsequent sea-level competition.

12. Hypoxic swim training is a misnomer and is of very little benefit.

13. Exercise in highly polluted air should be avoided. Any adaptation to such conditions is done at the expense of natural defense mechanisms.

REVIEW QUESTIONS

1. List and explain the four factors that increase oxygen dissociation during exercise. What venous percent saturation of oxygen ($SvO_2\%$) remains even under maximal exercise conditions?

2. Compare and contrast the pulmonary ventilation, external respiration, and internal respiration responses to short-term, light to moderate submaximal exercise; long-duration, heavy submaximal exercise; incremental exercise to maximum; and static exercise. Where known, explain the mechanisms for each response.

3. Should fitness participants and athletes be encouraged to practice entrainment as opposed to spontaneous breathing? Why or why not?

4. Explain exercise-induced hypoxemia (EIH) and discuss why it occurs only in highly trained elite athletes. Relate the factors responsible for EIH to the low incidence of respiratory training adaptations.

5. Prepare a flowchart of the physiological changes that occur as a result of acute exposure to altitude. How are these acute changes modified by acclimatization?

6. Defend or refute this statement: "Hypoxic training, whether achieved by training at altitude or breath holding, is beneficial to an athlete."

REFERENCES

1. Adams, W. C., E. M. Bernauer, D. B. Dill, & J. B. Bomar: Effects of equivalent sea-level and altitude training on $\dot{V}O_{2\,max}$ and running performance. *Journal of Applied Physiology.* 39(2):262–266 (1975).

2. Andrew, G. M., M. R. Becklake, J. S. Guleria, & D. V. Bates: Heart and lung functions in swimmers and nonathletes during growth. *Journal of Applied Physiology.* 32(2): 245–251 (1972).

3. Ashley, F., W. B. Kannel, P. D. Sorlie, & R. Masson: Pulmonary function: Relation to aging, cigarette habit and mortality; the Framingham Study. *Annals of Internal Medicine.* 82:739–745 (1975).

4. Asmussen, E.: Similarities and dissimilarities between static and dynamic exercise. *Circulation Research* (Suppl. I). 48(6):I-3–I-10 (1981).

5. Åstrand, I.: Aerobic work capacity in men and women with special reference to age. *Acta Physiologica Scandinavica* (Suppl. 169). 49:1–92 (1960).

6. Åstrand, P.-O.: *Experimental Studies of Physical Working Capacity in Relation to Sex and Age.* Copenhagen: Munksgaard (1952).

7. Åstrand, P.-O., T. E. Cuddy, B. Saltin, & J. Stenberg: Cardiac output during submaximal and maximal work. *Journal of Applied Physiology.* 19(2):268–274 (1964).

8. Åstrand, P.-O., L. Engstrom, B. O. Eriksson, P. Karlberg, I. Nylander, B. Saltin, & C. Thoren: Girl swimmers: With special reference to respiratory and circulatory adaption and gynecological and psychiatric aspects. *Acta Paediatrica* (Suppl.). 147:1–73 (1963).

9. Bachman, J. C., & S. M. Horvath: Pulmonary function changes which accompany athletic conditioning programs. *Research Quarterly.* 39(2):235–239 (1968).

10. Bar-Or, O.: *Pediatric Sports Medicine for the Practitioner: From Physiological Principles to Clinical Applications.* New York: Springer-Verlag, 1–65 (1983).

11. Bechbache, R. R., & J. Duffin: The entrainment of breathing frequency by exercise rhythm. *Journal of Physiology.* 272:553–561 (1977).

12. Becklake, M. R., H. Frank, G. R. Dagenais, G. L. Ostiguy, & C. A. Guzman: Influence of age and sex on exercise cardiac output. *Journal of Applied Physiology.* 20(5):938–947 (1965).

13. Berglund, E., G. Birath, J. Bjure, G. Grimby, I. Kjellmer, L. Sandqvist, & B. Söderholin: Spirometric studies in normal subjects. I. Forced expirograms in subjects between 7 and 70 years of age. *Acta Medica Scandinavica.* 173:185–206 (1963).

14. Bjure, J.: Spirometric studies in normal subjects. IV. Ventilatory capacities in healthy children 7–17 years of age. *Acta Paediatrica.* 52:232–240 (1963).

15. Blomqvist, C. G., & B. Saltin: Cardiovascular adaptations to physical training. *Annual Review of Physiology.* 45:169–189 (1983).

16. Bye, P. T. P., G. A. Farkas, & C. Roussos: Respiratory factors limiting exercise. *Annual Review of Physiology.* 45:439–451 (1983).

17. Caretti, D. M., P. C. Szlyk, & I. V. Sils: Effects of exercise modality on patterns of ventilation and respiratory timing. *Respiration Physiology.* 90:201–211 (1992).

18. Clanton, T. L., G. F. Dixon, J. Drake, & J. E. Gadek: Effects of swim training on lung and inspiratory muscle conditioning. *Journal of Applied Physiology.* 62(1):39–46 (1987).

19. Clark, J. M., F. C. Hagerman, & R. Gelfand: Breathing patterns during submaximal and maximal exercise in elite oarsmen. *Journal of Applied Physiology.* 55(2):440–446 (1983).

20. Clausen, J. P.: Effects of physical training on cardiovascular adjustments to exercise in man. *Physiology Reviews.* 57(4):779–815 (1977).

21. Comroe, J. H.: *Physiology of Respiration: An Introductory Text.* Chicago: Year Book Medical Publishers (1965).

22. Cooper, K. H.: *The New Aerobics.* New York: Bantam Books (1970).

23. Coyle, E. F., W. H. Martin III, D. R. Sinacore, M. J. Joyner, J. M. Hagberg, & J. O. Holloszy: Time course of loss of adaptations after stopping prolonged intense endurance training. *Journal of Applied Physiology: Respiratory, Environmental and Exercise Physiology.* 57(6):1857–1864 (1984).

24. Cordain, L., & J. Stager: Pulmonary structure and function in swimmers. *Sports Medicine.* 6:271–278 (1988).

25. Cordain, L., A. Tucker, D. Moon, & J. M. Stager: Lung volumes and maximal respiratory pressures in collegiate swimmers and runners. *Research Quarterly for Exercise and Sport.* 61(1):70–74 (1990).

26. Davies, C. T. M.: The oxygen-transporting system in relation to age. *Clinical Science.* 42:1–13 (1972).

27. Davies, C. T. M., P. E. DiPrampero, & P. Cerretelli: Kinetics of cardiac output and respiratory gas exchange during exercise and recovery. *Journal of Applied Physiology.* 32(5):618–625 (1972).

28. Dempsey, J. A.: Is the lung built for exercise? *Medicine and Science in Sports and Exercise.* 18(2):143–155 (1986).

29. Dempsey, J. A., & R. F. Fregosi: Adaptability of the pulmonary system of changing metabolic requirements. *American Journal of Cardiology.* 55:59D–67D (1985).

30. Dempsey, J. A., N. Gledhill, W. G. Reddan, H. V. Foster, P. G. Hanson, & A. D. Claremont: Pulmonary adaptation to exercise: Effects of exercise type and duration, chronic hypoxia and physical training. In P. Milvy (ed.), The Marathon: Physiological, Medical, Epidemiological, and Psychological Studies. *Annals of the New York Academy of Sciences.* 301:243–261 (1977).

31. DeVries, H. A., & G. M. Adams: Comparison of exercise responses in old and young men. II. Ventilatory mechanics. *Journal of Gerontology.* 27(3):349–352 (1972).

32. Dicker, S., G. K. Lofthus, N. W. Thorton, & G. A. Brooks: Respiratory and heart rate responses to tethered controlled frequency breathing swimming. *Medicine and Science in Sports and Exercise.* 12(1):20–23 (1980).

33. Donevan, R. E., W. H. Palmer, C. J. Varvis, & D. V. Bates: Influence of age on pulmonary diffusing capacity. *Journal of Applied Physiology.* 14(4):483–492 (1959).

34. Ekelund, L. G.: Circulatory and respiratory adaptation during prolonged exercise. *Acta Physiologica Scandinavica* (Suppl. 292). 70:1–38 (1967A).

35. Ekelund, L. G., & A. Holmgren: Central hemodynamics during exercise. *Circulation Research* (Suppl. 1). 20–21:1–33 (1967B).

36. Ericsson, P., & L. Irnell: Spirometric studies of ventilatory capacity in elderly people. In J. R. Edge, K. K. Pump, J. Arias-Stella, et al., *Aging Lung: Normal Function.* New York: MSS Information Corporation, 209–222 (1974).

37. Eriksson, B. O.: Physical training, oxygen supply and muscle metabolism in 11–13 year old boys. *Acta Physiologica Scandinavica* (Suppl.). 384:1–48 (1972).

38. Eriksson, B. O.: Effects of physical training on hemodynamic response during submaximal and maximal exercise in 11–13 year old boys. *Acta Physiological Scandinavica.* 87:27–39 (1973).

39. Fahey, T. D., A. D. Valle-Zuris, G. Oehlsen, M. Trieb, & J. Seymour: Pubertal stage differences in hormonal and hematological responses to maximal exercise in males. *Journal of Applied Physiology: Respiratory, Environmental and Exercise Physiology.* 46(4):823–827 (1979).

40. Ferris, B. G., D. O. Anderson, & R. Zickmantel: Prediction values for screening tests of pulmonary function. *American Review of Respiratory Diseases.* 91:252–261 (1965).

41. Fleck, S. J., & W. J. Kraemer: *Designing Resistance Training Programs.* Champaign, IL: Human Kinetics Publishers (1987).

42. Fringer, M. N., & G. A. Stull: Changes in cardiorespiratory parameters during periods of training and detraining in young adult females. *Medicine and Science in Sports.* 6(1):20–25 (1974).

43. Green, J. S., & S. F. Crouse: Endurance training, cardiovascular function and the aged. *Sports Medicine.* 16(5):331–341 (1993).

44. Grimby, G.: Respiration in exercise. *Medicine and Science in Sports.* 1(1):9–14 (1969).

45. Grover, R. F.: Adaptation to high altitude. In L. J. Folinsbee, J. A. Wagner, J. F., Borgia, B. L. Drinkwater, J. A. Gliner, & J. F. Bedi (eds.), *Environmental Stress: Individual Human Adaptations.* New York: Academic Press (1978).

46. Gurtner, H. P., P. Walser, & B. Fässler: Normal values for pulmonary hemodynamics at rest and during exercise in man. *Progress in Respiration Research.* 9:295–315 (1975).

47. Guyton, A. C.: *Textbook of Medical Physiology* (7th edition). Philadelphia: Saunders (1986).

48. Haffor, A. A., A. C. Harrison, & P. A. Catledge Kirk: Anaerobic threshold alterations caused by interval training in 11-year-olds. *Journal of Sports Medicine and Physical Fitness.* 30(1):53–56 (1990).

49. Hannon, J. P.: Comparative altitude adaptability of young men and women. In: L. J. Folinsbee, J. A. Wagner, J. F. Borgia, B. L. Drinkwater, J. A. Gliner, & J. F. Bedi (eds.), *Environmental Stress: Individual Human Adaptations.* New York: Academic Press (1978).

50. Hanson, P., A. Claremont, J. Dempsey, & W. Reddan: Determinants and consequences of ventilatory responses to competitive endurance running. *Journal of Applied Physiology: Respiratory, Environmental and Exercise Physiology.* 52(3):615–623 (1982).

51. Haymes, E. M., & C. L. Wells: *Environment and Human Performance.* Champaign, IL: Human Kinetics Publishers (1986).

52. Hill, A. R., J. M. Adams, B. E. Parker, & D. F. Rochester: Short-term entrainment of ventilation to the walking cycle in humans. *Journal of Applied Physiology.* 65(2):570–578 (1988).

53. Holmer, I., & L. Gullstrand: Physiological responses to swimming with a controlled frequency of breathing. *Scandinavian Journal of Sports Science.* 2(1):1–6 (1980).

54. Jain, S. K., & C. K. Gupta: Age, height, and body weight as determinants of ventilatory "norms" in healthy men above forty years age. In J. R. Edge, K. K. Pump, J. Arias-Stella et al., *Aging Lung: Normal Function.* New York: MSS Information Corporation, 190–202 (1974).

55. Jain, S. K., & C. K. Gupta: Lung function studies in healthy men and women over forty. In J. R. Edge, K. K. Pump, J. Arias-Stella, et al., *Aging Lung: Normal Function.* New York: MSS Information Corporation, 182–189 (1974).

56. Jasinskas, C. L., B. A. Wilson, & J. Hoare: Entrainment of breathing rate to movement frequency during work at two intensities. *Respiration Physiology.* 42:199–209 (1980).

57. Johnson, B. D., & J. A. Dempsey: Demand vs. capacity in the aging pulmonary system. In J. O. Holloszy (ed.), *Exercise and Sport Sciences Reviews.* 19:171–210 (1991).

58. Jones, N. L.: Exercise testing in pulmonary evaluation: Rationale, methods and the normal respiratory response to exercise. *New England Journal of Medicine.* 293(11):541–544 (1975).

59. Kao, F. F.: *An Introduction to Respiratory Physiology.* New York: American Elsevier (1974).

60. Kaufmann, D. A., E. W. Swenson, J. Fencl, & A. Lucas: Pulmonary function of marathon runners. *Medicine and Science in Sports.* 6(2):114–117 (1974).

61. Kay, J. D. S., E. Strange Petersen, & H. Vejby-Christensen: Breathing in man during steady-state exercise on the bicycle at two pedalling frequencies, and during treadmill walking. *Journal of Physiology.* 251:645–656 (1975).

62. Kenney, R. A.: *Physiology of Aging: A Synopsis.* Chicago: Year Book Medical Publishers (1982).

63. Koyal, S. N., B. J. Whipp, D. Huntsman, G. A. Bray, & K. Wasserman: Ventilatory responses to the metabolic acidosis of treadmill and cycle ergometry. *Journal of Applied Physiology.* 40(6):864–867 (1976).

64. Krahenbuhl, G. S., J. S. Skinner, & W. M. Kohrt: Developmental aspects of maximal aerobic power in children. In R. L. Terjung (ed.), *Exercise and Sport Sciences Reviews.* 13:503–538 (1985).

65. Lavoie, J.-M., & R. R. Montpetit: Applied physiology of swimming. *Sports Medicine.* 3:165–189 (1986).

66. Leff, A. R., & P. T. Schumacker: *Respiratory Physiology: Basics and Applications.* Philadelphia: Saunders (1993).

67. Leith, D. G., & M. Bradley: Ventilatory muscle strength and endurance training. *Journal of Applied Physiology.* 41(4):508–516 (1976).

68. Loat, C. E. R., & E. C. Rhodes: Relationship between the lactate and ventilatory thresholds during prolonged exercise. *Sports Medicine.* 15(2):104–115 (1993).

69. Maclennan, S. E., G. A. Silvestri, J. Ward, & D. A. Mahler: Does entrained breathing improve the economy of rowing? *Medicine and Science in Sports and Exercise.* 26(5):610–614 (1994).

70. Magel, J. R., & K. Lange Andersen: Pulmonary diffusing capacity and cardiac output in young trained Norwegian swimmers and untrained subjects. *Medicine and Science in Sports.* 1(3):131–139 (1969).

71. Mahler, D. A., C. R. Shuhart, E. Brew, & T. A. Stukel: Ventilatory responses and entrainment of breathing during rowing. *Medicine and Science in Sports and Exercise.* 23(2):186–192 (1991).

72. Malina, R. M., & C. Bouchard: *Growth, Maturation and Physical Activity.* Champaign, IL: Human Kinetics Publishers (1991).

73. McCafferty, W. B.: *Air Pollution and Athletic Performance.* Springfield, IL: Thomas (1981).

74. Mostyn, E. M., S. Helle, J. B. L. Gee, L. G. Bentivoglio, & D. V. Bates: Pulmonary diffusing capacity of athletes. *Journal of Applied Physiology.* 18(4):687–695 (1963).

75. Niinimaa, V., & R. J. Shepard: Training and oxygen conductance in the elderly. I. The respiratory system. *Journal of Gerontology.* 33(3):354–361 (1978).

76. Pardy, R. L., S. N. A. Hussain, P. T. Macklein: The ventilatory pump in exercise. *Clinics in Chest Medicine.* 5(1):35–49 (1984).

77. Paterson, D. H., T. M. McLellan, R. S. Stella, & D. A. Cunningham: Longitudinal study of ventilation threshold and maximal O_2 uptake in athletic boys. *Journal of Applied Physiology.* 62(5):2051–2057 (1987).

78. Pearce, D. H., & H. T. Milhorn: Dynamic and steady-state respiratory responses to bicycle exercise. *Journal of Applied Physiology: Respiratory, Environmental and Exercise Physiology.* 42(6):959–967 (1977).

79. Pollock, M. L., T. K. Cureton, & L. Greninger: Effects of frequency of training on working capacity, cardiovascular function, and body composition of adult men. *Medicine and Science in Sport.* 1(2):70–74 (1969).

80. Powers, S. K., & R. E. Beadle: Onset of hyperventilation during incremental exercise: A brief review. *Research Quarterly for Exercise and Sport.* 56(4):352–360 (1985).

81. Powers, S. K., D. Martin, & S. Dodd: Exercise-induced hypoxemia in elite endurance athletes: Incidence, causes and impact on $VO_{2\ max}$. *Sports Medicine.* 16(1):14–22 (1993).

82. Rasmussen, B., K. Klausen, J. P. Clausen, & J. Trap-Jensen: Pulmonary ventilation, blood gases, and blood pH after training of the arms or the legs. *Journal of Applied Physiology.* 38(2):250–256 (1975).

83. Ratzin Jackson, C. G., & B. J. Sharkey: Altitude, training, and human performance. *Sports Medicine.* 6:279–284 (1988).

84. Reid, J. G., & J. M. Thomson: *Exercise Prescription for Fitness*. Englewood Cliffs, NJ: Prentice-Hall (1985).

85. Reuschlein, P. S., W. G. Reddan, J. Burpee, J. B. L. Gee, & J. Rankin: Effect of physical training on the pulmonary diffusing capacity during submaximal work. *Journal of Applied Physiology*. 24(2):152–158 (1968).

86. Robinson, E. P., & J. M. Kjeldgaard: Improvement in ventilatory muscle function with running. *Journal of Applied Physiology: Respiratory, Environmental and Exercise Physiology*. 52(6):1400–1406 (1992).

87. Robinson, S.: Experimental studies of physical fitness in relation to age. *Arbeitsphysiologie*. 10:251–323 (1938).

88. Rowell, L. B.: Circulation. *Medicine and Science in Sports*. 1(1):15–22 (1969).

89. Rowell, L. B., H. L. Taylor, Y. Wang, & W. S. Carlson: Saturation of arterial blood with oxygen during maximal exercise. *Journal of Applied Physiology*. 19(2):284–286 (1964).

90. Rowland, T. W.: Developmental aspects of physiological function relating to aerobic exercise in children. *Sports Medicine*. 10(4):255–266 (1990).

91. Rowland, T. W., J. A. Auchmachie, T. J. Keenan, & G. M. Green: Physiologic responses to treadmill running in adult and prepubertal males. *International Journal of Sports Medicine*. 8(4):292–297 (1987).

92. Rowland, T. W., & G. M. Green: Physiological responses to treadmill exercise in females: Adult-child differences. *Medicine and Science in Sports and Exercise*. 20(5): 474–478 (1988).

93. Saltin, B.: Physiological effects of physical conditioning. *Medicine and Science in Sports*. 1(1):50–56 (1969).

94. Saltin, B., G. Bloomqvist, J. H. Mitchell, R. L. Johnson, K. Wildenthal, & C. B. Chapman: Response to exercise after bed rest and after training. *Circulation* (Suppl VII). 38(5):VII-1–VII-78 (1968).

95. Saris, W. H. M., A. M. Noordeloos, B. E. M. Ringnalda, M. A. Van't Hof, & R. A. Binkhorst: Reference values for aerobic power of healthy 4- to 18-year-old Dutch children: Preliminary results. In R. A. Binkhorst, H. C. G. Kemper, & W. H. M. Saris (eds.), *Children and Exercise XI*. Champaign, IL: Human Kinetics Publishers, 15:151–160 (1985).

96. Sawka, M. N., R. G. Knowlton, & R. M. Glaser: Body temperature, respiration, and acid-base equilibrium during prolonged running. *Medicine and Science in Sports and Exercise*. 12(5):370–374 (1980).

97. Seals, D. R., B. F. Hurley, J. Schultz, & J. M. Hagberg: Endurance training in older men and women. II. Blood lactate response to submaximal exercise. *Journal of Applied Physiology: Respiratory, Environmental, and Exercise Physiology*. 57(4):1030–1033 (1984).

98. Segal, S. S.: Convection, diffusion, and mitochondrial utilization of oxygen during exercise. In D. R. Lamb & C. V. Gisolfi (eds.), *Energy Metabolism in Exercise and Sport*. Dubuque, IA: Brown & Benchmark, 269–338 (1992).

99. Shapiro, W., C. E. Johnston, R. A. Dameron, & J. L. Patterson: Maximum ventilatory performance and its limiting factors. *Journal of Applied Physiology*. 19(2):197–203 (1964).

100. Shepard, R. J.: *Physical Activity and Aging*. Chicago: Year Book Medical Publishers, 40–44; 85–95 (1978).

101. Skinner, J. S., & T. H. McLellan: The transition from aerobic to anaerobic metabolism. *Research Quarterly for Exercise and Sport*. 51(1):234–298 (1980).

102. Slonim, N. B., & L. H. Hamilton: *Respiratory Physiology* (3rd edition). St. Louis: Mosby (1976).

103. Stanescu, S., Q. St. Dutu, Z. Jienescu, L. Hartia, N. Nicolescu, & F. Sacerdoteanu: Investigations into changes of pulmonary function in the aged. In J. R. Edge, K. K. Pump, &

J. Aris-Stella et al., *Aging Lung: Normal Function*.New York: MSS Information Corporation, 171–181 (1974).

104. Storstein, O., & A. Voll: New prediction formulas for ventilation measurements: A study of normal individuals in the age group 20–59 years. In J. R. Edge, K. K. Pump, & J. Aris-Stella et al., *Aging Lung: Normal Function*. New York: MSS Information Corporation, 156–170 (1974).

105. Turner, J. M., J. Mead, & M. E. Wohl: Elasticity of human lungs in relation to age. *Journal of Applied Physiology*. 25(6):664–671 (1968).

106. Vaccaro, P., & D. H. Clarke: Cardiorespiratory alterations in 9 to 11 year old children following a season of competitive swimming. *Medicine and Science in Sports*. 10(3):204–207 (1978).

107. Vaccaro, P., C. W. Zauner, & W. F. Updyke: Resting and exercise respiratory function in well trained child swimmers. *Journal of Sports Medicine and Physical Fitness*. 17:297–306 (1977).

108. Wagner, P. D.: Central and peripheral aspects of oxygen transport and adaptation with exercise. *Sports Medicine*. 11(3):133–142 (1991).

109. Walsh, M. L., & E. W. Banister: Possible mechanisms of the anaerobic threshold: A review. *Sports Medicine*. 5:269–302 (1988).

110. Wasserman, K.: Breathing during exercise. *New England Journal of Medicine*. 298(14):780–785 (1978).

111. Wasserman, K., A. L. VanKessel, & G. G. Burton: Interaction of physiological mechanisms during exercise. *Journal of Applied Physiology*. 22(1):71–85 (1967).

112. Wasserman, K., & B. J. Whipp: Exercise physiology in health and disease. *American Review of Respiratory Disease*. 112:219–249 (1975).

113. Whipp, B. J.: The hyperpnea of dynamic muscular exercise. In R. S. Hutton (ed.), *Exercise and Sport Science Reviews* (Vol. 5). Santa Barbara, CA: Journal Publishing Affiliates (1977).

114. Whipp, B. J., & S. A. Ward: Ventilatory control dynamics during muscular exercise in men. *International Journal of Sports Medicine*. 1:146–159 (1980).

115. Whipp, B. J., S. A. Ward, N. Lamarra, J. A. Davis, & K. Wasserman: Parameters of ventilatory and gas exchange dynamics during exercise. *Journal of Applied Physiology: Respiratory, Environmental and Exercise Physiology*. 52(6):1506–1513 (1982).

116. Wilmore, J. H., J. Royce, R. N. Girandola, F. I. Katch, & V. L. Katch: Physiological alterations resulting from a 10-week program of jogging. *Medicine and Science in Sports*, 2(1):7–14 (1970).

117. Younes, M., & G. Kivinen: Respiratory mechanics and breathing pattern during and following maximal exercise. *Journal of Applied Physiology: Respiratory, Environmental and Exercise Physiology*. 57(6):1773–1782 (1984).

118. Zauner, C. W., & N. Y. Benson: Physiological alterations in young swimmers during three years of intensive training. *Journal of Sports Medicine and Physical Fitness*. 21:179–185 (1981).

119. Zauner, C. W., M. G. Maksud, & J. Milichna: Physiological considerations in training young athletes. *Sports Medicine*. 8(1):15–31 (1989).

120. Zempel, C.: Hypoxic isn't: Exploding the myth. *Triathlete*. Nov/Dec 20–21 (1989).

121. Zwiren, L. D., K. J. Cureton, & P. Hutchinson: Comparison of circulatory responses to submaximal exercise in equally trained men and women. *International Journal of Sports Medicine*. 4:255–259 (1983).

4

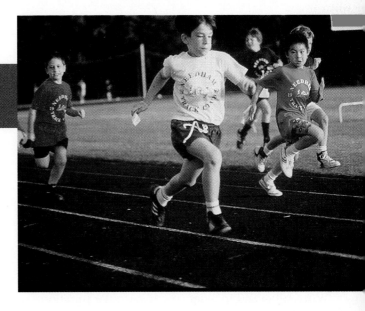

The Cardiovascular System

After studying the chapter, you should be able to:

- Explain the functions of the cardiovascular system.

- Identify the various components of the cardiovascular system.

- Distinguish among the vessels that comprise the vascular system, and compare the pressure, velocity, and resistance in each type of vessel.

- Explain how electrical excitation is spread through the conduction system of the heart.

- Explain the relationships among the electrical, pressure, contractile, and volume changes throughout the cardiac cycle.

- Calculate mean arterial pressure, total peripheral resistance, and cardiac output.

- Describe the hormonal mechanisms by which blood volume is maintained.

- Explain how the cardiovascular system is regulated.

- Describe the measurement of maximal oxygen consumption, cardiac output, stroke volume, heart rate, and blood pressure.

Introduction

Chapter 2 described how oxygen is taken into the body and made available for delivery to the cells of the body. The ability of the body to circulate oxygen (and other substances) depends upon the proper functioning of the cardiovascular system. In many ways the cardiovascular system and the respiratory system operate in a parallel fashion, since they have a common mission—to deliver oxygen to working muscles—and are driven by similar mechanisms. This chapter provides an overview of the cardiovascular system, discusses basic principles of cardiovascular dynamics, and outlines techniques currently used to assess cardiovascular function.

Overview of the Cardiovascular System

The *cardiovascular system* includes the heart, blood vessels, and blood. Its primary functions are (1) transporting oxygen and nutrients to the cells of the body and transporting carbon dioxide and waste products from the cells; (2) regulating body temperature, pH levels, and fluid balance; and (3) protecting the body from blood loss and infection. The heart is the pump that provides the force to circulate the blood throughout the vessels of the circulatory system. The blood vessels serve as conduits for the blood as it travels to the lungs to become oxygenated, to the digestive system to receive nutrients, and to the cells to deliver the oxygen and the nutrients. Blood is then returned to the heart to repeat the cycle. It is the blood that is primarily responsible for the majority of the transport that occurs within the cardiovascular system.

Figure 4.1 provides a schematic overview of the cardiovascular system. *Arteries* carry blood away from the heart, and *veins* return blood to the heart.

Intercalated Discs The junction between cardiac muscle cells that forms the mechanical and electrical connection between the two cells.

Syncytium The individual cells of the myocardium that function collectively as a unit during depolarization.

The *capillary beds* serve as the site of exchange for gases and nutrients between the blood and the tissues of the body.

The Heart

The heart is a hollow muscular organ located in the thoracic cavity. It weighs approximately 250–350 g and is 12–14 cm long, about the size of a clenched fist.[19] It serves as the double pump for the cardiovascular system. The heart muscle is referred to as the *myocardium.*

Macroanatomy of the Heart   The heart contains four chambers and is functionally separated into the right and left heart. The right side pumps blood to the lungs (pulmonary circulation), and the left side pumps blood to the entire body (systemic circulation). The two sides of the heart are separated by the intraventricular septum. The upper chambers, called *atria* (atrium is the singular), receive the blood; the lower chambers, called *ventricles,* eject blood from the heart (see Figure 4.2a). Blood is ejected from the right ventricle via the pulmonary artery and from the left ventricle via the aorta.

One-way valves control blood flow through the heart. The *atrioventricular (AV) valves* separate the atrium and ventricle on each side of the heart; specifically, the tricuspid valve separates the atrium and ventricle on the right side of the heart, and the bicuspid (or mitral) valve separates the atrium and ventricle on the left side of the heart. The *semilunar valves* control blood flow from the ventricles; specifically, the aortic semilunar valve allows blood to flow from the left ventricle into the aorta, and the pulmonary semilunar valve allows blood to flow from the right ventricle into the pulmonary artery.

Figure 4.2a depicts the chambers and valves of the heart and diagrams the flow of blood through the heart. Figure 4.2b summarizes the blood flow through the heart.

Microanatomy of the Heart   Cardiac muscle cells are both similar to and different from skeletal muscle cells. Both types of muscle cells are striated in appearance because they contain the contractile proteins, actin and myosin. The primary difference between cardiac and skeletal muscle cells is

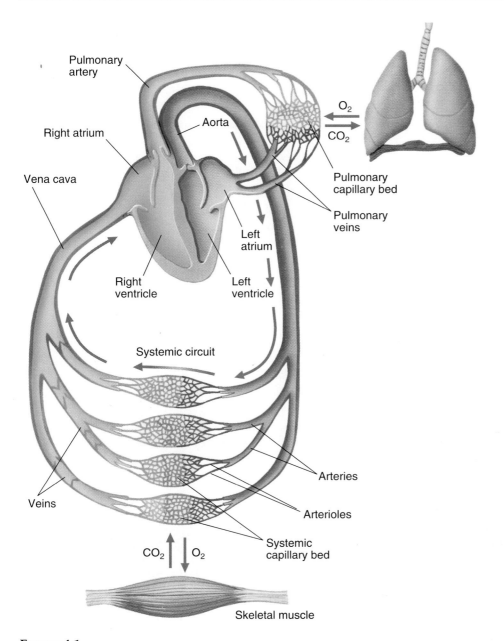

FIGURE 4.1

Overview of the Cardiovascular System

that cardiac muscle cells are highly interconnected. That is, the cell membranes of adjacent cardiac cells are functionally linked by **intercalated discs.** These junctions between cells form the electrical connection between two cells. This connection allows the electrical activity in one cell to pass to the adjacent cell. Thus, the individual cells of the myocardium function collectively; when one cell is stimulated electrically, the stimulation will spread cell to cell over the entire area. The result is that the cells of the myocardium function as a unit during depolarization, which is called a **syncytium.** There are two functional syncytia, atrial and ventricular, and each contracts as a unit.

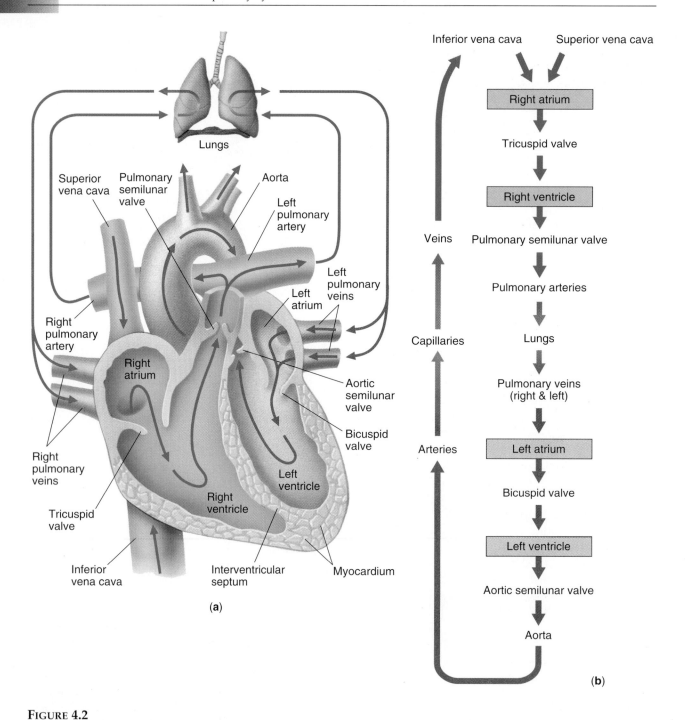

FIGURE 4.2

Blood Flow Through the Heart

The Heart as Excitable Tissue Cardiac muscle cells are excitable cells that contract when they become sufficiently depolarized and, as a result of contraction, produce force that ejects blood from the chambers. Individual myocardial cells function together to produce a coordinated contraction of the entire organ. The conduction system cells with the fastest spontaneous rate of depolarization are called the *pacemaker* cells and are located in the *sinoatrial* (SA) *node* in the right atria. As shown in Figure 4.3a, the excitation is spread from the SA node throughout the right atria by internodal tracts and to the left atria by Bachmann's bundle. Since the atrial and ventricular syncytia contract separately, an action potential in the atria does not lead directly to the contraction of cardiac cells in the ventricles. The signal is spread from the atria to the ventricles via the atrioventricular node (AV). Once the AV node is depolarized, the electrical signal continues down the specialized conduction system consisting of the bundle of His, the left and right bundle branches, and the Purkinje fibers. The electrical excitation then spreads out from the conducting system to excite all of the myocardial cells. Remember that the excitation is spread by the conduction system and cell-to-cell contact: The excitation is passed from cell to cell within the ventricles since the conduction system does not reach each individual cell.

As mentioned earlier, the cells of the SA node are considered the pacemaker cells of the heart because they have the fastest rate of depolarization under normal conditions. Cells in each area of the conduction system have their own inherent rate of depolarization. For the SA node the rate of depolarization is 70–80 times·min^{-1} in sedentary males and females. The AV node discharges at an intrinsic rate of 40–60 times·min^{-1}, and the Purkinje fibers at a rate of 15–40 times·min^{-1}.[13] In an individual with a diseased SA node, the AV node takes over the pacemaking. Thus, if the only thing you knew about an individual was that he or she had a heart rate of 40 b·min^{-1}, you could not tell whether the person was a highly trained endurance athlete, since endurance training results in a lowering of heart rate, or someone in need of an artificial pacemaker implant.

Electrocardiogram   An *electrocardiogram* (ECG) provides a graphic illustration of the electrical current generated by excitation of the heart muscle. Figure 4.3b presents an ECG tracing that is color-coded to match the conduction system in Figure 4.3a.[22]

The P wave in Figure 4.3b represents atrial depolarization, which causes atrial contraction. The spread of the electrical signal through the conduction system of the atria is indicated by green in Figures 4.3a and 4.3b. Repolarization of the atria is normally not detectable on an ECG. The electrical signal reaches the AV node at the end of the P wave (yellow). Excitation of the bundle of His and bundle

FIGURE 4.3

Conduction System of the Heart
Source: Modified from Netter[22].

branches (red) occur in the middle of the PR interval, followed by excitation of the Purkinje fibers (purple). Notice that excitation of the various portions of the conduction system requires very little time and that activation of the entire conduction system precedes the QRS complex. The QRS complex reflects depolarization of the muscle fibers in the ventricles, which occurs after the electrical signal has traveled through the specialized conduction system. The T wave reflects repolarization of the muscle fibers in the ventricles and leads to relaxation in preparation to start the cycle all over again.

Although the SA node can depolarize spontaneously, the firing of the SA node is influenced by neural and hormonal factors. Additionally, heart rate varies with age. Table 4.1 presents typical resting heart rate (HR) values in healthy individuals of various ages. Factors that affect heart rate are discussed in greater detail later in this chapter.

Cardiac Cycle   In order to successfully function as a pump, the heart must have alternating times of relaxation and contraction. The relaxation phase, called *diastole,* is the period when the heart fills with blood. The contraction phase, called *systole,* is the period when blood is ejected from the heart. The **cardiac cycle**—one complete sequence of contraction and relaxation of the heart—includes all events associated with the flow of blood through the heart and is marked by dramatic changes in pressure and blood volume. Figure 4.4 summarizes the position of the heart valves throughout the phases of the cardiac cycle and provides information regarding ventricular pressure (indicated by arrows) and volume (indicated by cavity size) at each phase.

The ventricular-filling period (VFP) (see Figure 4.4a) occurs when the ventricles are at rest (ventricular diastole) and the AV valves are open. The ventricles fill as blood is returned to the atria and flows down into the ventricles because of the force of gravity. Atrial contraction also pushes a small volume of additional blood into the ventricles at the end of diastole. Blood volume in the ventricles is greatest at the end of ventricular filling, but pressure remains relatively low because the ventricles are relaxed.

Systole (the contraction phase) is divided into two periods, the isovolumetric contraction period (ICP) and the ventricular ejection period (VEP). During the ICP (Figure 4.4b) both the AV valves and the semilunar valves are closed. Thus, blood volume in the ventricles remains constant despite the

high pressure generated by the contraction of the ventricular myocardium. Once pressure in the ventricles exceeds pressure in the aorta, the semilunar valves are forced open. Blood is then ejected from the ventricles, initiating the VEP and causing ventricular volume to decrease (see Figure 4.4c).

During the isovolumetric relaxation period (IRP) both the AV and the semilunar valves are closed (Figure 4.4d). Thus, ventricular volume is unchanged, and pressure is low because the ventricles are relaxed.

Figure 4.5 summarizes the cardiac cycle. This diagram integrates information about the electrocardiogram; the pressure in the left atrium, the left ventricle, and aorta; the left ventricular volume; the ventricular phase; the period of the cardiac cycle; and the position of the heart valves. Figure 4.5 begins arbitrarily during the VFP of ventricular diastole. The AV valves are open, allowing blood to flow from the atria into the ventricle; therefore, volume is increasing. As the atrium contracts (P wave), more blood is forced into the ventricle, causing a small increase in ventricular volume and ventricular pressure.

Following the QRS complex, there is an immediate and dramatic increase in ventricular pressure as the myocardium contracts. Notice, however, that the volume does not change until the pressure in the ventricle is greater than the pressure in the aorta and pulmonary artery, and the semilunar valves are forced open. This is the isovolumetric contraction period. Locate Point *A* on the graph of ventricular pressure in Figure 4.5. This is the point where pressure in the ventricle exceeds pressure in the arteries, and the aortic semilunar valves are forced open. Follow the dashed lines downward to the row for the semilunar valves in the chart at the bottom of the

TABLE 4.1 ▪ **Typical Resting Cardiovascular Values for Males and Females of Various Ages**

	Age of Males (yr)			Age of Females (yr)		
CARDIOVASCULAR VALUE	10–15	20–30	50–60	10–15	20–30	50–60
Heart rate HR (b·min^{-1})	82	75	80	85	75	80
Stroke volume SV (mL·b^{-1})	50	90	70	40	75	62
Cardiac output (L·min^{-1})	4.0	6.5	5.5	3.4	5.5	5.0

Sources: Astrand,[4] Fleg et al.,[11] Ogawa et al.,[21] and Spina et al.[30,31,32]

FIGURE 4.4

Periods of the Cardiac Cycle

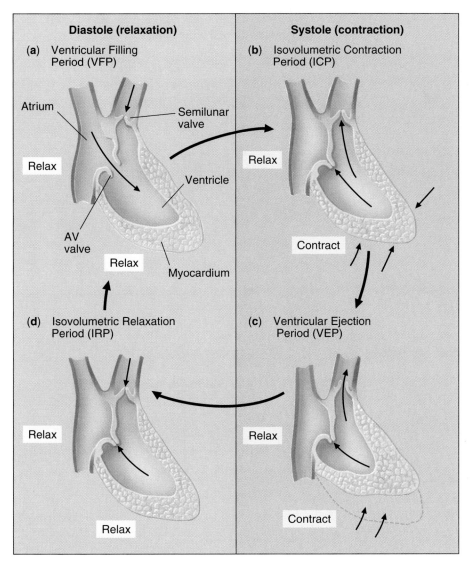

Diastole (relaxation)

(a) Ventricular Filling
Period (VFP)

Atrium

Semilunar
valve

Relax

Ventricle

Relax

AV
valve

Relax

Myocardium

(d) Isovolumetric Relaxation
Period (IRP)

Relax

Relax

Systole (contraction)

(b) Isovolumetric Contraction
Period (ICP)

Relax

Contract

(c) Ventricular Ejection
Period (VEP)

Relax

Contract

figure, and note that these valves are now opened. Also note that this dashed line coincides with the start of a rapid decrease in ventricular volume. Once the valves are open, blood is forced out of the ventricles; thus, blood volume in the ventricle decreases.

When pressure in the ventricles falls below pressure in the arteries, the semilunar valves close. Refer to Point *B* on the pressure curve of Figure 4.5 and again follow the dashed line downward, noting ventricular volume and valve position. As pressure continues to decrease, ventricular volume remains constant, because all the valves are closed and no

blood can enter or leave the ventricles (isovolumetric relaxation period).

Following the T wave, which signals ventricular relaxation, the ventricles again begin to fill with blood: The AV valves are open, and ventricular volume is increasing. This cycle of diastole followed by systole followed by diastole continues with each beat of the heart.

Cardiac Cycle One complete sequence of contraction and relaxation of the heart.

FIGURE 4.5

Summary of the Cardiac Cycle

The phases of the cardiac cycle are labeled as 1, which is the VFP; 2, which is the ICP (and ventricular volume is unchanged; 3, which is the VEP; and 4, which is the IRP (and ventricular volume is again unchanged).

Diastole provides time for the cardiac cells to relax and the ventricles to fill, thereby directly affecting the amount of blood that is pumped during the subsequent systole. Furthermore, it is during diastole that the myocardium is supplied with its blood supply, known as the *coronary circulation.*

Systole is the contraction period of the heart, first isometrically (ICP) and then dynamically (VEP). The volume of blood ejected from the ventricles determines the cardiovascular system's ability to meet the demands of the body. The volume of blood in the left ventricle at the end of diastole is termed **left ventricular end–diastolic volume (LVEDV)** and is labeled in Figure 4.5. Similarly, the volume of blood in the left ventricle at the end of systole is termed **left ventricular end–systolic volume (LVESV).** The amount of blood ejected from the heart with each beat is called **stroke volume (SV).**

Before going on to the next section, study Figures 4.4 and 4.5. Be sure that you understand what is happening with the ECG, with ventricular, atrial, and aortic pressure, with ventricular volume, and with the heart valves at each period of the cardiac cycle. Now, find your radial pulse and begin counting: 0, 1, 2, 3,. . . . All the events described in this section occur every time you feel a pulse, which is once every 0.8 sec, assuming you have a resting heart rate of 75 b · min^{-1}. **Heart rate (HR)** is thus defined as the number of cardiac cycles per minute, expressed as beats per minute (b · min^{-1}).

Stroke Volume   As mentioned previously, stroke volume (SV) is the volume of blood ejected from the ventricles with each beat, usually expressed in milliliters (mL). The amount of blood ejected from the heart is determined by three factors:

1.   The volume of blood returned to the heart (preload).

2.   The force of contraction (contractility).

3.   The resistance presented to the contracting ventricle (afterload).

The volume of blood returned to the heart is called **preload** and is critical to determining the amount of blood ejected from the heart (the heart cannot eject blood that is not there). Under resting conditions the heart ejects approximately 50–60% of the blood that is returned; this is known as the **ejection fraction (EF).** Figure 4.6 depicts changes in

the volume of blood in the ventricles throughout the cardiac cycle and defines specific volumes and capacities associated with the ventricles. The LVEDV is approximately 130 mL of blood under resting conditions. Following systole the LVESV is approximately 60 mL of blood. Stroke volume can then be calculated as

(4.1)   stroke volume (mL) = left ventricular end–diastolic volume (mL) – left ventricular end–systolic volume (mL)

or
$$SV = LVEDV - LVESV$$
$$130 \text{ mL} - 60 \text{ mL} = 70 \text{ mL}$$

Thus, 70 mL of blood was ejected from the heart at rest.

The ejection fraction (EF) can now be calculated from the information as follows:

(4.2)   ejection fraction (%) = stroke volume (mL) ÷ left ventricular end–diastolic volume (mL)

or
$$EF = \frac{SV}{LVEDV} \times 100$$

■ **EXAMPLE**

Calculate the ejection fraction for the previous example.
$$EF = [(70 \text{ mL}) \div (130 \text{ mL})] \times 100 = 54\% \quad ■$$

Left Ventricular End–Diastolic Volume (LVEDV) The volume of blood in the left ventricle at the end of diastole.

Left Ventricular End–Systolic Volume (LVESV) The volume of blood in the left ventricle at the end of systole.

Stroke Volume (SV) Amount of blood ejected from the ventricles with each beat of the heart.

Heart Rate (HR) The number of cardiac cycles per minute, expressed as beats per min (b · min^{-1}).

Preload Volume of blood returned to the heart.

Ejection Fraction (EF) The percentage of LVEDV that is ejected from the heart.

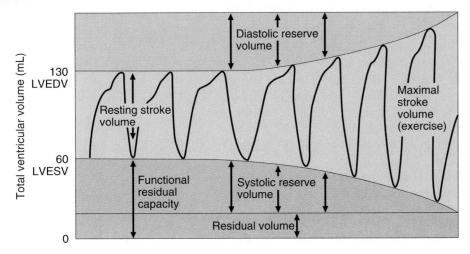

FIGURE 4.6

Subdivisions of Ventricular Volume

Source: G. A. Brecher and P. M. Galletti. Functional anatomy of cardiac pumping. In W. F. Hamilton (ed.), *Handbook of Physiology, Section 2: Circulation.* Washington, D. C.: American Physiological Society (1963). Reprinted by permission.

Notice in Figure 4.6 that the SV can increase by either an increased LVEDV (which encroaches into diastolic reserve volume) or decreased LVESV (which encroaches into systolic reserve volume) or a combination of the two. However, the entire blood volume cannot be ejected; thus, there is always a residual volume of blood in the heart.[8,9] Since the subdivisions of ventricular volume parallel those of the lungs, it may be helpful to refer back to Figure 2.4.

Functional residual capacity is equal to the residual volume and the systolic reserve volume. Total ventricular capacity is the sum of residual volume, systolic reserve volume, stroke volume, and diastolic reserve volume and represents the maximal amount of blood the ventricles can hold.

As the volume of blood returned to the heart (LVEDV) increases, the SV increases. This phenomenon is known as the Frank-Starling law of the heart. The relationship is shown in Figure 4.7. Box 4.1 is provided to ensure your understanding of this figure.

Contractility of the myocardium is determined primarily by neural innervation. Sympathetic nerve fibers cause an increase in contractility of the myocardium independent of the volume of blood returned to the heart.

The **afterload,** or the resistance presented to the contracting ventricle, is determined primarily by the blood pressure in the aorta. As blood pressure increases, resistance increases and less blood is ejected from the ventricles for any force of contraction—that is, stroke volume decreases as afterload increases. The stroke volume decreases in this way because the increased pressure in the aorta causes the semilunar valves to remain closed longer and to close sooner. The valve is thus open for less time, thereby causing a decrease in ejection time and a subsequent decrease in stroke volume. Table 4.1 presents typical values for stroke volume at rest in healthy individuals of various ages.

Contractility The force of contraction of the heart.

Afterload Resistance presented to the contracting ventricle.

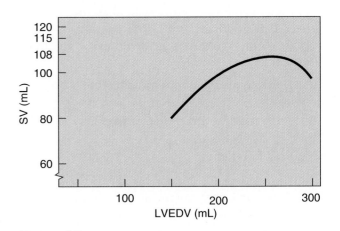

FIGURE 4.7

Frank-Starling Law of the Heart

Box 4.1 A Question of Understanding

Using Figure 4.6, answer the following questions:

1. What is the SV associated with an LVEDV of 150 mL? Of 200 mL? Of 250 mL?
2. What is the EF for each SV?

Box 4.2 A Question of Understanding

Using your knowledge of the determinants of cardiac output, perform the necessary calculations to determine the missing values.

	HR ($b \cdot min^{-1}$)	SV ($mL \cdot b^{-1}$)	$\dot{Q}$ ($L \cdot min^{-1}$)
Mike	80	90	
Sharon	60	120	
Kirk	122	146.5	
Don	72		6.34
Nora		98	5.68

Cardiac Output   **Cardiac output,** $\dot{Q}$, is the amount of blood pumped per unit of time, normally reported in liters per minute. It represents the total blood flow of the entire cardiovascular system and represents the body's ability to meet changing metabolic needs during rest and exercise. Cardiac output is calculated as:

(4.3)   cardiac output (mL · min⁻¹) = stroke volume (mL · b⁻¹) × heart rate (b · min⁻¹)

or $\qquad \dot{Q} = SV \times HR$

At rest the total blood volume (~5 L) is approximately equal to the cardiac output. Table 4.1 presents typical values for cardiac output at rest in healthy individuals of various ages.

■ EXAMPLE

Calculate $\dot{Q}$ for an individual with a HR of 64 b · min⁻¹ and an SV of 100 mL of blood.

$$\dot{Q} = SV \times HR = (100 \text{ mL} \cdot b^{-1}) \times (64 \text{ b} \cdot min^{-1})$$
$$= 6400 \text{ mL} \cdot min^{-1}$$

Since $\dot{Q}$ is usually reported in liters, this value is divided by 1000 and is reported as 6.4 L · min⁻¹. Notice that although SV is usually expressed as milliliters (mL), it is actually measured in milliliters per beat (mL · b⁻¹) since by definition SV must be per beat.   ■

Box 4.2 asks you to do some simple calculations to check your understanding of these formulas.

Coronary Circulation   The energy necessary for cardiac function is supplied through aerobic metabolism, which means that the heart is richly supplied with blood vessels to deliver oxy-

gen. The myocardial blood flow required to provide the necessary amount of oxygen at rest is about 250 mL · min⁻¹, which represents approximately 5% of the normal resting cardiac output.[27] The coronary circulation provides blood to the myocardium. Blood is supplied to the heart by two major coronary arteries, the right and left coronary artery, that originate at the root of the aorta. The left coronary artery divides into the left circumflex and anterior descending arteries. The right coronary artery divides into the marginal artery and the posterior interventricular artery. The myocardium is supplied with a dense distribution of arterioles and capillaries, approximately 3000 to 4000 capillaries per square millimeter of cardiac muscle.[12,27] The venous blood from the coronary circulation is returned to the right atrium via the coronary sinus.

Blood flow through the coronary circulation is affected greatly by the phase of the cardiac cycle. Figure 4.8 depicts coronary blood flow throughout the cardiac cycle. Because of the high intramyocardial pressure during systole, the coronary arteries are compressed, and blood flow to the myocardium is decreased, demonstrating that the myocardium receives the largest portion of its blood flow during diastole.[13]

The coronary circulation is very effective in the extraction of oxygen as the blood flows through the capillary beds. Under resting conditions 60–70% of the available oxygen is extracted.

Cardiac Output The amount of blood pumped per unit of time, in liters per minute.

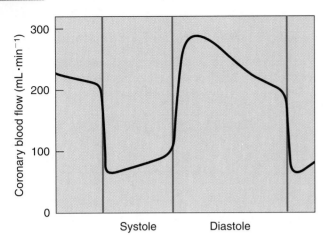

FIGURE 4.8

Coronary Blood Flow Through the Cardiac Cycle
Source: A. C. Guyton. *Textbook of Medical Physiology.* Philadelphia: Saunders (1991), p. 238. Modified and reprinted by permission.

Myocardial Oxygen Consumption Oxygen consumption is determined by oxygen extraction (a-vO$_2$ diff) and blood flow. Clearly, the metabolic demands of the myocardium are increased during exercise—that is, myocardial oxygen consumption increases during exercise. As mentioned previously (see Coronary Circulation), oxygen extraction of the coronary circulation is nearly optimal at rest (60–70%); thus, the increased myocardial oxygen consumption of the myocardium is supported almost entirely by increased blood flow to the myocardium.

The coronary blood flow must be regulated to meet the demands of the myocardium for oxygen. In addition to an increased heart rate, an increased blood flow is achieved by two mechanisms:

1. The greater force of myocardial contraction that results from exercise causes more blood to be forced into the coronary circulation, thus increasing blood flow and helping to meet the metabolic demands of the myocardium.

Blood Pressure (BP) The force exerted on the wall of the blood vessel by the blood as a result of contraction of the heart (systole) or relaxation of the heart (diastole).

2. By-products of cellular work cause vasodilation of the arterioles that supply the myocardium. Thus, as the heart works harder and produces more by-products, the arterioles dilate, which decreases resistance and effectively increases blood flow to support the work of the myocardium.

Myocardial oxygen consumption increases as heart rate increases. Since heart rate increases in relation to the intensity of exercise, so also does myocardial oxygen consumption.[14]

Myocardial oxygen consumption can be estimated from the *rate-pressure product* (RPP), which is the product of heart rate (HR) and systolic blood pressure (SBP):

(4.4)	rate-pressure product (units) = [systolic blood pressure (mmHg) × heart rate (b·min^{-1})] ÷ 100
or	RPP = (SBP × HR) ÷ 100

RPP provides a good estimate of myocardial oxygen consumption under a wide range of conditions, including dynamic and static exercise.

The Vascular System

The *vascular system* is composed of vessels that transport the blood throughout the body. Each portion of the vascular system has a specific structure and function that is related to the overall function of the cardiovascular system. The components of the vascular system are illustrated in Figure 4.9.

Arteries The arteries are thick-walled conduits that carry blood from the heart to the various organs (see Figure 4.9). They contain a large amount of elastic tissue that allows them to distend when blood is ejected during systole and to recoil during diastole. Blood flow in the arteries is pulsatile owing to the pumping action of the heart.

As the left ventricle ejects blood into the aorta, the blood stretches its elastic walls. **Blood pressure (BP)** is the force exerted on the wall of the blood vessel by the blood. The peak pressure is referred to as *systolic blood pressure* because it is essentially caused by the contraction of the heart (systole). During relaxation of the heart (diastole), the arterial walls

Vena cava
(3.0 cm)

Aorta
(2.5 cm)

Heart

Regulation of
blood flow

Veins
(3.0 cm)

Arteries
(0.5 cm)

Endothelial
cell

Capillaries
(6 μm)

Arterioles
(30 μm)

Smooth muscle

recoil, maintaining pressure on the blood that remains in the vessels. Thus, although the blood pressure drops during diastole, there is always some pressure in the arteries, and this pressure is known as *diastolic blood pressure* (DBP). *Mean arterial pressure* (MAP) represents the mean driving force of blood throughout the arterial system. Typical blood pressure values for males and females are given in Table 4.2.

Mean arterial pressure is determined by first calculating pulse pressure, which is equal to the difference between SBP and DBP (PP = SBP – DBP). Mean arterial pressure is then calculated as

(4.5a) mean arterial pressure (mmHg) = pulse pressure (mmHg) ÷ 3 + diastolic blood pressure (mmHg)

or $\quad MAP = \dfrac{PP}{3} + DBP$

MAP is not simply computed as the average of SBP and DBP because diastole lasts longer than systole and is thus weighted more heavily in the computation of MAP. This equation is generally accepted for calculating MAP during resting and recovery conditions. However, during exercise

TABLE 4.2 ▪ Typical Resting Blood Pressure Values for Males and Females of Various Ages

BLOOD PRESSURE VALUE	Age of Males (yr)			Age of Females (yr)		
	10–15	20–30	50–60	10–15	20–30	50–60
Systolic blood pressure, SBP (mmHg)	100	120	134	84	120	130
Diastolic blood pressure DBP (mmHg)	60	80	84	40	74	84
Mean arterial pressure MAP (mmHg)	73	93	97	55	88	92

Sources: Fleg et al.,[11] Ogawa et al.,[21] and Spina et al.[31,32]

MAP can be computed according to a modified equation:[25]

> **(4.5b)**   mean arterial pressure (mmHg) = pulse pressure (mmHg) ÷ 2 + diastolic blood pressure (mmHg)
>
> or $$MAP = \frac{PP}{2} + DBP$$

This formula provides a more accurate measurement of MAP during exercise conditions because it gives less weight to DBP. Although both systole and diastole time shorten owing to an increased heart rate, diastole shortens proportionally more.

Arterioles   The *arterioles,* also called **resistance vessels,** are smaller than the arteries and are the major site of resistance in the vascular system (see Figure 4.9). Because of the increased resistance in the arterioles, the pulsatile arterial blood flow becomes continuous before it reaches the capillaries. The arterioles are able to absorb the pulsatile force of the blood flow because of the large amount of elastic tissue they contain. The importance of the elastic tissue in absorbing force can be seen by considering an analogy of bouncing a basketball on a gymnasium floor or on a wrestling mat. The ball rebounds from the gym floor at an angle and height

> **Resistance Vessels** Another name for arterioles due to their ability to vasodilate and vasoconstrict; changing diameter allows them to control the flow of blood.

that is proportional to the force imparted by your muscle action. However, the same force will not produce much (if any) rebound from the wrestling mat. The elastic tissue in the walls of the arteries absorbs the energy from the pulsatile blood flow in a similar way that the mat absorbs energy from the basketball. In an individual with reduced elasticity, or hardening of the arteries (called arteriosclerosis), the arteries, like the gym floor, are not able to distend as readily and blood pressure is elevated.

The smooth muscle surrounding arterioles is innervated by sympathetic neurons. The smooth muscle is able to change the diameter of the vessel by the processes of *vasoconstriction* (contraction of smooth muscle, causing decreased vessel diameter) and *vasodilation* (relaxation of smooth muscle, causing increased vessel diameter). In fact, the vasoconstriction and vasodilation of the smooth muscles surrounding the arterioles is primarily responsible for determining blood flow distribution to various organs. For instance, if vasodilation occurs in the arterioles to the skeletal muscle of the legs, blood flow to this area increases. Likewise, if vasoconstriction occurs in the arterioles that supply the gastrointestinal tract, blood flow to this area decreases.

The degree to which a given arteriole vasodilates or vasoconstricts depends upon the balance of two mechanisms: local control and neural control. When tissue is metabolically active, it produces metabolic by-products that act locally to cause vasodilation, thereby increasing blood flow to the metabolically active area. In contrast, stimulation of the sympathetic nervous system generally causes vasoconstriction of arterioles.

Capillaries   The *capillaries* perform the ultimate function of the cardiovascular system: exchanging gases and nutrients between the blood and tissues. The walls of the capillaries are composed of a single layer of epithelial tissue called the *endothelium* (see Figure 4.11). The diameter of the capillaries is very small, often necessitating that the red blood cells pass through in single file. Within a single capillary, there is increased resistance to flow because of its small diameter.

Blood flow through the capillaries depends on the other vessels that make up the microcirculation. As shown in Figure 4.10, the *microcirculation* includes several vessels: arterioles, venules, arteriovenous anastomoses, metarterioles, and true capillaries.[33,36] The *anastomoses* are wide, connecting channels that act as shunts between the arterioles and venules. These vessels are particularly abundant in the skin and play an important role in thermoregulation. When the anastomoses are open, large volumes of blood can be directed to blood vessels close to the surface of the skin, facilitating heat dissipation.[33] The *metarteriole* is a short vessel that connects the arteriole with the venule, creating a shortcut through the capillary bed. The metarteriole gives rise to the capillaries. *True capillaries* vary in number depending upon the capillary bed and usually contain a precapillary sphincter, which controls the flow of blood into the true capillaries. These *sphincters* are smooth muscles that open and close in

response to local chemical conditions.[36] Thus, a capillary bed can be perfused with blood or be almost entirely bypassed, depending upon the needs of the tissue it supplies.

The exchange of gases and nutrients in the capillaries depends on diffusion. In order for a substance to diffuse from a capillary into a cell, it must cross two membranes: the endothelium of the capillary and the cell membrane. Substances pass from the capillary to the interstitial space by the process of diffusion. Movement from the interstitial space to the cell may occur by diffusion, or it may require carrier-mediated transport. The movement of gases and nutrients into and out of the capillaries depends upon the concentration gradient or pressure gradient of the substance or gas that is diffusing.

Fluids also pass through the capillary membrane. The movement of fluids is determined by two opposing forces: hydrostatic pressure and osmotic pressure. *Hydrostatic pressure* is created by blood pressure and acts to "push" fluid out of the capillaries. *Osmotic pressure,* caused by the larger concentration of proteins in the capillaries, acts to "pull" water into the capillaries. The net result of these opposing forces is the loss of approximately 3 L of fluid a day from the plasma into the interstitial spaces.[19] This fluid is returned to the blood via the lymphatic system. Any change in hydrostatic pressure (BP) or the osmolarity of the blood will

FIGURE 4.10

Anatomy of the Microcirculation

Smooth muscle

Arteriole

Precapillary sphincters

True capillary with single layer of endothelium

Anastomosis (shunt)

Metarteriole

Venule

alter fluid exchange between the blood and the interstitial fluid.

Venules   The venules are small vessels on the venous side of the vascular system. These vessels contain some smooth muscles that can influence capillary pressure. The venules and capillaries constitute the microcirculation where nutrient exchange occurs. Venules empty into the veins.

Veins   Veins, also called **capacitance vessels,** serve as low-resistance conduits that return blood to the heart (Figure 4.11). They contain smooth muscle innervated by the sympathetic nervous system; thus, they can also change their diameter. Contraction of smooth muscle around the veins is known as *venoconstriction*; relaxation of the veins is known as *venodilation.* Because of the ability of the veins to expand (distensibility), they are capable of pooling large volumes of blood—up to 60% of the total blood volume at rest—and are sometimes referred to as a blood reservoir. The amount of blood in the veins varies with posture and activity. If blood accumulates in the veins and is not returned to the right atrium, left ventricular end–diastolic volume decreases, with the result that stroke volume decreases. Conversely, if venoconstriction occurs, it can significantly increase left ventricular end–diastolic volume and thereby lead to an increase in stroke volume, according to the Frank-Starling law of the heart.

The skeletal muscle pump and the respiratory pump help to increase venous return by "massaging" blood back toward the heart. The one-way valves in the veins also help regulate venous pressure and are particularly helpful in counteracting the upright posture, because they prevent the backward flow of blood. Additionally, the increased sympathetic nervous activity during exercise helps to increase venous return via venoconstriction.

Capacitance Vessels Another name for veins, owing to their distensibility, which enables them to pool large volumes of blood and become reservoirs for blood.

Hematocrit The ratio of blood cells to total blood volume, expressed as a percentage.

Blood

Blood is the fluid that circulates through the heart and the vasculature, and it is responsible for the transport of nutrients and gases. Blood contains living blood cells suspended in a nonliving fluid matrix called plasma. Blood cells can be identified as erythrocytes (red blood cells, RBC) or leukocytes (white blood cells, WBC). Blood cells account for 38–45% of the total blood volume in adult females and 43–48% of the total blood volume in adult males. The ratio of blood cells to total blood volume is known as **hematocrit** and is usually expressed as a percentage.

As discussed in the respiratory section, it is the red blood cells (RBC) that transport oxygen from the lungs to the cells by binding the oxygen to the hemoglobin. Leukocytes are less numerous than erythrocytes, accounting for about 1% of total blood volume. However, these blood cells are essential to the body's defense against disease.

Plasma accounts for approximately 55% of the volume of blood. It is composed primarily of water, which accounts for 90% of its volume, and contains over 100 dissolved solutes, including proteins, electrolytes, and respiratory gases. The composition of plasma can vary greatly, depending upon the needs of the body. Plasma also plays an important role in thermoregulation, helping to distribute heat throughout the body.

This information can be practically applied, for example, to the effects of blood donation on an exerciser. One pint of blood (about 450–500 mL) is typically donated. Since total blood volume is approximately 5000 mL (5 L), the amount of blood donated results in roughly a 10% reduction in blood volume. This amount, however, will represent a greater percentage in small individuals with less blood (typically women). The blood plasma volume is reestablished in approximately 24 hr, whereas red blood cells are replaced in about six weeks. Given the reduction in plasma volume, it seems prudent for endurance athletes to avoid blood donation during the competitive phases of the training cycle. Training intensity may need to be slightly reduced pending complete RBC replacement for fitness participants or athletes who do donate blood. Also, strenuous activities should be avoided for 4–5 hr after giving blood to allow the body to replace the majority of the lost fluids. Plenty of water should be ingested following blood donation.

Hormonal Control of Blood Volume

As just discussed, blood volume is decreased following blood donation. It can also be decreased due to profuse sweating and/or dehydration. Blood volume varies considerably among individuals and is affected by fitness status and hydration level. Healthy adult men have an average blood volume of approximately 75 mL of blood per kg of body weight, or about 5–6 L of blood. Healthy adult women have approximately 65 mL of blood per kg of body weight, which equals 4–4.5 L of blood for the average size woman. Children typically have about 60 mL of blood per kg of body weight, with total volume varying depending on the size of the child.

Blood volume plays an important role in maintaining stroke volume, cardiac output, and blood pressure. Under normal conditions blood volume is maintained within physiological limits by homeostatic mechanisms involving the endocrine system and urinary system. The major hormones involved in maintaining blood volume are antidiuretic hormone (ADH), released from the posterior pituitary gland, and aldosterone, released from the adrenal cortex. Figure 4.11 outlines the hormonal mechanisms responsible for responding to a reduction in blood volume.

Plasma volume reduction causes a decrease in atrial and arterial pressure. This reduction is sensed by atrial baroreceptors (*atrial* means "in the atrium";

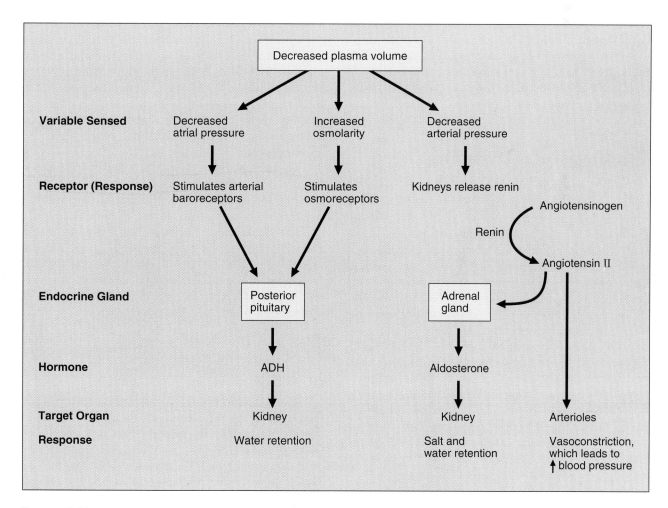

FIGURE 4.11

Hormonal Control of Blood Volume

baro means "pressure") and arterial receptors within the kidneys. Atrial baroreceptor activation leads to the release of ADH from the posterior pituitary gland, which causes the tubules of the kidneys to reabsorb water, thus increasing plasma volume.

A reduction in blood volume is also associated with an increase in plasma osmolarity. For example, with profuse sweating more water than solutes is lost; thus, the osmolarity of the blood increases. An increase in osmolarity of the blood stimulates osmoreceptors in the hypothalamus, which signals the posterior pituitary gland to release ADH. ADH causes the kidneys to retain water and thus leads to an increase in blood volume.

At the same time the receptors in the kidneys respond to a decrease in arterial pressure by releasing renin. Renin is an enzyme that is necessary for the conversion of angiotensinogen to angiotensin II. Angiotensin II then signals the adrenal cortex to release the hormone aldosterone. Aldosterone causes the kidneys to retain salt and water. Angiotensin II also has a vasoconstrictor effect on arterioles, thus helping to increase blood pressure.

Cardiovascular Dynamics

This section deals with the different components of the cardiovascular system and how they function together to meet the changing demands of the body. Essential to understanding this information is an appreciation for the vast amount of integration and interdependence within the cardiovascular system. Specifically, both the heart and the vasculature respond independently to various conditions but are interrelated since the response of the heart affects the vessels, and vice versa.

In differentiating the response of the heart and the vessels, we commonly refer to central and peripheral circulatory responses. *Central circulatory responses* are those directly related to the heart— heart rate, stroke volume, cardiac output, etc. *Peripheral circulatory responses* are those occurring in vessels—vasodilation, vasoconstriction, venous return, etc.

Resistance The factors that oppose blood flow.

Cardiac Output ($\dot{Q}$)

The volume of air or blood flow can be described by the basic formula presented in Chapter 2 (Equation 2.1, $F = \Delta P/R$). Applied to the cardiovascular system, this equation is

---

(4.6)   cardiac output (L · min^{-1}) = mean arterial blood pressure (mmHg) ÷ total peripheral resistance (mmHg · mL^{-1} · min^{-1})

or

$$\dot{Q} = \frac{MAP}{TPR}$$

In this formula, cardiac output represents the blood flow for the entire cardiovascular system, mean arterial pressure reflects the pressure gradient, and total peripheral resistance refers to the factors that oppose blood flow in the entire system. The equation should really use the difference in pressure (ΔP), that is, the difference between mean arterial pressure and the pressure in the right atrium (where blood is flowing to). However, since pressure in the right atrium is so low (less than 4 mmHg), it is considered negligible and is not usually given in the formula. Thus, the pressure used is simply mean arterial pressure.

Total peripheral resistance, or simply **resistance** (R), represents the factors that oppose blood flow. It is expressed in millimeters of mercury per milliliter per minute (mmHg · mL^{-1} · min^{-1}) or more simply as TPR units. The majority of the resistance in the vascular tree results from the friction against the vessel walls, and it varies depending upon the size of the vessel. The three primary factors that affect resistance and their mathematical relationship are described by Poiseuille's law, which states:

(4.7)

$$resistance = \frac{length \times viscosity}{(radius)^4}$$

Thus, the more viscous the blood is, the greater resistance to flow it provides. The longer the blood vessel, the greater the friction that will result between the walls of the vessel and the blood. However, under normal conditions vessel length and blood viscosity do not change substantially. The radius of the vessel, however, can change considerably owing to vasodilation or vasoconstriction. Furthermore, because the resistance is inversely related to the fourth power of the radius, a small change in vessel diameter can result in a large change in blood flow. Thus, vessel radius is by far the most important factor determining resistance to blood flow. Recall that vessel diameter is affected by local metabolic conditions and neural innervation.

Total peripheral resistance (TPR) can be calculated by rearranging the formula $\dot{Q}$ = MAP ÷ TPR to solve for TPR, provided that the flow rate ($\dot{Q}$) and blood pressure (MAP) are known. The formula for TPR becomes

> **(4.8)** total peripheral resistance (TPR units) = mean arterial blood pressure (mmHg) ÷ cardiac output (L·min⁻¹)
>
> or
> $$TPR = \frac{MAP}{\dot{Q}}$$

■ EXAMPLE

Assume that normal resting blood pressure is 110/80 (MAP = 90 mmHg), normal cardiac output is 5.4 L·min, and central venous pressure is zero. Calculate TPR for the entire cardiovascular system. The calculation is

$$TPR = \frac{MAP}{\dot{Q}} = \frac{90 \text{ mmHg}}{5.4 \text{ L} \cdot \text{min}} = 16.67 \text{ (TPR units)} \quad ■$$

This calculation can also be arranged to indicate that MAP is the product of $\dot{Q}$ and TPR. This equation then becomes

$$MAP = \dot{Q} \times TPR$$

Box 4.3 provides an example for you to work through to calculate TPR.

Principles of Blood Flow

Figure 4.12 presents the relationships among the cross-sectional area of the blood vessels, blood

---

Box 4.3 A Question of Understanding

Given the following information, calculate TPR.

SBP = 150 mmHg   DBP = 90 mmHg $\dot{Q}$ = 5.1 L·min⁻¹

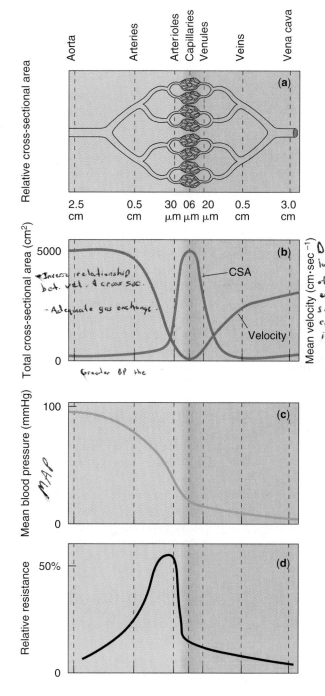

FIGURE 4.12

Relationships Among Cross-Sectional Area of Blood Vessels, Blood Pressure, and Resistance

Source: J. T. Shepherd and P. M. Vanhoutte. *The Human Cardiovascular System.* New York: Raven Press (1980). Reprinted by permission.

velocity, blood pressure, and resistance throughout the vascular system. The diameter of the various vessels is shown in Figure 4.12a, and the total cross-sectional area of the various vessels is shown in Figure 4.12b. Thus, although a single capillary is incredibly small, approximately 6 μm (see Figure 4.12a), there are so many capillaries that the total cross-sectional area far exceeds that of the other vessels. The blue curve in Figure 4.12b depicts the velocity of blood in the various vessels—that is, the rate of movement or speed at which blood flows. The velocity of a fluid in a closed system varies inversely with the total cross-sectional area at any given point. Therefore, the velocity of blood flow decreases dramatically in the capillaries. This decreased velocity allows adequate time for the exchange of respiratory gases and nutrients.

Figure 4.12c depicts the change in the mean blood pressure throughout the vascular system. The driving force for the blood is the contraction of the myocardium. Blood flows because of a pressure gradient. Thus, blood flows through the vascular tree because pressure is highest in the aorta and major arteries and lowest in the great veins and right atrium of the heart. Pressure continues to decrease as the blood travels further from the heart, reaching a low of approximately 4 mmHg in the right atrium. In fact, one-way venous valves and muscle and respiratory pump activity are needed to help return blood to the heart.

Resistance to blood flow is shown in Figure 4.12d. Notice that the majority of the resistance is encountered in the arterioles. As the blood enters the capillaries, the resistance decreases.

Regulation of the Cardiovascular System

The regulation of the cardiovascular system is accomplished by interrelated and overlapping mechanisms, including mechanical events, neural control, and neurohormonal control. Mechanical events, such as muscle action, influence venous return and thereby help regulate stroke volume and cardiac output. This regulation is particularly important during exercise. The neural and neurohormonal mechanisms of cardiovascular control are more complex and are discussed in detail in the following sections.

Neural Control

Three cardiovascular centers are located within the medulla oblongata of the brain stem (Figure 4.13). The cardioaccelerator and cardioinhibitor centers innervate the heart. As the names imply, the *cardioaccelerator center* sends signals, via sympathetic accelerator nerves, that cause the heart rate to increase and the force of contraction to strengthen. The *cardioinhibitor center,* also called the vagal nucleus, sends signals via the vagus nerve that result in a decreased heart rate.

The *vasomotor center* innervates the smooth muscles of the arterioles via sympathetic nerves. Activation of these sympathetic fibers results in a different response depending upon location of the arterioles. The arterioles that supply skeletal muscles vasodilate when stimulated, whereas the arterioles in visceral beds constrict under sympathetic influence. This response ensures that activation of the sympathetic nervous system increases blood flow to skeletal muscles and decreases blood flow in nonessential areas in situations where movement may be required. If all of the arterioles were to dilate during sympathetic stimulation, there would not be

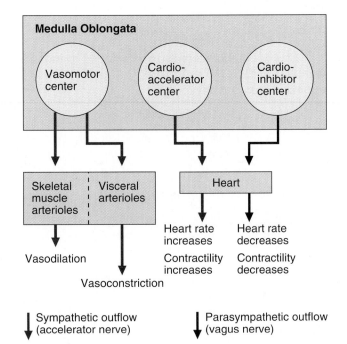

FIGURE 4.13

Neural Control of Cardiovascular Function

adequate blood volume or pressure to meet the circulatory demands of the body.

In summary, activation of sympathetic nervous outflow leads to increased heart rate, increased contractility, vasodilation in the arterioles of skeletal muscle and vasoconstriction in visceral arterioles. Activation of the parasympathetic nervous system leads to a decrease in each of the above. Table 4.3 summarizes these cardiovascular responses.

Anatomical Sensors and Factors Affecting Control of the Cardiovascular System

The cardiovascular centers—and therefore, the sympathetic and parasympathetic outflow from those centers—are influenced by several factors. These factors operate in a variety of circumstances, including exercise. Figure 4.14 schematically presents the most important factors influencing the cardiovascular centers. These factors are described in detail in the following subsections.

Higher Brain Centers

The cardiovascular medullary centers are influenced by several higher brain centers, including the cerebral cortex and the hypothalamus. Emotional influences arising from the cerebral cortex can affect cardiovascular function at rest. Additionally, input from the motor cortex, which is relayed through the hypothalamus, can influence cardiovascular function during exercise, leading to an increase in heart rate and vasodilation in active muscle. The influence of the cortex and hypothalamus on the cardiovascular centers

during exercise is often termed "central command," suggesting that the signal to alter cardiovascular variables comes from the central nervous system.

Body temperature also affects the cardiovascular centers through the influence of the hypothalamus. An increase in body temperature results in an increased heart rate, increased cardiac output, and vasodilation in the arterioles of the active muscles and skin.

Systemic Receptors

Systemic receptors are found in the great veins, the heart, and the arterial system. These receptors provide sensory information to the cardiovascular control centers that leads to reflex action.

Baroreceptors. Baroreceptors are located in the aorta and carotid bodies. These receptors are sensitive to an increase in mean arterial pressure and cause a reflex decrease in mean arterial pressure owing to a decrease in heart rate and, thus, cardiac output. The decrease in heart rate is mediated through an increased parasympathetic outflow and a simultaneous decrease in sympathetic outflow to the heart. This reflex control of blood pressure is called the *baroreceptor reflex.*

Since this reflex attempts to keep the mean arterial blood pressure down, you may wonder how anyone can become hypertensive or why mean arterial blood pressure goes up during exercise. In the first situation the action of the baroreceptors is mediated by a set point. If something causes the resting blood pressure to be elevated (and no one knows precisely what causes this elevation), the baroreceptors fire for about 24 hr, trying to bring the mean arterial pressure down. If they are unsuccessful, they simply reset at a level above the current value. In the case of exercise the relatively weak parasympathetic system is simply overwhelmed by the more powerful sympathetic system. The baroreceptor reflex is, however, very important in achieving recovery to baseline values after exercise.

Stretch Receptors. Stretch receptors are located in the right atrium of the heart and are stimulated by an increase in venous return. The signal is transmitted to the cardiovascular centers in the medulla, where they cause an increase in sympathetic outflow and a decrease in parasympathetic outflow. This results in an increased rate and force of

TABLE 4.3 ■ Summary of Cardiovascular Response to Stimulation of Sympathetic and Parasympathetic Activation

RESPONSE	SYMPATHETIC STIMULATION	PARASYMPATHETIC STIMULATION
Rate of contraction	↑	↓
Force of contraction	↑	↓
Excitability	↑	↓
Conductivity	↑	↓
Metabolism	↑	↓

Source: McNaught and Callauder.[20]

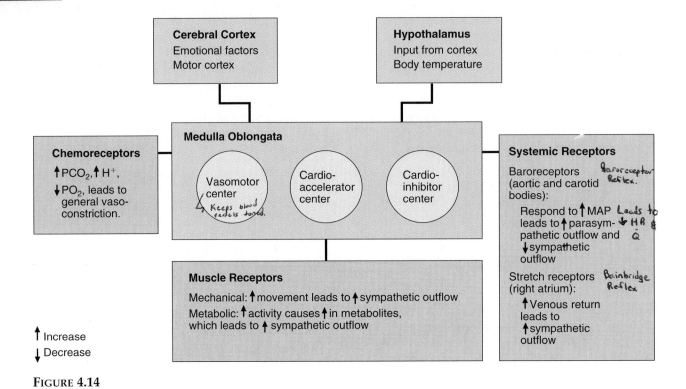

FIGURE 4.14

Factors Affecting Neural Control of Cardiovascular Function

contraction of the heart and leads to increased cardiac output. This sequence is called the *Bainbridge reflex.*

Chemoreceptors   *Chemoreceptors* are located in the aortic and carotid arteries. They are sensitive to arterial blood PO_2, PCO_2, and H^+. An increase in PCO_2 and H^+ or a decrease in PO_2 causes a reflex vasoconstriction of arterioles.

Muscle Joint Receptors   *Muscle receptors* include mechanical *(mechanoreceptors)* and metabolic *(metaboreceptors)* receptors. They are located in the joints and muscles, and they send impulses to the brain, where the impulses synapse with the cardiovascular centers. These receptors are stimulated by muscle contraction and lead to an increased rate and force of heart contraction and vasodilation in active muscle. Vasoconstriction occurs in inactive skeletal muscles.

Neurohormonal Control

The endocrine system also plays an important role in the regulation of the cardiovascular system. Con-

siderable control is exerted by components of the autonomic nervous system and the hormones of the adrenal medulla. The previous section discussed the influence of the sympathetic nervous system on the heart and the blood vessels. The sympathetic nervous system also innervates the adrenal medulla, causing the adrenal glands to release the hormones epinephrine and norepinephrine. These hormones circulate in the bloodstream and travel to the target organs, namely, the heart and the blood vessels. Generally, epinephrine and norepinephrine have the same effect on the target organs as the sympathetic nerve fibers innervating them.

In addition to the adrenal hormones, aldosterone and ADH are involved in maintaining blood volume and blood pressure as described in the section on blood volume.

Assessment of Cardiovascular Variables

The assessment and monitoring of cardiovascular variables is routine in sports and fitness settings.

The following variables are measured so that one can assess fitness, prescribe exercise, and monitor physiological responses to exercise. Most of these variables can be assessed at rest and during submaximal or maximal exercise.

Cardiac Output

Recall that cardiac output ($\dot{Q}$) is equal to the product of stroke volume and heart rate (Eq. 4.3). However, since stroke volume has historically been very difficult to measure, cardiac output has been calculated from another known relationship described by the **Fick equation.** This equation states that

(4.9) cardiac output ($mL \cdot min^{-1}$) = oxygen consumption ($mL \cdot min^{-1}$) ÷ arteriovenous oxygen difference ($mL \cdot dL^{-1}$)

or
$$\dot{Q} = \frac{\dot{V}O_2}{a\text{-}vO_2 \text{ diff}} \times 100$$

The direct determination of cardiac output via the Fick equation requires that oxygen consumption and arteriovenous oxygen difference both be measured. Many laboratories can directly measure oxygen consumption and this test is described thoroughly in Chapter 11. The assessment of arteriovenous oxygen difference is more problematic. This test requires a sample of arterial blood from an artery and a sample of mixed venous blood from the vena cava or right atrium.

Because cardiac output is difficult to measure directly without expensive laboratory equipment, it is often estimated from the relationship between cardiac output and oxygen consumption. Estimates of exercise cardiac output can be derived if oxygen consumption is known. This estimate is based on a mathematically established relationship between cardiac output and oxygen consumption. Cardiac output at light to moderate workloads (under 70% $\dot{V}O_2max$) can be calculated according to the following formulas:[3]

(4.10a) men: $y = 6.55 + 4.35x$

(4.10b) women: $y = 3.66 + 6.81x$

where y = predicted cardiac output (in liters per minute) and x = measured oxygen consumption (in

Box 4.4 A Question of Understanding

Calculate the estimated cardiac output for a woman who is cycling at an oxygen consumption of $2.0 \text{ L} \cdot min^{-1}$.

liters per minute). Box 4.4 provides an opportunity for you to do a sample calculation to check your understanding of this equation.

Stroke Volume

Advances in technology have made the assessment of stroke volume (SV) more readily available, particularly during exercise. Stroke volume can now be measured using Doppler echocardiography. **Doppler echocardiography** is a technique that calculates stroke volume from measurements of aortic cross-sectional area (CSA) and time-velocity integral (TVI) of the flow in the ascending aorta (see Figure 4.15). The formula is

(4.11) stroke volume (mL) = cross-sectional area (cm^2) × time-velocity integrals (cm)

or
$$SV = CSA \times TVI$$

Note that, for conversion purposes, $cm^3 = mL$.

Two-dimensional echocardiography is used to measure aortic diameter (Figure 4.15a). Cross-sectional area is then calculated from a geometric model using the following formula:

(4.12) cross-sectional area (cm^2) = diameter^2 (cm) × $\pi/4$

or
$$CSA = d^2 \times \frac{\pi}{4}$$

Doppler ultrasound is used to assess blood flow velocity in the ascending aorta (Figure 4.15b). From

Fick Equation An equation used to calculate cardiac output from oxygen consumption and arteriovenous oxygen difference (a-vO$_2$ diff).

Doppler Echocardiography A technique that calculates stroke volume from measurements of aortic cross-sectional area and time-velocity integrals in the ascending aorta.

FIGURE 4.15

Determination of Aortic Diameter and Blood Velocity
Ultrasound technician obtains aortic diameter (a) and Doppler waveforms from the suprasternal notch (b). Print-out of aortic diameter (c) and Doppler waveforms (d).

the Doppler waveforms a time-velocity integral is obtained.

■ **EXAMPLE**

Using the information provided in Figures 4.15c and d, calculate SV.
The calculations are

$$CSA = 2.57^2 \times \frac{\pi}{4} = 5.18 \text{ cm}^2$$

$$SV = (5.18 \text{ cm}^2) \times (25 \text{ cm}) = 129.5 \text{ mL} \qquad ■$$

Heart Rate

In a laboratory setting heart rate is often obtained by measuring the R-R interval from an ECG recording (see Figure 4.16). The first step is to calculate the distance the ECG paper travels in one minute based on the speed of the paper. The distance between cycles is then measured. Since you now know the number of cycles that occurred within the distance measured, you can solve for the $b \cdot min^{-1}$ by solving for X in the following equation:

FIGURE 4.16

ECG Used to Calculate Heart Rate

(4.13) HR $b \cdot min^{-1}$ = [number of beats ÷ distance the cycles occupy (mm)] = [$X\ b \cdot min^{-1}$ ÷ distance the paper travels in one minute ($mm \cdot min^{-1}$)]

■ EXAMPLE

Using the ECG strip in Figure 4.16, calculate the heart rate.

Step 1: Using the paper speed, calculate the distance the paper travels in one minute. Paper speed equals 25 $mm \cdot sec^{-1}$. Since there are 60 $sec \cdot min^{-1}$, 25 $mm \cdot sec^{-1}$ × 60 $sec \cdot min^{-1}$ = 1500 $mm \cdot min^{-1}$.

Step 2: Measure the distance between 4 cycles, which in this case is 125 mm.

Step 3: Since 4 cycles (1 box = 5 mm) occurred within the time period required for the ECG paper to travel 125 mm, you calculate how many beats will occur in one minute by solving for X in the equation:

$$\frac{4}{125} = \frac{X}{1500}$$

$$125X = 6000,\ X = 6000/125 = 48\ b \cdot min^{-1}\ \blacksquare$$

Heart rate can also be recorded by wireless telemetry, such as a heart rate watch. The transmitter is worn around the chest of the individual, and the heart rate signal is transmitted to a small receiver that looks very similar to a watch.

Heart rate is often measured during exercise to monitor exercise intensity. During most exercise sessions sophisticated and expensive heart rate–measuring devices are not available. Instead, heart rate is assessed by counting the pulse, sometimes called palpitation. The pulse can be counted at the carotid or radial artery. Each individual should receive instruction for and have practice in counting his or her pulse if it is to be used to accurately monitor exercise intensity.

To measure an exercise heart rate, the subject usually ceases exercise and finds the pulse as quickly as possible. The pulse count begins with zero and is counted for a set period of time, usually 6, 10, or 15 sec. This pulse count is then multiplied by 10, 6, or 4 to obtain a per-minute heart rate. Less than 1 min is used for counting because heart rate drops quickly following exercise; thus, the count must be obtained as quickly as possible.

Maximal Oxygen Consumption

Maximal oxygen consumption ($\dot{V}O_2max$) is the greatest amount of oxygen that the body can take in, transport, and utilize during heavy exercise. It is abbreviated as $\dot{V}O_2max$ to indicate the volume of oxygen consumed. The body relies on the respiratory system to bring in the oxygen from the environment, the cardiovascular system to transport the oxygen, and the cells to extract the oxygen and use it in the production of energy. Thus, the assessment of maximal oxygen consumption provides a means for quantifying the functional capacity of the entire cardiovascular system.

The limit of circulatory function is reached at the highest attainable oxygen consumption and, rearranging the Fick equation (Eq. 4.9), is expressed in the following equation:

(4.14a) maximal oxygen uptake ($mL \cdot kg \cdot min^{-1}$) = [maximal heart rate ($b \cdot min^{-1}$) × stroke volume (mL) × maximal arteriovenous oxygen difference ($mL \cdot 100\ mL^{-1}$)]

or $\dot{V}O_2max$ = (HR max) × (SV max) × (a-vO_2 diff max)

The equation may be simplified to

(4.14b) $\quad \dot{V}O_2\text{max} = (\dot{Q}\,\text{max}) \times (\text{a-v}O_2\,\text{diff max})$

Although $\dot{V}O_2$max can be calculated from the variables in Equation 4.14a, it is most often measured with laboratory equipment, namely, open-circuit indirect spirometry, also called metabolic equipment. The assessment of oxygen consumption is described in detail in Chapter 11. Because the delivery of oxygen is primarily limited by the cardiovascular system, $\dot{V}O_2$max is considered to be a cardiovascular variable, not a metabolic one; although it is often measured metabolically via open-circuit spirometry, it is impractical to obtain the cardiovascular variables necessary to compute $\dot{V}O_2$max. $\dot{V}O_2$max is often considered the single most important variable in describing an individual's fitness level.[5]

Factors Limiting $\dot{V}O_2$max At some point an individual can no longer continue to increase the intensity of the exercise load or to work at maximum effort because the body can no longer provide enough oxygen to support an additional load. But what specifically limits $\dot{V}O_2$max? Figure 4.17 summarizes possible limitations to oxygen consumption within the major systems involved in providing oxygen during exercise.

Many researchers report that skeletal muscles possess a greater ability to use oxygen than can be met by the respiratory and cardiovascular systems.[26,28] Not all researchers agree with this view, though, and some have proposed that failure of muscle performance may explain exhaustion during maximal exercise.[23]

Research evidence suggests that oxygen uptake is not limited by pulmonary ventilation in normal, healthy, nonelite athletes without exercise-induced hypoxemia (Chapter 3). Generally, the functional capacity of the respiratory system is considered to exceed the demands of maximal exercise.[26] The only respiratory variable likely to impose a limitation on oxygen transport is a-vO_2 diff. And, some physiologists consider it to be a cardiovascular variable (in addition to, or instead of, being a respiratory variable).

Thus, the cardiovascular system emerges as the primary system that limits $\dot{V}O_2$max in most individuals. Evidence for this conclusion is based on findings that $\dot{V}O_2$max can be achieved when only about 50% of the skeletal muscles are active (for example, the muscles of the legs during treadmill running). Even if additional muscle mass is added (perhaps arm work is added), little or no further increase in $\dot{V}O_2$ or cardiac output is achieved. The implication is that the heart is not capable of providing enough blood flow to support all the muscles of the body: Maximal cardiac output is needed to support 50% of the muscles that are active at $\dot{V}O_2$max.[26]

Possibly, the factors limiting $\dot{V}O_2$max vary with the fitness level of the individual. According to this hypothesis, in the untrained individual the respiratory capacity for gas exchange exceeds the cardiovascular system's capacity to deliver oxygen. A training program results in little change in the respiratory capacity but large changes in the cardiovascular capacity. Thus, in highly trained individuals the increased cardiovascular capacity may exceed the respiratory capacity.[10] In this case the respiratory system becomes the factor limiting $\dot{V}O_2$max.

Heritability of $\dot{V}O_2$max Genetics have been suspected as an important component in determining an individual's $\dot{V}O_2$max. Research studies confirm that genotype contributes to individual differences in $\dot{V}O_2$max, but estimates of the genetic influence determining $\dot{V}O_2$max are quite modest. The estimated genetic effect on $\dot{V}O_2$max expressed per kilogram of body weight is less than 40% of individual differences, and it is less than 25% when $\dot{V}O_2$max is expressed relative to fat-free mass.[7,18]

Genetic variation apparently accounts for a substantial fraction of the individual differences in the response to exercise training. Individual differences in sensitivity to exercise training are largely inherited differences, with some individuals being "high responders" and others being "low responders."[6,18] Different genetic sensitivity to exercise among individuals helps explain the individualization principle of training, which states that even when individuals engage in similar training programs, different results should be expected.

Field Tests of Cardiorespiratory Capacity ($\dot{V}O_2$max) Several techniques may be used to assess cardiorespiratory endurance and estimate cardiorespiratory capacity ($\dot{V}O_2$max). They include

Cardiovascular System

Central circulation
• Cardiac output (heart rate, stroke volume)
• Arterial blood flow
• Hemoglobin concentration

Peripheral circulation
• Flow to nonexercising regions
• Muscle blood flow
• Muscle capillary density
• Oxygen diffusion
• Oxygen extraction
• Hemoglobin-oxygen exchange

Respiratory System
• Oxygen diffusion
• Ventilation
• Alveolar ventilation: perfusion ratio
• Arteriovenous oxygen difference

Skeletal Muscle
• Enzymes and oxidative potential
• Energy stores and delivery
• Myoglobin
• Mitochondria size and number

FIGURE 4.17

Possible Limitation to Maximal Oxygen Consumption
Source: Modified from Rowell.[26]

submaximal cycle ergometer tests, step tests, and distance walks or runs. By far the most practical and inexpensive method, especially when large numbers of individuals must be measured and evaluated in a short period of time (such as in a school setting), is the distance run. Walking tests are often inaccurate for school-aged individuals, including college students, but they are recommended for testing the elderly or other very sedentary adults. Three tests will be presented here: the 1-mi walk/run, the progressive aerobic cardiovascular endurance run (PACER),[34] and the Rockport Fitness Walking Test (RFWT).[15]

Both the mile walk/run (FITNESSGRAM) and the RFWT cover the same distance. The mile test allows the individual to walk, if necessary; but the intent is to cover the distance as fast as possible, and that goal is best accomplished by running the entire distance. Thus, the individual is asked to perform at a high percentage of his or her maximal capacity for the entire duration of the test. The RFWT, on the other hand, is specifically designed for walking, although the fastest sustainable walking speed is the goal. Depending on the age and fitness level of the participant, this speed may or may not represent a high percentage of maximal aerobic capacity.

Unlike the previous tests, the PACER (developed in Europe by Léger and his colleagues) is a multistage fitness test adapted from the 20-m shuttle run.[16,17] It most closely resembles a graded exercise test that would be done on a treadmill in a laboratory setting. It begins with a light workload and progresses, by small increments, until the individual can no longer complete the required number of laps per minute. This test is run between two lines marked 20 m apart on a smooth unobstructed surface. Running from one line to the other constitutes one lap. The initial speed is set at $8.5 \text{ km} \cdot \text{hr}^{-1}$, and the individual should complete 7 laps in 1 min if that speed is to be achieved. Each minute the speed increases $0.5 \text{ km} \cdot \text{hr}^{-1}$. For the first 15 min the lap count is 7, 8, 8, 9, 9, 10, 10, 11, 11, 11, 12, 12, 13, 13, 13. Thus, this test does not require a sustained high-intensity effort but a gradual progression from submaximal to maximal effort. Pacing is accomplished by prerecorded music or beeps.[34]

The equations used to estimate maximal oxygen consumption from the RFWT and the PACER test are given in Appendix B. The estimate from the mile run is as follows:

(4.15) $\dot{V}O_2\text{max} = 0.21(\text{age} \times \text{sex}) - 0.84(\text{BMI})$
$- 8.41(\text{MT}) + 0.34(\text{MT}^2) + 108.94$
$\text{SEE} = 4.8 \text{ ml} \cdot \text{kg}^{-1} \cdot \text{min}^{-1}$

where age is the age of the individual in years; sex is 0 if female or 1 if male; BMI is the body mass index, which is weight (in kilograms) divided by height squared (in meters squared); MT is the time it takes the individual to run a mile (in minutes).

■ EXAMPLE

Estimate $\dot{V}O_2\text{max}$ given the following data.

age = 15 yr   sex = female   BMI = 24.3   MT = 8.75 min

The calculation is

$\dot{V}O_2\text{max} = (0.21)(15 \times 0) - (0.84)(24.3) - (8.41)(8.75)$
$+ 0.34(8.75^2) + 108.94 = 40.97 \text{ mL} \cdot \text{kg}^{-1} \cdot \text{min}^{-1}$ ■

Notice that the equation includes an indication of the standard error of the estimate (SEE). This

value means that as estimates, not measured values, the calculated results could be expected to vary from the measured value by that much. These errors are generally acceptable, ranging from 3 to $5 \text{ mL} \cdot \text{kg} \cdot \text{min}$. Norms are available for evaluation of the results of these field tests.[34]

Blood Pressure

In well-equipped laboratories and hospitals blood pressure can be measured directly by an intra-arterial transducer. A small transducer is inserted into the artery, and systolic blood pressure and diastolic blood pressure are recorded for every beat of the heart. Although this procedure provides valuable information, it is not practical for routine use owing to the dangers of the invasive procedure.

By far the most common method of obtaining blood pressure measurements is the *auscultation method*. The indirect method of auscultation uses a sphygmomanometer, as diagramed in Figure 4.18. This instrument consists of a cuff containing an inflatable bag and a mercury or aneroid manometer to measure pressure in the bag (Figure 4.18a). Blood pressure is determined in the following steps.

1. The subject is allowed to rest quietly while the arm is measured and a proper cuff size is selected (see Table 4.4). The blood pressure cuff is secured around the upper arm, and the stethoscope is placed just below the antecubital space over the brachial artery (see Figure 4.18a). The movement of the blood through the brachial artery at this point is not impeded. Therefore, the blood flow is laminar, and the pulse cannot be heard through the stethoscope.

2. The blood pressure cuff is then inflated to a pressure greater than systolic blood pressure (usually around 140 mmHg at rest), using the inflation bulb (Figure 4.18b). During this time no sound is detected when a person listens to the brachial artery with a stethoscope, because blood flow is occluded.

3. The pressure inside the cuff is slowly released (at the rate of 2 or 3 $\text{mmHg} \cdot \text{sec}^{-1}$), using the release valve attached to the inflation bulb. When the pressure within the cuff falls just below the systolic blood pressure, blood flows through the artery and can be heard through the stethoscope with each heartbeat. The sounds heard are re-

FIGURE 4.18

Assessment of Blood Pressure

ferred to as *Korotkoff sounds* and are created by the movement of blood through the partially compressed blood vessel. The pressure at which the first Korotkoff sound is heard represents the systolic blood pressure (see Figure 4.18c).

4. The pressure inside the cuff continues to be released; the Korotkoff sounds are heard clearly now (see Figure 4.18d). As the pressure contin-

ues to be released, there is a muffling of the Korotkoff sounds, which is taken to be the fourth Korotkoff sound and is called the first measure of diastolic blood pressure (DBP_1). The disappearance of the Korotkoff sounds represents the fifth Korotkoff sound and indicates the second measure of diastolic blood pressure (DBP_2). The pressure at the fifth Korotkoff sound (DBP_2) is

TABLE 4.4 ■ Guidelines for Type of Blood Pressure Cuff

SIZE (UPPER ARM CIRCUMFERENCE) (CM)	TYPE OF CUFF	BLADDER SIZE (CM)
33–47	Large adult	33 or 42 × 15
25–35	Adult	24 × 12.5
18–26	Child	21.5 × 10

Source: Adams.[2]

considered the best measure of diastolic blood pressure in normal adults at rest. However, DBP_1 is recommended for children, for adults during exercise, and for adults if DBP_2 is lower than 40 mmHg.[2]

SUMMARY

1. The primary functions of the cardiovascular system are transporting oxygen and nutrients to the cells of the body and transporting carbon dioxide and waste products from the cells; regulating body temperature, pH levels, and fluid balance; and protecting the body from blood loss and infection.

2. The heart is the muscular organ that serves as the pump for the cardiovascular system; the heart muscle is referred to as the myocardium.

3. The cells of the heart, called cardiac muscle cells, are functionally linked by intercalated discs. When one cell is depolarized, the stimulation spreads over the entire myocardium.

4. The heart has its own conduction system, consisting of the sinoatrial (SA) node, internodal fibers and Bachmann's bundle, the atrioventricular (AV) node, the bundle of His, the left and right bundle branches, and Purkinje fibers, all of which rapidly spread the electrical signal throughout the heart.

5. The cardiac cycle refers to the alternating periods of relaxation and contraction of the heart. The contraction phase is called systole, and the relaxation phase is called diastole. There are known relationships among the electrical, pressure, volume, and contractile events throughout the cardiac cycle.

6. The volume of blood ejected from the heart with each beat is known as stroke volume. The amount of blood ejected from the heart each minute is called cardiac output. Under resting conditions the heart ejects approximately 60% of the blood that is returned to it; this percentage represents the ejection fraction.

7. Blood pressure is the force exerted on the wall of the blood vessel by the blood it contains. Blood flow is the actual volume of blood flowing through a vessel, organ, or the entire circulation system per unit of time. Resistance is the opposition to blood flow created by the friction that the blood encounters.

8. Primary control of the cardiovascular system resides in the medulla oblongata (cardioaccelerator, cardioinhibitor, and vasomotor centers). Factors affecting these centers include:
- **(a)** Higher brain centers that exert conscious and unconscious control.
- **(b)** Baroreceptors that are sensitive to mean arterial pressure.
- **(c)** Stretch receptors that sense blood return to the right atrium.
- **(d)** Chemoreceptors that sense the PO_2, PCO_2, and H^+.

9. Maximal oxygen consumption ($\dot{V}O_2max$) is the highest amount of oxygen that the body can take in, transport, and utilize. The assessment of maximal oxygen consumption provides a means for quantifying the functional capacity of the entire cardiovascular system.

4 During max ex, blood flow → w/muscles
c 85%

Box 4.1 Answer

1. LVEDV = 150; SV ≈ 80 mL·b⁻¹
   LVEDV = 200; SV ≈ 100 mL·b⁻¹
   LVEDV = 250; SV ≈ 105 mL·b⁻¹

2. $EF = \dfrac{80}{150} = 53\%$

   $EF = \dfrac{100}{200} = 50\%$

   $EF = \dfrac{105}{250} = 42\%$

Box 4.2 Answer

	HR (b·min⁻¹)	SV (mL·b⁻¹)	$\dot{Q}$ (L·min⁻¹)
Mike	80	90	7.20
Sharon	60	120	7.20
Kirk	122	146.5	17.87
Don	72	88.05	6.34
Nora	58	98	5.68

5 Cardiac has color drifts

Box 4.3 Answer

$$PP = SBP - DBP = 150 - 90 = 60 \text{ mmHg}$$

$$MAP = \frac{PP}{3} + DBP = \frac{60}{3} + 90 = 110 \text{ mmHg}$$

$$TPR = \frac{MAP}{\dot{Q}} = \frac{110 \text{ mmHg}}{5.1 \text{ L} \cdot \text{min}^{-1}} = 21.57$$

Box 4.4 Answer

The calculation is

$$y = 3.66 + (6.81)(2.0 \text{ L} \cdot \text{min}^{-1}) = 17.28 \text{ L} \cdot \text{min}^{-1}$$

2 Cardiovasc changes in dramatically : response = B 1st 30 seconds

REVIEW QUESTIONS

1. Diagram the conduction system of the heart, and describe how activation of the SA node leads to contraction of the heart.

2. Describe the electrical events in the heart in relation to pressure in the left ventricle, the volume of blood in the left ventricle, and the position of the heart valves.

3. Identify the different vessels of the peripheral circulation, and describe the velocity and pressure in each. What accounts for the differences?

4. Describe the hormonal mechanisms by which the body attempts to compensate for a decrease in plasma volume.

5. Discuss the neurohormonal regulation of the cardiovascular system and the factors that affect such regulation.

6. Why is maximal oxygen consumption ($\dot{V}O_2$max) considered to be a cardiovascular variable?

7. What are the possible factors limiting maximal oxygen consumption? What are the most likely factors limiting it?

8. Explain the steps involved in attaining an accurate measurement of blood pressure.

3 ↑ % VO₂ → SV reach steady state ≈▲ 40-50%

REFERENCES

1. American College of Sports Medicine: *Resource Manual for Guidelines for Exercise Testing and Prescription.* Malvern, PA: Lea & Febiger (1993).

2. Adams, G. M.: *Exercise Physiology Laboratory Manual.* Dubuque, IA: Brown (1990).

3. Åstrand, P., T. E. Cuddy, B. Saltin, & J. Stenberg: Cardiac output during submaximal and maximal work. *Journal of Applied Physiology.* 19(2):268–274 (1964).

4. Åstrand, P.: Experimental Studies of Physical Working Capacity in Relation to Sex and Age. *University Microfilms International* (1952).

5. Åstrand, P. O., & K. Rodahl: *Textbook of Work Physiology.* New York: McGraw-Hill (1986).

6. Bouchard, C., F. T. Dionne, J. Simoneau, & M. R. Boulay: Genetics of aerobic and anaerobic performances. In J. O. Holloszy (ed.), *Exercise and Sport Sciences Reviews.* Baltimore: Williams & Wilkins (1992).

7. Bouchard, C., & L. Pérusse: Heredity, activity level, fitness, and health. In C. Bouchard, R. J. Shephard, & T. Stephens (eds.), Physical Activity, Fitness, and Health. *International Proceedings and Consensus Statement.* Champaign, IL: Human Kinetics Publishers (1994).

8. Brechar, G. A., & P. M. Galletti: Functional anatomy of cardiac pumping. In W. F. Hamilton (ed.), *Handbook of Physiology, Section 2: Circulation.* Washington, D.C.: American Physiological Society (1963).

9. Clark, D. H.: *Exercise Physiology.* Englewood Cliffs, NJ: Prentice-Hall (1975).

10. Dempsey, J. A.: Is the lung built for exercise? *Medicine and Science in Sports and Exercise.* 18(2):143–155 (1986).

11. Fleg, J. L., F. O'Connor, G. Gerstenblith, L. C. Becker, J. Clulow, S. P. Schulman, & E. G. Lakatta: Impact of age on the cardiovascular response to dynamic upright exercise in healthy men and women. *Journal of Applied Physiology.* 78(3):890–900 (1995).

12. Fox, S. I.: *Human Physiology.* Dubuque, IA: Brown (1990).

13. Guyton, A. C.: *Textbook of Medical Physiology.* Philadelphia: Saunders (1986).

14. Kitamura, K., C. R. Jorgensen, F. L. Gobel, H. L. Taylor, & Y. Wang: Hemodynamics correlates of myocardial oxygen consumption during upright exercise. *Journal of Applied Physiology.* 32:516–522 (1972).

15. Kline, G. M., J. P. Porcari, R. Huntermeister, P. S. Freedson, A. Ward, R. F. McCarron, J. Ross, & J. M. Rippe: Estimation of $\dot{V}O_2$max from a one-mile track walk, gender, age and body weight. *Medicine and Science in Sports and Exercise.* 19:253–259 (1987).

16. Léger, L. A., & J. Lambert: A maximal multistage 20-m shuttle run test to predict $\dot{V}O_2$max. *European Journal of Applied Physiology.* 49:1–12 (1982).

17. Léger, L. A., D. Mercier, C. Gadoury & J. Lambert: The multistage 20 metre shuttle run test for aerobic fitness. *Journal of Sports Sciences.* 6:93–101 (1988).

18. Malina, R. M., & C. Bouchard: *Growth, Maturation, and Physical Activity.* Champaign, IL: Human Kinetics Publishers (1991).

19. Marieb, E. N.: *Human Anatomy and Physiology.* Redwood City, CA: Benjamin/Cummings (1989).

20. McNaught, A. B., & R. Callander: *Illustrated Physiology.* New York: Churchill Livingstone (1983).

21. Ogawa, T., R. J. Spina, W. H., Martin, W. M. Kohrt, K. B. Schechtman, J. O. Holloszy, & A. A. Ehsani: Effects of aging, sex, and physical training on cardiovascular responses to exercise. *Circulation.* 86:494–503 (1992).

22. Netter, F. H.: *The CIBA Collection of Medical Illustrations.* New York: CIBA Pharmaceutical Company (1987).

23. Noakes, T. D.: Implications of exercise testing for prediction of athletic performance: A contemporary perspective. *Medicine and Science in Sports and Exercise.* 20(4):319–330 (1988).

24. Ramsbottom, R., J. Brewer, & C. Williams: A progressive shuttle run test to estimate maximal oxygen uptake. *British Journal of Sports Medicine.* 22(4):141–144 (1988).

25. Robinson, T. E., D. Y. Sue, A. Huszczuk, D. Weiler-Ravell, & J. E. Hansen: Intra-arterial and cuff blood pressure responses during incremental cycle ergometry. *Medicine and Science in Sports and Exercise.* 20(2):142–149 (1988).

26. Rowell, L. B.: *Human Cardiovascular Control.* New York: Oxford University Press (1993).

27. Rowell, L. B.: *Human Circulation Regulation During Physical Stress.* New York: Oxford University Press (1986).

28. Saltin, B., & P. D. Golnick: Skeletal muscle adaptability: Significance for metabolism on performance. In L. D. Peachey, R. H. Adrian, & S. R. Geigher (eds.), *Handbook of Physiology. Skeletal Muscle.* Bethesda, MD: American Physiological Society (1983).

29. Shepherd, J. T., & P. M. Vanhoutte: *The Human Cardiovascular System.* New York: Raven Press (1980).

30. Spina, R. J., T. Ogawa, W. H. Martin III, A. R. Coggan, J. O. Holloszy, & A. A. Ehsani: Exercise training prevents decline in stroke volume during exercise in young healthy subjects. *Journal of Applied Physiology.* 72(6):2458–2462 (1992).

31. Spina, R. J., T. Ogawa, W. M. Kohrt, W. H. Martin III, J. O. Holloszy, & A. A. Ehsani: Differences in cardiovascular adaptations to endurance exercise training between older men and women. *Journal of Applied Physiology.* 75(2):849–855 (1993).

32. Spina, R. J., T. Ogawa, T. R. Miller, W. M. Kohrt, & A. A. Ehsani: Effect of exercise training on left ventricular performance in older women free of cardiopulmonary disease. *American Journal of Cardiology.* 71:99–104 (1993).

33. Strand, F. L.: *Physiology: A Regulatory Systems Approach.* Dubuque, IA: Brown (1983).

34. The Prudential FITNESSGRAM®: Test Administration Manual. Dallas, TX: Cooper Institute for Aerobics Research (1992).

35. Wood, J. E.: The venous system. *Scientific American.* 218(1):86–96 (1968).

36. Vander, A. J., J. H. Sherman, & D. S. Luciano: *Human Physiology: The Mechanisms of Body Function.* New York: McGraw-Hill (1990).

5

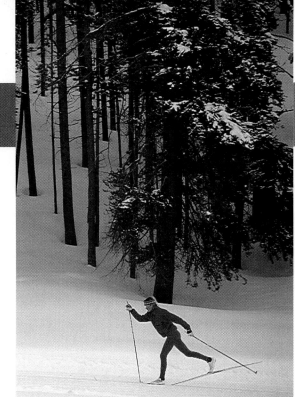

Cardiovascular Responses to Exercise

handwritten notes: chp 6

1.E 2.C 3.B 4.E 5 Central Cardiovascular adaptation

After studying the chapter, you should be able to:

- Graph and explain the pattern of response for the major cardiovascular variables during short-term, light to moderate, submaximal dynamic aerobic exercise.

- Graph and explain the pattern of response for the major cardiovascular variables during prolonged, heavy, submaximal dynamic aerobic exercise.

- Graph and explain the pattern of response for the major cardiovascular variables during dynamic, incremental exercise to maximum.

- Graph and explain the pattern of response for the major cardiovascular variables during dynamic resistance exercise.

- Graph and explain the pattern of response for the major cardiovascular variables during static exercise.

- Compare and contrast the response of the major cardiovascular variables to short-term, light to moderate submaximal dynamic aerobic exercise; dynamic aerobic incremental exercise to maximum; dynamic resistance exercise; and static exercise.

- Discuss the similarities and differences between the sexes in the cardiovascular response to the various classifications of exercise.

- Discuss the similarities and differences between young and middle-aged adults in the cardiovascular response to the various classifications of exercise.

Introduction

All types of human movement, no matter what the mode, duration, intensity, or pattern, require an expenditure of energy above resting values. Much of this energy will be provided through the use of oxygen. In order to supply the working muscles with the needed oxygen, the cardiovascular and respiratory systems must work together. The role of the respiratory system was detailed Chapter 3. This chapter will describe the parallel cardiovascular responses to dynamic aerobic activity, static, and dynamic resistance exercise.

Cardiovascular Responses to Dynamic Aerobic Exercise

Dynamic aerobic exercise requires more energy—and, hence, more oxygen (and thus the use of the term *aerobic,* with oxygen)—than either static or dynamic resistance exercise. How much oxygen is needed depends primarily on the intensity at which the activity is performed and secondarily on the duration of the activity. Like the discussion on respiration, this discussion will categorize the exercises performed as being short-term (5–10 min), light (30–49% of maximal oxygen consumption, $\dot{V}O_2$max) to moderate (50–74% of $\dot{V}O_2$max) submaximal exercise; prolonged (greater than 30 min), moderate-to-heavy submaximal (60–85% of $\dot{V}O_2$max) exercise; or incremental exercise to maximum.

Short-Term, Submaximal, Light- to Moderate-Intensity Exercise

At the onset of short-term, low- to moderate-intensity exercise there is a rapid increase in cardiac output ($\dot{Q}$) (see Figure 5.1a). This increase plateaus within the first 2 min of exercise, reflecting the fact that cardiac output is sufficient to transport the oxy-

Steady State A condition in which the energy expenditure provided during exercise is balanced with the energy required to perform that exercise and factors responsible for the provision of this energy reach elevated levels of equilibrium.

gen needed to support the metabolic demands of the activity. Cardiac output increases owing to an increase in both stroke volume (SV) (Figure 5.1b) and heart rate (HR) (Figure 5.1c). Both of these variables level off within 2 min.

During exercise of this intensity the cardiorespiratory system is able to meet the metabolic demands of the body; thus, the term **steady state** or steady rate is often used to describe this type of exercise. During steady state exercise, the exercise is performed at an intensity such that energy expenditure is balanced with the energy required to perform the exercise. The plateau evidenced by the cardiovascular variables (in Figure 5.1) indicates that a steady state has been achieved.

The increase in stroke volume results from an increase in venous return, which, in turn, increases the left ventricular end–diastolic volume (LVEDV) (preload). The increased preload stretches the myocardium and causes it to contract more forcibly in accordance with the Frank-Starling law of the heart described in Chapter 4. Contractility of the myocardium is also enhanced by the sympathetic nervous system, which is activated during physical activity. Thus, an increase in the left ventricular end–diastolic volume and a decrease in the left ventricular end–systolic volume (LVESV) account for the increase in stroke volume during light to moderate dynamic exercise.[55] Heart rate increases immediately at the onset of activity as a result of parasympathetic withdrawal. As exercise continues, further increases in heart rate are due to the action of the sympathetic nervous system.[59]

Systolic blood pressure (SBP) will rise in a pattern very similar to that of cardiac output: There is an initial rapid increase and a subsequent leveling off once steady state is achieved (Figure 5.1d). The increase in systolic blood pressure is brought about by the increase in cardiac output. Systolic blood pressure would be even higher if not for the fact that resistance decreases, thereby partially offsetting the increase in cardiac output. When blood pressure (BP) is measured intra-arterially, diastolic blood pressure (DBP) does not change. When it is measured by auscultation it either does not change or may go down slightly. Diastolic blood pressure remains relatively constant because of peripheral vasodilation, which facilitates blood flow to the working muscles. The small rise in systolic blood pressure and the lack of a significant change in dia-

FIGURE 5.1

Cardiovascular Responses to Short-Term, Light to Moderate Dynamic Aerobic Exercise

stolic blood pressure cause the mean arterial pressure (MAP) to rise only slightly, following the pattern of systolic blood pressure.

Resistance (R) decreases owing to vasodilation in the active muscles (Figure 5.1e). The vasodilation of vessels in the active muscles is brought about primarily by the influence of local chemical factors (lactate, K^+, and so on), which reflect increased metabolism. The decrease in total peripheral resistance (TPR) can be calculated using Equation 4.8:

$$TPR = \frac{MAP}{\dot{Q}}$$

■ **EXAMPLE**

Calculate TPR by using the following information from Figures 5.1a and 5.1d:

$$MAP = 110\,mmHg \qquad \dot{Q} = 15\,L \cdot min^{-1}$$

The computation is

$$TPR = \frac{110\,mmHg}{15\,L \cdot min^{-1}} = 7.33\ (R\ units)$$

Thus, TPR is 7.33 for light dynamic exercise.   ■

The decrease in resistance has two important implications. First, the vasodilation in the active muscle that causes the decrease in resistance has the effect of increasing blood flow to the active muscle, thereby increasing the availability of oxygen and nutrients. Second, the decrease in resistance keeps mean arterial pressure from increasing dramatically. The increase in mean arterial pressure is determined by the relative changes in resistance and cardiac output. Since cardiac output increases more than resistance decreases, mean arterial pressure increases during dynamic exercise. However, the increase in mean arterial pressure would be much greater if resistance did not decrease.

Myocardial oxygen consumption increases during dynamic aerobic exercise since the heart must do more work to pump an increased cardiac output to the working muscles. The rate-pressure product will increase in relation to increases in heart rate and systolic blood pressure, reflecting the greater myocardial oxygen demand of the heart during exercise (Figure 5.1f). Box 5.1 provides an example of a normal blood pressure response to exercise. Compute the resistance and rate-pressure product for this individual.

The actual magnitude of the change for each of the variables shown in Figure 5.1 depends on the workload, environmental conditions, and the genetic makeup and fitness level of the individual.

Blood volume decreases during dynamic aerobic exercise. Figure 5.2 shows the percent reduction of plasma volume during 30 min of moderate bicycle exercise (60–70% $\dot{V}O_2$max) in a warm environment.[23] The largest changes occur during the first 5 min of exercise, which is consistent with short-term exercise. Following the initial rapid decrease, plasma volume stabilizes. This rapid decrease in plasma volume suggests that it is fluid shifts, rather than fluid loss, that accounts for the initial decrease in plasma volume.[75] The magnitude of the decrease in plasma volume is dependent upon the intensity of exercise, environmental factors, and the hydration status of the individual.

Figure 5.3 illustrates the distribution of cardiac output at rest and during light exercise. Notice that cardiac output increases from 5.8 L · min⁻¹ to 9.4 L · min⁻¹ in this example (the increase in $\dot{Q}$ is illustrated by the increased size of the pie chart). The most dramatic change in cardiac output distribution with light exercise is the increased percentage (47%) and the actual amount of blood flow (4500 mL) that is directed to the working muscles. Skin blood flow

---

Box 5.1 A Question of Understanding

The following measurements were obtained on a 42-year-old man at rest and during light dynamic aerobic exercise, during heavy dynamic aerobic exercise, during maximal dynamic aerobic exercise, and during sustained static contractions at 50% MVC.

Condition	HR (b · min⁻¹)	SBP (mmHg)	DBP (mmHg)	$\dot{Q}$ (L · min⁻¹)
Rest	80	134	86	6
Light dynamic	130	150	86	10
Heavy dynamic	155	170	88	13
Maximal dynamic	180	200	88	15
Sustained static	135	210	100	8

Calculate MAP, TPR, and RPP.

FIGURE 5.2

Percent Reduction of Plasma Volume During 30 min Moderate Bicycle Exercise to Maximum

Source: S. M. Fortney, C. B. Wenger, J. R. Bove, & E. R. Nadel. Effect of blood volume on sweating rate and body fluids in exercising humans. *Journal of Applied Physiology.* 51 (6):1594–1600 (1981). Reprinted by permission.

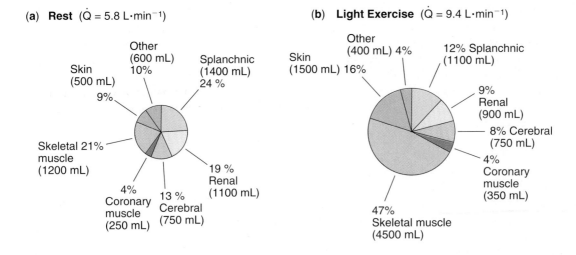

(a) Rest ($\dot{Q}$ = 5.8 L·min⁻¹)

Other (600 mL) 10%
Skin (500 mL) 9%
Splanchnic (1400 mL) 24 %
Skeletal 21% muscle (1200 mL)
4% Coronary muscle (250 mL)
13 % Cerebral (750 mL)
19 % Renal (1100 mL)

(b) Light Exercise ($\dot{Q}$ = 9.4 L·min⁻¹)

Other (400 mL) 4%
Skin (1500 mL) 16%
12% Splanchnic (1100 mL)
9% Renal (900 mL)
8% Cerebral (750 mL)
4% Coronary muscle (350 mL)
47% Skeletal muscle (4500 mL)

FIGURE 5.3

Distribution of Cardiac Output at Rest and During Light Exercise

Source: Data from Anderson.[3]

also increases to meet the thermoregulatory demands of exercise. The absolute amount of blood flow to the coronary muscle also increases although the percentage of cardiac output remains relatively constant. The absolute amount of cerebral blood flow remains constant which means that the percent of cardiac output distributed to the brain decreases. Both renal and splanchnic blood flow are modestly decreased during light exercise.

Prolonged, Heavy, Submaximal Dynamic Exercise

The cardiovascular responses to prolonged, moderate-to-heavy exercise (60–85% of $\dot{V}O_2$max) are shown in Figure 5.4. As for light to moderate workloads, cardiac output increases rapidly during the first minutes of exercise and is then maintained at a relatively constant level throughout exercise (Figure 5.4a). Notice, however, that the absolute value attained is higher during heavy exercise than it was during light to moderate exercise. The initial increase in cardiac output is brought about by an increase in both stroke volume and heart rate.

Stroke volume increases rapidly during the first minutes of exercise and plateaus at a maximal level after a workload of approximately 40–50% of $\dot{V}O_2$max has been achieved[7] (Figure 5.4b). Thus,

during work that requires more than 50% of $\dot{V}O_2$max, the stroke volume response is not intensity-dependent. Stroke volume remains relatively constant during the first 30 min of heavy exercise.

As for light to moderate exercise, the increase in stroke volume results from an increased venous return, leading to the Frank-Starling mechanism, and increased contractility owing to sympathetic nerve stimulation. Thus, changes in stroke volume occur because left ventricular end–diastolic volume increases and left ventricular end–systolic volume decreases.[55] Left ventricular end–diastolic volume increases because of the return of blood to the heart by the active muscle pump, increased venoconstriction (which decreases venous pooling, thereby increasing venous return), and increased cardiac output. Left ventricular end–systolic volume decreases owing to augmented contractility of the heart, which effectively ejects more blood from the ventricle, leaving a smaller residual volume.

However, if exercise continues beyond approximately 30 min, stroke volume gradually drifts downward although it remains elevated above resting values. The downward shift in stroke volume after approximately 30 min is most likely due to thermoregulatory stress and a redirection of blood to the cutaneous vessels in an attempt to dissipate heat.[59] This effectively reduces venous return

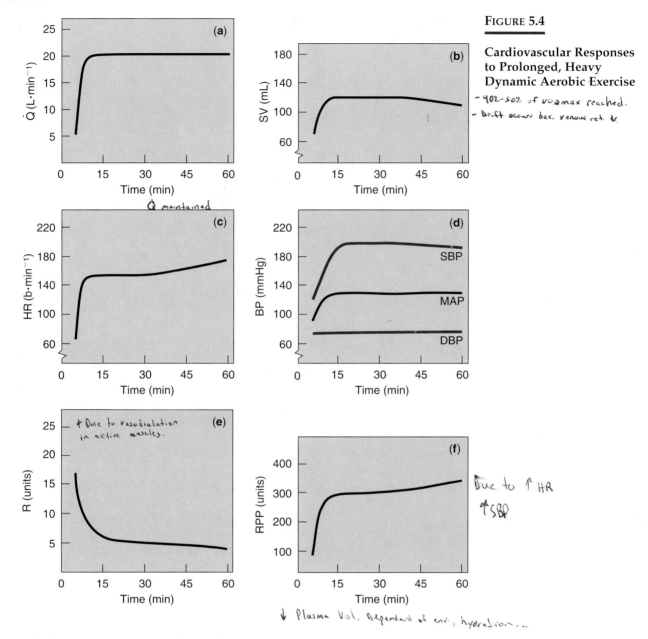

FIGURE 5.4

Cardiovascular Responses to Prolonged, Heavy Dynamic Aerobic Exercise

Handwritten notes on figure:
- 40%–50% of vo₂max reached.
- Drift occurs bec. venous ret. ↓
- Q̇ maintained
- ↑ Due to vasodialation in active muscles.
- Due to ↑ HR ↑ SBP
- ↓ Plasma Vol. Dependant of env, hydration...

and thus causes the slight reduction in stroke volume.

Heart rate increases sharply during the first 1–2 min of exercise, with the magnitude of the increase depending upon the intensity of exercise (Figure 5.4c). The increase in heart rate is brought about by parasympathetic withdrawal and activation of the sympathetic nervous system. After approximately 30 min of heavy exercise heart rate begins to drift upward. The increase in heart rate is proportional to the decrease in stroke volume, so cardiac output is maintained during exercise.

The changes observed in cardiovascular variables, notably in heart rate and stroke volume, during prolonged, heavy submaximal exercise without a change in workload are known as **cardiovascular drift.** Cardiovascular drift is probably associated with rising body temperature during prolonged exercise. The combination of exercise and heat stress produces competing regulatory demands—specifically, competition between skin and muscle

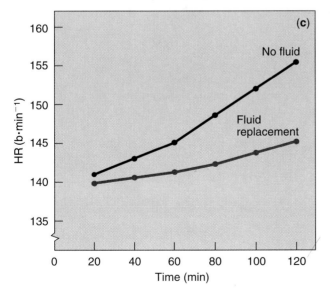

FIGURE 5.5

Cardiovascular Response to Prolonged, Heavy Exercise (70–76% $\dot{V}O_2$max) with and without Fluid Replacement

Source: M. T. Hamilton, J. G. Alonso, S. J. Montain, & E. F. Coyle. Fluid replacement and glucose infusion during exercise prevents cardiovascular drift. *Journal of Applied Physiology.* 71:871–877 (1985). Reprinted by permission.

for large fractions of cardiac output. Stroke volume decreases as a result of vasodilation, a progressive increase in the fraction of blood being directed to the skin in an attempt to dissipate heat from the body, and a loss of plasma volume.[57,67]

The magnitude of cardiovascular drift is heavily influenced by fluid ingestion. Figure 5.5 presents data from a study in which subjects cycled for 2 hr with and without fluid replacement.[28] Values are for minutes 20 through 120; thus, the initial increase in each of the variables is not shown in this figure. When subjects consumed enough water to completely replace the water lost through sweat, cardiac output remained nearly constant throughout the first hour of exercise and actually increased during the second hour (Figure 5.5a). Cardiac output was maintained in the fluid replacement trial because stroke volume did not drift downward (Figure 5.5b). Heart rate was significantly lower when fluid replacement occurred (Figure 5.5c). This information can be used by coaches and fitness leaders. If your clients exercise for prolonged periods, they must replace the fluids that are lost during exercise or performance will suffer.

Let us return to the cardiovascular responses illustrated in Figure 5.4. Systolic blood pressure increases rapidly during the first 1–2 min of exercise, with the magnitude of the increase dependent upon the intensity of the exercise (Figure 5.4d). Systolic blood pressure then remains relatively stable or drifts slightly downward as a result of continued vasodilation and a resultant decrease in resistance.[19]

Cardiovascular Drift The changes in observed cardiovascular variables that occur during prolonged, heavy submaximal exercise without a change in workload.

Diastolic blood pressure changes little with prolonged exercise in a thermoneutral environment. But it may decrease slightly when exercise is performed in a warm environment owing to increased vasodilation as a result of heat production. Because of the increased systolic blood pressure and the relatively stable diastolic blood pressure, mean arterial pressure increases modestly during prolonged activity. Again, as in light to moderate exercise, the magnitude of the increase in mean arterial pressure is mediated by a large decrease in resistance that accompanies exercise.

Resistance drops during prolonged heavy exercise (Figure 5.4e) because of vasodilation in active muscle and because of vasodilation in the cutaneous vessels in order to dissipate the heat produced by mechanical work.[57] Finally, since both heart rate and systolic blood pressure increase substantially during heavy work, the rate-pressure product increases markedly (Figure 5.4f). The initial increase in rate-pressure product occurs rapidly with the onset of exercise. An upward drift in rate-pressure product may occur after approximately 30 min of exercise as a result of heart rate increasing to a greater extent than systolic blood pressure decreases. The high rate-pressure product reflects the large amount of work the heart must perform to support heavy exercise.

During prolonged exercise, particularly if performed in the heat, there is continued loss of total body fluid owing to profuse sweating. Total body water loss during long-duration exercise varies from 900–1300 mL·hr^{-1}, depending upon work intensity and environmental conditions.[75] If fluid is not replaced during long-duration exercise, there is a continued reduction in plasma volume throughout exercise.

Figure 5.6 illustrates the distribution of cardiac output at rest and during heavy exercise. Notice that cardiac output increases from 5.8 L·min^{-1} at rest to 17.5 L·min^{-1} in this example. The most dramatic change in cardiac output distribution with heavy exercise is the dramatic increase in blood flow to the working muscle, which now receives 71% of cardiac output. Skin blood flow is also increased to meet the thermoregulatory demands of exercise. The absolute amount of blood flow to the coronary muscle again increases although the percentage of cardiac output remains relatively constant. The absolute amount of cerebral blood

FIGURE 5.6

Distribution of Cardiac Output at Rest and During Moderate Exercise
Source: Data from Anderson.[3]

(a) **Rest** ($\dot{Q}$ = 5.8 L·min^{-1})

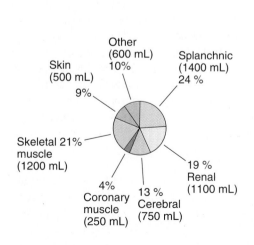

(b) **Heavy Exercise** ($\dot{Q}$ = 17.5 L·min^{-1})

flow remains constant which means that the percent of cardiac output distributed to the neural tissue decreases. Both renal and splanchnic blood flow are further decreased as exercise intensity increases.

Incremental Dynamic Exercise to Maximum

An incremental exercise to maximum bout consists of a series of progressively increasing work intensities that continue until the individual can do no more. The length of each work intensity (stage) varies from 1 to 3 min to allow for the achievement of a steady state, at least at the lower workloads.

Cardiac output increases in a rectilinear fashion and plateaus at maximal exercise (Figure 5.7a). The initial increase in cardiac output reflects an increase in stroke volume and heart rate; however, at workloads greater than 40–50% $\dot{V}O_2$max, the increase in cardiac output is achieved solely by an increase in heart rate. As shown in Figure 5.7b, in normally active individuals stroke volume increases initially and then plateaus at approximately 40–50% of $\dot{V}O_2$max.[7,31] Stroke volume may actually decrease slightly near the end of maximal exercise in untrained and moderately trained individuals.[26]

Figure 5.8 indicates the changes in left ventricular end–diastolic volume and left ventricular end–systolic volume that account for changes in stroke volume during progressively increasing exercise.[55] Left ventricular end–diastolic volume increases largely because of the return of blood to the heart by the active muscle pump and the increased sympathetic outflow to the veins causing venoconstriction and augmenting venous return. Left ventricular end–systolic volume decreases because of augmented contractility of the heart, which ejects more blood from the ventricle and leaves less in the ventricle.

Heart rate increases in a rectilinear fashion and plateaus at maximal exercise (Figure 5.7c). The myocardial cells are capable of contracting at over 300 b·min⁻¹ but rarely exceeds 210 b·min⁻¹ because a faster heart rate would not be of any benefit since there would be inadequate time for ventricular filling. Thus, stroke volume and ultimately cardiac output would be decreased. Consider the simple

analogy of a bucket brigade. Up to a certain point it is very useful to increase the speed of passing the bucket; however, there is a limit to this speed since there must be some time allowed for the bucket to be filled with water.

The maximal amount of oxygen an individual can take in, transport, and utilize ($\dot{V}O_2$max) is another variable that is usually measured during an incremental maximal exercise test (Figure 5.7d). Although $\dot{V}O_2$max is considered primarily a cardiovascular variable, it also depends upon the respiratory system, since it is defined as follows (Equation 5.1):

(5.1) $$\dot{V}O_2\text{max} = (\dot{Q}\text{ max}) \times (a\text{-}vO_2 \text{ diff max})$$

The changes in cardiac output during a maximal incremental exercise test have just been described (a rectilinear increase). The changes in the a-vO₂ diff were discussed in Chapter 3 (an increase plateauing at approximately 60% of $\dot{V}O_2$max). Reflecting these changes, oxygen consumption ($\dot{V}O_2$) also increases in a rectilinear fashion and plateaus at maximum ($\dot{V}O_2$max) during an incremental exercise test to maximum. The plateauing of $\dot{V}O_2$ is one of the primary indications that a true maximal test has been achieved.

The arterial blood pressure responses to incremental dynamic exercise to maximum are shown in Figure 5.7e. Systolic blood pressure increases during maximal exercise, often reaching values in excess of 200 mmHg in very fit individuals. The increase in systolic blood pressure is caused by the increased cardiac output, which outweighs the decrease in resistance. Systolic blood pressure and heart rate are two variables that are routinely monitored during an exercise test to ensure the safety of the participant. If either of these variables fails to rise with an increasing workload, cardiovascular insufficiency and an inability to adequately profuse tissue is a possibility, and the exercise test should stop.

Diastolic blood pressure typically remains relatively constant or may even decrease at high levels of exercise. Diastolic pressure remains relatively constant because of the balance of vasodilation in the vasculature of the active muscle and vasoconstriction in other vascular beds. Diastolic pressure is most likely to decrease when exercise is performed in a hot environment; under these conditions skin

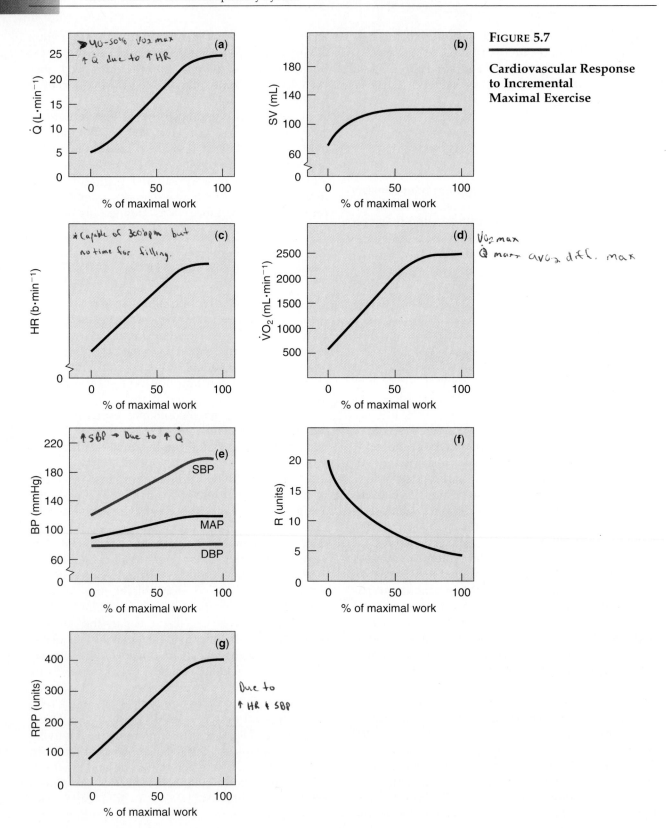

FIGURE 5.7

Cardiovascular Response to Incremental Maximal Exercise

Handwritten annotations:

(a) 40-50% VO₂ max ↑ Q̇ due to ↑HR

(c) * Capable of 300 bpm but no time for filling.

(d) VO₂ max; Q̇ max; avo₂ diff. max

(e) ↑SBP → Due to ↑Q̇

(g) Due to ↑HR & SBP

FIGURE 5.8

Changes in LVEDV and LVESV That Account for Change in SV During Incremental Exercise

Source: Based on data from Poliner et al.[55]

vessels are more dilated, and there is decreased resistance to blood flow.

An excessive rise in either systolic blood pressure (over 260 mmHg) or diastolic blood pressure (over 115 mmHg) indicates an abnormal exercise response and is also reason to consider stopping an exercise test or exercise session.[1] Individuals who exhibit an exaggerated blood pressure response to exercise are two to three times more likely to develop hypertension than those with a normal exercise blood pressure response.[2]

Resistance decreases rapidly with the onset of exercise and reaches its lowest level at maximal exercise (Figure 5.7f). Decreased resistance reflects maximal vasodilation in the active tissue in response to the need for increased blood flow that accompanies maximal exercise. Also, the large drop in resistance is important in keeping mean arterial pressure from exhibiting an exaggerated increase. Finally, the rate-pressure product increases in a rectilinear fashion throughout an incremental exercise test (Figure 5.7g), paralleling the increases in heart rate and systolic blood pressure.

The reduction in plasma volume seen during submaximal exercise is also seen in incremental ex-

ercise to maximum. Since the magnitude of the reduction depends upon the intensity of exercise, the reduction is greatest at maximal exercise. A decrease of 10–20% can be seen during incremental exercise to maximum.[75]

Considerable changes in blood flow occur during maximal incremental exercise. Figure 5.9 illustrates the distribution of cardiac output at rest and at maximal exercise. Maximum cardiac output in this example is 25 L · min^{-1}. Again, the most striking characteristic of this figure is the tremendous amount of cardiac output that is directed to the working muscles (88%). At maximal exercise skin blood flow is reduced in order to direct the necessary blood to the muscles. Renal and splanchnic blood flow also decrease considerably. Blood flow to the brain and cardiac muscle is maintained.

Table 5.1 summarizes the cardiovascular responses to exercise that have been discussed in these sections.

Upper-Body Versus Lower-Body Exercise

Upper-body exercise is routinely performed in a variety of industrial, agricultural, military, and sporting activities. Additionally, upper-body exercise in rehabilitative medicine is becoming increasingly popular for improving the health and fitness of individuals with spinal cord injuries.[64]

There are some important differences in the cardiovascular responses depending upon whether exercise is performed on an arm ergometer (using muscles of the upper body) or a cycle ergometer (using muscles of the lower body). When the oxygen consumption required to perform a submaximal workload is the same, cardiac output is similar for upper- and lower-body exercise (Figure 5.10a). However, the mechanism to achieve the required increase in cardiac output is not the same. As shown in Figures 5.10b and 5.10c, upper-body exercise results in a lower stroke volume and a higher heart rate at any given submaximal workload.[12,47,53] Systolic, diastolic, and mean arterial blood pressures (Figure 5.10d), total peripheral resistance (Figure 5.10e), and rate-pressure product (Figure 5.10f) are significantly higher in upper-body exercise than in lower-body exercise performed at the same oxygen consumption.

TABLE 5.1 ■ Cardiovascular Responses to Exercise*

	LIGHT- TO MODERATE-INTENSITY, SHORT-TERM SUBMAXIMAL EXERCISE[†]	HEAVY, LONG-DURATION[†] SUBMAXIMAL EXERCISE	INCREMENTAL-TO-MAXIMUM EXERCISE	STATIC EXERCISE	RESISTANCE EXERCISE
$\dot{Q}$	Increases rapidly; levels off at steady state within 2 min	Increases rapidly; levels off	Rectilinear increase with plateau at max	Modest increase[‡]	Modest increase[‡]
SV	Increases rapidly; levels off at steady state within 2 min	Increases rapidly; levels off; drifts downward	Increases initially; plateaus at 40–50% $\dot{V}O_2$max	Relatively constant[‡] at low workloads; decreases at high workloads	Little change, slight increase[‡]
HR	Increases rapidly; levels off at steady state within 2 min	Increases rapidly; levels off; drifts upward	Rectilinear increase with plateau at max	Modest increase	Increases progressively with number of reps
SBP	Increases rapidly; levels off at steady state within 2 min	Increases rapidly; levels off; may drift downward	Rectilinear increase with plateau at max	Marked increase	Increases progressively with number of reps[‡]
DBP	Shows no change	Shows no change	Shows no change	Marked increase	No change or increase[‡]
MAP	Increases rapidly; levels off at steady state within 2 min	Increases initially; little if any drift	Small rectilinear increase	Marked increase	Increases progressively with number of reps[‡]
TPR	Decreases rapidly; levels off	Decreases rapidly; levels off; may drift downward	Decreases sharply; levels off slightly	Decreases	[‡]
RPP	Increases rapidly; levels off at steady state within 2 min	Increases rapidly; levels off; drifts upward	Rectilinear increase with plateau at max	Marked increase	Increases progressively with number of reps[‡]

*Resting values are taken as baseline.
[†]The difference between leveling during the light to moderate short-term and heavy long-duration submaximal exercise responses is one of magnitude; that is, leveling occurs at a higher value with higher intensities.
[‡]Limited research data available.

There are several likely reasons for the differences in cardiovascular responses to upper-body and lower-body exercise. The elevated heart rate is thought to reflect a greater sympathetic stimulation during upper-body exercise.[9,17,47] Stroke volume is less during upper-body exercise than during lower-body exercise because of the absence of the skeletal muscle pump augmenting venous return from the legs. The greater sympathetic stimulation that oc-curs during upper-body exercise may also be partially responsible for the increased blood pressure and total peripheral resistance seen with this type of activity. Additionally, upper-body exercise is usually performed using an arm-cranking ergometer, which involves an isometric component since the individual must grasp the hand crank. Isometric tasks are known to cause exaggerated blood pressure responses.

(a) Rest $(\dot{Q} = 5.8 \text{ L·min}^{-1})$

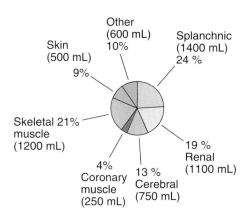

(b) Maximal Exercise $(\dot{Q} = 25 \text{ L·min}^{-1})$

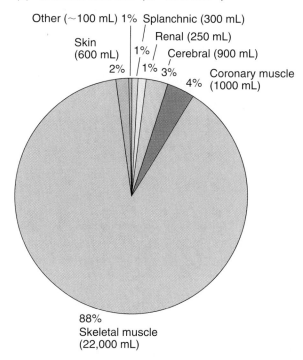

FIGURE 5.9

Distribution of Cardiac Output at Rest and During Maximal Exercise
Source: Data from Anderson.[3]

When maximal exercise is performed by using upper-body exercise, $\dot{V}O_2$max values are approximately 30% lower than when maximal exercise is performed by using lower-body exercise.[47,53] Maximal heart rate values for upper-body exercise are 90–95% of those achieved for lower-body exercise, and stroke volume is 30–40% less during maximal upper-body exercise. Maximal systolic blood pressure and the rate-pressure product are usually similar for both forms of exercise, but diastolic blood pressure is typically 10–15% higher during upper-body exercise.[47]

The different cardiovascular responses to a given level of exercise for upper-body work and lower-body work suggest that exercise prescriptions for arm work cannot be based on data obtained from testing with leg exercises. Furthermore, the greater cardiovascular strain associated with upper-body work must be kept in mind when one prescribes exercise for individuals with cardiovascular disease.

Sex Differences During Dynamic Aerobic Exercise

The pattern of cardiovascular responses to dynamic exercise is similar for both sexes, although the magnitude of the response may vary between the sexes for some variables. Differences in body size and structure are related to many of the differences in cardiovascular responses evidenced between the sexes.

Submaximal Exercise Females have a higher cardiac output than males during submaximal exercise when work is performed at the same *absolute workload*.[7,11,24] Females have a lower stroke volume and a higher heart rate than males during submaximal exercise when exercise is performed at the same absolute workload.[7] The lower stroke volume is due to the smaller heart size in females. The higher heart rate more than compensates for the lower stroke volume in females, resulting in the

enhanced venous ret. = ↑ SV

FIGURE 5.10

Cardiovascular Response to Incremental Maximal Upper-Body and Lower-Body Exercise

higher cardiac output seen at the same absolute workload. Thus, if a man and woman perform the same workout, the woman will typically be stressing the cardiovascular system to a greater extent.

This relative disadvantage to the woman results from several factors. First females typically are smaller than males; they have a smaller heart and less muscle mass. Second, they have a lower oxygen-carrying capacity than males. Finally, they typically have lower aerobic capacity ($\dot{V}O_2max$). Therefore, researchers commonly discuss exercise response in

terms of *relative workload*. That is, how do individuals compare when they are both working at the same percentage of their $\dot{V}O_2max$.

The importance of distinguishing between relative and absolute workloads when comparing males and females is shown in Figure 5.11. This figure compares the cardiovascular response of men and women to the same *absolute workload* (600 kgm · min⁻¹) on the left side of the graph and the same *relative workload* (50% of $\dot{V}O_2max$) on the right side of the graph. Cardiac output is higher in women during the same absolute workload. How-

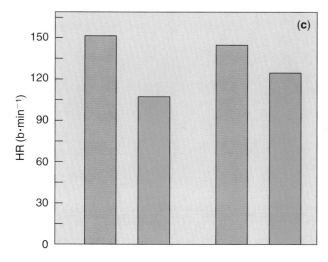

FIGURE 5.11

Comparison of Cardiovascular Responses of Men and Women to Submaximal Exercise

Source: Data from Astrand.[8]

ever, cardiac output (Figure 5.11a) is less for women when the same relative workload is performed. Stroke volume (Figure 5.11b) is lower in women than in men whether the workload is expressed on an absolute or relative basis. Notice that the values are very similar for both conditions, suggesting that stroke volume has plateaued as would be expected at 50% of $\dot{V}O_2$max in both conditions. The difference in heart rate between the sexes (Figure 5.11c) is smaller when exercise is performed at the same relative workload.

Males and females display the same pattern of response for blood pressure; however, males tend to have a higher systolic blood pressure than females at the same relative workloads.[42,51] Much of the difference in the magnitude of the blood pressure response is attributable to differences in resting systolic blood pressure. Diastolic blood pressure response to submaximal exercise is very similar for both sexes. Thus, mean arterial blood pressure is slightly greater in males during submaximal work at the same relative workload. The pattern of response for resistance is similar for males and females, although males typically have a lower resistance owing to their greater cardiac output. Males and females both exhibit cardiovascular drift during heavy, prolonged submaximal exercise.

Incremental Exercise to Maximum   The cardiovascular response to incremental exercise is similar for both sexes, although, again, there are differences in the maximal values attained. Maximal oxygen consumption ($\dot{V}O_2$max) is higher for males than for females. When $\dot{V}O_2$max is expressed in absolute values (liters per minute), males typically have values that are 40–60% higher than in females.[8,70] When differences in body size are considered and $\dot{V}O_2$max values are reported on the relative basis of body weight (in milliliters per kilogram per minute), the differences between the sexes decreases to 20–30%. If differences in body composition are considered and $\dot{V}O_2$max is expressed relative to fat-free mass (in milliliters per kilogram of fat-free mass per minute), the difference between the sexes is reduced to 0–15%.[70] Reporting $\dot{V}O_2$max relative to fat-free mass is important in terms of understanding the influence of adiposity and fat-free mass in determining $\dot{V}O_2$max. However, it is not a very practical way to express $\dot{V}O_2$max since, in reality, consuming oxygen in relation to only the fat-free

FIGURE 5.12

Distribution of $\dot{V}O_2$max for Males and Females

Source: C. L. Wells & S. A. Plowman. Sexual differences in athletic performance: Biological or behavioral? *Physician and Sports Medicine.* 11(8):52–63 (1983). Reprinted by permission.

mass is not an option. Individuals cannot leave their fat mass behind when exercising.

Figure 5.12 represents the distribution of $\dot{V}O_2$max values for males and females expressed per kilogram of weight and per kilogram of fat-free mass. This figure demonstrates the important point that there is considerable variability in $\dot{V}O_2$max for both sexes. Thus, although males generally have a higher $\dot{V}O_2$max than females, some females will have a higher $\dot{V}O_2$max than the average man.

Figure 5.13 shows the differences in $\dot{V}O_2$max, expressed in relative terms (Figure 5.13a) and absolute terms (Figure 5.13b) and body weight (Figure 5.13c) between the sexes across the age span. Differences in $\dot{V}O_2$max between the sexes is largely explained by differences in the size of the heart (and thus maximal cardiac output) and differences in the oxygen-carrying capacity of the blood.[49] Males have approximately 6% more red blood cells and 10–15% more hemoglobin than females; thus, males have a greater oxygen-carrying capacity than females.[9]

Males typically have maximal cardiac output values that are 30% higher than those of females.[77] Maximal stroke volume is higher for men, but the

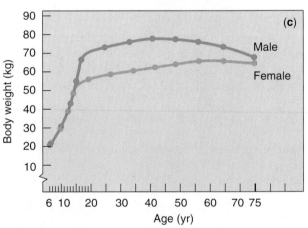

FIGURE 5.13

Maximal Oxygen Consumption ($\dot{V}O_2$max) and Weight for Males and Females from 6–75 Years

Source: E. Shvartz & R. C. Reibold. Aerobic fitness norms for males and females aged 6 to 75 years: A review. *Aviation, Space, and Environmental Physiology.* 61:3–11 (1990). Reprinted by permission.

increase in stroke volume during maximal exercise is achieved by the same mechanisms in both sexes.[71] Furthermore, if maximal stroke volume is expressed relative to body weight, there is no difference between the sexes. The maximal heart rate is similar for both sexes.

Males and females display the same pattern of blood pressure response; however, males attain a higher systolic blood pressure than females at maximal exercise.[42,51,76] Diastolic blood pressure response to maximal exercise is similar for both sexes. Thus, mean arterial blood pressure is slightly greater in males at the completion of maximal work. The pattern of response for resistance and rate-pressure product is the same for both sexes. Resistance is greatly reduced during maximal exercise in both sexes. Since the heart rate response is similar and since systolic blood pressure is greater in males, males tend to have a higher rate-pressure product at maximal exercise levels than do females.

Table 5.2 summarizes the differences between the sexes in cardiovascular variables at various exercise levels.

Responses of Children to Dynamic Aerobic Exercise

The responses of children to cardiovascular exercise are similar to the responses of adults. However, there are differences in the magnitude of the responses primarily because of differences in body size and structure.

Submaximal Exercise The pattern of cardiac output response to submaximal dynamic exercise is similar in children and adults, with cardiac output increasing rapidly at the onset of exercise and leveling off when steady state is achieved. However, children have a lower cardiac output than adults at all levels of exercise, primarily because children have a lower stroke volume than adults at any given level of exercise.[10,61] The lower stroke volume in children is compensated for, to some extent, by a higher heart rate. Stroke volume in girls is less than that in boys at all levels of exercise.[10]

The magnitude of the cardiovascular response depends upon the intensity of the exercise. Table 5.3 reports the cardiac output, stroke volume, and heart rate values of children 8–12 years old during treadmill exercise at 40%, 53%, and 68% of $\dot{V}O_2$max.[40] Both cardiac output and heart rate increase in response to increasing intensities of exercise. Stroke volume peaks at 40% of $\dot{V}O_2$max and changes little with increasing exercise intensity. This is consistent with the finding that stroke volume plateaus at 40–50% of $\dot{V}O_2$max in adults.[7]

Although the pattern of response in children is similar to that of adults, a careful review of Table 5.3 reveals that the values for cardiac output and stroke volume are much smaller in children. As children grow and mature, cardiac output and stroke volume increase at rest and during exercise. The heart rate response, on the other hand, is higher in the younger children.[10,14]

Systolic blood pressure in children increases during exercise, as it does in adults, and depends upon the intensity of the exercise. Boys tend to have a higher systolic blood pressure than girls.[42] The magnitude of the increase in systolic pressure at submaximal exercise is less in children than in

TABLE 5.2 ■ Cardiovascular Variables for Women When Compared to Men

VARIABLE	REST	ABSOLUTE, SUBMAXIMAL	RELATIVE, SUBMAXIMAL	INCREMENTAL, MAXIMAL
		Exercise Condition		
$\dot{V}O_2$max	—	—	—	Lower
$\dot{Q}$	Lower	Higher	?	Lower
SV	Lower	Lower	Lower	Lower
HR	Higher	Higher	Higher	Similar

Source: Wells.[77]

S
Δ
MAP
Res.

TABLE 5.3 ■ Cardiovascular Responses in Children to Submaximal Exercise of Various Intensities

	Intensity of Exercise (% $\dot{V}O_2$max)		
VARIABLE	**40%**	**53%**	**68%**
$\dot{Q}$ (L·min⁻¹)	6.7	7.6	8.5
SV (mL·b⁻¹)	53	51	49
HR (b·min⁻¹)	126	149	173

Source: Lussier and Buskirk.[40]

adults.[33,76] The failure of systolic blood pressure to reach adult levels is probably the result of lower cardiac output in children. As children mature, the increases in systolic blood pressure during exercise become greater. Diastolic pressure changes little during exercise but is lower in children than adults.[33,76]

Similar decreases in resistance occur in children as in adults, owing to vasodilation in working muscles. Myocardial oxygen consumption and, thus, rate-pressure product increase in children during exercise. However, the work of the heart reflects the higher heart rate and lower systolic blood pressure for children than for adults. Blood flow through the exercising muscle appears to be greater in children than in adults, resulting in a higher a-vO₂ diff and thereby compensating partially for the lower cardiac output.[61,62] Children appear to exhibit cardiovascular drift during heavy, prolonged exercise, just as adults do.[4]

Incremental Exercise to Maximum   The cardiovascular responses to incremental exercise to maximum are similar for children and adults; however, children achieve a lower maximal cardiac output and a lower maximal stroke volume. Maximal heart rate is higher in children than in adults.[14]

The maximal oxygen consumption that is typically attained by children between the ages of 6 and 18 yr is shown in Figure 5.14. As children grow, their ability to take in and utilize oxygen improves. This improvement represents dimensional and maturational changes—specifically, heart volume, maximal stroke volume, maximal cardiac output, blood volume and hemoglobin concentration, and a-vO₂ diff

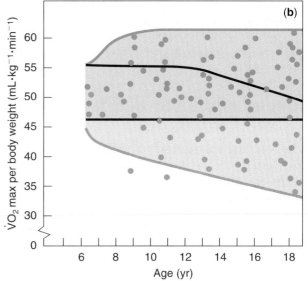

FIGURE 5.14

Maximal Oxygen Consumption ($\dot{V}O_2$max) of Children

(a) Changes in $\dot{V}O_2$max in children and adolescents during the ages of 6–18 are expressed in absolute terms. The dots represent means from various studies. The black center line approximates a mean from various studies, and the outer lines indicate normal variability in values. (b) Changes in $\dot{V}O_2$max in children and adolescents during the ages of 6–18 are expressed relative to body weight. The dots represent means from various studies. The lines indicate normal variability in reported values.

Source: O. Bar-Or. Physiologic principles to clinical applications. *Pediatric Sports Medicine for the Practitioner.* New York: Springer-Verlag (1983). Reprinted by permission.

increase and the maximal heart rate decreases as children grow.

The rate of improvement in absolute $\dot{V}O_2$max (expressed in liters per minute) is similar for boys and girls until approximately 12 yr of age (Figure 5.14a). Maximal oxygen uptake continues to increase in boys until the age of 18; it remains relatively constant in girls between the ages of 14 and 18 yr.

When $\dot{V}O_2$max is expressed relative to body weight (expressed in milliliters per kilogram of body weight per minute), it remains relatively constant throughout the years between 8 and 16 for boys (Figure 5.14b). However, there is a tendency for the $\dot{V}O_2$max expressed per kilogram of body weight per minute to decrease in girls as they enter puberty, and their adiposity increases (Figure 5.14b). As children mature, they also grow; and the developmental changes indicated previously are largely offset if $\dot{V}O_2$max is described per kilogram of body weight. Notice that in both parts of Figure 5.14 there is a large area of overlap for reported values of $\dot{V}O_2$max. This reflects the large variability in $\dot{V}O_2$max among children.

One major difference between children/adolescents and adults is the meaning of $\dot{V}O_2$max. In adults $\dot{V}O_2$max reflects both physiological function (cardiorespiratory power) and cardiovascular endurance (the ability to perform strenuous, large-muscle exercise for a prolonged period of time).[72] In children, $\dot{V}O_2$max is not as directly related to cardiorespiratory endurance as it is in adults.[10,34,61] Figure 5.15b shows performance as determined by the number of stages or minutes completed in the PACER test.[35] This progressive, aerobic cardiovascular endurance run (PACER) was fully described in Chapter 4. Recall that the higher the number, the better cardiorespiratory endurance is. Figure 5.15a shows that for boys the mean value of $\dot{V}O_2$max changes very little from age 6 to 18 yr. However, mean performance on the PACER test (Figure 5.15b) shows a definite linear improvement with age. The girls show the same trend as the boys prior to puberty; but thereafter, $\dot{V}O_2$max declines steadily and PACER performance plateaus. Similar results are seen in treadmill endurance times and other distance runs.[13] Thus, in general, endurance performance improves progressively throughout childhood, at least until puberty; but directly determined $\dot{V}O_2$max does not. Furthermore, at any given age the relationship between $\dot{V}O_2$max and endurance performance is weak.

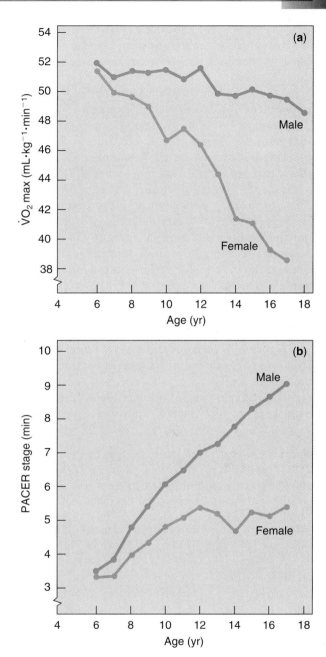

FIGURE 5.15

Maximal Oxygen Consumption ($\dot{V}O_2$max) and Endurance Performance in Children and Adolescents

Source: L. A. Leger, D. Mercer, C. Gadoury, & J. Lambert. The multistage 20 metre shuttle run test for aerobic fitness. *Journal of Sports Sciences.* 6:93–101 (1988). Modified and reprinted by permission.

The reason for the weak association between $\dot{V}O_2$max and endurance performance in young people is unknown. The most frequent suggestion is that children use more energy (require greater oxygen) at any submaximal pace than adults do. This phenomenon is called *running economy* and is fully discussed in the unit on metabolism. More important than the actual oxygen consumption at a set pace, however, may be the percentage of $\dot{V}O_2$max that value represents, and more so in children than adolescents.[44] Other factors that may impact endurance running performance in children and adolescents include body composition, particularly the percentage body fat component; sprint speed, possibly as a reflection of a high percentage of muscle fibers differentiated for speed and power; and various aspects of body size.[15,16,43,46] There is also the possibility that many children and adolescents are not motivated to perform exercise tests and so do not perform well despite high $\dot{V}O_2$max capabilities.

Figure 5.16 presents the arterial blood pressure response of children and adolescents to incremental maximal exercise. The blood pressure response is similar for children and adults; however, there are again age- or size-related quantitative differences.

TABLE 5.4 ■ Cardiovascular Responses to Maximal Exercise in Pre- and Postpubescent Children

	Boys		Girls	
VARIABLE	10 YR	15 YR	10 YR	15 YR
$\dot{Q}$ (L·min^{-1})	12	18	11	14
SV (mL·b^{-1})	60	90	55	70
HR (b·min^{-1})	200	200	200	200
$\dot{V}O_2$ (L·min^{-1})	1.7	3.5	1.5	2.0
SBP (mmHg)	144	174	140	170
DBP (mmHg)	65	65	65	65
MAP (mmHg)	105	110	103	117.5
R (units)	7.0	6.1	9.4	8.4
RPP (units)	290	350	280	340

Source: Astrand[8]; Rowland.[61]

For a given level of exercise a small child responds with a lower systolic and diastolic blood pressure than does an adolescent, and an adolescent responds with lower blood pressure than an adult. The lower blood pressure response in young children is consistent with their lower stroke volume response. Typically, boys have a higher peak systolic blood pressure than girls.[56,75] This difference too is most likely attributable to differences in stroke volume.

Table 5.4 reports typical cardiovascular responses to maximal exercise in pre- and postpubescent children.

Response of the Elderly to Dynamic Aerobic Exercise

Aging is associated with a loss of function in many systems of the body. Thus, aging is characterized by a decreased ability to respond to physiological stress.[68] There is considerable debate, though, about what portion of the loss of function that characterizes aging represents an inevitable age-related loss, what portion is related to disease, and what portion is attributable to the sedentary lifestyle that so often accompanies aging, since each causes similar decrements in function.

There are many examples of older adults who remain active into their later years and who perform

FIGURE 5.16

Blood Pressure Response of Children and Adolescents to an Incremental Exercise Test

Source: D. A. Riopel, A. B. Taylor, & A. R. Hohn. Blood pressure, heart rate, pressure-rate product and electrocardiographic changes in healthy children during treadmill exercise. *American Journal of Cardiology.* 44(4):697–704 (1979). Reprinted by permission.

amazing athletic feats. For example, Mavis Lindgren began an exercise program of walking when she was in her early sixties. She slowly increased her training volume and began jogging. At the age of 70 she completed her first marathon. In the next 12 years she raced in over fifty marathons.[52] Many studies of physical activity suggest that by remaining active in the older years, individuals can markedly reduce loss of cardiovascular function, even if they don't run a marathon.

Submaximal Exercise   At the same absolute submaximal workload cardiac output and stroke volume are lower in older adults, but heart rate is higher, when compared with those variables for younger adults. The pattern of systolic and diastolic pressure is the same for younger and older individuals. The difference in resting blood pressure is maintained throughout exercise, so that older individuals have a higher systolic, diastolic, and mean blood pressure at any given level of exercise.[51] The higher blood pressure response is related to a higher resistance in older individuals, resulting from a loss of elasticity in the blood vessels. Since heart rate and systolic blood pressure are higher for any given level of exercise in the elderly, myocardial oxygen consumption, and thus rate-pressure product, will also be higher in older individuals than in younger adults.

Incremental Exercise to Maximum
Maximal cardiac output is lower in older individuals than in younger adults. This results from a lower heart rate and a lower stroke volume. Maximal stroke volume decreases with advancing age, and the decline is of similar magnitude for both men and women, although women have a much smaller maximal stroke volume initially. Maximal heart rate decreases with age but does not vary significantly between the sexes. A decrease of approximately 10% per decade, starting at approximately 30 yr, has been reported for $\dot{V}O_2$max in sedentary adults.[6,30] Figures 5.13a and 5.13b depict the change in $\dot{V}O_2$max from childhood to age 75.

As with resting blood pressure, systolic and diastolic blood pressure responses to exercise are typically higher in older individuals than in younger individuals of similar training.[51] Maximal systolic blood pressure may be 20–50 mmHg higher in older individuals, whereas maximal diastolic blood pressure may be 15–20 mmHg higher. As a result of an elevated systolic and diastolic blood pressure, mean arterial blood pressure is considerably higher at maximal exercise in the elderly than in younger adults.

Total peripheral resistance decreases during dynamic exercise in the elderly, but not to the same extent that it does in younger individuals. This difference is another consequence of the loss of elasticity of the connective tissue in the vasculature that accompanies aging. Since the decrease in maximal heart rate for older individuals is greater than the increase in maximal systolic blood pressure when compared with those variables for younger adults, older individuals have a lower rate-pressure product at maximal exercise than younger individuals have. Table 5.5 presents typical cardiovascular values at maximal exercise in young and old adults of both sexes.

Cardiovascular Responses to Static Exercise

Static work occurs repeatedly during daily activities, such as lifting and carrying heavy objects, and is a common form of activity encountered in many occupational settings, particularly manufac-

TABLE 5.5 ■ Cardiovascular Responses to Maximal Exercise in Young and Older Adults

VARIABLE	Men		Women	
	25 YR	65 YR	25 YR	65 YR
$\dot{Q}$ (L·min^{-1})	25	16	18	12
SV (mL)	128	100	92	75
HR (b·min^{-1})	195	155	195	155
$\dot{V}O_2$ (L·min^{-1})	3.5	2.5	2.5	1.5
SBP (mmHg)	190	200	190	200
DBP (mmHg)	70	84	64	84
MAP (mmHg)	130	143	128	143
R (units)	5.2	8.9	7.1	11.9
RPP (units)	371	310	371	310

Source: Ogawa.[51]

turing jobs where lifting is common. Additionally, a large number of sports and recreational activities have a static component associated with their performance. For example, weight-lifting, rowing, and racquet sports all involve static exercise. The magnitude of the cardiovascular response to static exercise is affected by several factors, but most noticeably by the intensity of muscle contraction.

Intensity of Muscle Contraction

The cardiovascular response to static exercise depends upon the intensity of contraction, provided the contraction is held for a specified time period. The intensity of a static contraction is expressed as a percentage of maximal voluntary contraction (% MVC). Figure 5.17 illustrates the cardiovascular response to static contractions of the forearm (handgrip) muscles at 10, 20, and 50% MVC. Notice that at 10 and 20% MVC the contraction could be held for 5 min, but at 50% MVC the contraction could be held for only 2 min. Also note that the data presented in this figure are from handgrip exercises. Although the pattern of response appears to be similar for different muscle groups, the actual values may vary considerably depending upon the amount of active muscle involved.

Cardiac output increases during static contractions owing to an increase in heart rate, with the magnitude of the increase dependent upon the intensity of exercise. Stroke volume (Figure 5.17b) remains relatively constant during low-intensity contractions and decreases during high-intensity contractions. There is a marked increase in stroke volume immediately following the cessation of high-intensity contractions.[37,69] The reduction in stroke volume during high-intensity contractions is probably the result of both a decreased preload and an increased afterload. Preload is decreased because of high intrathoracic pressure, which compresses the vena cava and thus decreases the return of venous blood to the heart. Since arterial blood pressure is markedly elevated during isometric contractions (increased afterload), less blood will be ejected

at a given force of contraction. Heart rate (Figure 5.17c) increases during static exercise. The magnitude and the rate of the increase in heart rate depends on the intensity of contraction. The greater the intensity, the greater the heart rate response.

Static exercise is characterized by a rapid increase in both systolic pressure and diastolic pressure, termed the **pressor response**, which appears to be inappropriate for the amount of work produced by the contracting muscle.[37] Since both systolic and diastolic pressures increase in static exercise, there is a marked increase in mean arterial pressure (Figure 5.17d).[18,37,49,65,73] As in any muscular work, static exercise increases metabolic demands to the active muscle. However, in static work high intramuscular tension results in mechanical constriction of the blood vessels, which impedes blood flow to the muscle. The reduction in muscle blood flow during static exercise results in a buildup of local by-products of metabolism. These chemical by-products [H^+, adenosine diphosphate (ADP), and others] stimulate sensory nerve endings, which leads to a pressor reflex, causing a rise in mean arterial pressure (pressor response). This rise is substantially larger than the increase during dynamic exercise requiring similar energy expenditure.[5,29] Notice in Figure 5.17d that holding a handgrip dynamometer at 20% MVC for 5 min results in an increase of 30–35 mmHg in mean arterial pressure.

Resistance, indicated by TPR in Figure 5.17e, decreases during static exercise, although not to the extent seen in dynamic aerobic exercise. The failure of resistance to decrease markedly helps to explain the higher blood pressure response to static contractions. The high blood pressure generated during static contractions helps overcome the resistance to blood flow owing to mechanical occlusion. Since systolic blood pressure and heart rate both increase during static exercise, there is a large increase in myocardial oxygen consumption and rate-pressure product.

Blood Flow During Static Contractions

Blood flow to the working muscle is impeded during static contractions because of mechanical constriction of the blood vessel supplying the contracting muscle.[25,67] Figure 5.18 depicts blood flow in the quadriceps muscle when a 5% and 25% MVC contraction were held to fatigue. The 5% MVC load

Pressor Response The rapid increase in both systolic pressure and diastolic pressure during static exercise.

FIGURE 5.17

Cardiovascular Response to Varying Intensities of Handgrip Exercise

Source: Modified from A. R. Lind, S. H. Taylor, P. W. Humphreys, B. M. Kennelly, & K. W. Donald. The circulatory effects of sustained voluntary muscle contraction. *Clinical Science.* 27:229–244. Reprinted by permission of the Biochemical Society and Portland Press.

FIGURE 5.18

Blood Flow in the Quadriceps Muscle During Different Intensities of Contraction

Source: G. Sjogaard, G. Savard, & C. Juel. Muscle blood flow during isometric activity and its relation to muscle fatigue. *European Journal of Physiology.* 57:327–335 (1988). Reprinted by permission.

could be held for 30 min; the 25% load could be held for only 4 min. Quadriceps blood flow is greater during the 5% MVC, suggesting that at 25% MVC there is considerable impedance to blood flow. In fact, blood flow during the 25% MVC load was very close to resting levels despite the metabolic work done by the muscle. The response seen during recovery suggests that when contraction ceases, a mechanical occlusion to the muscle is released. The marked increase in blood flow compensates for the reduced flow during sustained contraction. The relative force at which blood flow is impeded varies greatly among different muscle groups.[36,38,60]

There is also mechanical constriction during dynamic exercise. However, the alternating periods of muscular contraction and relaxation that occur during rhythmical activity allow—and, indeed, encourage—blood flow, especially through the venous system.

Comparison of Dynamic Aerobic and Static Exercise Figure 5.19 compares the heart rate (5.19a) and blood pressure (5.19b) responses to fatiguing handgrip (static) exercise (30% MVC held to fatigue) and a maximal treadmill (dynamic aero-

FIGURE 5.19

Comparison of Heart Rate and Blood Pressure Response to Static and Dynamic Exercise

Source: A. Lind. Cardiovascular responses to static exercise. *Circulation.* XLI(2) (1970). Reproduced with permission. Copyright 1970 American Heart Association.

bic) test to fatigue. Dynamic exercise (treadmill) is characterized by a large increase in heart rate, which contributes to an increased cardiac output. It also shows a modest increase in systolic blood pressure and a relatively stable or decreasing diastolic blood pressure. Fatiguing static exercise (handgrip) is characterized by a modest increase in heart rate but a dramatic increase in blood pressure (press or response). Mean blood pressure increases as a result of increased systolic and diastolic blood pressure.

Table 5.1 summarizes cardiovascular responses to static exercise.

Sex Differences in Responses to Static Exercise

The heart rate response to static exercise (Figure 5.20a) is similar in males and females.[48] However, as shown in Figure 5.20b, when a group of young adult, healthy subjects held maximal contractions of the handgrip muscles for 2 min, the blood pressures reported for women were significantly lower than those reported for men.[48] Stroke volume and cardiac output responses in women during maximal iso-metric contraction of the finger flexors were similar to the responses observed in the men, but no direct comparisons between men and women were made for these variables.[69] There are no comparable data available for boys and girls.

Cardiovascular Responses to Static Exercise in Older Adults

Many studies have described the cardiovascular responses to static exercise in the elderly.[27,45,54,63,74] As an example, Figure 5.21 depicts the cardiovascular responses of young and old men to sustained hand-grip and leg extension exercise over a range of sub-maximal static workloads.[74] Note that cardiac output (Figure 5.21a) and stroke volume (Figure 5.21b) values are lower than normally reported owing to the measurement technique. However, concentrating on the relative differences between the responses of the young and older subjects reveals that cardiac output, stroke volume, and heart rate (Figure 5.21c) were lower for the older men than the younger men at each intensity. In contrast, blood pressure responses (Figures 5.21d and 5.21e) were higher for the older men at each intensity. As with dynamic aerobic exercise the differences in the cardiovascular responses between the two age groups are probably due to an age-related increase in resistance due to a loss of elasticity in the vascu-lature and a decreased ability of the myocardium to stretch and contract forcibly.[74] The rate-pressure product (Figure 5.21f) was higher for the younger subjects than for the older subjects at 30, 45, and 60% MVC. The small difference in rate-pressure product reflected a higher heart rate in younger sub-jects at each intensity of contraction, which was not completely offset by a lower systolic blood pressure in the younger subjects.

FIGURE 5.20

Heart Rate and Blood Pressure Response of Males and Females to Static Exercise

Source: J. E. Misner, S. B. Going, B. H. Massey, T. E. Ball, M. G. Bemben, & L. K. Essandoh. Cardiovascular response in males and females to sustained maximal voluntary static muscle con-traction. *Medicine and Science in Sports and Exercise.* 22(2):194–199 (1990). Reprinted by permission of Williams & Wilkins.

Cardiovascular Responses to Dynamic Resistance Exercise

Weight-lifting or resistance exercise includes a combination of dynamic and static contractions. Re-sistance exercise is a series of static contractions performed dynamically.[32,41] During dynamic resis-tance exercise there is a dissociation between the energy demand and the cardiorespiratory system.

FIGURE 5.21

Cardiovascular Response of Males by Age to Static Exercise

Source: M. D. VanLoan, et al. Age as a factor in the hemodynamic responses to isometric exercise. *Journal of Sports Medicine and Physical Fitness.* 29(3):262–268 (1989). Reprinted by permission.

In contrast, during dynamic endurance activity the cardiorespiratory system is directly tied to the use of oxygen for energy production. In part, the reason for this dissociation between oxygen use and cardiovascular response to resistance exercise is that much of the energy required for resistance exercise comes from anaerobic (without oxygen) sources. There are two other important differences between resistance exercise and dynamic exercise that affect

cardiovascular responses. First, there is less activation of the sympathetic nervous system during dynamic resistance exercise. Second, there is mechanical constriction of blood flow during resistance exercise because of the isometric nature of the contraction.

The magnitude of the cardiovascular response to resistance exercise depends upon the intensity of the load (the weight lifted) and the number of repe-

FIGURE 5.22

Cardiovascular Response to Fatiguing Resistance Exercise (concentric knee extension exercise)

Source: Based on data from Falkel et al.[20]

titions performed. Very little information exists about cardiac output and stroke volume during resistance exercise because of the problems of collecting the information. However, studies show that heart rate and blood pressure increase progressively during resistance exercise as more repetitions are completed.[21,22] For example, when subjects performed ten repetitions of three different weights (identified as light, moderate, and heavy), blood pressure was highest at the completion of the heaviest set.[79] Systolic blood pressure increased 16, 22, and 34% during the light, moderate, and heavy sets, respectively. Diastolic blood pressure, measured by ascultation, did not change significantly with any of the sets. There is disagreement about the diastolic blood pressure response to resistance exercise; some authors report an increase and others report no change.[21,22,79] These discrepancies may reflect differences in measurement techniques (namely, ascultation and intra-arterial assessment) and timing of the measurement. The cardiovascular response of children to resistance exercise is similar to that of adults, with heart rate and blood pressure increasing progressively throughout a set.[50]

A different pattern of response is seen when a given load is performed to fatigue. In this case the individual is performing maximal work regardless of the load. Figure 5.22 shows the cardiovascular response to leg extension exercise performed to fatigue. Subjects performed 50%, 80%, and 100% of their one repetition maximum (1 RM) as many times as they could, and cardiovascular variables were recorded at the end of each set.[20] Subjects could perform the 100% load only one time, of course; but they could perform the 80 and 50% loads an average of 8 and 15 times, respectively. Cardiac output at the completion of the set was highest when the lightest load was lifted for the greatest number of repetitions (Figure 5.22a).

The stroke volume achieved at the end of a set was similar for each condition (Figure 5.22b). Notice, however, that the stroke volume measures are all considerably less than stroke volume measures obtained during dynamic aerobic exercise. Thus, dynamic resistance exercise does not produce the stroke volume overload that dynamic endurance exercise does.[32,36]

Heart rate was highest after completion of the set using the lightest load and lifting it the greatest number of times (Figure 5.22c). Heart rate was lowest when the single repetition using the heaviest weight was performed. Heart rates between 130 and 160 b·min^{-1} have commonly been reported during resistance exercise.[32,36] There is some evidence that the heart rate and blood pressure attained at fatigue are the same when loads between 60 and 100% of 1 RM are used, regardless of the number of times the load can be performed.[50]

Blood pressure increases dramatically when resistance exercise is performed to fatigue.[22,41] Figure 5.23a shows the mean arterial blood pressure, measured intra-arterially, during a set of leg press exercises that represented 95% of one repetition maximum, and Figure 5.23b shows the heart rate during these exercises. In this study peak systolic blood pressure averaged 320 mmHg and peak diastolic blood pressure averaged 250 mmHg. The dramatic increase in blood pressure during dynamic resistance exercise results from the mechanical compression on the blood vessels and performance of the Valsalva maneuver (as explained in Chapter 3). Total peripheral resistance is higher during dynamic resistance exercise than during dynamic aerobic exercise due to the vasoconstriction caused by the pressor reflex. Myocardial oxygen consumption and, thus, the rate-pressure product can reach extremely high levels because of the tachycardia and exaggerated systolic blood pressure response. Dynamic resistance exercise causes large (about 15%) but transient decreases in plasma volume.[32]

A summary of cardiovascular responses to resistance exercise is included in Table 5.1.

FIGURE 5.23

Heart Rate and Blood Pressure Response to Resistance Exercise

Source: J. D. MacDougall, D. Tuxen, D. G. Sale, J. R. Moroz, & J. R. Sutton. Arterial blood pressure response to heavy resistance exercise. *Journal of Applied Physiology.* 58(3):785–790 (1985). Reprinted by permission.

SUMMARY

1. During short-term, light to moderate dynamic aerobic exercise, cardiac output, stroke volume, heart rate, systolic blood pressure, and rate-pressure product increase rapidly at the onset of exercise and reach steady state within approximately 2 min. Diastolic blood pressure remains relatively unchanged, and resistance decreases rapidly and then plateaus.

2. During prolonged, heavy dynamic aerobic exercise, cardiac output, stroke volume, heart rate, systolic blood pressure, and rate-pressure product increase rapidly. Once steady state is achieved, cardiac output remains relatively constant owing to the downward drift of stroke volume and the upward drift of heart rate. Systolic blood pressure and resistance may also drift downward during prolonged, heavy work. This cardiovascular drift is associated with rising body temperature.

3. During incremental aerobic exercise to maximum, cardiac output, heart rate, systolic blood pressure, and rate-pressure product increase in a rectilinear fashion with increasing workload. Stroke volume increases initially and then plateaus at a workload corresponding to approximately 40–50% of $\dot{V}O_2$max in normally active adults and children. Diastolic blood pressure remains relatively constant throughout an incremental exercise test.

Resistance decreases rapidly with the onset of exercise and reaches its lowest value at maximal exercise.

4. The decrease in resistance that accompanies dynamic aerobic exercise has two important implications. First, the decrease in resistance allows greater blood flow to the working muscles. Second, the decrease in resistance keeps blood pressure from rising excessively. The increase in cardiac output would produce a much greater rise in blood pressure if it were not for the fact that there is a simultaneous decrease in resistance.

5. Blood volume decreases during dynamic aerobic exercise. The majority of the decrease occurs within the first 10 min of activity and depends upon exercise intensity. A decrease of 10% of blood volume is not uncommon.

6. Stroke volume initially increases during dynamic aerobic exercise and then plateaus at a level that corresponds to 40–50% of $\dot{V}O_2$max. The increase in stroke volume results from changes in left ventricular end–diastolic volume and left ventricular end–systolic volume. Left ventricular end–diastolic volume increases primarily because the active muscle pump returns blood to the heart. Left ventricular end–systolic volume decreases owing to augmented contractility of the heart, thus ejecting more blood and leaving less in the ventricle.

7. The pattern of cardiovascular response is the same for both sexes. However, males have a higher cardiac output, stroke volume, and systolic blood pressure at maximal exercise. Additionally, males have a higher $\dot{V}O_2$max. Most of these differences are attributable to differences in body size and heart size between the sexes and to the greater hemoglobin concentration of males.

8. The pattern of cardiovascular response in children is similar to the adult response. However, children have a lower cardiac output, stroke volume, and systolic blood pressure at an absolute workload and at maximal exercise. Most of these differences are attributable to differences in body size and heart size.

9. As adults age, their cardiovascular responses change. Maximal cardiac output, stroke volume, heart rate, and $\dot{V}O_2$max decrease. Maximal systolic blood pressure, diastolic blood pressure, and mean arterial pressure increase.

10. Static exercise is characterized by modest increases in heart rate and cardiac output and exaggerated increases in systolic blood pressure, diastolic blood pressure and mean arterial pressure, known as the pressor response.

11. Dynamic resistance training results in an increase in heart rate and blood pressure, with each variable increasing progressively throughout a set.

Box 5.1 Answers

Condition	MAP (mmHg)	TPR (units)	RPP (units)
Rest	102*	17.5	107
Light dynamic	118†	12.0	195
Heavy dynamic	129†	10.2	263
Maximal dynamic	144†	9.8	360
Sustained static	155†	19.4	284

*Use Equation 4.5a.
†Use Equation 4.5b.

REVIEW QUESTIONS

1. Graph and explain the pattern of response for each of the major cardiovascular variables during short-term, light to moderate dynamic aerobic exercise. Explain the mechanisms responsible for each response.

2. Graph and explain the pattern of response for each of the major cardiovascular variables during prolonged, heavy dynamic aerobic exercise. Explain the mechanisms responsible for each response.

3. Graph and explain the pattern of response for each of the major cardiovascular variables during incremental aerobic exercise to maximum. Explain the mechanisms responsible for each response.

4. Graph and explain the pattern of response for each of the major cardiovascular variables during static exercise. Explain the mechanisms responsible for each response.

5. Graph and explain the pattern of response for each of the major cardiovascular variables during dynamic resistance exercise. Explain the mechanisms responsible for each response.

6. Discuss the change that occurs in total peripheral resistance during exercise, and explain its importance for blood flow and blood pressure. Why is resistance altered in older adults?

7. Describe the pressor response to static exercise, and explain the mechanisms by which blood pressure is elevated.

REFERENCES

1. American College of Sports Medicine: *Guidelines for Exercise Testing and Prescription* (5th edition). Philadelphia: Lea & Febiger (1995).

2. American College of Sports Medicine: Position stand: Physical activity, physical fitness, and hypertension. *Medicine and Science in Sports and Exercise. 25(10):1-X (1993).*

3. Anderson, K. L.: The cardiovascular system in exercise. In H. B. Falls (ed.), *Exercise Physiology.* New York: Academic Press (1968).

4. Asano, K., & K. Hirakoba: Respiratory and circulatory adaptation during prolonged exercise in 10–12 year-old children and adults. In J. Ilmarinen, & I. Valimaki (eds.), *Children and Sports.* Berlin: Springer-Verlag (1984).

5. Asmussen, E.: Similarities and dissimilarities between static and dynamic exercise. *Circulation Research* (Suppl. I). 48(6):3–10 (1981).

6. Astrand, I.: Aerobic work capacity in men and women with special reference to age. *Acta Physiologica Scandinavica* (Suppl. 169). 49:1–92 (1960).

7. Astrand, P., T. E. Cuddy, B. Saltin, & J. Stenberg: Cardiac output during submaximal and maximal work. *Journal of Applied Physiology* 19(2):268–274 (1964).

8. Astrand, P.: Experimental Studies of Physical Working Capacity in Relation to Sex and Age. *University Microfilms International* (1952).

9. Astrand, P. O., & K. Rodahl: *Textbook of Work Physiology.* New York: McGraw-Hill (1986).

10. Bar-Or, O.: Physiologic principles to clinical applications. *Pediatric Sports Medicine, for the Practitioner.* New York: Springer-Verlag (1983).

11. Becklake, M. R., H. Frank, G. R. Dagenais, G. L. Ostiguy, & C. A. Guzman: Influence of age and sex on exercise cardiac output. *Journal of Applied Physiology* 20(5):938–947 (1965).

12. Clausen, J. P.: Circulatory adjustments to dynamic exercise and effect of physical training in normal subjects and in patients with coronary artery disease. *Progressive Cardiovascular Disease.* 18:459–495 (1976).

13. Cumming, G. R., D. Everatt, & L. Hastman: Bruce treadmill test in children: Normal values in a clinic population. *American Journal of Cardiology.* 41:69–75 (1978).

14. Cunningham, D. A., D. H. Paterson, C. J. R. Blimkie, & A. P. Donner: Development of cardiorespiratory function in circumpubertal boys: A longitudinal study. *Journal of Applied Physiology: Respiratory Environment Exercise Physiology.* 56(2):302–307 (1984).

15. Cureton, K. J., T. A. Baumgartner, & B. McManis: Adjustment of 1-mile run/walk test scores for skinfold thickness in youth. *Pediatric Exercise Science* 3:152–167 (1991).

16. Cureton, K. J., R. A. Boileau, T. G. Lohman, & J. E. Misner: Determinants of distance running performance in children: Analysis of a path model. *Research Quarterly.* 48(2):270–279 (1977).

17. Davies, C. T. M., J. Few, K. G. Foster, & A. J. Sargeant: Plasma catecholamine concentration during dynamic exercise involving different muscle groups. *European Journal of Applied Physiology.* 32:195–206 (1974).

18. Donald, K. W., S. R. Lind, G. W. McNichol, P. W. Humphreys, S. H. Taylor, & H. P. Stauton: Cardiovascular responses to sustained (static) contractions. *Circulation Research* (Suppl. I). 15–32 (1967).

19. Ekelund. L. G., & A. Holmgren: Central hemodynamics during exercise. *Circulation Research* (Suppl. I). 33–43 (1967).

20. Falkel, J. E., S. J. Fleck, & T. F. Murray: Comparison of central hemodynamics between powerlifters and bodybuilders during resistance exercise. *Journal of Applied Sport Science Research* 6(1):24–35 (1992).

21. Fleck, S. J.: Cardiovascular adaptations to resistance training. *Medicine and Science in Sports and Exercise.* 20:S146–S151 (1988).

22. Fleck, S. J., & L. S. Dean: Resistance-training experience and the pressor response during resistance exercise. *Journal of Applied Physiology.* 63:116–120 (1987).

23. Fortney, S. M., C. B. Wenger, J. R. Bove, & E. R. Nadel: Effect of blood volume on sweating rate and body fluids in exercising humans. *Journal of Applied Physiology* 51(6):1594–1600 (1981).

24. Freedson, P., V. L. Katch, S. Sady, & A. Weltman: Cardiac output differences in males and females during mild cycle ergometer exercise. *Medicine and Science in Sports.* 11(1):16–19 (1979).

25. Freund, P. R., S. F. Gobbs, & L. B. Rowell: Cardiovascular responses to muscle ischemia in man, dependency on muscle mass. *Journal of Applied Physiology.* 45:762–767 (1979).

26. Gledhill, N., D. Cox, & R. Jamnik: Endurance athletes' stroke volume does not plateau: Major advantage is diastolic function. *Medicine and Science in Sports and Exercise.* 26:1116–1121 (1994).

27. Goldstraw, P. W., & D. J. Warren: The effect of age on the cardiovascular responses to isometric exercise: A test of autonomic function. *Gerontology.* 31:54–58 (1989).

28. Hamilton, M. T., J. G. Alonso, S. J. Montain, & E. F. Coyle: Fluid replacement and glucose infusion during exercise prevents cardiovascular drift. *Journal of Applied Physiology.* 71:871–877 (1991).

29. Hanson, P., & F. Nagle: Isometric exercise: Cardiovascular responses in normal and cardiac populations. *Cardiology Clinics.* 5(2):157–170 (1985).

30. Heath, G. W., J. M. Hagberg, Ali A. Ehsani, & J. O. Holloszy: A physiological comparison of young and older endurance athletes. *Journal of Applied Physiology.* 51:634–640 (1981).

31. Higginbotham, M. B., K. G. Morris, R. S. Williams, P. A. McHale, R. E. Coleman, & F. R. Cobb: Regulation of stroke volume during submaximal and maximal upright exercise in normal man. *Circulation Research.* 58:281–291 (1986).

32. Hill, D. W., & S. D. Butler: Haemodynamic responses to weightlifting exercise. *Sports Medicine.* 12(1):1–7 (1991).

33. James, F. W., S. Kaplan, C. J. Glueck, J. Y. Tsay, M. J. S. Knight & C. J. Sarwar: Responses of normal children and young adults to controlled bicycle exercise. *Circulation.* 61:902–912 (1980).

34. Krahenbuhl, G. S., J. S. Skinner, & W. M. Kohrt: Developmental aspects of maximal aerobic power in children. In R. L. Terjung (ed.), *Exercise and Sport Science Reviews.* 13: 503–538 (1985).

35. Leger, L. A., D. Mercer, C. Gadoury, & J. Lambert: The multistage 20 metre shuttle run test for aerobic fitness. *Journal of Sports Sciences.* 6:93–101 (1988).

36. Lewis, S. F., P. G. Snell, W. F. Taylor, M. Hamra, R. M. Graham, W. A. Pettinger, & C. G. Blomqvist: Role of muscle mass and mode of contraction in circulatory responses to exercise. *Journal of Applied Physiology.* 58(1):146–151 (1985).

37. Lind, A. R., S. H. Taylor, P. W. Humphreys, B. M. Kennelly, & K. W. Donald. The circulatory effects of sustained voluntary muscle contraction. *Clinical Science.* 27:229–244 (1964).

38. Lind, A. R., & G. W. McNichol: Circulatory responses to sustained handgrip contractions performed during other exercise. *Journal of Physiology.* 192:595–607 (1967).

39. Lind, A.: Cardiovascular responses to static exercise. *Circulation.* XLI(2): (1970).

40. Lussier, L., & E. R. Buskirk: Effects of an endurance training regimen on assessment of work capacity in prepubertal children. *Annals of the New York Academy of Sciences,* 734–777 (1977).

41. MacDougall, J. D., D. Tuxen, D. G. Sale, J. R. Moroz, & J. R. Sutton: Arterial blood pressure response to heavy resistance exercise. *Journal of Applied Physiology* 58(3):785–790 (1985).

42. Malina, R. M. & C. Bouchard: *Growth, Maturation and Physical Activity.* Champaign, IL: Human Kinetics Publishers (1991).

43. Mayhew, J. L., & P. B. Gifford: Prediction of maximal oxygen intake in preadolescent boys from anthropometric parameters. *Research Quarterly.* 46(3):302–311 (1975).

44. McCormack, W. P., K. J. Cureton, T. A. Bullock, & P. G. Weyand: Metabolic determinants of 1-mile run/walk performance in children. *Medicine and Science in Exercise in Sport and Exercise.* 23(5):611–617 (1991).

45. McDermott, D. J., W. J. Steikel, J. J. Barboriak, L. C. Kloth,& J. J. Smith: Effect of age on hemodynamic and metabolic response to static exercise. *Journal of Applied Physiology.* 37(6):923–926 (1974).

46. McVeigh, S. K., A. C. Payne, & S. Scott: The reliability and validity of the 20-meter shuttle test as a predictor of peak oxygen uptake in Edinburgh school children, ages 13 to 14 years. *Pediatric Exercise Science.* 7:69–79 (1995).

47. Miles, D. S., M. H. Cox, & J. P. Bomze: Cardiovascular responses to upper body exercise in normal and cardiac patients. *Medicine and Science in Exercise in Sport and Exercise.* 21(5):s126-s131 (1989).

48. Misner, J. E., S. B. Going, B. H. Massey, T. E. Ball, M. G. Bemben, & L. K. Essandoh: Cardiovascular response in males and females to sustained maximal voluntary static muscle contraction. *Medicine and Science in Sports and Exercise* 22(2):194–199 (1990).

49. Mitchell, J. H., B. Schibye, F. C. Payne III, & B. Saltin: Response of arterial blood pressure to static exercise in relation to muscle mass, force development and electromyographic activity. *Circulation Research* (Suppl. I). 48(6):70–75 (1981).

50. Nau, K. L., V. L. Katch, R. H. Beekman, & M. Dick II: Acute intra-arterial blood pressure response to bench press weight lifting in children. *Pediatric Exercise Science.* 2:37–45 (1990).

51. Ogawa, T., R. J. Spina, W. H. Martin, W. M. Kohrt, K. B. Schechtman, J. O. Holloszy, & A. A. Ehsani: Effects of aging, sex, and physical training on cardiovascular responses to exercise. *Circulation.* 86:494–503 (1992).

52. Nieman, D.: *Fitness and Sports Medicine.* Palo Alto, CA: Bull Publishing (1990).

53. Pendergast, D. R.: Cardiovascular, respiratory, and metabolic responses to upper body exercise. *Medicine and Science in Sport and Exercise.* 21(5):s122-s125 (1989).

54. Petrofsky, J. S. & A. R. Lind: Aging, isometric strength and endurance, and cardiovascular responses to static effort. *Journal of Applied Physiology.* 38(1):91–95 (1975).

55. Poliner, L. R., G. J. Dehmer, S. E. Lewis, R. W. Parkey, C. G. Blomqvist, & J. T. Willerson: Left ventricular performance in normal subjects: A comparison of the responses to exercise in the upright supine positions. *Circulation.* 62:528–534 (1980).

56. Riopel, D. A., A. B. Taylor, & A. R. Hohn: Blood pressure, heart rate, pressure-rate product and electrocardiographic changes in healthy children during treadmill exercise. *American Journal of Cardiology.* 44:697–704 (1979).

57. Rowell, L.: Human cardiovascular adjustments to exercise and thermal stress. *Physiological Reviews.* 54:75–159 (1974).

58. Rowell, L. B., H. J. Marx, R. A. Bruce, R. D. Conn, & F. Kusumi: Reductions in cardiac output, central blood volume, and stroke volume with thermal stress in normal men during exercise. *Journal of Clinical Investigation.* 45(11):(1966).

59. Rowell, L. B.: *Human Circulation: Regulation During Physical Stress.* New York: Oxford University Press (1986).

60. Rowell, L. B.: *Human Cardiovascular Control.* New York: Oxford University Press: (1993).

61. Rowland, T. W.: *Exercise and Children's Health.* Champaign, IL: Human Kinetics Publishers (1990).

62. Rowland, T. W., & G. M. Green: Physiological responses to treadmill exercise in females: Adult-child differences. *Medical Science Sports Exercise.* 20(5):474–478 (1988).

63. Sagiv, M., E. Goldhammer, E. G. Abinader, & J. Rudoy: Aging and the effect of increased after-load on left ventricular contractile state. *Medicine and Science in Sport and Exercise.* 20(3):281–284 (1988).

64. Sawka, M. N.: Upper body exercise: Physiology and practical considerations. *Medicine and Science in Sport and Exercise.* 21(5):s119-s120 (1989).

65. Seals, D. R., R. A. Washburn, & P. G. Hanson: Increased cardiovascular response to static contraction of larger muscle groups. *Journal of Applied Physiology.* 54(2):434–437 (1985).

66. Shvartz, E., & R. C. Reibold: Aerobic fitness norms for males and females aged 6 to 75 years: A review. *Aviation, Space, and Environmental Physiology.* 61:3–11 (1990).

67. Sjogaard, G., G. Savard, & C. Juel: Muscle blood flow during isometric activity and its relation to muscle fatigue. *European Journal of Physiology.* 57:327–335 (1988).

68. Skinner, J. S: *Exercise Testing and Exercise Prescription for Special Cases* (2nd edition). Philadelphia: Lea & Febiger (1993).

69. Smith, D. L., J. E. Misner, D. K. Bloomfield, & L. K. Essandoh: Cardiovascular responses to sustained maximal isometric contractions of the finger flexors. *European Journal of Applied Physiology.* 67:48–52 (1993).

70. Sparling, P. B.: A meta-analysis of studies comparing maximal oxygen uptake in men and women. *Research Quarterly for Exercise and Sport.* 51(3):542–542 (1980).

71. Sullivan, M. J., F. R. Cobb, & M. B. Higginbotham: Stroke volume increases by similar mechanisms during upright exercise in normal men and women. *American Journal of Cardiology.* 67: (1991).

72. Taylor, H. L., E. Buskirk, & A. Henshel: Maximal oxygen intake as an objective measure of cardio-respiratory performance. *Journal of Applied Physiology.* 8:73–80 (1955).

73. Tuttle, W. W., & S. M. Horvath: Comparison of effects of static and dynamic work on blood pressure and heart rate. *Journal of Applied Physiology.* 10(2):294–296 (1957).

74. VanLoan, M. D., B. H. Massey, R. A. Boileau, T. G. Lohman, J. E. Misner, & P. L. Best: Age as a factor in the hemodynamic responses to isometric exercise. *Journal of Sports Medicine and Physical Fitness.* 29(3):262–268 (1989).

75. Wade, C. E., & B. J. Freund: Hormonal control of blood volume during and following exercise. In C. V. Gisolfi, & D. R. Lamb (eds.), *Perspectives in Exercise Science and Sports Medicine.* 3 (1990).

76. Wanne, O. P. S., & E. Haapoja: Blood pressure during exercise in healthy children. *European Journal of Applied Physiology.* 58:62–67 (1988).

77. Wells, C. L.: *Women, Sport and Performance.* Champaign, IL: Human Kinetics Publishers (1985).

78. Wells, C. L., & S. A. Plowman: Sexual differences in athletic performance: Biological or behavioral? *Physician and Sports Medicine.* 11(8):52–63 (1983).

79. Wescott, W., & B. Howes: Blood pressure response during weight training exercise. *National Strength and Conditioning Association Journal.* January–February: 67–71 (1983).

6

Cardiorespiratory Training Principles and Adaptations

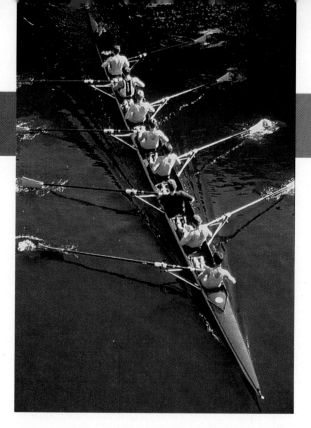

After studying the chapter, you should be able to:

- Discuss the application of each of the training principles to the development of a cardiorespiratory training program.

- Explain how the FIT principle is related to the overload principle.

- Differentiate among the methods used to classify exercise intensity.

- Calculate training intensity ranges by using the percentage of maximal heart rate, the percentage of heart rate reserve, and percentage of oxygen consumption methods.

- Discuss the merits of specificity of modality and cross training in bringing about cardiovascular adaptations.

- Identify central and peripheral cardiovascular adaptations that occur at rest, during submaximal exercise, and at maximal exercise following a dynamic endurance or dynamic resistance training program.

*I*ntroduction

Early scientific investigations leading to the development of training principles for the cardio-vascular system almost always had the improvement of physical fitness, operationally defined as an improvement of maximal oxygen consumption ($\dot{V}O_2$max), as the desired endpoint. Such studies formed the basis for the guidelines developed by the American College of Sports Medicine (ACSM), originally published in 1978[1] as "the recommended quantity and quality of exercise for developing and maintaining fitness in healthy adults" and revised in 1990[2] to "the recommended quantity and quality for exercise for developing and maintaining car-diorespiratory and muscular fitness in healthy adults." In the years between 1978 and 1990 these guidelines were increasingly applied not only to healthy adults intent on becoming more fit but also to individuals wishing solely to receive health bene-fits from exercise training. Although there is suf-ficient evidence to support the view that health benefits will accrue when fitness is improved, health and fitness are not the same thing. The quan-tity and quality of exercise required to develop or maintain cardiorespiratory fitness may not be (and probably is not) the same as that required to im-prove and maintain cardiorespiratory health.[2,50] Furthermore, most exercise science or physical edu-cation college majors and competitive athletes who want or need high levels of fitness can handle phys-ically rigorous and time-consuming training pro-grams. However, these programs carry the risk of injury and are often psychologically intimidating to those who are sedentary, elderly, or obese. Thus, what constitutes an optimal cardiovascular training program—which maximizes the benefit while min-imizing the time, effort, and risk—will vary with both the population and the intended goal.

This chapter addresses the application of the training principles to the development of **cardio-respiratory fitness**, defined as the ability to deliver and use oxygen during intense and prolonged exer-cise or work. The discussion relies heavily on the 1990 ACSM guidelines. These guidelines have been shown to be effective for a wide spectrum of the population. The (ACSM) recommendations for devising an aerobic training program are summa-rized below.

- *Mode:* Any activity that uses large muscle groups continuously in rhythmical fashion and is primarily aerobic.
- *Intensity:* 60–90% HR max; 50–85% HRR (heart rate reserve); 50–85% $\dot{V}O_2$max; 12–16 RPE (rat-ing of perceived exertion).
- *Duration:* 20–60 min continuous.
- *Frequency:* 3–5 days per week.

Note: Health benefits may be obtained from activi-ties at lower intensities if the accumulated (not nec-essarily continuous) duration is at least 30 min and the frequency is daily.

Where possible, we will cite variations for the upper and lower extremes in order to acknowledge that these guidelines do not represent a threshold below which no benefits are achieved. There is a point of diminishing return, where more exercise is not necessarily better; nevertheless, some activity is always better than no activity.

*A*pplication of the Training Principles

Specificity

Any activity that involves large muscle groups and is sustained for prolonged periods of time has the potential to increase cardiovascular fitness. Such modes of exercise include aerobics, bicycling, cross-country skiing, dancing (various forms), jogging, roller blading, rowing, speed skating, stair climbing or stepping, swimming, and walking. Sports in which the action is basically high-energy and non-stop, such as field hockey, lacrosse, and soccer, can also positively benefit the cardiovascular system.[2,81]

For the fitness participant the choice of exercise modalities should be based upon interest, availabil-ity, and risk of injury. If the activity is enjoyable to the individual, it is more likely that he or she will adhere to the program. Although jogging or run-ning may be the most time-efficient way to achieve

---

Cardiorespiratory Fitness The ability to deliver and use oxygen under the demands of intensive, prolonged exercise or work.

cardiovascular fitness, these activities are not enjoyable for many individuals, and they have a relatively high incidence of overuse injuries. Therefore, other options should be available in fitness programs.

Although many different modalities can improve cardiovascular function, the greatest improvements in performance occur in the modality that was used for training—that is, there is *modality specificity.* For example, individuals who train by swimming improve more in swimming than in running,[67] and individuals who train by bicycling improve more in cycling than running.[79,83] This modality specificity has two important practical applications. First, to determine whether an individual is improving, he or she should be tested in the modality that is used for training. Second, the more the individual is concerned with sports competition rather than fitness or rehabilitation, the more important the mode of exercise becomes. That is, the competitive rower, whether competing on open water or on an indoor ergometer, should do most of his or her training in that modality. Running, however, does seem to be less specific than most other modalities; running forms the basis of many sports other than track or road races.[79,83,98]

Having just emphasized the importance of modality specificity for competitive athletes, we must now make a case for cross training. Originally, the term *cross training* referred to the development or maintenance of muscle function in one limb by exercising the contralateral limb or upper limbs as opposed to lower limbs.[56,61,78] Such training remains important, especially in situations where one limb has been injured or placed in a cast. As used here, however, the term **cross training** means the development or maintenance of cardiovascular fitness by

Cross Training The development or maintenance of cardiovascular fitness by alternating between or concurrently training in two or more modalities.

Central Cardiovascular Adaptations Adaptations that occur in the heart and contribute to an increased ability to deliver oxygen.

Peripheral Cardiovascular Adaptations Adaptations that occur in the vasculature or the muscles that contribute to an increased ability to extract oxygen.

alternating between or concurrently training in two or more modalities. The interest in cross training comes from two primary sources. The first is the prevention of detraining in injured athletes, particularly those injuries associated with high-mileage running. The second is in the growth of multisport competitions such as biathlons and triathlons.

Theoretically, there is merit to the application of specificity and cross training to a training program. Any form of aerobic endurance exercise will affect both central and peripheral cardiorespiratory functioning. The central cardiovascular system is comprised of the heart and oxygen delivery components. **Central cardiovascular adaptations** are adaptations that occur in the heart and contribute to an increased ability to deliver oxygen. Central cardiovascular adaptations are the same regardless of modality provided the heart is stressed to the same extent. That is, central cardiovascular adaptations are the same regardless of whether the activity is running, skiing, or roller blading. Thus, many modalities can have the same overall training benefit by leading to central cardiovascular adaptations.

The peripheral cardiovascular system is involved in oxygen extraction in the musculature; and, which muscles are exercised does vary from modality to modality. **Peripheral cardiovascular adaptations** are adaptations that occur in the vasculature or the muscles that contribute to an increased ability to extract oxygen. Peripheral cardiovascular adaptations are specific to the modality and the specific muscles used in an exercise. For example, additional capillaries will be formed to carry oxygen to habitually active muscles but not to habitually inactive ones. Other factors within the exercising muscles such as mitochondrial density and enzyme activity will also impact upon the body's ability to reach a high $\dot{V}O_2$max. Specificity of modality operates because peripheral adaptations occur in the muscles that were trained. Thus, the specific activity—or closely related activities that mimic the muscle action of the primary sport—are needed to maximize peripheral adaptations. Examples of mimicking muscle action are side sliding or cycling for speed skating and water running in a flotation vest for jogging or running.

In one study endurance-trained runners were divided into three groups. One-third continued to train by running, one-third trained on a cycle ergometer, and one-third trained by deep water running. The intensity, frequency, and duration of workouts in each modality were equal. After six weeks, the $\dot{V}O_2max$ of all three groups had decreased slightly (approximately 4%), and performance in a 2-mi run had improved slightly (approximately 1%).[36] Thus, running performance was maintained by each of the modalities. On the other hand, arm ergometer training has not been shown to maintain training benefits derived from leg ergometer activity.[78] Apparently, then, the closer the activities are in terms of muscle action, the greater the potential benefit of cross training is.

Table 6.1 lists several situations, in addition to the maintenance of fitness when injured, where cross training may be beneficial.[60,75] Note that the multisport athlete may or may not be limited to the sports in which he or she is competing. For example, although a duathlete needs to train for both running and cycling, this training will have the benefits of both specificity and cross training. In addition, this athlete may also cross train by doing other activities such as roller blading or speed skating. Note also that cross training can be recommended at

TABLE 6.1 ■ Situations in Which Cross Training Is Beneficial

Reason	Fitness Participant	Competitive Athlete
Multisport participation		Preseason, in-season, off-season
Injury or rehabilitation; fitness maintenance	As needed	As needed
Inclement weather	As needed	As needed
Baseline or general conditioning	Always	Off-season
Recovery	After intense workout	After intense workout or competition
Prevention of boredom and burnout	Always	Active-rest phase

Source: Kibler & Chandler.[60]

any time for a fitness participant, but its value to a healthy competitive athlete is sporadic during the season and higher in the off-seasons.

Overload

Overload of the cardiovascular system is achieved by manipulating the intensity, duration, and frequency of the training bouts. These variables are easily remembered by the *FIT acronym* (F = frequency, I = intensity, and T = time or duration). However, as the most critical component, intensity will be discussed first.

Intensity   Intensity is very important in improving $\dot{V}O_2max$ both alone and in conjunction with duration. The intensity of an exercise may be described in relation to heart rate, oxygen consumption, or rating of perceived exertion (RPE). Laboratory studies typically use percentage $\dot{V}O_2max$, but heart rate and RPE are more practical for individuals anywhere. Fortunately, there is a direct relationship between heart rate and $\dot{V}O_2max$ responses, so the results from one can be applied to the other.

Figure 6.1a shows the relationship between change (Δ) in $\dot{V}O_2max$ and exercise intensity. At exercise levels greater than 100% (supramaximal exercise), where the amount of training decreases, improvement falls somewhat. Interval training, in which the individual alternates work and rest intervals, permits greater amounts of exercise to be completed at 90–100% $\dot{V}O_2max$ and, therefore, results in the greatest improvement in $\dot{V}O_2max$. However, the rate of improvement may be higher with continuous, nonstop effort. Adaptation at submaximal workloads is not as intensity-dependent.

Table 6.2 includes techniques used to classify intensity and suggested percentages for activity that varies from very light to very heavy.[82] Note that these percentages and classifications are intended to be used when the exercise duration is 20–60 minutes.

Heart Rate Methods.   Exercise intensity can be expressed either as a percentage of maximal heart rate (% HR max) or as a percentage of heart rate reserve (% HRR). Both techniques, which are explained in succeeding paragraphs, require that maximal heart rate be known or estimated. The

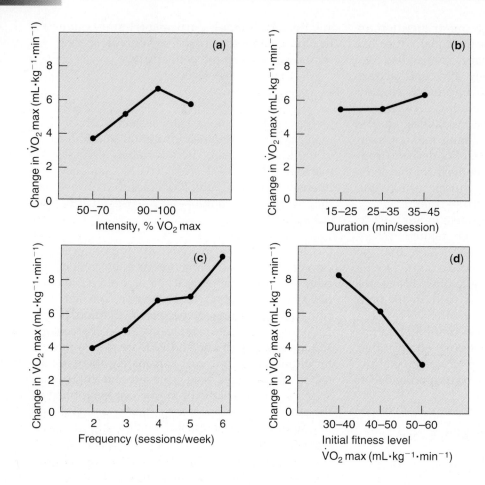

FIGURE 6.1

Changes in $\dot{V}O_2$max Based on Frequency, Intensity, and Duration of Training and on Initial Fitness Level

Source: H. A. Wenger and G. J. Bell. The interactions of intensity, frequency and duration of exercise training in altering cardiorespiratory fitness. *Sports Medicine.* 3:346–356 (1986). Reprinted by permission Adis International, Inc.

TABLE 6.2 ▪ Classification of Intensity of Exercise Based on 20 to 60 Minutes of Endurance Training

CLASSIFICATION OF INTENSITY	Relative Intensity		RATING OF PERCEIVED EXERTION
	% HR MAX	% $\dot{V}O_2$MAX OR % HRR	
Very light	35%	30%	10
Light	35–59%	30–49%	10–11
Moderate	60–79%	50–74%	12–13
Heavy	80–89%	75–84%	14–15
Very heavy	90%	85%	16

Source: M. L. Pollock & J. H. Wilmore. *Exercise in Health and Disease.* Philadelphia: Saunders (1990). Reprinted by permission.

methods are most accurate if the maximal heart rate is actually measured during a maximal graded exercise test. However, if such a test cannot be performed, maximal heart rate can be estimated by using the following general age-dependent formula:

(6.1a)   maximal heart rate (b · min⁻¹) = 220 − age (yr)

For obese individuals the following equation is more accurate:[68]

(6.1b)   maximal heart rate (b · min⁻¹) = 200 − [0.5 × age (yr)]

■ EXAMPLE

For a 28-yr-old female with a normal body composition, find her predicted or estimated HR max.

The calculation is

HR max = 220 − age = 220 − (28 yr) = 192 b · min⁻¹

If the female is obese, her estimated maximal heart rate is

HR max = 200 − (0.5 × age) = 200 − (0.5 × 28 yr)
= 186 b · min⁻¹

Because these values are estimated values, based on population averages, there will be wide variability. The estimated value may either overestimate or underestimate the true HR max by as much as 10–12 b · min⁻¹.[68]   ■

Once a maximal heart rate is available, the % HR max may be calculated as follows:

1. Determine the desired intensity of the workout.
2. Use Table 6.2 to find the % HR max associated with the desired exercise intensity.
3. Multiply the percentages (as decimals) times the HR max.

■ EXAMPLE

Determine the target HR training range for the non-obese 28-yr-old woman in the previous example who wants to perform a moderate workout.

1. Since the desired intensity for this example is a moderate workout, you would consult Table 6.2 and determine that a moderate workout ranges from 60–79% HR max.
2. Multiply the percentages (as decimals) times the HR max.

maximal heart rate (b · min⁻¹)	192	192
desired intensity (decimal)	× .6	× .79
target training range (to closest b · min⁻¹)	115	152

Thus a HR of 115 b · min⁻¹ represents 60% of HR max and a HR of 152 b · min⁻¹ represents 79% of HR max. So, in order to be exercising between 60 and 79% of HR max, which represents a moderate workload, this individual should keep her heart rate between 115 and 152 b · min⁻¹.   ■

It is always best to provide the potential exerciser with a target range rather than just a lower threshold heart rate. In fact, the term *threshold* may be a misnomer since no particular percentage has been shown to be a minimally necessary threshold stimulus for all individuals in all situations.[50] Additionally, a range allows for the heart rate drift that occurs in exercise after about 30 min and for variations in weather, terrain, fluid replacement and other influences on the individual. The upper limit can serve as a boundary against overexertion.

Alternatively, a target heart rate range can be calculated as a percentage of heart rate reserve (% HRR). This technique of calculating training heart rate is also called the *Karvonen method*. It involves a little more mathematics but has the added advantage of taking resting heart rate into consideration. The steps are as follows:

1. Determine the heart rate reserve (HRR) by subtracting the resting heart rate from the maximal heart rate.

(6.2)   Heart rate reserve (b · min⁻¹) = maximal heart rate (b · min⁻¹) − resting heart rate (b · min⁻¹)

or   HRR = HR max − RHR

The resting heart rate is best determined when the individual is truly resting, such as immediately upon awakening in the morning. Heart rates taken prior to an exercise test are anticipatory, not resting, and will be abnormally high.

2. Determine the desired intensity of the workout.

3. Use Table 6.2 to find the % HRR associated with the desired exercise intensity.

4. Multiply the percentages (as decimals) for the upper and lower exercise limits by the HRR.

5. Add RHR to these numbers.

■ EXAMPLE

Determine the appropriate HR range for a moderate workout for a 28-year-old using the HRR method; assuming a RHR of 80 b·min⁻¹.

1. Determine the (HRR):

$$192 \text{ b·min}^{-1} - 80 \text{ b·min}^{-1} = 112 \text{ b·min}^{-1}$$

2. Determine the desired intensity of the workout. Again, using Table 6.2, 50–74% of HRR corresponds to a moderate workout. This reinforces the point that the % HR max does not equal % HRR.

3. Multiply the percentages (as decimals) for the upper and lower exercise limits by the HRR. Thus:

HRR	112	112
desired intensity (decimal)	× .5	× .74
	56	83

4. Add RHR as follows:

target HR training range (b·min⁻¹)	56	83
	+ 80	+ 80
	136	163

Thus, a HR of 136 b·min⁻¹ represents 50% of HRR and a HR of 163 b·min⁻¹ represents 74% of HRR. So, in order to be exercising between 50 and 74% of HRR, which represents a moderate workload, this individual should keep her heart rate between 136 and 163 b·min⁻¹. ■

This heart rate range (136–163 b·min⁻¹), although still moderate, is different from the one calculated by using % HR max because of the influence of resting the heart rate.

Work through the problem presented in Box 6.1, paying careful attention to the influence of resting heart rate in determining the training heart rate range when using the Karvonen method.

Box 6.1 A Question of Understanding

Calculate the target HR range for a light workout for two individuals, using the % HR max and % HRR methods and the following information.

	Age	RHR
Lisa	50	62
Susie	50	82

Since maximal heart rate is age-dependent, declining in a rectilinear fashion with advancing age, the heart rate, calculated by either the maximal heart rate or heart rate reserve method, needed to achieve a given intensity level will decrease with age. Figure 6.2 exemplifies these decreases for light, moderate, and heavy exercise using the percent of heart rate reserve method.

FIGURE 6.2

Age-Related Changes in Training Heart Rate Ranges Based on the Karvonen Method

Note: Calculations are based on RHR = 80 b·min⁻¹, HR max = 220 – age.

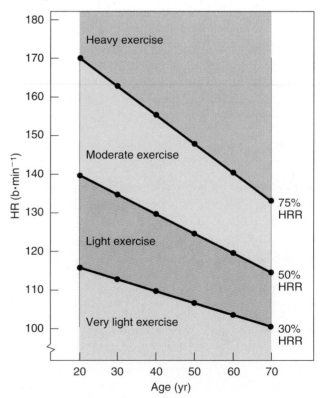

Oxygen Consumption/% $\dot{V}O_2$max Methods. In a laboratory setting where an individual has been tested for $\dot{V}O_2$max and equipment is available for monitoring $\dot{V}O_2$ during training bouts, any selected % $\dot{V}O_2$max may be used directly based on desired intensity. The following steps are used to calculate training intensity using this method.

1. Determine the desired intensity of the workout.

2. Use Table 6.2 to find the % $\dot{V}O_2$max associated with the desired exercise intensity.

3. Multiply the percentage (as a decimal) of the desired intensity times the $\dot{V}O_2$max.

4. Because oxygen drifts, as does heart rate, the load will probably have to be adjusted to a lower workload if exercise continues for longer than 30 minutes. Set values (e.g., 70%), instead of ranges, are typically used in this situation.

■ EXAMPLE

Determine the $\dot{V}O_2$ that corresponds to a moderate workout intensity for an individual with a $\dot{V}O_2$max of 43 ml·kg^{-1}·min^{-1}.

1. Based on Table 6.2 it is determined that a moderate workout corresponds to 50–74% of $\dot{V}O_2$max. For this example, we have selected 70% of $\dot{V}O_2$max.

2. Multiply the percentage (as a decimal) times the $\dot{V}O_2$max.

$\dot{V}O_2$max (ml·kg^{-1}·min^{-1}).	43
desired intensity	× .7
target training intensity (ml·kg·min^{-1})	30

Thus, this individual would work at a workload that elicited an oxygen consumption of approximately 30 ml·kg^{-1}·min^{-1} in order to achieve a moderate workout. If the workout is to continue for more than 30 minutes the workload may be adjusted downward. ■

Basing the intensity of a workout on % $\dot{V}O_2$max is not a very practical option since most do not have access to the needed equipment. However, the technique is modifiable for individuals who wish to use it.

Look closely again at Table 6.2. Note that the column for % $\dot{V}O_2$max is also the column for % HRR. That is, any given % HRR represents an equivalent % $\dot{V}O_2$max. Thus, an individual who is working at 50% HRR is also working at 50% $\dot{V}O_2$max. Therefore, heart rate can be used to indicate oxygen consumption when an individual is training or competing.

Research indicates that the % HRR/%$\dot{V}O_2$max relationship holds for the weight-bearing activities of treadmill running, simulated skiing, and stair-stepping but not aerobic dance. The relationship also does not hold for non-weight-bearing modalities such as arm and leg ergometry and rowing.[64,76]

Table 6.3 provides information on how long running can be continued at a specific percentage of maximal oxygen consumption. Boxes 6.2 and 6.3 provide two examples of how this information (Table 6.2) can be used in training and in a running competition. Take the time now to work through the situations described in the boxes.

Rating of Perceived Exertion Methods. The third way that intensity can be prescribed is based on the RPE scales, which are given in Table 6.4.[10] The RPE response to graded exercise corresponds closely to cardiovascular and metabolic variables and is considered a valid and reliable indicator of the level of exertion during steady-state exercise.[3] The 6–19 scale on the left in the table is most frequently used in exercise prescription; the values that correspond to % HR max, % HRR, or % $\dot{V}O_2$max are provided in Table 6.4.

The classification of exercise intensity and the corresponding relationships between % HR max, % $\dot{V}O_2$max, % HRR, and RPE presented in Table 6.2 have been derived from and are intended for use

TABLE 6.3 ■ Time a Selected % $\dot{V}O_2$max Can Be Sustained During Running

% $\dot{V}O_2$MAX	TIME (MIN)
100	8–10
97.5	15
90	30
87.5	45
85	60
82.5	90
80	120–210

Source: Daniels & Gilbert.[24]

Box 6.2 A Question of Understanding

Four friends from work meet at the track for a noon time workout. The physiological characteristics are as follows. (The estimated $\dot{V}O_2$max values have been calculated from a 1-mi running test.)

Individual	Age (yr)	Estimated $\dot{V}O_2$max mL·kg⁻¹·min⁻¹	Resting HR (b·min⁻¹)
Janet	23	52	60
Jeff	35	64	48
Mark	22	49	64
Gail	28	56	58

The following oxygen requirements have been calculated for a given speed based on the equations that are presented in Appendix B.

Speed (mph)	Oxygen Requirement (mL·kg⁻¹·min⁻¹)
5	30.3
6	35.7
7	41.0
8	46.4
9	51.7
10	57.1

The friends wish to do a moderate workout and run together. Assume temperate weather conditions.

1. At what speed should they be running?
2. What heart rate should be achieved by each runner at that pace?

Check your answers with the ones provided at the end of the chapter.

with land-based activities in moderate environments. The relationships between RPE and % HR max and RPE and % $\dot{V}O_2$max are more variable for different modalities than the relationship between % HR max and % $\dot{V}O_2$max, but not enough to invalidate the use of RPE.[94] In addition, exercise in a hot environment alters the relationship among HR, $\dot{V}O_2$max, and RPE. For instance, HR is higher for a given $\dot{V}O_2$ or RPE when exercise is performed in hot environments.

Box 6.3 A Question of Understanding

Pat plans to run the 10-km run at the Corn Fest. Her estimated $\dot{V}O_2$max from the PACER test is 48 mL·kg⁻¹·min⁻¹. Other pertinent physiological characteristics for Pat follow.

Body weight	145 lb (65.9 kg)
Resting heart rate	62 b·min⁻¹
Age	33 yr
Finishing time goal	45–69 min

Pat owns and will be wearing a heart rate monitor. What heart rate range should she aim for (assuming reasonable weather conditions) to allow her to achieve her target time?

For activities performed in water, postural and pressure changes shift the blood volume centrally and necessitate adjustments in blood pressure, cardiac output, resistance, and respiration. Although there is a large variation among individuals in the magnitude of change in the cardiovascular system, the most consistent changes are lower submaximal HR (8–12 b·min⁻¹) at any given $\dot{V}O_2$, a lower HR max, and a lower $\dot{V}O_2$max when exercise is performed in the water. A greater reliance on anaerobic metabolism is evident, and the RPE is higher at the same workload used on land.[93] The lower HR is probably a compensation for the increased stroke volume that occurs when blood is shifted centrally. As a result, the HR prescription should be about 10% lower for water workouts than for land-based workouts. Thus, if an individual would normally work out at 75% HR max on land, the prescription for an equivalent workout in the water should be 65% HR max. This change should effectively reduce the RPE as well.

Regardless of the method chosen to prescribe exercise intensity, it is important to consider three factors.

1. Exercise intensity should generally be prescribed within a range regardless of the method used (the exception to this being steady-state exercise that is performed while $\dot{V}O_2$ is being

TABLE 6.4 ■ Scales for Ratings of Perceived Exertion

ORIGINAL RPE SCALE		NEW RATIO RPE SCALE	
6		0	Nothing at all
7	Very, very light	0.5	Very, very weak
		1	Very weak
8		2	Weak
9	Very light	3	Moderate
10		4	Somewhat strong
11	Fairly light	5	Strong
12		6	
13	Somewhat hard	7	Very Strong
		8	
14		9	
15	Hard	10	Very, very strong
16			Maximal
17	Very hard		
18			
19	Very, very hard		

Source: Borg.[10]

monitored). Many activities will require different levels of exertion throughout the activity. This is particularly true of games and athletic activities, but it also applies to activities like jogging and bicycling where changes in terrain can greatly affect exertion. In addition, a range allows for the cardiovascular drift that occurs during prolonged exercise.

2. Exercise intensity must be considered in conjunction with duration and frequency.
   a. Intensity cannot be prescribed without regard to duration. These two variables are inversely related: In general, the more intense an activity is, the shorter its duration should be.
   b. The appropriate intensity of exercise also depends on the fitness level of the individual and, to some extent, on the point the individual has reached in his or her fitness program. Individuals should begin an exercise program at a low exercise intensity and grad-

ually increase intensity until the desired level is achieved.

3. Using heart rate or perceived exertion to monitor training sessions, rather than merely time over distance, allows the influence of weather, terrain, and surfaces and the way the individual is responding to be taken into account in the assessment of adaptation to a training program.

Duration As shown in Figure 6.1b, improvements in $\dot{V}O_2$max can be achieved when exercise is sustained for durations of 15–45 min.[97] Slightly greater improvements are achieved from the longer sessions (35–45 min) than from shorter sessions (either 15–25 or 25–35 min). Indeed, greater improvements in $\dot{V}O_2$max can be achieved if the sessions are long (35–45 min) and the intensity low (50–90%) than if the sessions are short (25–35 min) and the intensity high (90–100%). Apparently, the total volume of work done is more important in determining cardiorespiratory adaptations than either intensity or duration of the exercise considered individually. This is good news, since the risk of injury is lower in low-intensity, long-duration activity than in high-intensity, short-duration activity; and the compliance rate is higher. Thus, most adults' fitness programs should emphasize moderate- to heavy-intensity workouts (60–90% HR max; 50–85% HRR or $\dot{V}O_2$max) for a duration of 20–60 min.[2]

This does not mean that exercise sessions of less than 20 min are not valuable either in terms of $\dot{V}O_2$max or health benefit, or that the 20 min must be accumulated during one exercise session. An accumulation of 30 min of activity spread throughout the day may be sufficient to achieve health benefits. For example, two groups of adult males participated in a walk-jog program at 65–75% HR max, for five days per week for eight weeks.[27] The only variation between the groups was that one did the 30-min workout continuously and the other participated in 10-min sessions at three different times throughout the day. Both groups increased their $\dot{V}O_2$max significantly (although the 30-min consecutive group did so to a greater extent) and lost equal amounts of weight— an important health benefit.

Thus, for the individual who claims he or she does not have time to exercise, the suggestion of a 10-min walk in the morning (perhaps to work or taking the kids to school), at noon (to a favorite restaurant and back), and in the evening (perhaps walking home from work or taking the kids for a walk) might make it easier for the person to achieve a total of 30 min of activity. Once again, some activity is better than no activity, especially if the goal is health benefits rather than improved performance.

A recognition of the benefit of split sessions is particularly important for those in a rehabilitation program and for children. The injured person may simply not be able to exercise for a long period of time, but short bouts may be possible if they are spread throughout the day. Children tend to be sporadic exercisers by nature, and getting them to exercise continuously for 20 min is often difficult.[18] Since many elementary schools only have physical education classes scheduled for 20 min, a program of running for 20 min would mean the children would do nothing else, which is not pedagogically sound. Thus, some portion of each class should be devoted to fitness development, and the children should be encouraged to be active outside school.

Frequency   If the total work done or the number of exercise sessions is held constant, there is basically no difference in the improvement of $\dot{V}O_2$max over 2, 3, 4, or 5 days.[81] However, when these conditions are not adhered to, there does seem to be an advantage to more frequent training. As seen in Figure 6.1c, the improvement in $\dot{V}O_2$max is proportional to the number of training sessions per week.[97] In general, training less than 2 days per week does not result in improvements in $\dot{V}O_2$max. Likewise, further improvement in $\dot{V}O_2$max is not meaningful if exercise participation is increased from 4 to 5 days a week. Although there is the potential for further improvement in $\dot{V}O_2$max if a 6th day of training is added, a 6th day is not generally recommended for those pursuing fitness goals because of a higher incidence of injury and fatigue. The optimal frequency for all intensities appears to be 4 days per week.

The ACSM recommendation for healthy individuals is a frequency of 3–5 days per week. However, individuals with very low fitness levels may wish to start a program of only 2 days per week if they are attempting to meet the ACSM intensity and duration guidelines or to be active daily in less-intense and shorter-duration bouts of exercise. Athletes in training may feel compelled to train 6 days per week as a way of increasing the total training volume. In this case "easy" and "hard" days should be interspersed. Cross training may also be employed.

Individualization

Fitness programs should be individualized to the participant. Not only will individual goals vary, but also individuals will respond to and adapt to exercise differently. One of the major determinants of the individual's response is genetics, which was discussed in Chapter 3. Another major determinant is initial fitness level. Figure 6.1d clearly shows that independent of frequency, intensity, or duration, the greatest improvements in $\dot{V}O_2$max occur in the those individuals with the lowest initial-fitness level. Thus, both absolute and relative increases in $\dot{V}O_2$max are inversely related to initial fitness level. Although improvements in $\dot{V}O_2$max are smallest in highly fit individuals, at this level small changes may have a significant influence on performance (that is, many athletic events are won by fractions of a second).

The initial fitness level generalization also applies to health benefits. Health benefits are greatest when a person moves from a low-fitness to a moderately fit category. This progress can be accomplished by most sedentary individuals if they participate in a regular, low-to-moderate–endurance exercise program.[50]

Adaptation

Adaptation can be categorized into several stages. The initial stage usually lasts four to six weeks, although this duration varies considerably among individuals. This stage should include low-level aerobic activities that cause a minimum of muscle soreness or discomfort. In fact, it is often prudent to begin an exercise program at an intensity lower than the desired exercise range. The duration of the aerobic exercise session should be at least 10 min and should gradually be increased. For individuals with very low levels of fitness a discontinuous training program may be warranted, wherein the individual completes several repetitions of exercise, each lasting 2–5 min.[3] Frequency may vary from short, light daily activity to longer exercise sessions two or three times per week.

Adaptation has occurred when the same amount of work can be accomplished in less time, when the same amount of work can be accomplished with less physiological disruption, when the same amount of work can be accomplished with a lower perception of fatigue or exertion, or when more work can be accomplished. During the improvement stage of a training program, significant improvements in physiological function indicate that the body is adapting to the stress of the training program. When adaptation occurs, the individual must increase his or her workload in order to continue to improve.

Progression

Once adaptation occurs, the workload must be increased if further improvement is desired. The workload can be increased by manipulating the frequency, intensity, and duration of the exercise. Increasing any of these variables will effectively increase the volume of exercise and will thus provide the overload necessary for further adaptation. The rate of progression depends on the individual's needs or goals, fitness level, health status, and age.

The improvement stage of a training program typically lasts for four to five months and is characterized by more rapid progression: Intensity is increased to the target level and duration is increased consistently every two to three weeks.[3] For an individual with a low fitness level the progression from a discontinuous activity to a continuous activity should occur first. Then the duration of the activity should be increased to 20–30 min. Frequency can then be increased. Intensity should be the last variable to be increased.

The principles of adaptation and progression are intertwined. Adaptation and progression may repeat themselves several times until the desired level of fitness or performance is achieved. Each time an exercise program is modified, there will be a period of adaptation that may be followed by further progression if desired.

Maintenance

Athletes tend to vary their training levels according to an active rest phase, off-season, preseason, and in-season schedule, with the active rest and in-season phases being the times when they can shift to a maintenance schedule. For the rehabilitation or fitness participant, maintenance typically begins after the first six months of training. Achieving the maintenance stage indicates that the individual has reached a personally acceptable level of cardiorespiratory fitness and is no longer interested in increasing the conditioning load.[3]

Once a desired level of aerobic fitness has been attained, this level can be maintained by either continuing the same volume of exercise or by decreasing the volume of training, as long as intensity is maintained. Figure 6.3 shows the results of research that investigated changes in $\dot{V}O_2$max with 10 weeks of relatively intense interval training and a subsequent 15-week reduction in training frequency (6.3a), duration (6.3b), or intensity (6.3c).[53,54,55] When training frequency was reduced from 6 days per week to 4 or 2 days per week and intensity and duration were held constant, training-induced improvements in $\dot{V}O_2$max were maintained. Similarly, when training duration was reduced from 40 to 26 or 13 min, improvements in $\dot{V}O_2$max were maintained. However, when intensity was reduced by two-thirds, improvements in $\dot{V}O_2$max were not maintained. These results indicate that intensity plays a primary role in maintaining cardiovascular fitness. Thus, although total volume of exercise is important in the attainment of a given fitness level, intensity is important in the maintenance of the achieved fitness level. During the maintenance phase of a training program, cross training becomes particularly beneficial, especially on days when a high-intensity workout is not called for.

Retrogression/Plateau/Reversibility

At one or more points in the training process an individual will fail to improve (plateau) or will exhibit a performance or physiological decrement (retrogression), despite progression of the training program. When a pattern of nonimprovement occurs, it is important to check for other signs of overtraining (see Chapter 1). A shift of training emphasis or the inclusion of more easy days is then warranted. Remember that a reduction in the frequency of training does not necessarily lead to detraining and may actually enhance performance.

If training is discontinued for any reason, detraining will occur. This principle, often referred to as the *reversibility concept*, holds that when a training

FIGURE 6.3

Effects of Reducing Exercise Frequency, Intensity, and Duration on Maintenance of $\dot{V}O_2$max

(a) improvements in $\dot{V}O_2$max during 10 weeks of training (bicycling and running) for 40 minutes a day, 6 days a week were maintained when training intensity and duration were maintained, but the frequency was reduced from 6 days a week to 4 or even 2 days per week. (b) $\dot{V}O_2$max was maintained when frequency of training and intensity were maintained, but training duration was reduced to 13 minutes. $\dot{V}O_2$max continued to improve when training duration was reduced to 26 minutes. (c) $\dot{V}O_2$max was maintained when frequency and duration were maintained and intensity was reduced by one-third. $\dot{V}O_2$max was not maintained when training was reduced by two-thirds.

Source: Hickson & Rosenkoetter[53]; Hickson et al.[54]; Hickson et al.[55]

program is stopped or reduced, the bodily systems readjust in accordance with the decreased physiological stimuli. Increases in $\dot{V}O_2$max with low- to moderate-exercise programs are completely reversed when training is stopped. Values of $\dot{V}O_2$max decrease rapidly during a month of detraining, followed by a slower rate of decline during the second and third month.[9]

Figures 6.4a–6.4d depict the time course for detraining for several cardiovascular variables in highly trained individuals who became sedentary. Notice that there is a decline in $\dot{V}O_2$max by almost 15% during the 84 days of detraining. However, this study did not measure $\dot{V}O_2$max before training; thus, we cannot conclude that $\dot{V}O_2$max returned to baseline values (as happens with low to moderate levels of training). In fact, the $\dot{V}O_2$max of these previously highly trained individuals was significantly higher following 84 days of detraining (50.8 mL · kg^{-1} · min^{-1}) than the $\dot{V}O_2$max of age matched untrained individuals (43.3 mL · kg^{-1} · min^{-1}).[19] The stroke volume and cardiac output of the trained subjects decreased during the 84 days of detraining (Figures 6.4c and 6.4d), reaching values that were similar to those for untrained individuals.

The higher $\dot{V}O_2$max in detrained athletes than in untrained subjects is due to an augmented ability of the muscles to extract oxygen, as evidenced by a greater capillary density in the trained athletes than

1st week & 3 weeks later have the most decreased VO2 max.

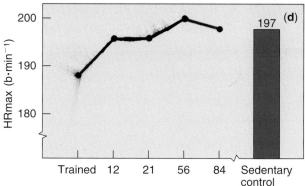

FIGURE 6.4

Effects of Detraining on Highly Conditioned Athletes

Source: E. F. Coyle, W. H. Martin, D. R. Sinacore, M. J. Joymer, J. M. Hagberg, & J. O. Holloszy. Time course of loss of adaptations after stopping prolonged intense endurance training. *Journal of Applied Physiology.* 57:1857–1864 (1984). Reprinted by permission.

in the sedentary controls. The reduction of stroke volume observed with detraining is largely a result of reduced blood volume, which occurs with detraining, and not a deterioration of heart function.[20] The cardiovascular changes with detraining appear to be the same for males and females.[29]

Warm-Up and Cool-Down

A warm-up period allows the body to adjust to the cardiovascular demands of exercise. At rest the skeletal muscles receive about 15–20% of the blood pumped from the heart; during moderate exercise they receive approximately 70% of cardiac output. This increased blood flow is important in warming the body since the blood carries heat from the metabolically active muscle to the rest of the body.

A warm-up period of 5–10 min should precede the conditioning portion of an exercise session.[3] The warm-up should gradually increase in intensity until the desired intensity of training is achieved. For many activities the warm-up period simply continues into the aerobic portion of the exercise session. For example, if an individual is going for a noontime run and wants to run at an 8-min-mi pace, he may begin with a slow jog for the first few minutes (say a 10-min-mi pace), increase to a faster pace (say a 9-min-mi pace), and then proceed into the desired pace (the 8-min-mi pace).

A warm-up period has the following beneficial effects on cardiovascular function.

- It increases blood flow to the active skeletal muscles.
- It increases blood flow to the myocardium.
- It increases the dissociation of oxyhemoglobin.
- It leads to earlier sweating, which plays a role in temperature regulation.
- It may reduce the incidence of abnormal rhythms in the conduction system of the heart

(arrhythmias), which can lead to abnormal heart function.[6]

The cool-down period should follow the conditioning period of the exercise session. The primary cardiovascular advantage to a cool-down period is that it prevents venous pooling and thus reduces the risk of fainting by keeping the muscle pump active when the venous system is dilated immediately after strenuous exercise.

Cardiovascular Adaptations to Endurance Training

Regular physical activities result in improvements in cardiovascular function, which is most readily demonstrated by an increase in the functional capacity of the cardiovascular system (that is,

an increase in $\dot{V}O_2max$). The magnitude of the improvement is determined by the training program—specifically by the frequency, intensity, and duration of the exercise and the initial-fitness status of the individual. Changes in cardiovascular function are evident at rest, during submaximal exercise, and during maximal exercise.

Figure 6.5 provides an overview of the cardiovascular system with numbers added to indicate sites where cardiovascular adaptations occur as a result of endurance training. The following subsections refer to that numerical sequence.

Cardiac Dimensions (1a)

Cardiac dimensions and mass increase with endurance training.[58,59,65] These changes are associated with high cardiac outputs during sustained dynamic aerobic exercise. Endurance training ex-

FIGURE 6.5

Sites of Cardiovascular Adaptations to Endurance Training

2 Blood volume

Venous system

RA

LA

RV

LV

Arterial system

4 $\dot{V}O_2max$

5 BP

1a Cardiac dimensions

1b Coronary blood flow

3a $\dot{Q}$

3b SV

3c HR

8 RPP

6 Total peripheral resistance

7 Muscle blood flow

Capillaries

poses the heart to conditions of increased ventricular filling, with subsequent high stroke volume and cardiac output. This chronic exposure to high levels of ventricular filling (large left ventricular end–diastolic volume) is known as *volume overload*.[71] Chronic volume overload results in an increased left ventricular end–diastolic diameter[58,59] and left ventricular mass.[12,65]

Coronary Blood Flow (1b)

Endurance training results in an increase in the size of the coronary vascular bed.[8] This increase in capillarization may be related to an increase in heart weight as a result of training.[86] Although there is some evidence that exercise training can lead to the development of *coronary collateral circulation,* defined as the ability to supply areas of the myocardium with blood through small new growth anastomoses, this finding is suspect in humans.[13,32,37] There is better evidence that coronary collateral circulation is caused by myocardial hypoxia that occurs with coronary artery disease.[101] One of the difficulties in determining the extent to which exercise training affects coronary collateral circulation is the inability to distinguish the effects of disease states and a sedentary lifestyle.

The internal diameter of the coronary arteries also may be increased by endurance training. Several studies (including the classic autopsy report of Clarence DeMar, winner of seven Boston marathons) have shown that habitual exercise is related to a larger cross-sectional arterial size. DeMar's arteries were reportedly two to three times normal size.[23] Conversely, a study that compared ultramarathoners with sedentary individuals did not show any difference in the internal diameter of the coronary arteries in the two groups at rest.[51] However, the capacity of the coronary arteries to dilate was two times greater in the marathoners than in the sedentary individuals (13.2 mm^2 versus 6 mm^2). The ability to dilate arteries while exercising may be even more important than the resting diameter, since the myocardial demand for oxygen is low during rest and high during exercise, as evidenced by the low rate-pressure product (RPP) seen at rest and the high RPP during exercise.

Blood Volume (2)

Blood volume increases as a result of endurance training. Highly trained endurance athletes have a 20–25% larger blood volume than untrained subjects. The increase in blood volume is primarily due to an expansion of plasma volume. This training-induced increase in blood volume has been reported for both males and females and appears to be independent of age.[15] Changes in plasma volume occur soon after the initiation of an endurance training program, with changes between 8 and 10% occurring within the first week,[14] followed by a plateauing of plasma volume. For up to ten days of training an expansion of plasma volume accounts for changes in blood volume, with little or no change in red blood cell mass.[14,15]

Tests of hematocrit and hemoglobin concentration during this time period are often low, since the red blood cells and hemoglobin are diluted by the larger plasma volume. At times this condition has been labeled as *sports anemia,* but this term is a misnomer, since the number of red blood cells is the same or may actually be increased above pretraining levels. Thus, this condition represents no reason for alarm and may be beneficial. The lower hematocrit as a result of elevated plasma volume and normal or slightly elevated number of red blood cells means that the blood is less viscous, which decreases resistance to flow and facilitates the transportation of oxygen.

After one month of training the increase in blood volume is distributed more equally between increases in plasma volume and red blood cell mass.[15,16] Blood volume and plasma volume return to pretraining levels when exercise is discontinued. Figure 6.6 depicts these changes in blood volume, plasma volume, and red blood cell volume during eight days of exercise training and after seven days of cessation of exercise.

Cardiac Output (3a)

Resting cardiac output is not changed following a training program; however, it is achieved by a larger stroke volume and a lower heart rate.[85] Cardiac output at an absolute submaximal workload is decreased or unchanged with training.[4,69] Maximal cardiac output is increased at maximal levels of exercise following an endurance exercise training program (Figure 6.7a). The increase in cardiac output seen at maximal exercise is the result of an increase in stroke volume, since maximal heart rate does not change with training. The magnitude of the increase

FIGURE 6.6

Changes in Blood Volume as a Result of Training and Detraining

Source: V. A. Convertino, P. J. Brock, L. C. Keil, E. M. Bernauer, & J. E. Greenleaf. Exercise training-induced hypervolemia: Role of plasma albumin, renin, and vasopressin. *Journal of Applied Physiology.* 48:665–669 (1980). Reprinted by permission.

depends on the level of training. Elite endurance athletes may have cardiac output values in excess of $35 \text{ L} \cdot \text{min}^{-1}$.

Stroke Volume (3b)

As shown in Figure 6.7b, endurance training results in an increased stroke volume at rest, during submaximal exercise, and during maximal exercise. The increase in stroke volume results from increased plasma volume, increased cardiac dimensions, increased venous return, and an enhanced ability of the ventricle to stretch and accommodate increased venous return.[69,90] Since several of these are structural changes, they will exert their influence whether the individual is resting or working.

It has traditionally been assumed that the pattern of stroke volume response during incremental work to maximum, described as an initial rectilinear rise that plateaus at about 40–50% of $\dot{V}O_2$max, was similar regardless of training status. However, as shown in Figure 6.8, evidence now suggests that stroke volume does not plateau in *highly trained* ($68.6 \text{ mL} \cdot \text{kg}^{-1} \cdot \text{min}^{-1}$) endurance athletes.[42] Enhanced ventricular filling (increased LVEDV) and emptying (decreased LVESV) both contribute to the augmented stroke volume in these highly trained athletes, although ventricular filling appears to have the greater influence.

Heart Rate (3c)

Resting heart rate is lower following endurance training (Figure 6.7c). Although **bradycardia** is technically defined as a resting heart rate of less than 60 $\text{b} \cdot \text{min}^{-1}$, the term is sometimes used to mean the reduction in resting heart rate that occurs as a result of exercise training. Bradycardia is one of the classic and most easily assessed indicators of training adaptation. The heart rate response to an absolute submaximal amount of work is significantly reduced following endurance training. Maximal heart rate is unchanged or slightly decreased (2–3 $\text{b} \cdot \text{min}^{-1}$) with endurance training.[34,85]

Bradycardia A heart rate less than 60 $\text{b} \cdot \text{min}^{-1}$.

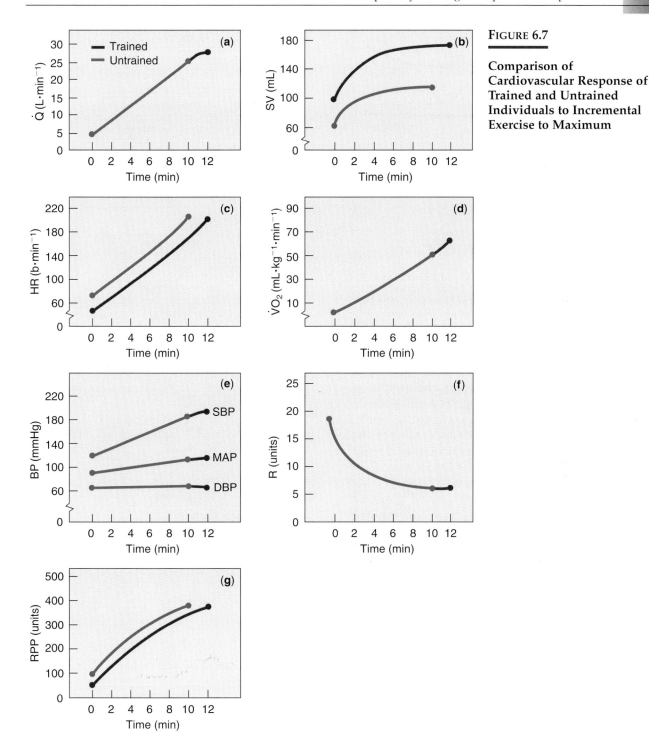

FIGURE 6.7

Comparison of Cardiovascular Response of Trained and Untrained Individuals to Incremental Exercise to Maximum

Maximal Oxygen Consumption (4)

Maximal oxygen consumption ($\dot{V}O_2$max) increases as a result of endurance training (Figure 6.7d). The magnitude of the increase depends upon the type of program followed. Improvements of 5–30% are commonly reported, with improvements of 15% routinely found for training programs that meet the

FIGURE 6.8

Stroke Volume Response in Trained and Untrained Subjects

Source: N. Gledill, D. Cox, & R. Jamnik. Endurance athletes' stroke volume does not plateau: Major advantage is diastolic function. *Medicine and Science in Sports and Exercise.* 26:1116–1121 (1994). Modified and reprinted by permission of Williams & Wilkins.

recommendations of the ACSM.[2] There are rapid improvements in $\dot{V}O_2$max during the first two months of an endurance training program. Following this period, improvements continue to occur, but at a slower rate. This pattern appears to be independent of gender and is consistent over a wide age range, although elderly individuals may take longer to adapt to endurance training.[2,21,87]

The improvement in $\dot{V}O_2$max is the result of central and peripheral cardiovascular adaptations. Recall that $\dot{V}O_2$max can be calculated as the product of cardiac output and arteriovenous oxygen difference (a-vO_2 diff) (equation 4.14b). Increased maximal cardiac output as a result of endurance training was discussed in a previous subsection, and it represents a central adaptation that supports the training-induced improvement in $\dot{V}O_2$max. The a-vO_2 diff reflects oxygen extraction by the working tissue and thus represents a peripheral adaptation that supports the improvement in $\dot{V}O_2$max (see Chapter 3). The changes in cardiac output are a more consistent training adaptation than the changes in a-vO_2 diff.

Figure 6.9 presents a compilation of data regarding $\dot{V}O_2$max of various athletic groups.[99] Several conclusions can be drawn from this graph. First, even in the athletic population the male-female difference is maintained, with males generally having a greater $\dot{V}O_2$max than females. Second, there is considerable variability in $\dot{V}O_2$max among

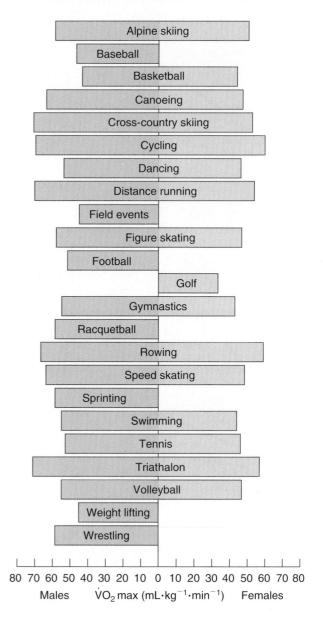

FIGURE 6.9

Average $\dot{V}O_2$max of Male and Female Athletes in Selected Sports

Source: Based on data from Wilmore & Costill.[99]

athletes. Third, $\dot{V}O_2$max is related to the demands of the sport. Athletes whose performance depends on the ability of the cardiovascular system to sustain dynamic exercise consistently have higher $\dot{V}O_2$max values than athletes whose sport performance is based primarily on motor skills, such as baseball. What is unclear from Figure 6.9 is the relative influence of genetics and training in determining an individual's $\dot{V}O_2$max. Genetics sets the upper limit on the $\dot{V}O_2$max that can ultimately be achieved by any individual. Thus, although all individuals are able to increase $\dot{V}O_2$max with training, an individual with a greater genetic potential is more likely to excel at sports that require a high $\dot{V}O_2$max. Furthermore, individuals differ in their sensitivity to training, in part because of different genetic makeup.[11]

Blood Pressure (5)

As indicated in Figure 6.7e and as most studies report, there is little or no change in arterial blood pressure (SBP, DBP, MAP) at rest, during submaximal exercise, or during maximal exercise in normotensive individuals following an endurance training program.[87] However, because the maximal amount of work that can be done increases with exercise training, a trained individual is capable of doing more work. Thus maximal systolic blood pressure may be higher for this individual at maximal exercise. This difference is usually small between sedentary and normally fit individuals.

Total Peripheral Resistance (6)

Resistance is unchanged at rest or during an absolute submaximal workload following a training program (Figure 6.7f). However, a further reduction in total peripheral resistance occurs in athletes at maximal exercise. For this reason, athletes can generate significantly higher cardiac outputs at similar arterial pressures during maximal exercise. Much of the additional decrease in the total peripheral resistance at maximal exercise is due to the increased capillarization of the skeletal muscle.[8]

Muscle Blood Flow (7)

Muscle blood flow is unchanged at rest following exercise training. Active muscle blood flow increases during maximal exercise as a result of endurance training. The effect of endurance training on muscle blood flow at submaximal levels is unclear.[4]

Rate-Pressure Product (8)

Myocardial oxygen consumption, indicated by the rate-pressure product, is lower at rest and during

TABLE 6.5 ■ Cardiovascular Adaptations to Dynamic Aerobic Exercise

	REST	ABSOLUTE SUBMAXIMAL EXERCISE	MAXIMAL EXERCISE
$\dot{Q}$	Unchanged	Decreased or unchanged	Increased
SV	Increased	Increased	Increased
HR	Decreased	Decreased	Unchanged
SBP	Little or no change	Little or no change	Little or no change
DBP	Little or no change	Little or no change	Little or no change
MAP	Little or no change	Little or no change	Little or no change
$\dot{V}O_2$	—	—	Increased
TPR	Unchanged	Unchanged	Decreased
RPP	Decreased	Decreased	Unchanged

submaximal exercise following endurance training (Figure 6.7g). This result reflects the greater efficiency of the heart, since fewer contractions are necessary to eject the same amount of blood during submaximal exercise following an endurance training program.[69] Since maximal heart rate is unchanged and systolic blood pressure is either unchanged or increases slightly with exercise training, it follows that the maximal rate-pressure product is unchanged or increases slightly following a training program. Table 6.5 summarizes the training adaptations that occur within the cardiovascular system as a result of a dynamic aerobic exercise program.

Sex Differences in Adaptations

Research evidence suggests that there are no differences between the sexes in central or peripheral adaptations to endurance training. Both sexes exhibit similar cardiovascular adaptations at rest, during submaximal exercise, and at maximal exercise.[28,70] Maximal cardiac output is higher in both sexes owing to an increased stroke volume following training; however, the absolute value achieved by a woman is less than that attained by a similarly trained man.

When males and females of similar fitness level train at the same frequency, intensity, and duration, there are no differences in the relative increase in $\dot{V}O_2$max.[63,70] As shown earlier in Figure 5.12, there is considerable overlap in $\dot{V}O_2$max between the sexes. Thus, a well-trained female may have a higher $\dot{V}O_2$max than a sedentary or even normally active male; however, a female will always have a lower $\dot{V}O_2$max than a similarly trained male.

The blood pressure (SBP, DBP, MAP) response to exercise is unchanged following an endurance training program for both sexes. Males and females show the same adaptations in total peripheral resistance and rate-pressure product. The effects of endurance training on cardiovascular variables at maximal exercise are reported in Table 6.6 for the two sexes. In summary, the trainability of females does not differ from that of their male counterparts, and similar benefits can and should be gained by regular activity by both sexes.[49] However, the absolute values achieved for maximal oxygen consumption, cardiac output, and stroke volume will generally be lower in females owing to their smaller body size and heart size.

Adaptations in Children

There is relatively little information available regarding cardiovascular adaptations in children and adolescents as a result of endurance training, especially in children of a very young age. However, it has been documented that endurance training re-

TABLE 6.6 ■ Comparison of Cardiovascular Responses to Maximal Exercise in Sedentary and Trained Young Adults (20–30 yr)

VARIABLE	Men		Women	
	SEDENTARY	TRAINED	SEDENTARY	TRAINED
$\dot{Q}$ max (L·min^{-1})	22	30	16	20
SV max (mL·b^{-1})	115	155	80	105
HR max (b·min^{-1})	195	195	195	195
$\dot{V}O_2$max (mL·kg^{-1}·min^{-1})	50	65	37	52
SBP (mmHg)	200	200	190	190
DBP (mmHg)	70	70	66	66
MAP (mmHg)	135	135	128	128
R (units)	6.1	4.5	8.0	6.4
RPP (units)	390	390	370	370

sults in an increase in left ventricular mass and heart volume in children, as it does in adults.[7,44] The increase in heart size is associated with an increase in resting stroke volume,[47] a decrease in resting heart rate, but no change in cardiac output.[35] Research also suggests an increased blood volume and hemoglobin level in young endurance athletes compared with sedentary children.[62,100] There has been some speculation that children are more likely to respond to endurance training at a certain age or maturity level, but no level or age has yet been clearly identified.[22,77,84]

At submaximal levels of exercise cardiac output is unchanged or slightly decreased in youngsters after endurance training.[7,91] This result is due to an increase in submaximal stroke volume and a decrease in heart rate.[7,66] Neither systolic nor diastolic blood pressure changes significantly as a result of endurance training during submaximal work.[66]

At maximal work, cardiac output increases in children and adolescents as a result of endurance training. This result is due to an increased maximal stroke volume and stable maximal heart rate.[35,66]

Children and adolescents in a wide variety of training programs, in either school or community-based settings, have consistently shown improvements in endurance performance. Such improvements have occurred whether endurance performance was measured as an increase in the workload performed (longer treadmill times or distances run, more distance covered in a set amount of time, higher work output on a bicycle ergometer, or longer rides at the same load setting) or as a faster time for a given distance.[17,25,26,30,31,45,46,73,88] Given the lack of association between endurance performance and $\dot{V}O_2$max in children, it should come as no surprise that endurance performance improvements are not always accompanied by a comparable improvement in $\dot{V}O_2$max.[25,26] Furthermore, although children and adolescents who participate in organized athletic activities have higher $\dot{V}O_2$max values than those who do not engage in such activities, the relationship between measures of physical activity (such as self-report questionnaires, heart rate monitoring, and motion detection devices) and measures of $\dot{V}O_2$max is generally only low to moderate.[72,95]

Because of these findings, researchers have hotly debated whether children and adolescents could improve $\dot{V}O_2$max as a result of training. At this time the consensus is that children can improve $\dot{V}O_2$max values; the key to this adaptation lies in the training program being of sufficient intensity, duration, and frequency. Precisely what constitutes an adequate intensity for the exercise prescription of children and adolescents is unknown, but intensities recommended for adults appear to be effective. For these intensities, improvements of 10–15% in $\dot{V}O_2$max are typical.

Adaptations in the Elderly

Elderly males and females respond to endurance exercise training with adaptations similar to those seen in younger adults.[48,52,74] Left ventricular wall thickness and myocardial mass are greater in elderly athletes than in elderly sedentary individuals, although these training adaptations may not be as pronounced or as quickly achieved as in younger adults.[43,52,74]

Left ventricular–end diastolic volume and ejection fraction increase as a result of endurance training in older individuals. These changes lead to an enhancement of myocardial contractile function, especially the Frank-Starling mechanism, and assist in maintaining cardiac outputs in the active elderly.[43]

Resting cardiac output is unchanged as a result of endurance training in the elderly. Elderly athletes with an extensive history of endurance training consistently show lower resting heart rates than their sedentary counterparts. However, short-term training programs sometimes show the expected decrease in resting heart rates and sometimes do not. Resting stroke volume typically increases, but the increase is generally small.[43]

As for normotensive individuals of other ages, endurance training does not affect systolic blood pressure, diastolic blood pressure, or mean arterial blood pressure at rest in elderly people. Both hemoglobin levels and blood volume increase in the elderly as a result of endurance training as does the density of capillaries supplying blood to the active musculature.[43]

Most training studies indicate that no change occurs in cardiac output during any given submaximal workload. The components of cardiac output, however, often change reciprocally with the expected decrease in heart rate and increase in stroke volume. Again, the stroke volume changes tend to be small and do not always reach statistical significance. Submaximal values for systolic blood pressure, mean arterial blood pressure, and total peripheral resistance are lower in elderly athletes than in nonathletes and decrease as a result of endurance training.[43]

Maximal cardiac output may be increased by exercise training in elderly individuals. This increase is completely accounted for by an increase in maximal stroke volume, since maximal heart rate is unchanged. The reported effects of endurance training on blood pressures and systematic vascular resistance are inconsistent, although the majority of the evidence suggests no change in these variables.[43]

The results of training status on cardiovascular responses to maximal exercise in the elderly, including $\dot{V}O_2$max, are shown in Table 6.7 for both men and women. $\dot{V}O_2$max is higher in trained than in untrained elderly. Thus, training programs can result in increases in $\dot{V}O_2$max in the elderly. The magnitude of the increase in $\dot{V}O_2$max depends upon the initial-fitness level of the individual and the training program followed. Research suggests, though, that healthy, elderly untrained males and females can improve their $\dot{V}O_2$max by 15–30% with training.[48,74,87]

One study using a short-duration exercise program (nine weeks) of endurance training reported that a low-intensity exercise prescription (30–45% HRR) was as effective as a high-intensity exercise prescription (60–75% HRR) in eliciting improvements in $\dot{V}O_2$max.[5] However, a one-year training program found that six months of training at low in-

tensities (40% HRR) resulted in a 10.5% improvement in $\dot{V}O_2$max. When the training program was progressively changed to a high-intensity program (85% HRR) and the duration was extended, the elderly subjects increased their $\dot{V}O_2$max by another 16.5%. This research suggests that elderly individuals respond to exercise training in much the same way that younger individuals do.

When initiating a training program with elderly people, it is important to begin at low intensities to avoid injury. However, significant improvements in function can be gained by low-intensity programs. After individuals become accustomed to the program, the training program can be upgraded to an intense training program if desired. Note that the rate of adaptation, though, may be slower in older individuals.[2]

Although elderly athletes are more similar to younger individuals than to their sedentary counterparts, and training programs tend to show that the same beneficial changes occur in the elderly that occur in younger subjects, exercise training does not stop the effects of aging on the cardiovascular system. At best, exercise training can only lessen the age-related losses in cardiovascular function that occur with age. This conclusion is exemplified in Figure 6.10, where the average rate of decline in $\dot{V}O_2$max is shown for both an active, highly fit (HF) group of females and a relatively sedentary, low-fitness (LF) comparison group.[79] The first thing to notice is that the HF group had higher $\dot{V}O_2$max val-

TABLE 6.7 ■ **Comparison of Cardiovascular Responses to Maximal Exercise in Sedentary and Trained Elderly Individuals (60–70 yr)**

	Men		Women	
VARIABLE	SEDENTARY	TRAINED	SEDENTARY	TRAINED
$\dot{Q}$ max (L·min^{-1})	16	19.4	12	15
SV max (mL)	100	125	75	90
HR max (b·min^{-1})	155	155	155	155
$\dot{V}O_2$max (mL·kg^{-1}·min^{-1})	28	48	22	35
SBP (mmHg)	190	190	190	190
DBP (mmHg)	84	84	84	84
MAP (mmHg)	138	138	138	138
R (units)	8.6	7.3	11.5	9.2
RPP (units)	290	290	290	290

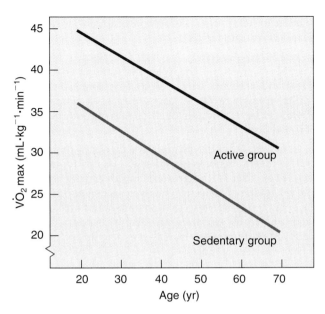

ues than the LF group in every decade. Indeed, the active 45-yr-old group had $\dot{V}O_2$max values that equaled those of the inactive 20-yr-olds. Second, $\dot{V}O_2$max expressed per kilogram of body weight declined with age, and the rate of decline was similar in the two groups.

Cardiovascular Adaptations to Dynamic Resistance Training

Low-volume dynamic resistance training (few repetitions and low weight) has not been shown to make any consistent or significant changes in cardiovascular variables. Thus, the changes described in the following sections depend upon high-volume (high–total workload) dynamic resistance training programs.[92]

Cardiac Dimensions

Dynamic resistance-trained athletes often have increased left ventricular wall and septal thicknesses,

although this is not a consistent finding in short-term training studies.[59,65,71] When the increase in wall thickness is reported relative to body surface area or lean body mass, the increase is greatly reduced or even nonexistent.[38] The increase in wall thickness results from the work the heart must do to overcome the high arterial pressures (increased pressure afterload) encountered during resistance training, and it depends on the training intensity and volume.

Stroke Volume and Heart Rate

Resting stroke volume in highly trained dynamic resistance athletes has been reported to be greater than normal and not different from normal.[33,40] Since stroke volume is so seldom measured during resistance activities, the changes that occur in the stroke volume response to resistance activities as a result of training are not known.[89]

Highly trained dynamic resistance athletes have average or below average resting heart rates.[92] Heart rate at a specified submaximal workload is lower following resistance training.[39]

Blood Pressure

Dynamic resistance-trained athletes do not have elevated resting blood pressures, provided that they are not chronically overtrained, do not have greatly increased muscle mass, or are not using anabolic steroids. This information contradicts the popular misconception that resistance-trained individuals have a higher resting blood pressure than endurance-trained or untrained individuals. Indeed, most scientific investigations report that highly trained resistance athletes have average or lower-than-average systolic and diastolic blood pressures.[40] Resistance-trained individuals also exhibit a lower blood pressure response to the same relative workload of resistance exercise than untrained individuals, even though the trained individuals are lifting a greater absolute load.

Dynamic resistance training has not been shown to consistently lower blood pressure in hypertensives. Therefore, resistance training is not recommended as the only exercise modality for hypertensives unless it is in the form of circuit training. *Circuit training* relies on high repetitions, low loads, and short rest periods set up in a series of stations. A supercircuit integrates aerobic endurance activities between the stations.

The rate-pressure product, which reflects myocardial oxygen consumption, is decreased at rest following strength training, during weight lifting or circuit training, and during aerobic exercise to which a resistance component has been added (such as holding hand weights while walking).[40,92] Researchers have suggested that these results occur because of a reduction in peripheral resistance.

Maximal Oxygen Consumption

Small increases (4–9%) in $\dot{V}O_2$max have been reported following circuit training and Olympic-style weight-lifting programs.[41,92] However, other studies have failed to identify any increase in $\dot{V}O_2$max with resistance training.[57] $\dot{V}O_2$max probably doesn't change much because of the low percentage of $\dot{V}O_2$max that is achieved during a resistance training program. Weight training may impact the central cardiovascular variables as described earlier (that is, resulting in a reduced resting heart rate), but it does not enhance peripheral cardiovascular adaptations (that is, a-vO_2 diff). Thus, individuals should not rely on resistance training programs to improve cardiorespiratory fitness; instead, a dynamic resistance training program should be used in conjunction with a dynamic endurance training program.

Owing to a lack of research data, nothing definitive can be said about sex differences in cardiovascular adaptations to resistance training or about adaptations in children and the elderly.

SUMMARY

1. What constitutes an optional cardiovascular training program depends on the age and health status of the individual and the goal of the program.

2. Any activity that involves large muscle groups and is sustained for prolonged periods of time has the potential to increase cardiovascular fitness. The choice of exercise modalities should be based upon interest, availability, and low risk of injury.

3. Training using different exercise modalities causes the same overall benefits by leading to central cardiovascular adaptations. However, peripheral cardiovascular adaptations are specific to the muscles being exercised.

4. Intensity is very important in improving maximal oxygen consumption ($\dot{V}O_2$max) both alone and in conjunction with duration. Intensity can be prescribed in relation to heart rate, oxygen consumption, or rating of perceived exertion (RPE).

5. The American College of Sports Medicine (ACSM) recommends the following training goals to develop and maintain cardiorespiratory fitness in healthy adults: frequency of 3–5 days per week; intensity of 60–90% HRmax; duration of 20–60 min of continuous aerobic activity.

6. The absolute and relative increases in $\dot{V}O_2$max and the health benefits are inversely related to initial fitness level. That is, the greatest improvements in fitness and health benefits occur when very sedentary individuals begin a regular, low- to moderate-endurance exercise program. Thus, meaningful health benefits can be achieved with minimal increases in activity or fitness by those who need it most.

7. Training intensity is the most important factor in maintaining cardiovascular fitness.

8. Endurance training results in an increase in cardiac dimensions, mass, and the size of the coronary vascular bed. The internal diameter of the coronary arteries may also increase as result of training. More importantly, the arteries are more distensible during exercise as a result of training.

9. Endurance training results in an increase in blood volume, with highly trained endurance athletes having 20–25% greater blood volume than untrained subjects. Changes in plasma volume occur early in a training program, with changes between 8 and 10% occurring within the first week. Early changes (one month) are due almost entirely to increases in plasma volume, whereas increases in red blood cells and hemoglobin occur later.

10. Cardiac output at rest and at an absolute submaximal workload is unchanged following an endurance training program. However, cardiac output at the same relative workload and at maximal exercise is greater following an endurance training program.

11. Stroke volume is greater at rest, at submaximal exercise (absolute and relative workloads), and at maximal exercise following an endurance training program.

12. Heart rate is lower at rest and during an absolute submaximal workload following endurance training. It is unchanged at the same relative submaximal workload and at maximal exercise.

13. There is little or no change in blood pressure at rest, during submaximal exercise, or during maximal exercise in normotensive individuals following an endurance training program.

14. $\dot{V}O_2$max increases as a result of endurance training; improvements of 15% are routinely reported with training programs that meet the recommendations of ACSM.

Box 6.1 Answer

% HRmax method:

Lisa:

estimated HR max = $220 - 50 = 170 \text{ b} \cdot \text{min}^{-1}$

training HR = $170 \times 0.35 = 59 \text{ b} \cdot \text{min}^{-1}$

training HR = $170 \times 0.59 = 100 \text{ b} \cdot \text{min}^{-1}$

On the basis of the % HR max method, a light exercise for Lisa elicits a heart rate between 59* and 100 b·min^{-1}.

Susie:

estimated HR max = $220 - 50 = 170 \text{ b} \cdot \text{min}^{-1}$

training HR = $170 \times 0.35 = 59 \text{ b} \cdot \text{min}^{-1}$

training HR = $170 \times 0.59 = 100 \text{ b} \cdot \text{min}^{-1}$

On the basis of the % HR max method, a light exercise for Susie elicits a heart rate between 59* and 100 b · min^{-1}.

% HRR method:

Lisa:

estimated HR max = $220 - 50 = 170 \text{ b} \cdot \text{min}^{-1}$

training HHR = $[(170 - 62) \times 0.30] + 62$
$= 94 \text{ b} \cdot \text{min}^{-1}$

training HRR = $[(170 - 62) \times 0.49] + 62$
$= 115 \text{ b} \cdot \text{min}^{-1}$

On the basis of the % HRR method, a light exercise for Lisa elicits a heart rate between 94 and 115 b · min^{-1}.

Susie:

estimated HR max = $220 - 50 = 170 \text{ b} \cdot \text{min}^{-1}$

training HRR = $[(170 - 82) \times 0.30] + 82$
$= 109 \text{ b} \cdot \text{min}^{-1}$

training HRR = $[(170 - 82) \times 0.49] + 82$
$= 125 \text{ b} \cdot \text{min}^{-1}$

On the basis of the % HRR method, a light exercise for Susie elicits a heart rate between 109 and 125 b · min^{-1}.

*Obviously a person cannot be working at less than his or her RHR, but this means that any activity above the resting level to the upper level can be done and would be beneficial for this person.

Box 6.2 Answers

1. A moderate workout represents 50–74% $\dot{V}O_2$max or HRR.

Individual	50%	74%
Janet	52 mL·kg^{-1}·min^{-1}	52 mL·kg^{-1}·min^{-1}
	× 0.5	× 0.74
	26 mL·kg^{-1}·min^{-1}	38.5 mL·kg^{-1}·min^{-1}
Jeff	64 mL·kg^{-1}·min^{-1}	64 mL·kg^{-1}·min^{-1}
	× 0.5	× 0.74
	32 mL·kg^{-1}·min^{-1}	47.4 mL·kg^{-1}·min^{-1}
Mark	49 mL·kg^{-1}·min^{-1}	49 mL·kg^{-1}·min^{-1}
	× 0.5	× 0.74
	24.5 mL·kg^{-1}·min^{-1}	36.3 mL·kg^{-1}·min^{-1}
Gail	56 mL·kg^{-1}·min^{-1}	56 mL·kg^{-1}·min^{-1}
	× 0.5	× 0.74
	28 mL·kg^{-1}·min^{-1}	41.4 mL·kg^{-1}·min^{-1}

5 mph is too low for Jeff. 9 and 10 mph are too high for everyone. 8 mph is moderate only for Jeff. 7 mph is moderate only for Jeff and Gail. 6 mph falls within the moderate range for all runners.

2. In order to determine the anticipated heart rate during the 6 mph run, you must first determine what percent $\dot{V}O_2$max (as a fraction) each individual is working at. Refer back to Box 6.2 to find the $\dot{V}O_2$max for each individual and the oxygen cost of running 6 mph. Divide $\dot{V}O_2$max by the oxygen cost of the 6 mph pace to find the % $\dot{V}O_2$max for each person.

Janet

$$\frac{\dot{V}O_2 \text{ 6 mph}}{\dot{V}O_2\text{max}} \quad \frac{35.7 \text{ mL} \cdot \text{kg}^{-1} \cdot \text{min}^{-1}}{52 \text{ mL} \cdot \text{kg}^{-1} \cdot \text{min}^{-1}} = 0.687$$

Jeff

$$\frac{\dot{V}O_2 \text{ 6 mph}}{\dot{V}O_2\text{max}} \quad \frac{35.7 \text{ mL} \cdot \text{kg}^{-1} \cdot \text{min}^{-1}}{64 \text{ mL} \cdot \text{kg}^{-1} \cdot \text{min}^{-1}} = 0.558$$

Mark

$$\frac{\dot{V}O_2 \text{ 6 mph}}{\dot{V}O_2\text{max}} \quad \frac{35.7 \text{ mL} \cdot \text{kg}^{-1} \cdot \text{min}^{-1}}{49 \text{ mL} \cdot \text{kg}^{-1} \cdot \text{min}^{-1}} = 0.728$$

Gail

$$\frac{\dot{V}O_2 \text{ 6 mph}}{\dot{V}O_2\text{max}} \quad \frac{35.7 \text{mL} \cdot \text{kg}^{-1} \cdot \text{min}^{-1}}{56 \text{ mL} \cdot \text{kg}^{-1} \cdot \text{min}^{-1}} = 0.638$$

(continued)

Box 6.2 Answers *(continued)*

These percentages (as fractions) can then be used in the HRR equation.

Janet	Jeff	
220	220	
−23	−35	Age (yr)
197	185	Predicted HR max (b·min⁻¹)
−60	−48	RHR (b·min⁻¹)
137	137	
× 0.687	× 0.558	% V̇O₂max = % HRR
94	76.5	(b·min⁻¹)
+ 60	+ 48.0	RHR (b·min⁻¹)
154	124.5 = 125	Exercise HR (b·min⁻¹)

Mark	Gail	
220	220	
−22	−28	Age (yr)
198	192	Predicted HR max (b·min⁻¹)
−64	−58	RHR (b·min⁻¹)
134	134	
× 0.728	× 0.638	% V̇O₂max = % HRR
97.6	85.4	(b·min⁻¹)
+ 64.0	+ 58.0	RHR (b·min⁻¹)
161.6 = 162	143.4 = 143	Exercise HR (b·min⁻¹)

Box 6.3 Answers

From Table 6.3 it is determined that Pat should be able to sustain between 85 and 87.5% V̇O₂max for the time span or 45–59 min.

220			
−33			
187 b·min⁻¹	Predicted HR max		
−62 b·min⁻¹	RHR		
125 b·min⁻¹	HRR	125 b·min⁻¹	
× 0.85	%V̇O₂max	× 0.875	
106 b·min⁻¹		109 b·min⁻¹	
+62 b·min⁻¹		+62 b·min⁻¹	
168 b·min⁻¹		171 b·min⁻¹	

Thus, Pat should aim for a heart rate of 168–171 b·min⁻¹ once she reaches a steady state.

REVIEW QUESTIONS

1. How is overload manipulated to bring about cardiorespiratory adaptation?

2. Differentiate between central and peripheral cardiovascular adaptations.

3. Compare and contrast cardiac output, stroke volume, heart rate, and blood pressure adaptations to endurance training at rest and during submaximal and maximal exercise.

4. Discuss the impact of an individual's initial-fitness level on expected improvements in fitness and health-related benefits.

5. Describe the physiological benefits of a warm-up and a cool-down period.

6. Explain the changes in blood volume that occur as a result of an endurance training program.

7. Compare and contrast cardiovascular adaptations to dynamic endurance and dynamic resistance training.

REFERENCES

1. American College of Sports Medicine: Position stand on the recommended quantity and quality of exercise for developing and maintaining fitness in healthy adults. *Medicine and Science in Sports and Exercise.* 10(3):vii–x (1978).

2. American College of Sports Medicine: Position stand on the recommended quantity and quality of exercise for developing and maintaining cardiorespiratory and muscular fitness in healthy adults. *Medicine and Science in Sports and Exercise.* 22:256–274 (1990).

3. American College of Sports Medicine: *Guidelines for Exercise Testing and Prescription* (5th edition). Philadelphia: Lea & Febiger (1995).

4. Astrand, P. O., & K. Rodahl: *Textbook of Work Physiology.* New York: McGraw-Hill (1986).

5. Badenhop, D. T., P. A. Cleary, S. F. Schaal, E. L. Fox, & R. L. Bartels: Physiological adjustments to higher- or lower-intensity exercise in elders. *Medicine and Science in Sports and Exercise.* 15(6):496–502 (1983).

6. Barnard, R. J., G. W. Gardner, N. V. Diasco, R. N. MacAlpin, & A. A. Kattus: Cardiovascular responses to sudden strenuous exercise—Heart rate, blood pressure and ECG. *Journal of Applied Physiology.* 34:833–837 (1973).

7. Bar-Or, O.: *Pediatric Sports Medicine for the Practitioner.* New York: Springer-Verlag (1983).

8. Blomqvist, C. G., & B. Saltin: Cardiovascular adaptations to physical training. *Annual Review of Physiology.* 45:169 (1983).

9. Bloomfield, S., & E. F. Coyle: Bedrest, detraining, and retention of training-induced adaptations. In American College of Sports Medicine (ed.), *Resource Manual for Guidelines for Exercise Testing and Prescription.* Philadelphia: Lea & Febiger (1993).

10. Borg, B. A. V.: Psychophysical bases of perceived exertion. *Medicine and Science in Sports and Exercise.* 14(5):377–381 (1982).

11. Bouchard, C., & L. Persusse: Heredity, activity level, fitness, and health. In C. Bouchard, R. J. Shephard, & T. Stephens (eds.), *Physical Activity, Fitness, and Health, International Proceedings and Consensus statement.* Champaign, IL: Human Kinetics Publishers (1994).

12. Cohen, J. L., & K. R. Segal: Left ventricular hypertrophy in athletes: An exercise-echocardiographic study. *Medicine and Science in Sports and Exercise.* 17:695–700 (1985).

13. Connor, J. F., F. LaCamera, E. J. Swanick, M. J. Oldham, D. W. Holzaepfel, & O. Lyczkowskyj: Effects of exercise on coronary collateralization—Angiographic studies of six patients in a supervised exercise program. *Medicine and Science in Sports.* 8(3):145–151 (1976).

14. Convertino, V. A., P. J. Brock, L. C. Keil, E. M. Bernauer, & J. E. Greenleaf: Exercise training–induced hypervolemia: Role of plasma albumin, renin, and vasopressin. *Journal of Applied Physiology.* 48:665–669 (1980).

15. Convertino, V. A.: Blood volume: Its adaptation to endurance training. *Medicine and Science in Sports and Exercise.* 23:1338–1348 (1991).

16. Convertino, V. A., G. W. Mack, & E. R. Nadel: Elevated central venous pressure: A consequence of exercise training-induced hypervolemia? *American Journal of Physiology.* 29:R273–R277 (1991).

17. Cooper, K. H., J. G. Purdy, A. Friedman, R. L. Bohannon, R. A. Harris, & J. A. Arends: An aerobics conditioning program for the Fort Worth, Texas, School District. *Research Quarterly.* 46:345–380 (1975).

18. Corbin, C. B., & R. P. Pangrazi: Toward an understanding of appropriate physical activity levels for youth. *Physical Activity and Fitness Research Digest.* 1(8): (1994).

19. Coyle, E. F., W. H. Martin, D. R. Sinacore, M. J. Joymer, J. M. Hagberg, & J. O. Holloszy: Time course of loss of adaptations after stopping prolonged intense endurance training. *Journal of Applied Physiology.* 57:1857–1864 (1984).

20. Coyle, E. F., M. K. Hemmert, & A. R. Coggan: Effects of detraining on cardiovascular responses to exercise: Role of blood volume. *Journal of Applied Physiology.* 60:95–99 (1986).

21. Cunningham, D. A., & J. S. Hill: Effect of training on cardiovascular response to exercise in women. *Journal of Applied Physiology.* 39:891–895 (1975).

22. Cunningham, D. A., D. H. Paterson, & C. J. R. Blinkie: The development of the cardiorespiratory system in growth and development. In R. A. Boileau (ed.), *Advances in Pediatric Sport Sciences* (Vol. 1). Champaign, IL: Human Kinetics Publishers, 85–116 (1984).

23. Currens, J. G., & P. D. White: Half century of running: Clinical, physiologic and autopsy findings in the case of Clarence De Mar, "Mr. Marathoner." *New England Journal of Medicine.* 265:988–993 (1961).

24. Daniels, J., & J. Gilbert: *Oxygen Power: Performance Tables for Distance Runners.* Tempe, AZ: Author (1979).

25. Daniels, J., & N. Oldridge: Changes in oxygen consumption of young boys during growth and running training. *Medicine and Science in Sports.* 3:161–165 (1971).

26. Daniels, J., N. Oldridge, F. Nagle, & B. White: Differences and changes in VO$_2$ among young runners 10 to 18 years of age. *Medicine and Science in Sports.* 10:200–203 (1978).

27. De Busk, R. F., U. Hakanssan, M. Sheehan, & W. L. Haskell: Training effects of long versus short bouts of exercise. *American Journal of Cardiology.* 65:1010–1013 (1990).

28. Drinkwater, B. L.: Women and exercise: Physiological aspects. *Exercise and Sport Sciences Reviews.* 12:21–52 (1984).

29. Drinkwater, B. L., & S. M. Horvath: Detraining effects on young women. *Medicine and Science in Sports and Exercise.* 4:91–95 (1972).

30. Ducan, B., W. T. Boyce, R. Itami, & N. Puffengarger: A controlled trial of a physical fitness program for fifth grade students. *Journal of School Health.* 53:467–471 (1983).

31. Dwyer, T., W. E. Coonan, D. R. Leitch, B. S. Hetzel, & R. A. Boghurst: An investigation of the effects of daily physical activity on the health of primary school students in South Australia. *International Journal of Epidemiology.* 12:308–313 (1983).

32. Eckstein, R. W.: Effects of exercise and coronary heart narrowing on coronary collateral circulation. *Circulation Research.* 5:230–235 (1957).

33. Effron, M. B.: Effects of resistance training on left ventricular function. *Medicine and Science in Sports and Exercise.* 21:694–697 (1989)

34. Ekblom, B., P. O. Astrand, B. Saltin, J. Stenberg, & B. Wallstrom: Effect of training on circulatory response to exercise. *European Journal of Applied Physiology.* 24:518–528 (1968).

35. Eriksson, B. O., & G. Koch: Effects of physical training on hemodynamic response during submaximal and maximal exercise in 11 to 13 year old boys. *Acta Physiological Scandinavia.* 87:27–39 (1973).

36. Eyestone, E. D., G. Fellingham, J. George, & A. G. Fisher: Effect of water running and cycling on maximum oxygen consumption and 2-mile run performance. *American Journal of Sports Medicine.* 21(1):41–44 (1993).

37. Ferguson, F. J., R. Petitclerc, G. Choquette, L. Chaniotis, P. Gauthier, R. Hout, C. Allard, L. Jankowski, & L. Campeau: Effect of physical training on treadmill exercise capacity, collateral circulation and progression of coronary disease. *American Journal of Cardiology.* 34:764–769 (1974).

38. Fleck, S. J.: Cardiovascular adaptations to resistance training. *Medicine and Science in Sports and Exercise.* 20:S146–S151 (1988).

39. Fleck, S. J. & L. S. Dean: Resistance-training experience and the pressor response during resistance exercise. *Journal of Applied Physiology.* 63:116–120 (1987).

40. Fleck, S. J.: Cardiovascular responses to strength training. In P. V. Komi (ed), *Strength and Power in Sport.* Champaign, IL: Human Kinetics Publishers, 305–319 (1988).

41. Gettman, L. R: Circuit weight-training: A critical review of its physiological benefits. *The Physician and Sports Medicine.* 9(1):44–59 (1981).

42. Gledhill, N., D. Cox, & R. Jamnik: Endurance athletes' stroke volume does not plateau: Major advantage is diastolic function. *Medicine and Science in Sports and Exercise.* 26:1116–1121 (1994).

43. Green J. S., & S. F. Crouse: Endurance training, cardiovascular function and the aged. *Sports Medicine.* 16(5): 331–341 (1993).

44. Greenen, D. L., T. B. Gilliam, D. Crowley, C. Moorehead-Steffens, & A. Rosenthal: Echocardiographic measures in 6 to 7 year old children after an 8 month exercise program. *American Journal of Cardiology.* 49:1990–1995 (1982).

45. Goode, R. C., A. Virgin, T. T. Romet, P. Crawford, J. Duffin, T. Palland, & Z. Woch: Effects of a short period of physical activity in adolescent boys and girls. *Canadian Journal of Applied Sport Sciences.* 1:241–250 (1976).

46. Graunke, J. M., S. A. Plowman, & J. R. Marett: Evaluation of a fitness based physical education curriculum for the high school freshman. *Illinois Journal of Health, Physical Education, Recreation and Dance.* 27:24–27 (1990).

47. Gutin, B., N. Mayers, J. A. Levy, & M. V. Herman: Physiologic and echocardiographic studies of age-group runners. In E. W. Brown & C. F. Branta (eds.), *Competitive Sports for Children and Youth*. Champaign IL: Human Kinetics Publishers, 115–128 (1988).

48. Hagberg, J. M., J. E. Graves, M. Limacher, D. R. Woods, S. H. Leggett, C. Cononie, J. J. Gruber, & M. L. Pollock: Cardiovascular responses of 70- to 79-yr-old men and women to exercise training. *Journal of Applied Physiology*. 66:2589–2594 (1989).

49. Hanson, J. S., & W. H. Nedde: Long-term physical training effect in sedentary females. *Journal of Applied Physiology*. 37:112–116 (1974).

50. Haskell, W. L.: Health consequences of physical activity: Understanding and challenges regarding dose response. *Medicine and Science in Sports and Exercise*. 26(6): 649–660 (1994).

51. Haskell, W. L., C. Sims, J. Myll, W. M. Bortz, F. G. St. Goar, & E. L. Alderman: Coronary artery size and dilating capacity in ultra distance runners. *Circulation*. 87(4): 1076–1082 (1993).

52. Heath, G. W., J. M. Hagberg, A. A. Ehsani, & J. O. Holloszy: A physiological comparison of young and older endurance athletes. *American Physiological Society*. 51(3): 634–640 (1981).

53. Hickson, R. C., & M. A. Rosenkoetter: Reduced training frequencies and maintenance of increased aerobic power. *Medicine and Science in Sports and Exercise*. 13:13–16 (1981).

54. Hickson, R. C., C. Foster, M. L. Pollock, T. M. Galassi, & S. Rich: Reduced training intensities and loss of aerobic power, endurance, and cardiac growth. *Journal of Applied Physiology*. 58:492–499 (1985).

55. Hickson, R. C., C. Kanakis, J. R. Davis, A. M. Moore, & S. Rich: Reduced training duration effects on aerobic power, endurance, and cardiac growth. *Journal of Applied Physiology*. 53(1): 225–229 (1982).

56. Housh, D. J., & T. J. Housh: The effects of unilateral velocity—Specific concentric strength training. *Journal of Orthopaedic and Sports Physical Therapy*. 17(5):252–260 (1993).

57. Hurley, B. F., D. R. Seals, A. A. Ehsani, L. J. Cartier, G. P. Dalsky, J. M. Hagberg, & J. O. Holloszy: Effects of high-intensity strength training on cardiovascular function. *Medicine and Science in Sports and Exercise*. 16(5):483–488 (1984).

58. Huston, T. P., J. C. Puffer, & W. MacMillan: The athletic heart syndrome. *New England Journal of Medicine*. 313:24–32 (1985).

59. Keul, J., H. H. Dickhuth, G. Simon, & M. Lehmann: Effect of static and dynamic exercise on heart volume, contractility, and left ventricular dimensions. *Circulation Research*. 48:I162–I170 (1981).

60. Kibler, W. B., & T. J. Chandler: Sport-specific conditioning. *American Journal of Sports Medicine*. 22(3):424–432 (1994).

61. Kilmer, D. D., M. A. McCrory, N. C. Wright, S. G. Aitkens, & E. M. Bernaver: The effect of a high resistance exercise program in slowly progressive neuro-muscular disease. *Archives of Physical Medicine and Rehabilitation*. 75(5):560–563 (1994).

62. Koch, G., & L. Rocher: Total amount of hemoglobin, plasma and blood volumes, and intravascular protein masses in trained boys. In K. Berg & B. O. Erickson (eds.), *Children and Exercise IX*. Baltimore: University Park Press, 109–115 (1980).

63. Lewis, D. A., E. Kamon, & J. L. Hodgson: Physiological differences between genders. Implications for sports conditioning. *Sports Medicine*. 3:357–369 (1986).

64. Londeree, B. R., T. R. Thomas, G. Ziogas, T. D. Smith, & Q. Zhang: % VO_2max versus % HR max regressions for six modes of exercise. *Medicine and Science in Sports and Exercise*. 27:458–461 (1995).

65. Longhurst, J. C., A. R. Kelly, W. J. Gonyea, & J. H. Mitchell: Chronic training with static and dynamic exercise: Cardiovascular adaptation and response to exercise. *Circulation Research*. 48:I171 (1981).

66. Lussier, L., & E. R. Buskirk: Effects of an endurance training regimen on assessment of work capacity in prepubertal children. *Annals of the New York Academy of Sciences*, 734–747 (1977).

67. Magel, J. R., G. F. Foglia, W. D. McArdle, B. Gutin, G. S. Pechar, & F. I. Katch: Specificity of swim training on maximum oxygen uptake. *Journal of Applied Physiology*. 38(1):151–155 (1975).

68. Miller, W. C., J. P. Wallace, & K. E. Eggert: Predicting max HR and the HR-VO_2 relationship for exercise prescription in obesity. *Medicine and Science in Sports and Exercise*. 25:1077–1081 (1993).

69. Mitchell, J. H., & P. Raven: Cardiovascular adaptation to physical activity. In C. R. Bouchard, R. J. Shepard, & T. Stephens (eds.), *Physical Activity, Fitness, and Health: International Proceedings and Consensus Statement*. Champaign, IL: Human Kinetics Publishers, 286–301 (1994).

70. Mitchell, J. H., C. Tate, P. Raven, F. Cobb, W. Kraus, R. Moreadith, M. O'Toole, B. Saltin, & N. Wenger: Acute response and chronic adaptation to exercise in women. *Medicine and Science in Sports and Exercise* (Suppl.). 24(6):258–265 (1992).

71. Morganroth, J., B. J. Maron, W. L. Henry, & S. E. Epstein: Comparative left ventricular dimensions in trained athletes. *Annals of Internal Medicine*. 82:521 (1975).

72. Morrow, J. R., & P. S. Freedson: Relationship between habitual physical activity and aerobic fitness in adolescents. *Pediatric Exercise Science*. 6:315–329 (1994).

73. Mosellin, R., & U. Wasmund: Investigations on the influence of a running-training program on the cardiovascular and motor performance capacity in 53 boys and girls of a second and third primary school class. In O. Bar-Or (ed.), *Pediatric Work Physiology: Proceedings of the Fourth International Symposium*. Natanya, Israel: Wingate Institute (1973).

74. Ogawa, T., R. J. Spina, W. H. Martin, W. M. Kohrt, K. B. Schechtman, J. O. Holloszy, & A. A. Ehsani: Effects of aging, sex, and physical training on cardiovascular responses to exercise. *Circulation*. 86:494–503 (1992).

75. O'Toole, M.: Prevention and treatment of injuries to runners. *Medicine and Science in Sports and Exercise* (Suppl.). 24(9):S360–S363 (1992).

76. Parker, S. B., B. F. Hurley, D. P. Hanlon, & P. Vaccaro: Failure of target heart rate to accurately monitor intensity during aerobic dance. *Medicine and Science in Sports and Exercise*. 21(2):230–234 (1989).

77. Pate, R. R., & D. S. Ward: Endurance exercise trainability in children and youth. In W. A. Grana, K. A. Lombardo, B. J. Sharkey, & J. A. Stone (eds.), *Advances in Sports Medicine and Fitness*. 3:37–55 (1990).

78. Pate, R. R., R. D. Hughes, J. V. Chandler, & J. L. Ratliffe: Effects of arm training on retention of training effects derived from leg training. *Medicine and Science in Sports*. 10(2):71–74 (1978).

79. Pechar, G. S., W. D. McArdle, F. I. Katch, J. R. Magel & J. Deluca: Specificity of cardiorespiratory adaptation to bicycle and treadmill training. *Journal of Applied Physiology.* 36(6):753–756 (1974).

80. Plowman, S. A., B. L. Drinkwater & S. M. Horvath: Age and aerobic power in women: A longitudinal study. *Journal of Gerontology.* 34(4):512–520 (1979).

81. Pollock, M. L.: The quantification of endurance training programs. In J. H. Wilmore (ed.), *Exercise and Sport Sciences Reviews.* 1:155–188 (1973).

82. Pollock M. L., & J. H. Wilmore: *Exercise in Health and Disease.* Philadelphia: Saunders (1990).

83. Roberts, J. A., & J. W. Alspaugh: Specificity of training effects resulting from programs of treadmill running and bicycle ergometer riding. *Medicine and Science in Sports.* 4(1):6–10 (1972).

84. Rowland, T. W.: *Exercise and Children's Health.* Champaign IL: Human Kinetics Publishers (1990).

85. Saltin, B.: Physiological effects of physical conditioning. *Medicine and Science in Sports.* 1:50–56 (1969).

86. Schaible, T. F., & J. Schever: Cardiac function in hypertrophied hearts from chronically exercised female rats. *Journal of Applied Physiology.* 50:1140–1145 (1981).

87. Seals, D. R., J. M. Hagberg, B. F. Hurley, A. A. Ehsani, & J. O. Holloszy: Endurance training in older men and women. *Journal of Applied Physiology.* 57(4):1024–1029 (1984).

88. Siegel, J. A., & T. G. Manfredi: Effects of a ten month fitness program on children. *The Physician and Sports Medicine.* 12:91–97 (1984).

89. Sjogaard, G., G. Savard, & C. Juel: Muscle blood flow during isometric activity and its relation to muscle fatigue. *European Journal of Applied Physiology.* 57:327–335 (1988).

90. Smith, M. L., & J. H. Mitchell: Cardiorespiratory adaptations to exercise training. In American College of Sports Medicine (ed.), *Resource Manual for Guidelines for Exercise Testing and Prescription.* Philadelphia: Lea & Febiger (1993).

91. Soto, K. I., C. W. Zauner, & A. B. Otis: Cardiac output in preadolescent competitive swimmers and in untrained normal children. *Journal of Sports Medicine.* 23:291–299 (1983).

92. Stone, M. H., S. J. Fleck, N. T. Triplett, & W. J. Kraemer: Health- and performance-related potential of resistance training. *Sports Medicine.* 11(4):210–231 (1991).

93. Svedenhag, J., & J. Seger: Running on land and in water: Comparative exercise physiology. *Medicine and Science in Sports and Exercise.* 24(10):1155–1160 (1992).

94. Thomas, T. R., G. Ziogis, T. D. Smith, Q. Zhang, & B. R. Londeree: Physiological and perceived exertion responses to six modes of submaximal exercise. *Research Quarterly for Exercise and Sport.* 66:239–246 (1995).

95. Vaccaro, P., & A. Mahon: Cardiorespiratory responses to endurance training in children. *Sports Medicine.* 4:352–363 (1987).

96. Wells, C. L., & S. A. Plowman: Sexual differences in athletic performance: Biological or behavioral? *The Physician and Sports Medicine.* 11(8): 52–63 (1983).

97. Wenger, H. A., & G. J. Bell: The interactions of intensity, frequency and duration of exercise training in altering cardiorespiratory fitness. *Sports Medicine.* 3:346–356 (1986).

98. Wilmore, J. H., J. A. Davis, R. S. O'Brien, P. A. Vodak, G. R. Walder, & E. A. Amsterdam: Physiological alterations consequent to 20-week conditioning programs of bicycling, tennis, and jogging. *Medicine and Science in Sports and Exercise.* 12(1):1–8 (1980).

99. Wilmore, J. H., & D. L. Costill: *Training for Sport and Activity: The Physiological Basis of the Conditioning Process* (3rd edition). Dubuque, IA: Brown (1988).

100. Zauner, C. W., M. G. Maksud, & J. Melichna: Physiological considerations in training young athletes. *Sports Medicine.* 8:15–31 (1989).

101. Zoll, P. M., S. Wessler, & M. J. Schlesinger: Interarterial coronary anastomoses in the human heart with particular reference to anemia and relative anoxia. *Circulation.* 4:797–815 (1951).

7

Thermoregulation

After studying the chapter, you should be able to:

- Identify environmental factors that affect human thermoregulation and be able to use indices of heat stress and windchill to assess the risk associated with exercise under various conditions.

- Describe thermal balance and discuss factors that contribute to heat gain and heat loss.

- List and define the mechanisms by which heat is lost from the body.

- Identify the factors that influence heat exchange between an individual and the environment.

- Describe the challenges facing the cardiovascular system when exercise is performed in a hot environment and in a cold environment.

- Differentiate between the different types of heat illness in terms of symptoms, causes, and first-aid.

- Identify ways in which an exercise leader can prevent heat and cold injuries and illness.

Introduction

Human thermoregulatory responses rely heavily on the cardiovascular system to maintain body temperature. This chapter will address the issue of exercise in environmental extremes, emphasizing the role of the cardiovascular system in mediating the body's response to exercise under such conditions.

Exercise in Environmental Extremes

Exercise in conditions of environmental extremes can present a serious challenge to the thermoregulatory and cardiovascular systems of the body. If the cardiovascular system is unable to meet the concurrent demands of supplying adequate blood to the muscles and maintaining thermal balance, heat illness may ensue. Heat illness covers a spectrum of disorders from heat cramps to life-threatening heat exhaustion. Cold conditions can also pose problems. If an exerciser is unprepared or inadequately clothed for exercise in cold environments, heat loss can exceed heat production, leading to cold-induced injury.

Exercise professionals have a responsibility to understand the problems associated with exercise in extreme environmental conditions because they may affect an individual's performance or place an exerciser at risk for injury or illness. An understanding of the body's response to extreme environmental conditions provides a basis for minimizing performance decrements and avoiding injury or illness in those who train and compete in adverse conditions.[34]

Basic Concepts

If you are to understand the body's response to exercise in different environments, you must first understand basic environmental measures and the way that body temperature is assessed.

Measurement of Environmental Conditions

Environmental conditions that affect human thermoregulation are ambient temperature (T_{amb}), rela-

FIGURE 7.1

Heat Stress Index

Source: Modified from Armstrong & Hubbard.[2]

[1]Low risk: Use discretion, especially if unconditioned or unacclimatized; little danger of heat stress for acclimatized individuals who hydrate adequately.
[2]Moderate risk: Heat-sensitive and nonacclimatized individuals may suffer; avoid strenuous activity in the sun; take adequate rest periods and replace fluids.
[3]High risk: Extreme heat stress conditions exist; consider canceling all exercise.

tive humidity, and wind speed. Ambient temperatures are most often measured with a mercury thermometer. **Relative humidity** indicates the moisture in the air relative to how much moisture, or water vapor, can be held by the air at any given ambient temperature. Thus, 70% humidity means that the air contains 70% of the moisture that it is capable of holding. The **heat stress index** is a scale used to determine the risk of heat stress from measures of ambient temperature and relative humidity (see Figure 7.1).

Relative Humidity The moisture in the air relative to how much moisture, or water vapor, can be held by the air at any given ambient temperature.

Heat Stress Index A scale used to determine the risk of heat stress from measures of ambient temperature and relative humidity.

Wind speed affects the amount of heat lost from the body and is used in the calculation of the wind-chill factor (see Table 7.1). The *windchill* is derived from the wind speed and the ambient temperature, and it reflects the temperature equivalent if wind were not a factor. For instance, if it is 20°F and the windspeed is 15 mi·hr^{-1}, the windchill factor is –5°F. This windchill factor means that a person will lose as much heat and feel as cold as he or she would if it were –5°C and there were no wind.

Measurement of Body Temperature

Exercise physiologists differentiate temperatures at different portions of the body, most commonly using *core* (T_{co}) and *skin temperature* (T_{sk}). Even this distinction is simplistic, since core temperature and skin temperature will each vary depending on the specific site that is measured. Core temperature is normally maintained within fairly narrow limits of approximately 36.1–37.8°C.[19] Skin temperatures, however, are considerably cooler, averaging approximately 33.3°C. They are also more variable, since they are greatly influenced by environmental conditions.

Measurements of body temperature are most commonly obtained from a thermometer placed in the oral cavity. However, this method is affected by many factors, including breathing rate and fluid ingestion, and it is not the method of choice among physiologists. Core temperature is most accurately assessed by measuring the temperature of the blood as it enters the right atrium or measuring esophageal temperatures. These are invasive procedures, however, and are not practical for routinely measuring core temperature. Therefore, rectal temperatures (T_{re}) are often used in laboratory settings to assess core body temperature.

Although rectal temperature is a reliable way to measure body temperature, it is not applicable for

TABLE 7.1 ▪ Wind Chill Index

WIND SPEED (MI·HR^{-1})	Thermometer Reading*										
	50	40	30	20	10	0	–10	–20	–30	–40	–50°F
5	48	37	27	16	6	–5	–15	–26	–36	–47	–57
10	40	28	16	4	–9	–24	–33	–46	–58	–70	–83
15	36	22	9	–5	–18	–32	–45	–58	–72	–85	–99
20	32	18	4	–10	–25	–39	–53	–67	–82	–96	–110
25	30	16	0	–15	–29	–44	–59	–74	–88	–104	–118
30	28	13	–2	–18	–33	–48	–63	–79	–94	–109	–125
35	27	11	–4	–20	–35	–41	–67	–82	–98	–113	–129
40	26	10	–6	–21	–37	–53	–69	–85	–100	–115	–132

Low risk | Moderate risk | High risk

Low Risk: Use discretion; little danger if properly clothed.

Moderate Risk: Postpone exercise if possible. Proper clothing is essential. Individuals at risk should take added precautions against overexposure.

High Risk: There is great danger from cold exposure; consider canceling all exercise.

Source: Vogel, Jones, & Rock.[33]

*Note that this table uses °F; see Appendix A for conversion.

mass testing, nor is it routinely used to assess temperatures in exercise participants or athletes. Despite the importance of the assessment of body temperature in the prevention and treatment of heat illness, there is no readily available, accurate, and convenient way of assessing core temperature in many situations, including athletic events. Often practitioners must rely on oral temperatures despite problems associated with this method. Other times medical personnel will obtain rectal temperatures. And in some instances tympanic membrane temperatures (T_{tym}) may be assessed although it is not clear that tympanic thermometry can actually detect exercise-induced heat stress.

Skin temperatures are not routinely measured in field settings, but they are important, because they determine the amount of heat that will be exchanged with the environment. Heat moves down a thermal gradient. Therefore, more heat will be lost from the body when the body is considerably hotter than the environment (larger gradient) than when the two temperatures are similar (smaller gradient). In the same way, more heat will be gained by the body when the environment is considerably hotter than the body. Skin temperatures are assessed via thermocouples attached to the skin.

Thermal Balance

The temperature of the body is the result of a balance between heat gain and heat loss (Figure 7.2). Although heat can be gained from the environment, the majority of heat is typically produced by the body as a result of metabolic activity. Heat is a by-product of cellular respiration; at rest the body liberates approximately 60–75% of the energy from aerobic metabolism as heat (see Chapter 11). The minimum energy required to meet the metabolic demands of the body at rest is called *basal metabolic rate* (BMR) or *resting metabolic rate* (RMR) and accounts for a large proportion of heat production.

The ingestion of food increases the body's production of heat and is known as *thermogenesis* (see Chapter 15). Also, any muscular activity will increase heat production, including activity related to muscle tone and posture; activities of daily living

FIGURE 7.2

Thermal Balance

Normal range in body temperature

36   37°C   38

Environmental
• Radiant
• Conductive
• Convective

Metabolic
• BMR/RMR
• Thermogenesis
• Muscular activity
  –Postural
  –ADL
  –Exercise

Heat Gain

Evaporative
Radiant
Conductive
Convective

Heat Loss

Thermal balance

(ADL), such as showering or getting to and from classes; and planned exercise. Since metabolism is greatly increased during physical activity, heat production is also increased dramatically.

Heat can be exchanged (gained or lost) from the body by four processes: radiation, conduction, convection, and evaporation. The effectiveness of these processes depends on environmental conditions—namely, ambient temperature, relative humidity, and wind speed.

Radiant heat loss occurs through the emission of electromagnetic heat waves to the environment and depends upon the thermal gradient between the body and the environment. When the environmental temperature equals skin temperature, no heat is lost through radiation. If the environmental temperature exceeds skin temperature, radiation will add to the heat load of the body.

Conduction involves the direct transfer of heat from one molecule to another. In terms of human temperature regulation conduction involves warming molecules of air and other surfaces in contact with the skin. The effectiveness of conductive heat loss is determined by the thermal gradient between the skin and the molecules in contact with the skin and by the thermal properties of the molecules in contact with the skin. Because water can absorb and conduct heat much better than air, submersion in water is an effective way to lower the body temperature.

Convective heat loss depends on the movement of the molecules in contact with the skin. When there is a breeze, heat loss is enhanced, because the warmer molecules are moved away from the skin. Thus the thermal gradient is maintained so that more heat can be lost by conduction.

Evaporation is the conversion of liquid into vapor. The evaporation of unnoticed water from the skin, called *insensible perspiration*, contributes to heat dissipation under resting conditions. The evaporation of sweat is a major mechanism for cooling the body under exercise conditions. Sweat is a hypotonic solution (99% water) derived from plasma and released from eccrine glands located throughout the body but concentrated on the forehead, hands, and feet.[19]

During heavy exercise the sweat rate of an individual can increase dramatically. Sweat rates vary considerably among individuals, depending upon genetics and fitness level. For any one individual

sweat rate depends upon environmental conditions, exercise intensity, fitness level, degree of acclimatization, and hydration status. Figure 7.3 provides an estimation of hourly sweating rates for running at various speeds under different environmental conditions.[26,29] Notice how common it is for sweating rates to exceed $1 \text{ L} \cdot \text{hr}^{-1}$ of sweat. Clearly, this water loss will lead to a decrease in total body water and plasma volume and will result in deleterious effects on cardiovascular function if fluid is not replaced.

The evaporation of sweat represents the primary defense against heat stress. Sweating itself does not cool the body; the sweat must be evaporated. The evaporation of sweat produces a cooling of the body because energy is needed to convert the liquid sweat into a vapor, and this energy is extracted from the immediate surroundings. The amount of energy needed for the evaporation of sweat can be quantified: 580 kcal of heat energy is released for each liter of water that is vaporized.[4]

When the body is in thermal balance, the amount of heat produced and the amount of heat lost are equal. So if they are added, the sum is equal to zero, and body temperature is constant. This can be explained by the following formula:[38]

(7.1)	$M \pm R \pm C \pm K - E = 0$

where M is metabolic heat production, R is radiant heat exchange, C is convective heat exchange, K is conductive heat exchange, and E is evaporative heat loss.

The plus or minus sign for radiant, convective, and conductive processes indicates that heat can be lost or gained by the body through these mechanisms. When the environment is hotter than the skin temperature, heat is gained by the body (a plus sign in the equation). When skin temperature is higher than the environment temperature, heat is lost from the body (a negative sign in the equation). Evaporation cannot add to the heat load of the body. This mechanism can only dissipate heat; thus, there is only a negative sign in the equation for evaporation.

Heat Exchange

The exchange (transfer) of heat between the body and the environment occurs by the mechanisms just

FIGURE 7.3

Estimated Sweating Rate at Various Running Speeds

Source: M. N. Sawka & K. B. Pandolf. Effects of body water loss on physiological function and exercise performance. In C. V. Gisolfi & D. R. Lamb (eds.), *Perspectives in Exercise Science and Sports Medicine. Vol 3: Fluid Homeostasis During Exercise.* Carmel, IN: Cooper Publishing Group. 97–151 (1993). Reprinted by permission.

described: conduction, convection, radiation, and evaporation. Heat exchange is represented schematically in Figure 7.4. These four mechanisms are important in dissipating heat to the environment under most conditions. However, under certain conditions—namely, high ambient temperatures—conduction, convection, and radiation may actually add heat to the body.

The effectiveness of heat exchange between an individual and the environment is affected by five factors:

1. The thermal gradient
2. The relative humidity
3. Air movement
4. The degree of direct sunlight
5. The clothing worn by the individual

The greater the difference between two temperatures—called the *thermal gradient*—the greater the heat loss is from the warmer of the two. Typically,

the body is warmer than the environment, so heat moves down its thermal gradient to the environment. More heat is lost on cooler days because the thermal gradient is greater.

High humidity decreases evaporative heat loss from the body since the air is already largely saturated with water vapor. Relative humidity is the primary factor that determines the effectiveness of evaporative cooling.[34]

Air movement increases convective heat loss from the skin to the environment. Thus, on windy days more heat is lost from the body.

Direct sunlight can add considerably to the radiant heat load of an individual. Conversely, shade or cloud cover can often provide significant relief from heat.

Clothing can also influence the effectiveness of heat transfer with the environment. In cold weather,

FIGURE 7.4

Mechanisms of Heat Exchange and Percentage of Heat Loss

Source: Modified from Gisolfi & Wenger.[15]

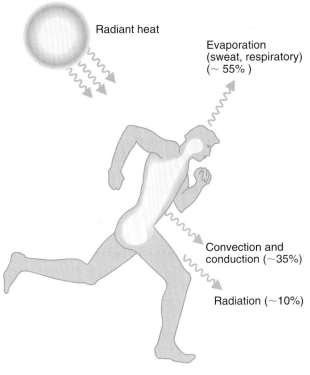

Radiant heat

Evaporation (sweat, respiratory) (~ 55%)

Convection and conduction (~35%)

Radiation (~10%)

Metabolic heat production

clothing protects against excessive heat loss. However, clothing can also interfere with heat dissipation in hot weather by decreasing convective heat loss. Clothing that is lightweight, nonrestrictive, and light in color promotes heat loss; heavy, dark clothing interferes with the dissipation of heat. Football uniforms, especially the protective padding, are an example of heavy, restrictive clothing. Helmets, in particular, limit heat loss by encapsulating the head. The color of the clothing is also a consideration. Dark colors absorb light and thereby add to the radiant heat load; light colors reflect light. Thus, dark-colored uniforms can contribute to the heat stress of athletes as they play on a synthetic field that radiates heat in the hot fall sun. Short shirts and the use of mesh materials are attempts to aid in heat dissipation under these conditions.

Heat Exchange During Exercise

Heat production and heat transfer occur by the same mechanisms during exercise as they do at rest. However, during exercise the total body metabolism may increase to 15–20 times the resting rate.[26] Under these conditions metabolic heat production may increase to an extent that heat production is greater than heat dissipation; thus, the body will store heat and body temperature will increase.

All of the factors discussed previously apply to heat exchange during exercise. The major change in the thermal balance equation during exercise is the dramatic increase in metabolic heat production. Metabolic heat from the muscles is transported to the core of the body by the blood. Heat is also transferred to the skin and exchanged with the environment by conduction, convection, radiation, and evaporation. During exercise heat production typically exceeds heat loss, so that heat is stored and body temperature rises, a condition known as hyperthermia.

Figure 7.5 depicts the relative importance of the heat exchange mechanisms during 60 min of cycling exercise (900 kgm · min⁻¹) at various ambient temperatures. Total heat loss remains relatively constant across a wide range of ambient temperatures. The fact that metabolic heat production exceeds the total heat loss accounts for the increase in temperature that is observed with exercise. Although total heat loss remains relatively constant, it is achieved by different mechanisms at different ambient tem-

FIGURE 7.5

Mechanisms of Heat Loss During Exercise at Different Ambient Temperatures

M = metabolic heat production, THL = total heat loss, R + C = heat loss by radiation and conduction, E = heat loss by evaporation. Exercise was performed for 60 min at workload of 900 kpm · min⁻¹ at each ambient temperature. Notice that the metabolic heat produced and the total heat loss (and thus the heat storage) is constant over a wide range of temperatures although it is achieved via different mechanisms. Evaporative heat loss becomes increasingly important as ambient temperature increases.

Source: C. V. Gisolfi & C. B. Wenger. Temperature regulation during exercise: Old concepts, new ideas. *Exercise and Sport Sciences Reviews.* 12:339–372 (1984). Reprinted with permission by Williams & Wilkins.

peratures. At high temperatures evaporative heat loss dominates, and radiant and convective heat losses become less effective.

Exercise in the Heat: Cardiovascular Demands

There are several interrelated problems that the cardiovascular system faces under hyperthermic conditions. First, there is a competition for blood flow between the skin and the muscles. The muscles need increased blood flow to meet the demands of metabolic activity, and the skin needs increased blood flow to dissipate heat from the core of the body. The combined needs of the skin and muscle for blood flow may exceed the cardiac output. Second, vasodilation in the cutaneous vessels effectively decreases venous return, thus decreasing stroke volume. Therefore, cardiac output may be reduced at a time when the demands for flow are greatest.[23] Third, the body must maintain an adequate blood pressure to perfuse the vital organs, including brain, kidneys, and liver. The ability to maintain blood pressure is challenged by widespread vasodilation in the skeletal muscle beds and cutaneous vessels, thus decreasing total peripheral resistance. Fourth, there is a reduction in plasma volume, which contributes to the reduction in cardiac output.

As seen in Figure 7.6a, during short-term, light submaximal exercise cardiac output increases to a similar degree whether exercise is performed in a hot or a thermoneutral environment.[24] However, cardiac output in a hot environment is achieved by a higher heart rate and a lower stroke volume than in a thermoneutral environment. The reduction in stroke volume occurs because of vasodilation in the cutaneous vessels, which decreases central venous volume. Mean arterial pressure is similar to or slightly lower in hot environments than in thermoneutral environments because of vasoconstriction in the kidneys and digestive tract. During light exercise in a hot environment rectal temperature is similar to values achieved in a thermoneutral environment.[28]

During prolonged, heavy submaximal exercise in the heat the increase in cardiac output is less than when exercise is performed in a thermoneutral environment (see Figure 7.6). The failure of cardiac output in hot environments to reach levels attained under thermoneutral conditions during heavy exercise reflects a progressive reduction in stroke volume as the severity of exercise increases. The higher heart rate seen under hot conditions is not able to compensate for the reduction in stroke volume during heavy exercise in hot conditions. Thus, cardiac output is lower in hot conditions.

During prolonged, heavy submaximal exercise in the heat vasoconstriction occurs in the digestive and renal areas in an attempt to maintain mean arterial blood pressure. In fact, vasoconstriction may result in ischemia and even tissue damage under severe conditions.[23] The regulatory mechanisms that maintain blood pressure are stressed by the excessive

FIGURE 7.6

Cardiovascular Responses to Hot or Thermoneutral Conditions

Source: L. B. Rowell. Human cardiovascular adjustments to exercise and thermal stress. *Physiological Reviews.* 54:75–159 (1974). Reprinted by permission.

water loss that occurs through profuse sweating (see Figure 7.3). If this fluid is not replaced, stroke volume, cardiac output, and blood pressure will decrease. Additionally, performance will suffer, and heat illness will be increasingly likely.

Maximal cardiac output is lower during incremental exercise to maximum when performed under hot conditions than thermoneutral conditions. This decrease results from a lower stroke volume, since maximal heart rate is unchanged, although maximal heart rate may occur earlier when exercise is performed in the heat. The estimated distribution of cardiac output during an incremental exercise test performed under neutral and hot conditions is presented in Figure 7.7.

When exercise is performed in the hot environment, it cannot be performed for as long as in cooler conditions. Consequently, $\dot{V}O_2$max is lower in the hot environment (Figure 7.7b). Cardiac output increases during exercise in both conditions. However, cardiac output at $\dot{V}O_2$max is less when exercise is performed in the hot environment, presumably because blood is displaced in cutaneous veins, thus decreasing venous return and stroke volume. Blood flow to the active skeletal muscles increases throughout exercise in both conditions. However, skeletal muscle blood flow represents a smaller proportion of total blood flow in the hot environment than in the thermoneutral environment, because skin blood flow accounts for a larger portion of the blood flow. At $\dot{V}O_2$max in the hot condition visceral blood flow is severely reduced in an effort to support the muscles with adequate blood flow and maintain blood pressure. The lower cardiac output and the decrease in blood flow when maximal exercise is performed in a hot environment both contribute to a lower $\dot{V}O_2$max.

Factors Affecting Cardiovascular Response to Exercise in the Heat

Several factors affect an individual's response to exercise in the heat. This section will discuss four of

> **Acclimatization** The adaptive changes that occur when an individual undergoes prolonged or repeated exposure to a stressful environment; these changes reduce the physiological strain produced by such an environment.

FIGURE 7.7

Distribution of Cardiac Output During Incremental Exercise in Thermoneutral (25.6°C) and Hot (43.3°C) Conditions
Source: Modified from Rowell.[23]

them: acclimatization, cardiovascular fitness, body composition, and hydration level.

Acclimatization **Acclimatization** refers to adaptive changes that occur when an individual undergoes prolonged or repeated exposure to a stressful environment; these changes reduce the physio-

FIGURE 7.8

Comparison of Rectal Temperature, Heart Rate, and Sweat Loss in Acclimated and Unacclimated Individuals During Prolonged Exercise

Source: Based on data in Wyndham.[40]

logical strain produced by such an environment. Acclimatization to heat is accomplished by repeated exposure to heat sufficient to increase core body temperature and elicit moderate to profuse sweating.[37] Light to moderate exercise in the heat for 1–2 hr a day can lead to positive adaptations within a few days.

Acclimatization to heat involves three underlying mechanisms:

1. Cardiovascular changes occur that decrease heart rate and cardiovascular strain at a given level of exercise in the heat.

2. Sweating patterns are altered such that sweating begins earlier.

3. There is a higher sweating rate for a given core temperature that can be maintained for longer periods of time.[36]

Figure 7.8 presents changes in rectal temperature, heart rate, and sweating rate during 4 hr of exercise before and after acclimatization.[36] These data reinforce the point that the benefits of heat acclimatization are lowered thermal and cardiovascular strain. Proper acclimatization ensures that individuals can perform longer and more safely in the heat.

Fitness Level   Aerobic fitness improves an individual's thermoregulatory function and heat tolerance.[36] Endurance training results in a lower resting core temperature, a larger plasma volume, an earlier onset of sweating, and a smaller decrease in plasma volume during exercise.[12,37] Therefore, individuals who are aerobically fit are better able to handle the cardiovascular demands associated with exercise in hot conditions than sedentary individuals. High-intensity, interval training in thermoneutral conditions also decreases the time required for acclimatization to exercise in a hot environment.[10]

Body Composition   Excessive body fat is a liability in terms of thermoregulation during exercise in the heat. Greater adiposity contributes to heat stress by two primary mechanisms. First, it interferes with the dissipation of heat; body fat acts to insulate the core. Second, body fat adds to the metabolic cost of activity by adding weight to the body that must be moved. Heat illness is more common in overweight individuals and more likely to be fatal to these individuals.[16]

Hydration Level An individual's level of hydration has a large impact on exercise tolerance and on the cardiovascular responses to prolonged exercise in the heat. Body water accounts for 65–70% of the total body mass of an average adult. During prolonged exercise in the heat profuse sweating leads to large losses of total body water and a reduction in plasma volume if fluid is not replaced.[35] The loss of plasma volume has negative effects on the thermoregulatory and cardiovascular systems and contributes to performance decrements and heat illness. Figure 5.5 presented the differences in cardiovascular responses to prolonged exercise with and without fluid replacement. When fluid was replaced, cardiac output and stroke volume could be maintained throughout exercise. However, when water was not replaced, there was a considerable downward drift in stroke volume and an upward drift in heart rate.

Thirst is an inadequate mechanism to fully replace the fluid lost during exercise. Even when unlimited access to water is provided, individuals will not voluntarily consume enough water to replace water loss, and a relative state of dehydration occurs. **Voluntary dehydration** refers to the exercise-induced dehydration that develops despite an individual's access to unlimited water. Thus, the coach or exercise leader needs to encourage participants to consume water beyond what thirst dictates. Experts recommend that 400–500 mL of water be ingested prior to activity and that another 200–400 mL be consumed every 15–30 min of activity.[20, 34] Thus, regardless of acclimatization or fitness level, an individual must be well hydrated prior to and during exercise in a warm environment.[11, 27]

Voluntary Dehydration Exercise-induced dehydration that develops despite an individual's access to unlimited water.

Sex Differences in Exercise Response in Heat

The majority of scientific evidence suggests that the response of individuals to exercise in a hot environment depends more upon the state of their cardiovascular system than upon their sex.[12, 30, 31] Early studies suggested that women experienced more heat strain than men when both performed the same absolute work. However, these studies failed to control for differences in aerobic fitness levels. That is, the women were working at a higher percentage of maximal effort, and core temperature response to exercise is related more to relative exercise intensity than absolute intensity.[3,12] More recent studies that have matched subjects for fitness level, body size, body fat, and degree of heat acclimatization have found few thermoregulatory differences between the sexes, particularly if the phase of the menstrual cycle was controlled.[31]

There does appear to be a difference between the sexes in sweating response. Males begin sweating at a lower core temperature and have a greater sweat rate in humid conditions than similarly trained females.[5,12] Whether this difference is an asset or a liability to males is unknown. Some researchers have argued that males are inefficient and wasteful in terms of sweat production and that females have the advantage of sweating less and, thus, decreasing blood volume to a lesser extent.[6, 39] Others counter that higher sweat rates might be advantageous in situations where evaporative heat loss is important.[14] Although the sweating response is slightly different in males and females, heart rate and core temperature responses to exercise in the heat are similar.[13] Heat acclimatization produces similar results in both sexes.[13]

One of the confounding factors that needs to be considered regarding the thermoregulatory response of females is the phase of the menstrual cycle. Several studies have reported that core temperature is greater, at rest and during exercise, during the luteal phase of the menstrual cycle (days 14–28).[22,30]

Exercise Response of Older Adults in the Heat

Cardiac output increases above resting levels during exercise in the heat for both young and older individuals. However, at higher workloads the increase in cardiac output is not as great when exercise is performed in the heat as when it is performed under thermoneutral conditions (see Figure 7.6). The increase in cardiac output during exercise in a hot environment is less in older persons than in younger individuals of similar fitness levels.[18] Furthermore, it appears that young people increase cardiac output by augmenting heart rate, but older individuals increase cardiac output by increasing stroke volume.[18] This result helps explain why differences exist in cardiac output at higher workloads; apparently, there is a limit to the extent to which older individuals can increase stroke volume.

Exercise-induced reductions in plasma volume are greater in older individuals than in young individuals when they exercise in hot and humid conditions. When exercising at the same relative workload, young and older individuals demonstrate similar changes in systolic, diastolic, and mean arterial blood pressure. There is no difference in core temperature between young and older individuals when they exercise in the heat. Acclimatization to heat results in similar changes in older individuals and in young people.[21]

Exercise Response of Children in the Heat

There are several age-related differences in thermoregulatory responses that place children at a disadvantage compared with adults when they exercise in the heat.[7, 9] Table 7.2 summarizes the cardiovascular responses of children, relative to adults, during exercise in the heat. As discussed in Chapter 5, children have a lower cardiac output than adults at any given level of oxygen consumption. This lower cardiac output proves to be a detriment for children exercising in the heat because of the demands for increased blood flow during exercise-induced heat stress. Children also have a smaller plasma volume than adults from which to draw fluids. Thus, they have a reduced sweating capacity compared with that of adults. This is true when sweat rate is reported in absolute values, per surface area, and per sweat gland. Additionally, the temperature at which sweating begins is lower in children than in adults.[7]

As a result of these differences in responses, children have a shorter tolerance time for exercise

TABLE 7.2 ■ Responses of Children Relative to Adults to Exercise in the Heat

CHARACTERISTIC	RESPONSE OF CHILDREN COMPARED WITH RESPONSE OF ADULTS
Cardiac output/O_2 uptake	Lower
Metabolic heat of locomotion	Higher
Sweating rate	Lower
Sweating threshold	Higher
Exercise tolerance time	Lower
Rise in core temperature	Faster
Acclimatization to heat	Slower

Source: Modified from Bar-Or.[7]

performed in the heat and experience a faster increase in core temperature when dehydration is a factor than adults. Thus, special concerns exist when children and adults exercise together in hot environments. Activity should be restricted for children to 30 min or less if the thermal conditions represent moderate or high risk (see Figure 7.1).

Children need a long and gradual acclimatization program to ensure that they are physiologically prepared for exercise in the heat.[25] Children subjectively feel acclimatized before physiological acclimatization has occurred, and thus, they are likely to try to do too much too soon.

Heat Illness

The magnitude of cardiovascular stress placed on the body by exercise in the heat was addressed by Rowell.[23]

> Probably the greatest stress ever imposed on the human cardiovascular system is the combination of exercise and hyperthermia. Together these stresses can present life-threatening challenges, especially in highly motivated athletes who drive themselves to extremes in hot environments.[23]

When the cardiovascular system is unable to meet the thermoregulatory and metabolic demands of the body, heat illness ensues. **Heat illness** represents a spectrum of disorders that range in intensity and severity from mild cardiovascular and central nervous system disruptions (for instance, hypotension and fainting) to severe cell damage, including the brain, kidney, and liver (heatstroke).[17] Heat illness may manifest itself in a number of ways; from least to most serious, heat illness can be categorized as heat cramps, heat syncope, heat exhaustion, and heatstroke.

Heat Cramps   *Heat cramps* are an acute disorder consisting of brief, recurrent, and excruciating pain in the voluntary muscles of the legs, arms, or abdomen. Typically, the muscles have recently been engaged in intense physical activity. Heat cramps may result from a fluid-electrolyte imbalance.

Heat Syncope   *Heat syncope* is a temporary disorder characterized by circulatory failure due to pooling of blood in the peripheral veins and the subsequent decrease in ventricular filling, which leads to a decrease in cardiac output.[36] Thus, the individual feels light-headed and may faint. Heat syncope occurs most often when individuals perform strenuous and unaccustomed exercise or when they perform exercise during a sudden rise in temperature and/or humidity.[17] Moving the individuals to a cooler location and having them rest in a recumbent position is the appropriate first aid treatment for heat syncope.

Heat Exhaustion   *Heat exhaustion* is characterized by a rapid and weak pulse, fatigue, weakness, profuse sweating, psychological disorientation, and fainting. The skin is often pale and clammy, and body temperature is near normal or moderately elevated (usually below 39.5°C). Heat exhaustion is caused by an acute fluid loss and the inability of the cardiovascular system to adequately compensate for the concurrent demands of muscle and skin blood flow.

Children may be more susceptible to heat exhaustion because they have a smaller plasma pool

from which to decrease fluids. Thus, they have a potential for greater deficiency of peripheral blood supply during strenuous activity in the heat than adults.[41]

Individuals suffering from heat exhaustion should be moved to a cool place, given fluids, and encouraged to lie down. In severe cases of heat exhaustion a person may require intravenous administration of fluids and electrolytes.

Heatstroke   *Heatstroke* is a serious medical emergency; it is characterized by elevated skin and core temperatures (core temperature may exceed 40°C), tachycardia (rapid heart rate), vomiting, diarrhea, hallucinations, and coma. Since sweating has stopped, the skin is usually dry, hot, and red. Heatstroke represents a failure of the thermoregulatory mechanisms; thus, core temperature increases rapidly to dangerous levels. If heatstroke is suspected, the individual should be cooled as quickly as possible (using water, ice, or a fan) and medical personnel notified immediately. Heat stroke is a life-threatening medical emergency.

Prevention   Although exercise professionals should be able to recognize and respond to heat illness, they should preferably prevent heat injuries by using sound judgment and observing some basic recommendations. The American College of Sports Medicine (ACSM) has published a position stand, "The Prevention of Thermal Injuries During Distance Running,"[1] that outlines strategies to decrease thermal injuries during road races. The following list provides basic recommendations for people who exercise in hot environments.[34]

1. Allow adequate time for acclimatization (10–14 days).

2. Exercise during cooler parts of the day (early morning or evening).

3. Limit or defer exercise if the heat stress index is in the high-risk zone (see Figure 7.1)

4. Adequately hydrate prior to exercise and replace fluid loss during exercise. Monitor daily body weight changes closely, since they reflect acute water loss.

5. Wear clothing that is light in color and loose fitting, with large areas of skin exposed to the air to enhance evaporation.

Heat Illness A spectrum of disorders that range in intensity and severity from mild cardiovascular and central nervous system disruptions to severe cell damage, including the brain, kidney, and liver.

*E*xercise in the Cold

Cold weather can cause significant injuries to individuals who are unprepared or inadequately equipped for exercise training or competition. Although cold-related injuries are less common than heat-related injuries, they can be serious. The most common instances of individuals' exercising in the cold are in sporting events and wilderness experiences. Sporting events include winter sports such as skiing and ice skating and athletic contests such as football. During most of these activities hypothermia is not a major threat, because individuals typically have proper clothing, are producing a great deal of metabolic heat, and have access to shelter if it is necessary. Wilderness activities, such as hiking and backpacking, present more risk because exposure can often be prolonged.

Exposure to cold results in several physiological responses that alter thermal balance: Heat production increases and heat loss is minimized. Heat production increases owing to nonshivering thermogenesis, shivering thermogenesis, and exercise metabolism. *Nonshivering thermogenesis* refers to increased metabolic heat production from sources other than muscular contraction. Circulating hormones—namely, catecholamines, glucocorticoids, and thyroxine—increase metabolic rate during cold exposure.[32] Muscular tensing without noticeable shivering accounts for over 30% of the increase in heat liberation in response to cold exposure.[32] This response is sometimes called *preshivering*. Shivering can also contribute significantly to heat production. Exercise significantly increases metabolic heat.

To a large extent, cool temperatures are useful as a means of dissipating the large amount of heat produced by exercise. Very often, individuals who are exposed to the cold will voluntarily increase muscular activity as a means of increasing heat production, thus feeling more comfortable. Heat loss is minimized by widespread vasoconstriction, which decreases blood flow to the periphery in an attempt to maintain core temperature.

Despite the compensatory mechanisms, there are situations in which heat loss exceeds heat production and body temperature drops. When an individual is exposed to cold environments and heat loss is greater than heat production, serious injuries can result. The two most common cold-induced injuries of concern to exercise professionals are hypothermia and frostbite.[34]

Cold-Induced Injuries

Hypothermia, defined as a core temperature less than 35°C, is a lowering of the body temperature to the point that it affects normal function.[9] This condition is potentially fatal. The lowering of body temperature occurs when heat loss exceeds heat production. The magnitude of heat loss is affected by temperature, wind speed, and how wet the individual becomes. The windchill chart (Table 7.1) takes into account the combined effects of temperature and windchill and should be consulted before activity is performed in the cold.

Heat production increases greatly during exercise. Thus, hypothermia is seldom a concern provided that the exerciser is properly clothed and is not exposed to the environment for prolonged periods of time. However, during long-term events, like a marathon, hypothermia may occur owing to a reduction in heat production and an increase in heat loss. For instance, many runners will run the second half of a race at a slower pace; thus, heat production will decrease. At this time the runner may also have removed some clothing, because of greater heat production earlier in the run, and may be wet due to accumulated sweat, thus increasing the rate of conductive heat loss.

As body temperature decreases, physical signs of hypothermia can be observed. Early signs of hypothermia include a depression of heart rate, respiration, and reflexes. Mild hypothermia is marked by a loss of judgment and an inability to reason. The person often complains of being cold and focuses attention on getting warm. As hypothermia progresses, fine motor skills are affected, and speech may become slurred. Severe hypothermia is characterized by agitation and inappropriate behavior.[34] Mild hypothermia can be managed by warming the individual with blankets and warm beverages. However, moderate and severe cases of hypothermia should be treated by medical personnel. Since a person suffering from hypothermia often has an impaired ability to reason, the person should not be left alone.

Frostbite is the consequence of water crystallization within tissues that causes cellular dehydration and leads to tissue destruction.[34] Insufficiently insulated skin can be frostbitten, leading to permanent circulatory damage and possible amputation. Activities that involve speed (such as running, skiing, and cycling) can create windchill conditions that increase the likelihood of frostbite.

Prevention

The prevention of injury is preferable to the treatment of injury. To avoid injury, individuals should exercise in appropriate clothing. Windproof and water-repellent outer garments are necessary. The layering of loose-fitting clothing is more advantageous than a single layer of heavy, bulky clothes. The layer next to the skin should be a material that wicks moisture away from the skin. Cotton should not be worn next to the skin since it holds moisture that will draw body heat away from the body.

Exercisers should consider warming up inside, but just to the point where they begin to sweat so that they aren't wet when they go outside. If possible, they should run into the wind first and return with the wind at their back. Exercisers should also avoid periods in which there is a decrease in metabolic heat production that is not compensated for by additional clothing or by leaving the cold environment. For instance, the cool-down period at the end of exercise is potentially dangerous because the exerciser has now decreased heat production, although heat loss will remain high. Additionally, the exerciser may be fatigued, which would further exacerbate the condition. Thus, the exerciser should consider cooling down inside as well as warming up inside.

Factors Influencing Cold Tolerance

Body size and composition are important factors influencing an individual's response to cold exposure. Body fat provides protection against heat loss and can thus be advantageous when an individual is exposed to cold.[32] Since women on average have a greater percentage of body fat than men, they may tolerate cold better. Since children have a larger surface area per kilogram of body weight, they have a greater rate of heat loss in the cold than adults. To compensate for this loss, children have a greater degree of vasoconstriction in the periphery to protect core temperature. This compensatory factor, however, increases the risk of frostbite in the extremities.[9] Children also cool faster in water because of their higher surface area and smaller amount of subcutaneous fat than adults. Thus, special attention should be paid when children are swimming on cool days or when water temperatures are cool.

SUMMARY

1. Environmental conditions that affect human thermoregulation are ambient temperature (T_{amb}), relative humidity, and wind speed. The heat stress index assesses the risk of thermal injury from measures of ambient temperature and relative humidity. The windchill index assesses the risk of cold-induced injury from wind speed and ambient temperature.

2. The temperature of the body is the result of a balance between heat gain and heat loss. The major contributor of heat gain is heat produced by the body as a result of metabolic heat production. Heat can be lost from the body by four processes: radiation, conduction, convection, and evaporation.

3. The evaporation of sweat is the primary defense against heat stress. 580 kcal of heat energy is released for each liter of water that is vaporized.

4. The effectiveness of heat exchange depends on the thermal gradient, relative humidity, air movement, degree of direct sunlight, and clothing worn.

5. There are several interrelated problems that challenge the cardiovascular system under hyperthermic conditions.
   (a) There is a competition for blood flow between the skin and the muscles.
   (b) Vasodilation in the cutaneous vessels effectively decreases venous return and, thus, stroke volume.
   (c) Adequate blood pressure must be maintained to perfuse the vital organs.
   (d) There is a reduction in plasma volume, which contributes to the reduction in cardiac output.

6. An individual's response to exercise is influenced by the degree of acclimatization, cardiovascular fitness, body composition, and hydration level.

7. Scientific evidence suggests that the response of males and females to exercise in a hot environment is similar, although males appear to have a greater sweat rate.

8. Children are at greater risk of heat stress than adults when exercising in hot environments.

9. When the cardiovascular system is unable to meet the thermoregulatory and metabolic demands of the body, heat illness ensues. Heat illness represents a spectrum of disorders that range in intensity and severity; it

includes heat cramps, heat syncope, heat exhaustion, and heatstroke.

10. During exercise in the cold heat loss may exceed heat production. When heat loss is greater than heat production, serious injuries can result. The two most common cold-induced injuries of concern to exercise professionals are hypothermia and frostbite.

REVIEW QUESTIONS

1. Diagram the thermal balance that is typically maintained at rest. Indicate how this balance is altered during exercise in hot and cold environments.

2. Identify the factors that influence heat exchange, and discuss how each factor facilitates or impedes the transfer of heat to and from the body.

3. Describe the cardiovascular response to incremental exercise in a hot environment. Explain why these responses occur.

4. What is the importance of acclimatization? How much time is needed for acclimatization to occur?

5. Explain the influence of hydration level on an individual's response to exercise in the heat. What is necessary to maintain adequate hydration during exercise?

6. Discuss the effects of fitness level and body composition on an individual's response to exercise in the heat.

7. Provide a definition, cause, and treatment for each of the following: heat cramps, heat syncope, heat exhaustion, and heatstroke.

8. Identify ways in which the likelihood of heat illness can be minimized.

9. Explain the underlying cause of hypothermia and frostbite. Suggest ways in which these conditions can be prevented.

REFERENCES

1. American College of Sports Medicine: Position stand: The prevention of thermal injuries during distance running. *Medicine and Science in Sports and Exercise.* 19(5):529–533 (1987).

2. Armstrong, L. E., & R. W. Hubbard: High and dry. *Runners World.* June:38–45 (1985).

3. Astrand, P.: Experimental Studies of Physical Working Capacity in Relation to Sex and Age. *University Microfilms International* (1952).

4. Astrand, P. O., & K. Rodahl: *Textbook of Work Physiology.* New York: McGraw-Hill (1986).

5. Avellini, B. A., E. Kamon, & J. T. Krajewski: Physiological responses of physically fit men and women to acclimation to humid heat. *Journal of Applied Physiology.* 49:254–261 (1980).

6. Avellini, B. A., Y. Shapiro, K. B. Pandolf, N. A. Pimental, & R. F. Goldman: Physiological responses of men and women to prolonged dry heat exposure. *Aviation Space Environmental Medicine.* 51:1081–1085 (1980).

7. Bar-Or, O.: Children and physical performance in warm and cold environments. In R. A. Boileau (ed.), *Advances in Pediatric Sport Sciences. Vol. 1: Biological Issues.* Champaign, IL: Human Kinetics Publishers, 117–130 (1984).

8. Bar-Or, O.: Children's responses to exercise in hot climates: Implications for performance and health. *Sports Science Exchange.* 7(2): (1994).

9. Bar-Or, O., & T. Baranowski: Physical activity, adiposity, and obesity among adolescents. *Pediatric Exercise Science.* 6(4):348–360 (1994).

10. Cohen, J. S., & C. V. Gisolfi: Effects of interval training on work-heat tolerance of young women. *Medicine and Science in Sports and Exercise.* 14:46–52 (1982).

11. Coyle, E. F., & S. J. Montain: Thermal and cardiovascular responses to fluid replacement during exercise. In C. V. Gisolfi, D. R. Lamb, & E. R. Nadel (eds.), *Perspectives in Exercise Science and Sports Medicine. Vol. 6: Exercise, Heat, and Thermoregulation.* Indianapolis: Benchmark Press, 179–213 (1993).

12. Drinkwater, B. L.: Women and exercise: Physiological aspects. *Exercise and Sport Sciences Reviews.* 12:21–52 (1984).

13. Frye, A. J., & E. Kamon: Sweating efficiency in acclimated men and women exercising in humid and dry heat. *Journal of Applied Physiology.* 54:972–977 (1983).

14. Frye, A. J., & E. Kamon: Responses to dry heat of men and women with similar aerobic capacities. *Journal of Applied Physiology.* 50:65–70 (1981).

15. Gisolfi, C. V., & C. B. Wenger: Temperature regulation during exercise: Old concepts, new ideas. *Exercise and Sport Sciences Reviews.* 12: 339–372 (1984).

16. Henshell, A.: Obesity as an occupational hazard. *Canadian Journal of Public Health.* 58:491–497 (1967).

17. Hubbard, R. W., & L. E. Armstrong: The heat illnesses: Biochemical ultrastructural and fluid-electrolyte considerations. In K. B. Pandolf, M. N. Sawka, & R. R. Gonzalez (eds.), *Human Performance Physiology and Environmental Medicine at Terrestrial Extremes.* Dubuque, IA: Brown & Benchmark, 305–360 (1988).

18. Kenney, W. L., & R. K. Anderson: Responses of older and younger women to exercise in dry and humid heat without fluid replacement. *Medicine and Science in Sports and Exercise.* 20:155–160 (1988).

19. Marieb, E. N.: *Human Anatomy and Physiology.* Redwood City, CA: Benjamin/Cummings (1992).

20. Nieman, D.C.: *Fitness and Sports Medicine: An Introduction.* Palo Alto, CA: Bull Publishing (1990).

21. Pandolf, K. B., B. S. Cadarette, M. N. Wawka, A. J. Young, R. P. Francesconi, & R. R. Gonzalez: Thermoregulatory responses of matched middle-aged and young men during dry-heat acclimation. *Journal of Applied Physiology.* 65(1):65–71 (1988).

22. Pivarnik, J. M., C. J. Marichal, T. Spillman, & J. R. Marrow, Jr.: Menstrual cycle phase affects temperature regulation during endurance exercise. *Journal of Applied Physiology.* 72:543–548 (1992).

23. Rowell, L. B.: *Human Circulation Regulation During Physical Stress.* New York: Oxford University Press (1986).

24. Rowell, L. B.: Human cardiovascular adjustments to exercise and thermal stress. *Physiological Reviews.* 54:75–159 (1974).

25. Rowland, T. W.: *Exercise and Children's Health.* Champaign, IL: Human Kinetics Publishers (1990).

26. Sawka, M. N., & K. B. Pandolf: Effects of body water loss on physiological function and exercise performance. In C. V. Gisolfi & D. R. Lamb (eds.), *Perspectives in Exercise Science and Sports Medicine. Vol. 3: Fluid Homeostasis During Exercise.* Indianapolis: Benchmark Press, 1–38 (1990).

27. Sawka, M. N., & C. B. Wenger: Physiological responses to acute exercise-heat stress. In C. V. Gisolfi, D. R. Lamb, & E. R. Nadel (eds.), *Perspectives in Exercise Science and Sports Medicine. Vol. 6: Exercise, Heat, and Thermoregulation.* Indianapolis: Benchmark Press, 97–151 (1993).

28. Seals, D. R.: Influence of aging on autonomic-circulatory control at rest and during exercise in humans. In C. V. Gisolfi, D. R. Lamb, & E. R. Nadel (eds.), *Perspectives in Exercise Science and Sports Medicine. Vol. 6: Exercise, Heat, and Thermoregulation.* Indianapolis: Benchmark Press, 257–297 (1993).

29. Shapiro, Y., K. B. Pandolf, & R. F. Goldman: Predicting sweat loss response to exercise, environment and clothing. *European Journal of Applied Physiology.* 48:83–96 (1982).

30. Stephenson, L. A., & M. A. Kolka: Thermoregulation in women. *Exercise and Sport Sciences Reviews.* 21: 231–262 (1993).

31. Stephenson, L. A., & M. A. Kolka: Effect of gender, circadian period and sleep loss on thermal responses during exercise. In K. B. Pandolf, M. N. Sawka, & R. R. Gonzalez (eds.), *Human Performance Physiology and Environmental Medicine at Terrestrial Extremes.* Dubuque, IA: Brown & Benchmark, 267–304 (1988).

32. Toner, M. M., & W. D. McArdle: Physiological adjustments of man to the cold. In K. B. Pandolf, M. N. Sawka, & R. R. Gonzalez (eds.), *Human Performance Physiology and Environmental Medicine at Terrestrial Extremes.* Dubuque, IA: Brown & Benchmark, 361–400 (1988).

33. Vogel, J. A., B. H. Jones, & P. B. Rock: Environmental considerations in exercise testing and training. In S. N. Blair, P. Painter, R. R. Pate, L. K. Smith, & C. B. Taylor (eds.), *American College of Sports Medicine Resource Manual for Guidelines for Exercise Testing and Prescription.* Philadelphia: Lea & Febiger (1988).

34. Vogel, J. A., P. B. Rock, B. H. Jones, & G. Havenith: Environmental considerations in exercise testing and training. In J. L. Durstine, A. C. King, P. L. Painter, J. L. Roctman, L. D. Zwiren, & W. L. Kenney (eds.), *American College of Sports Medicine Resource Manual for Guidelines for Exercise Testing and Prescription* (2nd edition). Philadelphia: Lea & Febiger (1993).

35. Wade, C. E., & B. J. Freund: Hormonal control of blood volume during and following exercise. In C. V. Gisolfi & D. R. Lamb (eds.), *Perspectives in Exercise Science and Sports Medicine. Vol. 3: Fluid Homeostasis During Exercise.* Indianapolis: Benchmark Press, 201–246 (1990).

36. Wenger, C. B.: Human heat acclimatization. In K. B. Pandolf, M. N. Sawka, & R. R. Gonzalez (eds.), *Human Performance Physiology and Environmental Medicine at Terrestrial Extremes.* Dubuque, IA: Brown & Benchmark, 153–198 (1988).

37. Werner, J.: Temperature regulation during exercise: An overview. In C. V. Gisolfi, D. R. Lamb, & E. R. Nadel (eds.), *Perspectives in Exercise Science and Sports Medicine. Vol. 6: Exercise, Heat, and Thermoregulation.* Indianapolis: Benchmark Press, 49–79 (1993).

38. Winslow, C. E. A., A. P. Gagge, & L. P. Herrington: Influence of air movement upon heat losses from clothed human body. *American Journal of Physiology.* 127:505 (1939).

39. Wyndham, C. H., J. F. Morrison, & C. G. Williams: Heat reaction of male and female Caucasians. *Journal of Applied Physiology.* 20:357–364 (1965).

40. Wyndham, C. H., N. B. Strydom, J. F. Morrison, C. G. Williams, G. A. G. Bredell, M. J. E. Von Rahden, L. D. Holdsworth, C. H. Van Graan, A. J. Van Resnburg, and A. Munro: Heat reactions of Caucasians and Bantu in South Africa. *Journal of Applied Physiology.* 19:598–606 (1964).

41. Zwiren, L. D.: Children and exercise. In R. J. Shephard & H. S. Miller (eds.), *Exercise and the Heart in Health and Disease.* New York: Dekker, 105–163 (1992).

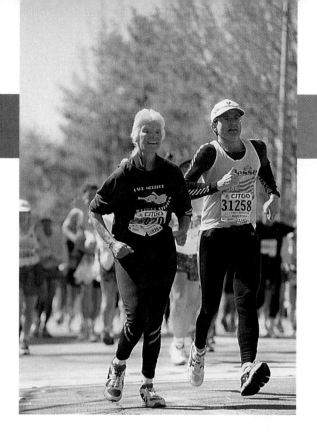

8

Cardiorespiratory System in Health and Disease

After studying the chapter, you should be able to:

- Identify the cardiovascular risk factors and classify them as major risk factors that can or cannot be modified, contributing risk factors, or nontraditional risk factors.

- Describe the relationship between each risk factor and cardiovascular disease. Identify how exercise training impacts on each of the risk factors.

- Differentiate between the immune response to moderate aerobic exercise and exhaustive exercise.

- Respond to the question: Does exercise increase or decrease the likelihood of illness?

- Describe the role of physical activity in the life of an individual infected with HIV.

Introduction

Earlier in this unit a distinction was made between the application of the training principles for the achievement of health and for the achievement of fitness. The health factor of primary concern is cardiovascular disease. Cardiovascular disease includes, but is not limited to, coronary heart disease (which can lead to myocardial infarctions or heart attacks), cerebrovascular disease (which can lead to strokes), hypertension, congestive heart failure, atherosclerosis and aneurysms, peripheral vascular diseases (which can lead to a claudication severe calf pain during walking), and rheumatic heart diseases. Coronary heart disease (CHD) is the most prevalent of the subdivisions of cardiovascular disease.[4] Additionally, the cardiovascular system is interrelated with the immune system, which protects against illness and infection. This chapter will explore the relationships between physical activity and cardiovascular disease and between physical activity and immune function.

Physical Activity and Cardiovascular Risk Factors

Between 1980 and 1990 the total number of deaths from cardiovascular disease declined steadily in males from 510,000 per year to 450,000 per year. For females the death rate increased from 490,000 per year in 1980 to about 502,000 in 1988 and then decreased to approximately 478,000 per year in 1990. Although this downward trend in the number of deaths per year is encouraging, it still means that cardiovascular disease is the number one cause of death in the United States. This is true for both males and females and for all races (white, African American, Hispanic, Asian, and Native American). Someone dies from cardiovascular disease every 34 sec in the United States alone.[4]

> **Risk Factor** An aspect of personal behavior or lifestyle, an environmental exposure, or an inherited characteristic that has been shown by epidemiological evidence to predispose an individual to the development of a specific disease.

Although the vast majority of these deaths (83%) occur in individuals over the age of 65, many individuals under the age of 65 have cardiovascular disease or acute heart attacks that do not immediately result in death. For example, 5% of all heart attacks occur in individuals under the age of 40, and 45% occur in people under the age of 65. Thus, old age increases the possibility of death from cardiovascular disease, but being young is not an automatic protection from impairment or death. Nor is being female a protection against cardiovascular disease, as the figures cited earlier emphasize. In fact, the actual number of deaths from cardiovascular disease was higher in females than in males from 1984 to 1990. This result, however, is at least partially a reflection of a higher population of females than males. When prorated per 100,000 population, the age-adjusted death rates show that men do have a higher rate of death from cardiovascular disease than women. At the same time, though, women who have had heart attacks are more likely to die from them within a few weeks to a year, or to suffer a second heart attack, than men who have had heart attacks.[4]

If the data are further subdivided by sex and race, the order from highest to lowest death rate is black males, white males, black females, and white females. Figures are unavailable for the other races.[4] The economic cost of cardiovascular disease, including all medical care and lost productivity resulting from disability, was estimated to be $128 million in 1994.[3]

Because of the statistics just listed, age, race, and sex are considered to be risk factors for coronary heart disease. A **risk factor** is defined as an aspect of personal behavior or lifestyle, an environmental exposure, or an inherited characteristic that has been shown by epidemiological evidence to predispose an individual to the development of a specific disease.[11] Table 8.1 lists various classifications of risk factors for coronary heart disease.[3] Note that the three factors already identified, along with heredity, constitute risk factors that cannot be changed. The point at which age becomes a risk factor for males is 45 yr; it is 55 yr for females, or the time of menopause without estrogen replacement. Heredity is interpreted as a family history (parent or sibling) with premature (less than 55 yr of age if male; less than 65 yr of age if female) cardiovascular disease or death from cardiovascular disease, especially heart attack or stroke. A family history of diabetes melli-

TABLE 8.1 ■ Coronary Heart Disease Risk Factors

FACTORS THAT CANNOT BE CHANGED	MAJOR FACTORS THAT CAN BE MODIFIED	OTHER CONTRIBUTING FACTORS THAT CAN BE MODIFIED	SELECTED NONTRADITIONAL FACTORS
Age	Cholesterol-lipid fractions	Diabetes mellitus	Apolipoproteins $\downarrow$ Apo-A1
Heredity	Cigarette smoking	Obesity	$\uparrow$ Apo-B
Race	Hypertension	Stress	Fibrinogen levels and fibrinolytic activity
Sex	Physical inactivity		

Increased = $\uparrow$, decreased = $\downarrow$.

tus, hypertension, and/or high cholesterol levels (hyperlipidemia) also increases the risk of coronary heart disease.

The other risk factors are, to some degree, modifiable through diet, exercise, medication, or other lifestyle changes. This section will discuss each of these risk factors, with major emphasis on the four primary factors and the role of physical activity or exercise training in modifying each. Each risk factor acts independently and will be discussed separately; but, in fact, many are also interrelated and act jointly. Furthermore, the list of nontraditional factors could be much longer, since the traditional factors predict only slightly more than 50% of the incidence of coronary heart disease.

Major Modifiable Risk Factors

Cholesterol-Lipid Fractions *Lipids,* or fats, are by definition water-insoluble substances. They may be classified as simple (or neutral) fats, compound fats, or derived fats. The primary simple fat is triglyceride. Compound fats are combinations of a neutral fat and another substance such as phosphate (phospholipid), glucose (glucolipid), or protein (lipoprotein). Derived fats originate from simple and compound fats. Chief among them is **cholesterol,** a derived fat that is essential for the body, but may be detrimental in excessive amounts.

Combining fats with another substance makes the compound water-soluble, and it is through such compounds—specifically **lipoproteins**—that fat is transported in the bloodstream. The protein portions of lipoproteins are called **apolipoproteins.**

Five types of lipoproteins circulate in blood, namely chylomicrons, very low density lipoproteins, intermediate-density lipoproteins, low-density lipoproteins, and high-density lipoproteins. *Chylomicrons* are microscopic fat particles formed after digestion that enter the blood stream via the lymphatic system. Triglycerides and some cholesterol are transported in the blood, from the small intestines or liver to adipose tissue or muscle for storage or use as fuel, by chylomicrons and *very low density lipoproteins* (VLDL). The VLDL from which the triglyceride has been removed is degraded into *an intermediate-density lipoprotein* (IDL), which in turn is converted in the liver to a **low-density lipoprotein (LDL).** LDL is composed of protein, a small portion of triglyceride, and a large portion of cholesterol. LDL transports 60–70% of the total cholesterol in the body to all cells except liver cells. The major apolipoprotein of LDL is called *Apo-B.*

Cholesterol A derived fat that is essential for the body but may be detrimental in excessive amounts.

Lipoprotein Water-soluble compound composed of apolipoprotein and lipid components that transport fat in the bloodstream.

Apolipoprotein The protein portion of lipoproteins.

Low-Density Lipoprotein (LDL) A lipoprotein in blood plasma composed of protein, a small portion of triglyceride, and a large portion of cholesterol whose purpose is to transport cholesterol to the cells.

If more cholesterol is made available to the cells than is needed, and an area of injury is present in the wall of the artery, the process of atherosclerosis begins. It is important to distinguish *atherosclerosis* from *arteriosclerosis.* **Arteriosclerosis** encompasses the natural aging changes that occur in blood vessels—namely, thickening of the wall, loss of elastic connective tissue, and hardening of the vessel wall. **Atherosclerosis** is a pathological process that results in the buildup of *plaque* (composed of connective tissue, smooth muscle cells, cellular debris, and cholesterol) inside the blood vessels. Ultimately, the buildup of plaque, often in conjunction with a blood clot, will obstruct blood flow. The primary sites of plaque growth are the aorta and the carotid, coronary, femoral, and iliac arteries. Depending on the amount of obstruction, the result can be pain (angina pectoris in the heart or claudication in the legs) or a heart attack or stroke.

High-density lipoprotein (HDL) is a lipoprotein in blood plasma composed primarily of protein and a minimum of cholesterol or triglyceride. The purpose of HDL is to transport cholesterol from the tissues to the liver. HDL carries cholesterol away from the tissue to the liver, where the cholesterol can be broken down and eliminated in the bile. There is also some speculation that HDL may block or in some way interfere with the deposition of cholesterol in the arterial wall lining. The major apolipoprotein of HDL is called *Apo-A1.*[49]

Whether triglycerides (and the associated VLDLs) represent a risk factor by themselves—that is, whether they act as an independent risk factor—is unknown. Chylomicrons are not thought to be atherosclerotic. There is abundant evidence, however, that an elevated total cholesterol (TC) level is independently and directly related to the incidence of CHD. A classification system for TC is presented in Table 8.2.[5,23] In the United States, an adult level of 240 mg·dL^{-1} represents twice the risk as a value of 200 mg·dL^{-1}. Therefore, these values have been taken as representing high-risk and acceptable levels, respectively. They apply to all adults regardless of age or sex. (The information on children will be considered later.) The term *hyperlipidemia* (excessive fat in the blood) is commonly used to describe this risk factor.

Not only is the total amount of cholesterol important, but also the fractions of LDL and/or HDL in that total are important. High levels of LDL and/or Apo-B are positively related to CHD. High levels of HDL and/or Apo-A1 are inversely related to CHD. Desirable levels of LDL are 130 mg·dL^{-1} or less. Desirable levels of HDL are 35 mg·dL^{-1} or more. An HDL level greater than or equal to 60 mg·dL^{-1} is actually so good that it is said to be a negative risk factor. Some consider a decrease in Apo-A1 and/or an increase in Apo-B to be independent risk factors.[57,60] However, specific levels have not been agreed upon and so the apolipoproteins are considered here to be nontraditional risk factors.

Cross-sectional studies in adults have generally shown that active individuals have lipid profiles indicating a reduced risk for CHD. This result is true at least as far as TC (lower in more active) and HDL (higher in more active) are concerned. However, there is little, if any, difference in LDL levels between active and inactive individuals. Cross-sectional studies, however, are by their very design difficult to interpret, since the element of self-

---

Arteriosclerosis The natural aging changes that occur in blood vessels—namely thickening of the walls, loss of elastic connective tissue, and hardening of the vessel wall.

Atherosclerosis A pathological process that results in the buildup of plaque inside the blood vessels.

High-Density Lipoprotein (HDL) A lipoprotein in blood plasma composed primarily of protein and a minimum of cholesterol or triglyceride whose purpose is to transport cholesterol from the tissues to the liver.

TABLE 8.2 ■ **Classification of Total Blood Cholesterol Levels**

Category	Level for Children and Adolescents (mg·dL^{-1})	Level for Adults (mg·dL^{-1})
Acceptable	< 170	< 200
Borderline	170–199	200–239
High	≥ 200	≥ 240

Sources: National High Blood Pressure Education Program;[32] Rowland.[43]

selection is always a danger. Perhaps individuals who have a good cholesterol profile are simply more likely to be active. This problem can be overcome by the use of training studies. In general, exercise training studies have supported a reduction in TC levels, but often not to statistically significant levels. Likewise, LDL levels have not shown significant reductions as a result of exercise training. On the other hand, all studies with a duration of greater than 12 weeks and a training volume of the equivalent of at least 15 km · week^{-1} of running have shown a significant increase in HDL levels.[60]

The direct impact of exercise training on the process of atherosclerosis has been difficult to document in humans. However, in a 1992 study one group of patients was placed on a low-fat diet (less than 20% of total calories; less than 200 mg of cholesterol) and a high-intensity daily exercise program (75% HR max). This study showed that 32% of the subjects experienced a regression in their coronary atherosclerotic lesion, 45% stayed the same, and only 23% exhibited a progression in their lesions. These figures were significantly better than the changes in the control group, who were advised to eat less fat and exercise but were left to their own initiatives. Other studies have supported this tendency.[16,24,45,49,60]

Although the results from exercise training studies are not as conclusive as might be desired, they are sufficient for the National Institutes of Health to support the statement that "the appropriate use of physical activity is considered an essential element in the nonpharmacologic therapy of elevated serum cholesterol."[57] Physical activity, of course, is to be used in conjunction with a low-fat diet and weight loss.

Cigarette Smoking   Nearly 20% of the deaths from cardiovascular disease can be directly attributed to cigarette smoking.[4] Breathing secondhand smoke also increases the risk of heart disease.[3] The chemicals in cigarettes, particularly nicotine, stimulate the sympathetic nervous system, causing an acute increase in heart rate and blood pressure, thus making the heart work harder. The carbon monoxide produced binds with hemoglobin, thus reducing oxygen transport. The atherosclerotic process is accelerated because smoking injures the arterial wall lining, increases the levels of circulating TC, and decreases the amount of HDL.

Smoking also causes blood platelets to adhere to each other, speeds up the rate of internal blood clotting, and makes the clots that do form tougher to dissolve. Prostacyclin, which is partially responsible for blood vessel dilation, is decreased. Capillaries and small arteries constrict and may spasm shut. Thus, the possibility of a thrombis (clot) or an embolism (moving clot) blocking an artery already narrowed by atherosclerosis is enhanced.

Narrowing of blood vessels to the arms and legs also makes smokers vulnerable to peripheral vascular disease, which may lead to gangrene and amputation. Certain life-threatening arrythmias of the heartbeat can also occur. Thus, smoking both operates independently and contributes to other CHD risk factors.[3,11,49,60]

The relationship between exercise training and smoking is only indirect. One study of over 3000 individuals showed a consistent and statistically significant inverse relationship between the number of cigarettes smoked and the level of physical activity in both males and females.[12] Another study (a random sampling of Peachtree Road Race runners) indicated that 85% of both men and women had never smoked. In addition, 81% of the men and 75% of the women who had smoked when they began running had since stopped. Only 1% of the men and 2% of the women who were nonsmokers began to smoke after beginning to run.[23] Although these results are encouraging, there is no direct cause-and-effect relationship. Most of you probably know someone who is active or a good athlete who also smokes. Individuals must make a conscious decision to not smoke.

Hypertension   One in every four American adults has *hypertension*.[4] The various stages of hypertension are presented in Table 8.3. These values are applicable to both sexes and all races throughout the entire adult life span. Note that the cutoff for defining **hypertension**, or high blood pressure, is 140/90 mmHg but readings between 130/85 and 140/90 mmHg represent values where lifestyle modifications should begin. All stages of hypertension are associated with an increased risk of

---

Hypertension High blood pressure, defined as values equal to or greater than 140/90 mmHg.

TABLE 8.3 ▪ Classification of Blood Pressure for Adults, Children, and Adolescents

CATEGORY	SYSTOLIC (mmHg)	DIASTOLIC (mmHg)
Adults (≥ 19 yr)		
Normal	<130	<85
High Normal	130–139	85–89
Hypertension		
Stage I (mild)	140–159	90–99
Stage II (moderate)	160–179	100–109
Stage III (severe)	180–209	110–119
Stage IV (very severe)	≥210	≥120
Children (3–12 yr)*		
Mild-moderate	≥130	≥86
Severe	≥144	≥96
Adolescents†		
Mild-moderate	≥144	≥90
Severe	≥160	≥104

*Values less than the 90th percentile for age and sex can be considered normal, and values between the 90th and 95th percentile abnormal.

†Values at or above the 95th percentile for age and sex indicate hypertension.

cardiovascular disease. The higher the stage of hypertension, the higher the risk of CHD is and the more aggressive the monitoring and treatment need to be.[32]

Ninety to 95% of the cases of hypertension have no known cause. Such hypertension is called *primary* or *essential hypertension*. However, for hypertension to occur, either cardiac output ($\dot{Q}$) or total peripheral resistance (TPR), or both, must be elevated. The most likely scenario is a transient increase in $\dot{Q}$ followed by an elevation in TPR that attempts to decrease $\dot{Q}$ and is itself sustained. The resultant high blood pressure may injure the artery linings and begin the process of atherosclerosis.[17]

The role of exercise training in the treatment of moderate hypertension is well substantiated by research. Individuals who are at high risk for developing hypertension—because of either genetics, body composition, primary disease status, or exaggerated blood pressure response to acute exercise—can reduce the risk by participating in an endurance

training program. Most, albeit not all, hypertensive individuals in well-designed and controlled studies have decreased both systolic and diastolic pressures by about 10 mmHg with aerobic endurance exercise programs. Light to moderate exercise (40–60% $\dot{V}O_2max$) has been shown to be equal to or better than higher-intensity programs.

Most studies have found that blood pressure responds quickly to exercise training. That is, the reduction in blood pressure occurs within three weeks to three months after the start of the training, often does not become fully normalized, and does not reduce further with continued training. If the training is stopped, the resting blood pressure returns to the elevated level. It may be that at least part of the reduction in blood pressure is a function of each individual exercise session rather than a permanent training adaptation, for even single sessions of submaximal exercise result in a reduced blood pressure for 1–9 hr postexercise.[2,17] That is, blood pressure exhibits a last-bout or augmented last-bout effect rather than a chronic adaptation to training. This means that maintenance of the training program is essential for keeping blood pressure lowered. These training changes seem to occur across the age spectrum of 15–79 yr and apply equally to males and females,[3] although females generally demonstrate a greater reduction in blood pressure than males who follow a similar training program.[2,17]

Dynamic aerobic endurance exercise training can also benefit individuals with severe or very severe hypertension. In this case, however, pharmacological therapy should be initiated first and then an exercise program added. Such a sequencing leads to a further reduction in blood pressure and ultimately a decreased reliance on antihypertensive medication.[2,17]

The pressor response accompanying dynamic resistance training has always been of great concern, and individuals with hypertension have historically been discouraged from doing weight lifting. Studies on resistance exercise, however, have failed to substantiate an adverse effect on blood pressure. At the same time, dynamic resistance training (with the exception of circuit weight training) has not consistently been shown to lower blood pressure in individuals with hypertension. Therefore, although the cardiovascular changes elicited by endurance training are more desirable than the changes brought about by resistance training, dynamic resistance training can be done by hypertensives as part of a comprehensive training program. Strength training should not be the only exercise program, though, and it is best if added after two or three months of typical aerobic endurance training.[2,17,51,52]

Physical Inactivity   Figure 8.1 shows the relationship between level of physical activity or fitness ($\dot{V}O_2$max) on the horizontal axis and the CHD mortality odds ratio on the vertical axis.[19] The odds ratio was computed by dividing the rate of deaths from CHD for more active or more fit individuals by the rate of death for the least active or least fit individuals. A definite inverse relationship is shown in the graph. That is, the more active or fit individuals have lower odds of death from CHD than the least active or least fit individuals. Of course, the relationship is not a perfect one and offers no guarantee for any given individual, but physical activity does tip the odds in a favorable direction for the population as a whole. Additional evidence suggests that even individuals with documented CHD can benefit from physical activity and reduce their likelihood of additional heart attacks or sudden death.

The degree of risk for those who are active, about twice that of those without the risk factor, is approximately the same for physical inactivity as for systolic hypertension, cigarette smoking, and hyperlipidemia. However, the number of individuals who are sedentary is substantially more than the

number possessing the other risk factors. Only about 10% of Americans report exercising daily for at least 30 min. Therefore, potentially more benefit overall could be achieved by increasing the activity level of U.S. citizens than by changing any other single risk factor.[4,11,16]

The mechanisms by which physical activity achieves its protective effect are many and varied. Some are independent and a direct result of the adaptive changes that occur in the cardiovascular system and its neural control that were documented earlier in this unit. For example, the increases in parasympathetic tone and decreases in sympathetic response will lower the resting and exercise heart rates in physically active individuals. These changes also will enhance the electrical stability of the myocardial cells, reducing the risk of potentially fatal conduction system defects and coronary vessel spasms. Other mechanisms are indirect and linked to the different risk factors.[11] The impact of physical activity or exercise training is briefly summarized in Table 8.4.

One of the most important facts about activity or exercise training is that the greatest health benefits occur when very sedentary individuals increase their endurance activity levels even minimally. The magnitude of health benefit becomes less as the intensity or amount of activity increases. Thus, as the text pointed out in the section on training principles (Chapter 6), for the achievement of physical fitness or performance in endurance sports, the most important element is training intensity. However, if the goal is one of health benefit, training volume (duration and frequency at a light to moderate intensity) is most important.[19]

Contributing Modifiable Risk Factors

Diabetes Mellitus   *Diabetes mellitus* is a complex metabolic disorder characterized by the inability to effectively use carbohydrates (glucose intolerance). *Type I diabetes* typically occurs in young individuals whose insulin-producing Beta cells in the pancreas fail. Thus, an external source of insulin must be supplied. *Type II diabetes* typically occurs in overweight or obese adults over the age of 40 yr. In such individuals, especially early in the progression of the disease, insulin may be produced in sufficient or even excessive amounts. However, there is a diminished sensitivity to the circulating insulin,

FIGURE 8.1

Relationship Between Activity Level and Mortality from Coronary Heart Disease

Source: W. S. L. Haskell. Health consequence of physical activity: Understanding and challenges regarding dose response. *Medicine and Science in Sports and Exercise.* 26(6):649–660 (1994). Reprinted by permission of Williams & Wilkins.

TABLE 8.4 ▪ Summary of Impact of Physical Activity or Exercise Training on Modifiable CHD Risk Factors

RISK FACTOR	IMPACT
Cholesterol-lipid fractions	↑ HDL fraction ↓ TC (maybe)
Cigarette smoking	Indirect
Hypertension	↓ SBP; ↓ DBP (incomplete normalization)
Physical inactivity	Directly eliminates
Diabetes mellitus	↑ glucose tolerance ↑ insulin sensitivity
Obesity	↓ Body fat
Stress	Unknown on hostility component of type A behavior; TABP may ↓
Fibrinogen levels and fibrinolytic activity	↓ fibrinogen levels ↑ fibrinolytic activity

Note: The impact is the same for children, adolescents, and adults except for stress and fibrinogen level and fibrinolytic activity, where insufficient information is available.

Increased = ↑, Decreased = ↓.

especially in the skeletal muscles and liver. Thus, Type II diabetics are, at least initially, noninsulin-dependent. Among the multitude of pathological complications resulting from diabetes is an acceleration of atherosclerosis, impaired myocardial contraction, and poor peripheral perfusion.[18]

One of the acute effects of submaximal dynamic endurance exercise is an increase in noninsulin-dependent uptake of glucose into the active skeletal muscle. This effect continues postexercise while the depleted stores of glucose (as glycogen) are restored. Additionally, an increased insulin sensitivity has been shown as a result of exercise training studies. These changes are transient and rely on a constant pattern of exercise. However, they are often sufficient to permit a reduction in the amount of daily insulin that needs to be injected in Type I diabetics. Regular exercise training, along with body weight or fat loss, has been shown to restore near-normal glucose tolerance and to increase insulin sensitivity in individuals with Type II diabetes.[18]

The use of exercise training for individuals with diabetes requires close monitoring and should be done in conjunction with medical personnel. Individuals with diabetes, especially Type I individuals, often exhibit abnormal blood pressure and other cardiovascular responses to exercise. Insulin injection (amount and site that avoids working muscles) and carbohydrate ingestions must be carefully adjusted to prevent the exercising diabetic from developing hypoglycemia.[18]

Obesity   The relationship between obesity and CHD is both independent of and interrelated with the other cardiovascular risk factors of hyperlipidemia and depressed HDL levels, hypertension, physical inactivity, and diabetes mellitus. Weight and/or fat reduction will improve the level of each and every one of these risk factors. The relationship between exercise training and body weight or body fat reduction is detailed in the metabolic unit of this text (Chapter 15).

Stress   Stress is probably the most controversial of the CHD risk factors. Many factors affect how stress impacts an individual, and these factors are difficult to identify and measure. How any given stressor is perceived will depend not just on the stressor but also on characteristics of the individual being stressed. For example, what vulnerabilities does the individual have, or what coping strategies are available to the individual?

The response to the stressor will vary on the basis of the individual's psychological and physiological level of reactivity. For example, among the acute physiological responses to fear or anger, mediated through the neural and hormonal systems, are an increase in heart rate, blood pressure, respiratory rate, and blood viscosity, and a decrease in clotting time and the breakdown of fats for use as a fuel. In the short-term these responses, if appropriate to the level of need, are good. After all, the individual might have to fight (and, if wounded, would need to clot blood quickly to prevent too great a loss of blood) or flee (and have sufficient energy and oxygen-carrying capacity to do so). However, if they are excessive, or if they become chronic, these responses form a possible mechanism for the development of hypertension, atherosclerosis, thrombogenesis, and clinical heart disease.

The consequences of both the stressor and the response to the stressor can also vary, from extremely positive and health enhancing to illness or injury or, ultimately, death. That is, such things as adaptation to exercise training for an improved fitness level can enhance health. On the other hand, as has been documented in several cases, bad news can precipitate sudden death from a heart attack in susceptible individuals.[11,25,40]

The type of stress primarily implicated in cardiovascular disease is psychosocial or emotional stress and not physical stress. Although life events, daily hassles, and occupational stresses, among other factors, have been considered in studies of stress, most emphasis has been placed on behavioral patterns known as Type A and Type B. The **type A behavior pattern (TABP)** is characterized by hard-driving competitiveness; time urgency, haste, and impatience; a workaholic lifestyle; and hostility. The **type B behavior pattern (TBBP)** is characterized by relaxation without guilt and no sense of time urgency.

Research in the 1970s showed a positive relationship between Type A behavior and CHD. Research in the 1980s and 1990s, however, seems to pinpoint only the hostility component. As a psychological concept, hostility includes cynicism, anger, mistrust, and aggression. Without hostility, the other Type A personality traits are now thought to be relatively benign.[25,40]

There have been only three studies to date on the impact exercise training has on TABP, and none of them isolated the component of hostility. Two of the three did show, however, a decrease in TABP with dynamic endurance exercise training. These studies involved both higher-intensity and longer-duration exercise than the study that showed no significant response.[25]

On the other hand, an acute bout of exercise is well established as an effective stress management technique. Thus, as with the influence of exercise on several of the other risk factors, it may be the short-term last-bout effect rather than the long-term chronic adaptation that is most important.[7]

Selected Nontraditional Risk Factors

Fibrinogen and Fibrinolytic Activity   As previously mentioned, one of the major dangers of the buildup of atherosclerotic plaque is that a clot might form and block the already narrowed blood vessel. *Fibrinogen* is a protein present in blood plasma that, under the proper physiological circumstances, is converted into *fibrin* threads that form the basis of a blood clot. In addition, fibrino-

gen increases blood platelet aggregation and blood viscosity. Thus, high levels of fibrinogen increase the likelihood of internal clot formation. Much of the relationship between smoking and CHD and some of the association between psychological stress and CHD may be mediated through plasma fibrinogen levels.[29]

Fibrinolytic activity, conversely, refers to the breakdown of the fibrin clots. Therefore, an enhanced fibrinolytic activity could potentially reduce the risk of clots and, hence, CHD.

A single bout of exercise has no documented effect on fibrinogen levels. There is only weak evidence from one study that dynamic endurance exercise training decreases fibrinogen level in older (over 60 yr) but not younger (24–36 yr) males.[53] Conversely, a single session of dynamic aerobic endurance exercise (but not static exertion) has consistently been shown to increase fibrinolytic activity.[14] The change is greater in active than in sedentary individuals, and high-intensity exercise produces more change than moderate-intensity exercise. The effect of exercise training is less certain, with only minimal evidence that training enhances fibrinolytic activity.[13,15,55,56,60]

Children and the Cardiovascular Risk Factors

The concern about cardiovascular disease risk factors for children is not that children exhibit clinical cardiovascular disease but that cardiovascular disease is a lifelong process that begins in childhood. Therefore, if risk factors can be prevented, modified, or counteracted in childhood, it may be possible to prevent or at least delay or reduce the severity of cardiovascular problems in adulthood.

In relation to physical activity the intent is to establish patterns of participation in children that

---

Type A Behavior Pattern (TABP) Behavior that is characterized by hard-driving competitiveness; time urgency, haste, and impatience; a workaholic lifestyle; and hostility.

Type B Behavior Pattern (TBBP) Behavior associated with characteristics of relaxation without guilt and no sense of time urgency.

will continue into and throughout adulthood. To a large extent, the success of this strategy depends upon a phenomenon called *tracking*. In this context **tracking** means that a characteristic is maintained, in terms of relative rank, over a long time span or even a lifetime. The easiest nonrisk factor to relate tracking to is height. Children in the upper percentiles of height at a very young age tend to maintain that position and be taller than average adults. Thus, in relation to children, it is important to be able to determine the presence or absence of the modifiable risk factors, the tracking strength of the risk factors, and the impact of physical activity and exercise training on both the short-term risk factor reductions and long-term lifestyle modifications.[42,44]

Cholesterol-Lipid Fractions

At birth total cholesterol levels are approximately 70 mg·dL^{-1} with 35 mg·dL^{-1} of that total being HDL. During the first few weeks of life that level rises rapidly to between 100 and 150 mg·dL^{-1}. By 2 yr and until adulthood the average value for males is about 160 mg·dL^{-1} and for females about 165 mg·dL^{-1} with HDL levels of between 50 and 55 mg·dL^{-1}. At puberty males show a decline of HDL and females a decline in LDL values.[57] In general, cholesterol levels do track from childhood to adulthood, but not all children with high juvenile levels of cholesterol will have elevated adult levels. In one study 43% of the children who had cholesterol values above the 90th percentile also had adult values above the 90th percentile and 81% had values above the 50th percentile.[5,30]

Values that represent acceptable, borderline, and high-risk levels for children are included in Table 8.2.[57] As for adults, high TC, high-LDL, and low-HDL levels have been found to be related to the magnitude of early atherosclerotic lesions. Autopsy reports have confirmed that early signs of atherosclerosis are present in children as young as 3 yr and frequently evident by age 10. Poor lipid profiles often run in families owing to both shared genetics and common lifestyle factors.[57] Insufficient evidence is available regarding the role of the apolipoproteins in children.

As with adults, cross-sectional studies have consistently reported that trained adolescents have higher HDL values than untrained adolescents but that TC levels do not differ with training status. Other studies have found similar, but less consistent, evidence between active and inactive children. The few short-term (8–12 weeks) aerobic exercise training studies that have investigated lipid changes in children and adolescents have found no significant changes in blood lipid profiles following training. The impact of dynamic resistance training on lipid levels in children and adolescents has not been adequately addressed.[5]

Cigarette Smoking

An estimated 2.2 million U.S. adolescents, 12–17 yr old, smoke. Every day another 3000 young people begin to smoke. Seventy-five percent of adult smokers started smoking before age 18, and 90% started smoking prior to age 21.[4] Thus, smoking definitely tracks from adolescence to adulthood. The physiological effects and the indirect relationship between activity and smoking are the same no matter what the age of the smoker.

One study of Finnish youth showed that over a 6-yr span, with individuals who were 12, 15, and 18 yr old at the beginning of the study, higher activity levels were related to less smoking in both boys and girls. Almost half of those who were sedentary smoked, but only about 10% of those who were active smoked.[41] A primary goal of physical education professionals must be to encourage an active lifestyle and discourage the onset of smoking in children and adolescents.[57]

Hypertension

Hypertension is evident in children as young as 6 yr of age. Between 6 and 17 yr of age as many as 2.8 million children are estimated to be hypertensive.[4] Table 8.3 gives systolic and diastolic values taken to represent normal, high-normal, and hypertensive blood pressures.[46] Note that in children these values are lower than in adults. The change in blood pressure with growth (age 2–18) is presented in Figure 8.2.[33] Since blood pressure changes so much with age, it may be better to use those values higher than the 90th percentile, especially at younger ages,

> **Tracking** A phenomenon in which a characteristic is maintained, in terms of relative rank, over a long time span or even a lifetime.

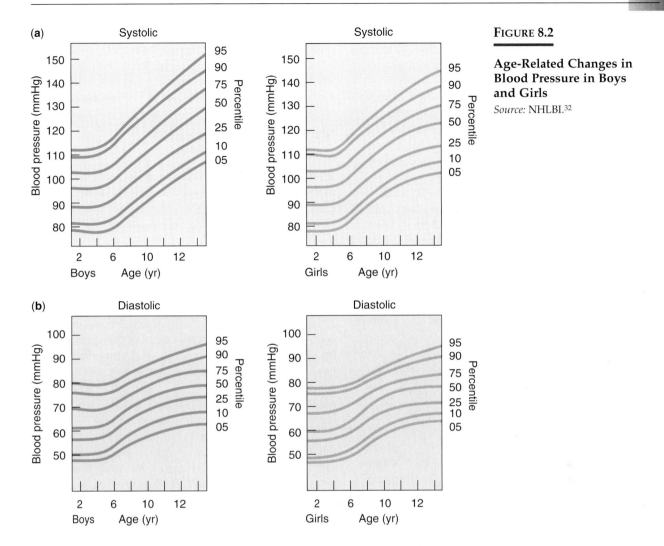

FIGURE 8.2

Age-Related Changes in Blood Pressure in Boys and Girls

Source: NHLBI.[32]

as the criterion for hypertension rather than the absolute values presented in Table 8.3.

Although childhood blood pressures do not predict adult blood pressures, there is a definite tendency for both systolic and diastolic blood pressures to track from childhood to adulthood. In one study children with blood pressures at the 90th percentile had three times the risk of having high adult systolic blood pressure and twice the risk of having high adult diastolic blood pressure as those whose childhood values were at the 50th percentile.[30]

Results from dynamic aerobic endurance training studies show consistent reductions in both systolic and diastolic blood pressure in hypertensive children, although, as with adults, these reductions rarely achieve normal blood pressure levels. Dynamic resistance training used by itself, in one reported study, did not bring about a reduction in either systolic or diastolic pressure. However, when weight training was instituted after a period of aerobic endurance training that resulted in reduced blood pressures, the reduction in blood pressure was maintained with just the weight training. Therefore, as with adults, the best procedure is to begin young hypertensives on a dynamic endurance activity regimen and add resistance training several months later, if desired.[1]

Physical Inactivity

At least as important as the level of physical fitness achieved and the amount of physical activity engaged in is the establishment of a physically active lifestyle in young people. That is, the health outcomes depend more on the constancy of physical activity throughout life than on any changes that may occur as a result of exercise training. One cannot deposit the benefits of physical activity into a fitness bank to withdraw at a later date. Furthermore, genetics has a definite impact on fitness scores. It is a hard but sad truth that some individuals will score high on fitness tests without doing any activity, but others who are very active may never achieve high fitness scores. It is the pattern of consistent activity that is most important for both types of individuals and everyone in between.

Significant tracking of physical activity was observed in a Finnish study of both boys and girls, with 44% remaining active from age 12 to 18 years, from 15 to 21 years, and from 18 to 24 years. Physical inactivity tracked even better, with 57% remaining inactive over the 6 years of the study. Those who remained active had better risk factor profiles than their inactive counterparts. That is, they smoked less (as mentioned earlier), were less fat, had higher HDL cholesterol and lower TC values, and exhibited favorable differences in insulin levels. They also consumed a healthier diet, which would, of course, have affected these results. Further tracking evidence to older ages is needed.[41]

Diabetes Mellitus

Children with Type I diabetes are at risk of prematurely developing atherosclerosis. Furthermore, Type I diabetes tracks into adulthood. The importance and cautions of physical activity and exercise training to Type I diabetics was discussed in the section on adults but are also applicable here.

Obesity

Close to 25% of all American children are obese. The number increased from the 1960s to the 1980s and has shown no signs of reversing.[57] Unfortunately, obesity does show evidence of tracking. Obese children are at an increased risk of becoming obese adults. Also, obese children are at greater risk for health problems, including those that relate to CHD. As for adults, the relationship between exercise training and body weight or body fat reduction is detailed

> **Immune System** A precisely ordered system of cells, hormones, and chemicals that regulate susceptibility to, severity of, and recovery from infection and illness.

in the metabolic unit of this text (Chapter 15). In general, obese adolescents appear to be less active than nonobese adolescents. In children, as well as in adults, aerobic exercise training has been shown to reduce body fat and/or increase fat-free mass.[6]

Stress, Fibrinogen, and Fibrinolytic Activity

Insufficient information is available on these factors in children and adolescents to link them directly to CHD risk or establish the influence of physical activity or exercise training on these factors.

Immune System, Exercise Training, and Illness

Exercise training has many health benefits; often active individuals, perhaps yourself included, claim they feel better and are healthier than their sedentary friends. They claim these benefits not just because they have altered their risk factors for major diseases, but also because they have experienced fewer colds, flu, sore throats, and other common illnesses. On the other hand, it is not unusual to hear that an Olympic or professional athlete has gotten out of a sick bed to compete or isn't competing because of illness, not injury. So which is it? Does exercise training make an individual more resistant to infections or illness, or does exercise training make the most fit individuals the most susceptible to infection? To answer these questions, we must explore the relationship between exercise training and the immune system. In addition, the role of exercise and exercise training in individuals with known infections is of concern (whether it be a simple cold or HIV/AIDS). Should they or should they not be active?

A definitive response to each of these questions is not yet possible. This section, however, will provide what is known about the functioning of the immune system, explore the acute immune response to exercise, consider adaptations in the immune system that occur as a result of exercise training, and, finally, address beneficial and detrimental influences of exercise on immune function and disease susceptibility.

Immune Response

Humans are constantly exposed to bacteria, viruses, and parasites that are capable of causing serious disease. The fact that we are not normally overcome by these foreign invaders is a testimony to the importance and efficiency of the body's defense mechanisms, comprised primarily of the immune system. The **immune system** is a complex yet precisely ordered system of cells, hormones, and chemicals that regulate susceptibility to, severity of, and recovery from infection and illness.[31] *Immunology* is the study of the physiological responses by which the body destroys or neutralizes foreign matter.[58]

The immune system can be functionally divided into two separate, but interrelated, branches: the innate (nonspecific) and the adaptive (specific) branches. The *innate branch* protects against foreign substances or cells without having to recognize them. It is nonselective; thus, it provides the first line of defense, along with intact epidermal and mucosal membranes, against microbial invasion. In contrast, the *adaptive branch* of the immune system requires that the immune cells recognize a foreign material and react specifically and selectively to destroy it. Figure 8.3 provides a summary of the immune system, with cells represented as circular structures and processes represented by arrows.[28,48] Proteins present in the blood, which are activated in an immune response, are shown in boxes.

Much of the difficulty in understanding the immune system stems from the terminology and the

FIGURE 8.3

Overview of Immune System
Source: Modified from Marieb[28] and Smith.[48]

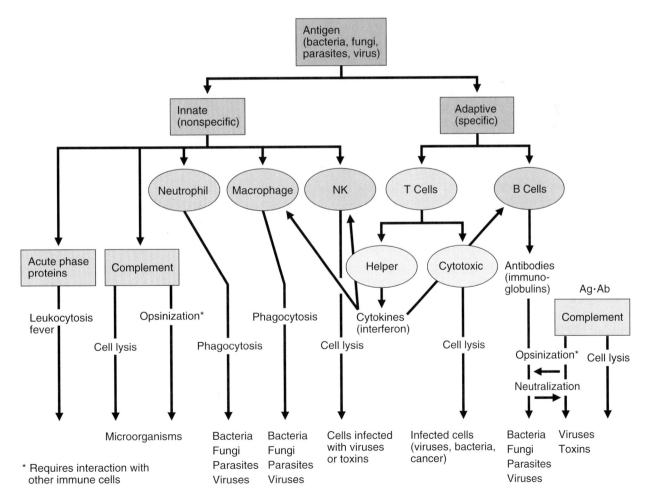

extensive interactions among the various components of the immune system. Table 8.5 provides an overview of the various cells involved in the immune response, the circulating molecules that are either present in the blood or secreted from an immune cell or infected body cell, and the processes by which the immune system combats foreign invaders. Once a foreign substance, an *antigen,* enters the body, the innate and adaptive immune responses are activated. The exact cells and molecules that are used to combat the invader depend primarily on the type of antigen present. There are often several types of cells that are activated to combat a single type of antigen.

Much of the interaction between the adaptive and innate immune system can be attributed to the central role of the *macrophages.* These cells are phagocytes; they engulf and destroy antigens through the process of *phagocytosis.* Additionally, they present the antigen to the adaptive immune cells, thereby activating an adaptive immune response. Macrophages can also secrete *cytokines,* which are chemical messengers that communicate with various cells. *Neutrophils* are innate immune cells that destroy antigens by the process of phagocytosis and represent the first line of defense against infectious agents. *Natural killer (NK) cells* are innate immune cells that destroy foreign invaders by *lysing* their cell membranes. NK cells are associated with the development and progression of cancer and acute and chronic viral infections, including HIV infection.[38]

Complement is a group of proteins that circulates in the blood stream and becomes activated when an antigen is present. Complement may be activated by either the adaptive or innate branches of the immune system, but the response is the same. Activation of the complement system leads to cell lysis of the antigen and *opsinization,* a process of "coating" the membrane of the antigen, which then enhances phagocytic killing by other cells of the immune system. *Acute phase proteins* (APP) are proteins that collectively increase leukocytosis (the production of white blood cells) and fever. These proteins play an important role in tissue repair following muscle cell damage.

The primary cells of the adaptive immune branch are the B and T lymphocytes, known as *B cells* and *T cells.* Both of these cells require exposure to and recognition of a specific foreign invader (antigen) before they can mount an immune response. Daughter cells of the B cells produce spe-

cific antibodies (also know as immunoglobulins [Igs]) in response to a specific antigen. Antibodies then bind specifically to the antigen. This binding promotes destruction of the antigen through opsinization, lysis, and *neutralization.*

There are different subsets of T cells: cytotoxic, helper, and suppressor. Cytotoxic T cells are responsible for antigen destruction, killing cells directly through lysis. Helper T cells, also called CD4 cells because of the receptors they bear on their membrane, play an important function in the immune response. They release chemical mediators that direct the function of several other cells. Suppressor T cells are regulatory cells that inhibit helper and cytotoxic T cells.

Effect of Exercise on Immune Response

An acute bout of exercise causes an immune response. The immune response depends upon the intensity and duration of activity. Studies consistently find that moderate exercise enhances immune function and that recovery to baseline values occurs shortly after exercise. In contrast, severe exercise is associated with an enhanced immune function followed by a suppression of cell activity. This pattern has been observed for NK cells, lymphocytes, neutrophils, and eosinophils.[37]

Innate Defense Mechanisms Moderate exercise leads to an increased number and activity of neutrophils, whereas heavy exercise suppresses neutrophil counts for at least 24 hr.[47] Similarly, moderate exercise increases the number, percentage, and activity of NK cells, and the increased activity may persist for 24 hr.[35,47] Exhaustive exercise, however, is associated with a reduction in NK cell activity that may last for hours to days.[47] The different responses seen during moderate versus heavy, exhaustive exercise may be related to the hormonal response to exercise, which is also intensity-dependent.[48] The depressed levels of NK cells following strenuous exercise is a likely explanation of the vulnerability to acute infection that is associated with high-level competition and chronic overtraining (see Chapter 1).[47]

The phagocytic activity of some macrophages appears to be enhanced by exercise, although this is not a universal finding.[26,48] There is also evidence that exercise increases the secretion of cytokines from macrophages.[26] The few studies that have been con-

TABLE 8.5 ■ Summary of Cells, Molecules, and Processes Involved in the Immune Response

BRANCH OF IMMUNE SYSTEM	PROCESSES	CELLS	MOLECULES
Innate and adaptive	*Lysis* is the killing of a cell via destruction of the cell membrane. *Phagocytosis* is the process of engulfing and digesting an antigen.	*Macrophages* are immune cells that (1) phagocytize pathogens, (2) present parts of the engulfed antigen on its plasma membrane to activate the T cell response, and (3) secretes cytokines. They are important in both the innate and adaptive immune responses.	*Complements* are groups of approximately 20 plasma proteins. When activated, they lyse microorganisms, enhance phagocytosis, and enhance the inflammatory response. Complements may be activated and function in either the innate or adaptive immune response. *Cytokines* are chemicals released from sensitized T cells (lymphokines) and activated macrophages (monokines) to help regulate the immune response.
Innate		*Natural killer* (NK) cells are innate immune cells that destroy virus-infected and cancerous body cells by cell lysis. *Neutrophils* are innate immune cells that phagocytize pathogens.	*Acute phase proteins (APPs)* are blood proteins produced in the liver that function in the innate immune response. APPs are important in the response to infection and inflammation.
Adaptive	*Neutralization* is a process that occurs when antibodies block the binding site on antigens so that they cannot bind to tissues and cause damage. *Opsinization* is the process of coating the membrane of an antigen, making it easier for phagocytes to adhere to and engulf the antigen.	*B cells* are lymphocytes that are part of the adaptive immune response and are responsible for the production of antibodies to a specific antigen. *T cells* are lymphocytes that are responsible for cell-mediated responses of the adaptive immune system. There are three classes of T cells: cytotoxic T cells, which destroy virus-infected and cancer cells directly via cell lysis; helper T cells (CD4 cells), regulatory cells that influence the activity of cytotoxic T cells, B cells, NK, and macrophages; and suppressor T cells, which slow or stop the T and C cells once the infection is controlled.	*Antibodies* are proteins produced by B cells to attack antigens. *Antigens* are substances capable of provoking an immune response.

ducted suggest that little or no changes occur in circulating levels of complement as a result of exercise.[26]

Acute phase proteins are elevated in the plasma following prolonged exercise of light to heavy intensity, and they remain elevated for days.[26,37] Acute phase protein levels are also influenced by a combination of intensity and duration. Elevation of the acute phase proteins lasts for several days and is believed to be involved in promoting clearance of damaged tissue and setting the stage for repair and growth.[37]

Adaptive Defense Mechanisms   Exercise results in an increased number of circulating lymphocytes (B and T cells) and changes in the relative proportion of the B and T cells. The number of lymphocytes increases in relation to exercise intensity.[26] The T cell response to exercise is determined by the duration and intensity of exercise; T cells increase in response to short-term, intense exercise but are unchanged or decrease during long-term exercise of moderate to high intensity.[26] The number of B cells increases dramatically during exercise and rapidly returns to baseline values following the cessation of activity.[26]

Exercise does not appear to alter the concentrations of the major classes of antibodies in the serum. In contrast, salivary levels of immunoglobulin are decreased during exercise.[26] The exercise-induced decrease in salivary immunoglobulin offers a theoretical explanation for the high incidence of upper respiratory tract infections (URTI) among highly trained athletes, since adaptive immunoglobulin in the saliva and mucosal linings inhibits viral and bacterial attachment to the walls of the respiratory system.

Hormonal Control of Immune Response to Exercise

As stated previously, moderate exercise enhances immune function and the cells of the immune system return to resting levels soon after exercise. On the other hand, severe exhaustive exercise is associated with an enhanced immune function that is followed by a suppression of cell activity.

The biphasic response observed following severe exercise probably depends upon hormones, specifically, epinephrine and cortisol. During exercise at greater than 60% of $\dot{V}O_2$max, epinephrine and cortisol levels in the blood begin to increase

rapidly, reaching their highest level following maximal exercise. Epinephrine is associated with a substantial increase in the number of lymphocytes in the blood. Cortisol causes an increase in the number of neutrophils but a decrease in the number of lymphocytes. Immediately following exercise, the blood concentrations of epinephrine fall rapidly to pre-exercise levels, whereas cortisol levels remain elevated for 2 hr or more. Thus, researchers hypothesize that following intense exercise epinephrine is responsible for the increase in circulating lymphocytes, and the longer-acting cortisol is responsible for the prolonged increase in neutrophils and the decrease in lymphocytes.[37]

Training Adaptations

The resting immune system of moderately trained aerobic athletes is usually within normal parameters.[37,47] There is evidence, though, that moderately conditioned athletes may have an enhanced NK cell activity. The exercise response is similar in aerobically fit and sedentary individuals, although NK cell count may be greater in fit individuals.[47] Individuals who engage in excessive exercise may have a decreased neutrophil functioning capacity, serum complement, and salivary immunoglobulin.[37,47]

Although there have been few well-controlled research studies documenting the longitudinal effect of exercise training programs of various intensities on immune function, it appears that moderate training enhances immune function. In contrast, excessive training may give rise to a cumulative disturbance of immune function, which manifests itself as illness.[47]

Selected Interactions of Exercise and Immune Function

Exercise, the Immune System, and Upper Respiratory Tract Infection

Many people believe that individuals who exercise regularly are less likely to acquire a cold or the flu, while others believe that highly trained, competitive athletes are more susceptible to upper respiratory tract infections (URTI). This section provides scientific evidence to suggest that both positions may be correct. It appears that the relationship between exercise and URTI is mediated by exercise intensity.[33,35]

A J-shaped model of relationship between exercise intensity and risk of URTI (see Figure 8.4) has been proposed to explain the risk of URTI infections among exercisers.[35] This model suggests that a moderate exercise session is beneficial but exhaustive exercise may be detrimental. This J-shaped model is consistent with the open-window model presented in Figure 8.5, which integrates information about the effect of exercise on immune cells and the impact it has on incidence of infection. The J-shaped model hypothesizes that the increase in NK cells during a moderate exercise session enhances immune function, which provides some level of protection against disease and results in less infections. Severe exercise, however, is associated with an increase in NK cells during activity but followed by a period of immunosuppression. Researchers hypothesize that the lower NK cell activity that occurs postexercise creates a period of an open window, during which time microbial agents can establish an infection. Probably many of the symptoms of overtraining reflect immunosuppression, and immunosuppression may be responsible for other negative effects evidenced during overtraining.

Moderate exercise, then, appears to enhance immune function and may play an important role in determining an individual's susceptibility to infection. There is insufficient evidence, however, to recommend any given laboratory test of immune func-

FIGURE 8.4

J-Shaped Model of Relationship Between Exercise Intensity and URTI

Source: D. C. Nieman, The effects of moderate exercise training on natural killer cells and acute upper respiratory tract infections. *International Journal of Sports Medicine.* 111:467–473 (1990). Reprinted by permission of Williams & Wilkins.

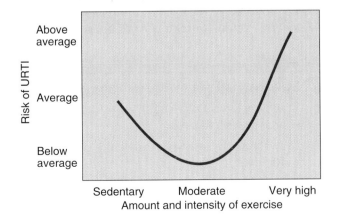

FIGURE 8.5

The "Open Window" Hypothesis

The open window is a period after severe exercise when NK cell activity decreases. During this period, microbial agents can establish an infection.

Source: Adapted from B. K. Pedersen, & H. Ullum. NK cell response to physical activity: Possible mechanisms of action. *Medicine and Science in Sports and Exercise.* 26(2):140–146 (1994). Reprinted by permission of Williams & Wilkins.

tion to ascertain whether an individual is at high risk for an infectious episode from overtraining or psychological stress.

Since endurance athletes often do not have the option of training moderately, the following precautions can help lessen the risk of URTI in competitive endurance athletes.[9,21,37] The following guidelines also suggest when exercise training is and is not appropriate. The precautions are as follows:

1. Eat a well-balanced diet. Improper nutrition can compound the negative influence of heavy exertion on the immune system.

2. Minimize other life stresses. Psychological stress may be additive.

3. Avoid overtraining and chronic fatigue. Get plenty of rest, and space vigorous workout and race events as far apart as possible.

4. Get a flu shot. Flu shots are especially important for athletes competing in the winter.

5. Avoid excessive muscular soreness. Soreness may require immune system involvement, which could decrease its ability to ward off viruses.

6. Try to avoid being around sick people.

The guidelines for stopping training are as follows:

1. Maintain training if the URTI is only minor, without a systemic infection (fever, aching

muscles, extreme fatigue, swollen glands), or just stop for a couple of days. Use decongestants during the day and antihistamines at night.

2. If the URTI has the positive systemic infection signs listed above, stop training for two to four weeks. If training is not stopped, viral cardiomyopathy or severe viral infection may result.

3. If symptoms are above the neck (runny or stuffy nose, scratchy throat), begin sessions with short or light activity. If symptoms worsen, stop; if symptoms lessen, continue. If symptoms are below the neck (muscle ache, vomiting, diarrhea, fever), stop training until the symptoms go away.

Exercise, the Immune System, and Cancer

The NK cells and macrophages are important cells in the innate immune system involved in the defense against the development and spread of malignancies.[59] Acute dynamic aerobic physical exercise causes an increase in these cells. Therefore, there is a theoretical, but largely undocumented, link between physical activity and cancer. Furthermore, epidemiological studies have found a relationship between physical activity and cancer.[8,50] Physical activity is associated with lower prevalence and mortality rates for cancers involving the colon, breast, prostate, and lung. The mechanisms responsible for the effects of exercise on cancer are unknown but may include a better overall lifestyle for the exercisers, lower body fat, decreased stool transit time, and enhancement of antioxidant enzyme systems.[59]

NK cells are known to be important in the control of tumor metastases.[22] Exercise training enhances NK activity and thus may play a role in the control of tumor metastasis.

Macrophages represent an important group of cells because of the central role they play in resistance to infection, surveillance against cancer, and the regulation of adaptive immunity. However, the impact of exercise-induced changes in macrophage function on defense against cancer is just beginning to be studied.[59]

Exercise, the Immune System, and AIDS

Acquired immune deficiency syndrome (AIDS) is a disease caused by the human immunodeficiency virus (HIV) and characterized by severe CD4 cell depletion. Current estimates suggest that 10–12 million people are infected with HIV worldwide.[9] This virus infects the CD4-bearing T cells (helper T cells), which orchestrate much of the immune response of the body. As the infection progresses, there is greater depletion of the CD4 cells, leading ultimately to immunodysregulation.[9] HIV infection is considered a chronic disease involving three stages:[39]

1. *Healthy carrier:* During this stage the virus infects relatively few CD4-bearing cells and is not clinically detectable except by blood testing. An individual may remain in this stage for up to 10 yr. These individuals are viral carriers and potentially infectious despite the absence of outward signs of infection.

2. *Symptomatic infections:* Mild symptoms of HIV infection, such as fatigue, intermittent fever, and weight loss, become evident during this phase. The CD4 count is further diminished.

3. *AIDS:* Severe CD4 cell depletion and the presence of major complications resulting from opportunistic infection or malignancy. At this stage of the disease the entire health of the individual is compromised.

During the early stages of the disease, when individuals are asymptomatic, moderate aerobic exercise training appears to be a useful strategy; some evidence suggests that exercise training may delay the progression of the disease.[9] These data may reflect the immune benefits of exercise training (increased number of CD4 cells) and/or psychological benefits of exercise training.[9,26] Furthermore, evidence suggests that exercise may be a safe activity throughout the course of the disease.

On the basis of research to date, some broad recommendations for exercise training can be made.[9] In general, before initiating an exercise program, all HIV-infected individuals should follow these guidelines:

1. Have a complete physical examination.

2. Discuss exercise plans with a physician and/or exercise specialist.

3. Comply with ACSM testing and prescription guidelines.

Healthy asymptomatic, HIV-positive individuals should follow these guidelines:

1. Continue unrestricted exercise activity.

2. Continue with competition.

3. Avoid overtraining.

Individuals in the stage defined as symptomatic infection should follow these steps:

1. Continue exercise training.

2. Terminate competition.

3. Avoid exhaustive exercise.

Individuals diagnosed as having AIDS should follow these guidelines:

1. Remain physically active.

2. Continue exercise training on a symptom-limited basis.

3. Avoid strenuous exercise.

4. Reduce or curtail exercise during acute illness.

SUMMARY

1. Cardiovascular disease is a major cause of death in the United States; in 1990 almost 1 million people died of cardiovascular disease.

2. Cardiovascular risk factors are classified as non-modifiable (age, heredity, race, and sex); major modifiable (hyperlipidemia, cigarette smoking, hypertension, physical inactivity); contributing modifiable (diabetes mellitus, obesity, stress); and nontraditional (apolipoproteins, fibrin level, fibrinolytic activity).

3. Triglycerides and a small amount of cholesterol are transported from the small intestines or liver to adipose tissue or muscles by chylomicrons and very low density lipoproteins (VLDL).

4. VLDLs are degraded into intermediate-density lipoproteins (IDL), which, in turn, are converted to low-density lipoproteins (LDL) in the liver. LDL transports 60–70% of the total cholesterol (TC) in the body to all cells except liver cells.

5. High-density lipoproteins (HDL) may block cholesterol uptake at the cellular or tissue level. HDL definitely carry cholesterol away from the sites of deposit to the liver, where the cholesterol can be broken down and eliminated in the bile.

6. Arteriosclerosis is characterized by a thickening of the arterial wall, loss of elastic connective tissue, and hardening of the vessel wall.

7. Atherosclerosis is a pathological process that results in the buildup of plaque (composed of connective tissue, smooth muscle cells, cellular debris, and cholesterol) inside the vessel. The buildup of plaque obstructs blood flow. Depending on the amount of obstruction, the result can be pain, a heart attack, or a stroke.

8. Active individuals generally have lipid profiles that indicate a reduced risk for coronary heart disease (CHD).

9. The atherosclerotic process is accelerated in individuals who smoke cigarettes, because smoking injures the arterial wall lining, increases the levels of circulating TC, and decreases the amount of HDL. Smoking also causes blood platelets to adhere to each other, speeds up the rate of internal blood clotting, and makes the clots that do form tougher to dissolve.

10. Individuals who are at high risk for developing hypertension can reduce the risk by participating in an endurance training program. Most hypertensive individuals experience decreased blood pressure as a result of an aerobic endurance exercise program.

11. Only about 10% of Americans report exercising daily for at least 30 min. Therefore, potentially more benefit overall could be achieved by increasing the activity level of U.S. citizens than by changing any other single CHD risk factor.

12. The immune system can be functionally divided into the innate and the adaptive branches. The innate branch protects against foreign substances or cells without having to recognize them. The adaptive branch of the immune system requires that the immune cells recognize a foreign material and react specifically and selectively to destroy it.

13. Moderate exercise leads to an increase in the number and activity of neutrophils; an increase in the number, percentage, and activity of NK cells; an increase in phagocytic activity and secretion of cytokines from macrophages; an increase in the number of acute phase proteins; and an increase in the number of B and T cells.

14. Exhaustive exercise is associated with a reduction in NK cell activity and a decrease in lymphocytes, neutrophils, and eosinophils.

15. The depressed levels of NK cells following strenuous exercise is a likely explanation of the vulnerability to acute infection that is associated with high-level competition and chronic overtraining.

16. Hormonal control of the immune response is mediated primarily by the action of epinephrine and cortisol.

17. Severe exercise training is associated with immunosuppression and an increased risk of URTI.

18. Physical activity is associated with lower prevalence and mortality rates for cancers involving the colon, breast, prostate, and lung.

19. Exercise training appears to be beneficial to individuals infected with the HIV virus.

REVIEW QUESTIONS

1. Identify risk factors that cannot be changed, and discuss their relationship with cardiovascular disease.

2. Identify the major risk factors that can be modified, and discuss their relationship with cardiovascular disease.

3. Identify contributing factors that can be modified, and discuss their relationship with cardiovascular disease.

4. Identify nontraditional risk factors, and discuss their relationship with cardiovascular disease.

5. What is the impact of exercise training on each CHD factor?

6. What is the importance of identifying cardiovascular disease risk factors in children?

7. Graphically present the two branches of the immune system, emphasizing how the two branches work together.

8. Describe the immune response to moderate aerobic exercise and to an exhaustive exercise bout.

9. Differentiate between the training adaptations of the immune system to a moderate training program and to overtraining.

10. Describe the relationship between exercise and the incidence of URTI.

11. Describe the relationship between physical activity levels and the risk of various cancers.

12. Describe the role of physical activity in the life of an individual infected with the HIV.

REFERENCES

1. Alpert, B. S., & J. H. Wilmore: Physical activity and blood pressure in adolescents. *Pediatric Exercise Science.* 6(4):361–380 (1994).

2. American College of Sports Medicine: Position stand: Physical activity, physical fitness, and hypertension. *Medicine and Science in Sports and Exercise.* 25(10):I–IX (1993).

3. American Heart Association: *Heart and Stroke Facts.* Dallas: Author (1994).

4. American Heart Association: *Heart and Stroke Facts: 1994 Statistical Supplement.* Dallas: Author (1993).

5. Armstrong, N., & B. Simons-Mortan: Physical activity and blood lipids in adolescents. *Pediatric Exercise Science.* 6(4):381–405 (1994).

6. Bar-Or, O., & T. Baranowski: Physical activity, adiposity, and obesity among adolescents. *Pediatric Exercise Science.* 6(4):348–360 (1994).

7. Berger, B. G.: Coping with stress: The effectiveness of exercise and other techniques. *Quest.* 46:100–119 (1994).

8. Blair, S. N., & H. C. Minocha: Physical fitness and all-cause mortality: A prospective study of healthy men and women. *Journal of the American Medical Association.* 262: 2395–2401 (1989).

9. Brenner, I. K. M., P. N. Shek, & R. J. Shephard: Infection in athletes. *Sports Medicine.* 17(2):86–107 (1994).

10. Calabrese, L. H., & A. LaPerriere: Human immunodeficiency virus infection, exercise and athletics. *Sports Medicine.* 15(1):6–13 (1993).

11. Caspersen, C. J. & G. W. Heath. The risk factor concept of coronary heart disease. In J. L. Durstine, A. C. King, P. L. Painter, J. L. Roitman, L. D. Zwireu, & W. L. Kenney (eds.), *American College of Sports Medicine: Resource Manual for Guidelines for Exercise Testing and Prescription* (2nd edition). Philadelphia: Lea & Febiger (1993).

12. Dannenberg, A. L., J. B. Keller, P. W. F. Wilson, & W. P. Castelli: Leisure time physical activity in the Framingham offspring study. *American Journal of Epidemiology.* 129:76–88 (1989).

13. Davis, G. L., C. F. Abildgaard, E. M. Bernauer, & M. Brittan: Fibrinolytic and hemostatic changes during and after maximal exercise in males. *Journal of Applied Physiology.* 40(3):287–292 (1976).

14. Drygas, W. K.: Changes in blood platelet function, coagulation, and fibrinolytic activity in response to moderate, exhaustive, and prolonged exercise. *International Journal of Sports Medicine.* 9:67–72 (1988).

15. Ferguson, E. W., L. L. Bernier, G. R. Bauta, J. Yu-Yahiro, & E. B. Schoomaker: Effects of exercise and conditioning on clotting and fibrinolytic activity in men. *Journal of Applied Physiology.* 62(4):1416–1421 (1987).

16. Froelicher, V. F.: Exercise, fitness, and coronary heart disease. In C. Bouchard, R. J. Shephard, T. Stephens, J. R. Sutton, & B. D. McPherson (eds.), *Exercise, Fitness, and Health: A Consensus of Current Knowledge.* Champaign, IL: Human Kinetics Publishers, 429–451 (1990).

17. Hagberg, J. M.: Exercise, fitness and hypertension. In C. Bouchard, R. J. Shephard, T. Stephens, J. R. Sutton, & B. D. McPherson (eds.), *Exercise, Fitness, and Health: A Consensus of Current Knowledge.* Champaign, IL: Human Kinetics Publishers (1990).

18. Hanson, P.: Pathophysiology of chronic diseases and exercise. In J. L. Durstine, A. C. King, P. L. Painter, J. L. Rostman, L. K. Zwireu, & W. L. Kenney (eds.), *American College of Sports Medicine Resource Manual for Guidelines for Exercise Testing and Prescription* (2nd edition). Philadelphia: Lea & Febiger, 187–196 (1993).

19. Haskell, W. L., C. Sims, J. Myll, W. M. Bortz, F. G. St. Goar, & E. L. Alderman: Coronary artery size and dilating capacity in ultra distance runners. *Circulation.* 87(4):1076–1082 (1993).

20. Haskell, W. S. L.: Health consequence of physical activity: Understanding and challenges regarding dose response. *Medicine and Science in Sports and Exercise.* 26(6):649–660 (1994).

21. Heath, G. W., C. A. Macera, & D. C. Nieman: Exercise and upper respiratory tract infections: Is there a relationship? *Sports Medicine.* 14(6):353–365 (1992).

22. Hoffman-Goetz, L.: Exercise, natural immunity, and tumor metastasis. *Medicine and Science in Sports and Exercise.* 26(2):157–163 (1994).

23. Koplan, J. P., K. E. Powell, R. K. Sikes, R. W. Shirley, & C. C. Campbell: An epidemiological study of the benefits and risks of running. *Journal of the American Medical Association.* 248:3118–3121 (1982).

24. LaFontaine, T.: Preventing the progression of or reversing coronary atherosclerosis. *American College of Sports Medicine Certified News.* 4(3):1–6 (1994).

25. Landers, D. M.: Performance, stress, and health: Overall reaction. *Quest.* 46:123–135 (1994).

26. Mackinnon, L. T.: *Exercise and Immunology.* Champaign, IL: Human Kinetics Publishers (1992).

27. Mackinnon, L. T.: Current challenges and future expectations in exercise immunology: Back to the future. *Medicine and Science in Sports and Exercise.* 26(2):191–194 (1994).

28. Marieb, E. N.: *Human Anatomy and Physiology.* Redwood City, CA: Benjamin/Cummings (1995).

29. Meade, T. W., S. Mellows, M. Brozovic, G. J. Miller, R. R. Chakrabart, W. R. S. North, A. P. Haines, Y. Stirling, J. P. Imeson, & S. G. Thompson: Haemostatic function and ischaemic heart disease: Principle results of the Northwick Park heart study. *Lancet.* 2:533–587 (1986).

30. Mahoney, L. T., R. M. Lauer, J. Lee, & W. R. Clarke: Factors affecting tracking of coronary heart disease risk factors in children: The Muscatine study. In Hyperlipidemia in Childhood and the Development of Atherosclerosis. *Annals of the New York Academy of Sciences.* 623:120–132 (1991).

31. Nash, M. S.: Exercise and immunology. *Medicine and Science in Sports and Exercise.* 26(2):125–127 (1994).

32. National High Blood Pressure Education Program: National Institutes of Health; National Heart, Lung, and Blood Institute: *The Fifth Report of the Joint Committee on Detection, Evaluation, and Treatment of High Blood Pressure.* Washington, D.C. (1993).

33. National Heart, Lung, and Blood Institute's Task Force on Blood Pressure Control in Children: Report of the task force on blood pressure control in children. *Pediatrics Supplement.* 59(5):797–820 (1977).

34. Nieman, D. C., L. M. Johanssen, J. W. Lee, & K. Arabatzis. Infectious episodes in runners before and after the Los Angeles Marathon. *Journal of Sports Medicine and Physical Fitness.* 30:316–328 (1990).

35. Nieman, D. C., A. R. Miller, D. A. Henson, B. J. Warren, G. Gusewitch, B. J. Johnson, J. M. Davis, D. E. Butterworth, & S. L. Nehlsen-Cannarella: Effects of high- vs moderate-intensity exercise on natural killer activity. *Medicine and Science in Sports and Exercise.* 25(10):1126–1134 (1993).

36. Nieman, D. C., S. L. Nehlsen-Cannarella, P. A. Markoff, et al.: The effects of moderate exercise training on natural killer cells and acute upper respiratory tract infections. *International Journal of Sports Medicine.* 11:467–473 (1990).

37. Nieman, D. C.: Exercise, upper respiratory tract and the immune system. *Medicine and Science in Sports and Exercise.* 26(2):128–139 (1994).

38. Pedersen, B. K., & H. Ullum. NK cell response to physical activity: Possible mechanisms of action. *Medicine and Science in Sports and Exercise.* 26(2):140–146 (1994).

39. Phair, J. D.: The natural history of HIV infection. In M. A. Sande & P. A. Volberding (eds.), *The Medical Management of AIDS.* Philadelphia: Saunders (1990).

40. Plowman, S. A.: Stress, hyperactivity, and health. *Quest.* 46:78–99 (1994).

41. Raitakari, O. T., K. V. K. Porkka, S. Taimela, R. Telama, L. Rasaneu, & J. S. A. Viikari: Effects of persistent physical activity and inactivity on coronary risk factors in children and young adults: The cardiovascular risk in young Finns study. *American Journal of Epidemiology.* 140(3):195–208 (1994).

42. Rowland, T. W.: Influence of physical activity and fitness on coronary risk factors in children: How strong an argument? *Pediatric Exercise Science.* 3(3):189–191 (1991).

43. Rowland, T. W.: *Exercise and Children's Health.* Champaign, IL: Human Kinetics Publishers (1990).

44. Rowland, T. W. & P. S. Freedson: Physical activity, fitness, and health in children: A close look. *Pediatrics.* 93(4):669–672 (1994).

45. Schuler, G., R. Hainbrecht, G. Schlierf, J. Niebauer, K. Haver, J. Neumann, E. Hoberg, A. Drinkmann, F. Bacher, M. Grunze, & W. Kubler: Regular physical exercise and low-fat diet: Effects on progression of coronary artery disease. *Circulation.* 86:1–11 (1992).

46. Scott, C. B.: Blood pressure and exercise. *American College of Sports Medicine Certified News.* 3(2):1–5 (1993).

47. Shephard, R. J., S. Rhind, & P. N. Shek: The impact of exercise on the immune system: NK cells, interleukins 1 and 2, and related responses. In J. O. Holloszy (ed.), *Exercise and Sport Sciences Reviews.* Baltimore: Williams & Wilkins (1995).

48. Smith, J. A.: Guidelines, standards, and perspectives in exercise immunology. *Medicine and Science in Sports and Exercise.* 27(4):497–506 (1995).

49. Squires, R. W. & W. L. Williams: Coronary atherosclerosis and acute myocardial infarction. In J. L. Durstine, A. C. King, P. L. Painter, J. L. Roctman, L. D. Zwiren, & W. L. Kenney (eds.), *American College of Sport Medicine Resource Manual for Guidelines for Exercise Testing and Prescription* (2nd edition). Philadelphia: Lea & Febiger, 129–150 (1993).

50. Sternfeld, B.: Cancer and the protective effect of physical activity: The epidemiological evidence. *Medicine and Science in Sports and Exercise.* 24:1195–1209 (1992).

51. Stewart, K. J.: Weight training in coronary artery disease and hypertension. *Progress in Cardiovascular Disease.* 35(2):159–168 (1992).

52. Strand, F.: Physiology: A Regulatory Systems Approach. New York: Macmillan (1978).

53. Stratton, J. R., W. L. Chandler, R. S. Schwartz, M. D. Cerqueira, W. C. Levy, S. E. Kahn, V. G. Larson, K. C. Cain, J. C. Beard, & I. B. Abrass: Effects of physical conditioning on fibrinolytic variables and fibrinogen in young and old healthy adults. *Circulation.* 83:1692–1697 (1991).

54. Summary of the Second Report of the National Cholesterol Education Program (NCEP): Expert panel on detection, evaluation and treatment of high blood cholesterol in adults (adult treatment panel II). *Journal of American Medical Association.* 269(23):3015–3023 (1993).

55. Szymanski, L. M. & R. R. Pate: Effects of exercise intensity, duration, and time of day on fibrinolytic activity in physically active men. *Medicine and Science in Sports and Exercise.* 26(9):1102–1108 (1994).

56. Szymanski, L. M., R. R. Pate, & J. L. Durstine: Effect of maximal exercise and venous occlusion on fibrinolytic activity in physically active and inactive men. *Journal of Applied Physiology.* 77(5):2305–2310 (1994).

57. U.S. Department of Health and Human Services, Public Health Service, National Institutes of Health: Report of the expert panel on blood cholesterol levels in children and adolescents. *National Institutes of Health Publication.* No. 91-2732 (1991).

58. Vander, A. J., J. H. Sherman, & D. S. Luciano: *Human Physiology.* New York: McGraw-Hill (1990).

59. Woods, J. A., & J. M. Davis: Exercise, monocyte/macrophage function, and cancer. *Medicine and Science in Sports and Exercise.* 26(2):147–157 (1994).

60. Wood, P. D., & M. L. Stefanick: Exercise, fitness, and atherosclerosis. In C. Bouchard, R. J. Shephard, T. Stephens, J. R. Sutton, & B. D. McPherson (eds.), *Exercise, Fitness, and Health: A Consensus of Current Knowledge..* Champaign, IL: Human Kinetics Publishers, 409–423 (1990).

Metabolic System

9

Energy Production

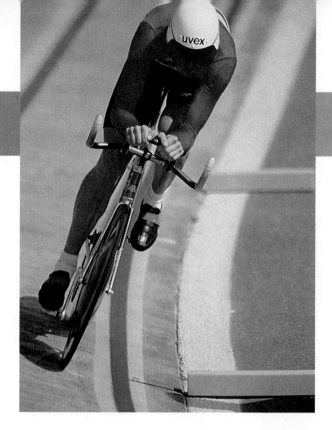

After studying this chapter, you should be able to:

- Describe the role of ATP.

- Summarize the processes of cellular respiration for the production of ATP from carbohydrate, fat, and protein fuel substrates.

- Calculate the production of ATP from glucose or glycogen, fatty acid, and amino acid precursors.

- Describe the goals of metabolic regulation during exercise.

- Explain how the production of energy is regulated by intracellular and extracellular factors.

- Compare the relative use of carbohydrate, fat, and protein fuel substrates on the basis of intensity and duration of exercise.

Introduction

Most individuals eat at least three meals a day. Despite the wide variation in content of those meals and despite the societal or psychological attributes that might be attached to them, physiologically eating is necessary to provide the energy that is essential for all cellular—and hence bodily—activity. In order to provide this energy, food must be transformed into chemical energy.

The total of all energy transformations that occur in the body is called **metabolism.** If the energy is used to build tissues—as when amino acids are combined to form proteins that make up muscle—the process is called *anabolism.* If the energy is produced from the breakdown of foodstuffs and stored so that it is available to do work, the process is called *catabolism.*

It is catabolism that is of primary importance in exercise metabolism. Here the interest is in providing energy to support muscle activity, whether a little or a lot of muscle mass is involved or the exercise is light or heavy, submaximal or maximal. In providing this needed energy the human body follows the *first law of thermodynamics*, which states that energy is neither created nor destroyed, but only changed in form. Figure 9.1 is a schematic representation of this law and the changes in form representing catabolism. Potential chemical energy—or fuel—is ingested as food. Carbohydrates, fats, and protein can all be used as fuels although they are not used equally by the body in that capacity. The chemical energy produced from the food fuel is stored as **adenosine triphosphate** (ATP). The ATP then transfers its energy to energy-requiring physiological functions, such as muscle contraction during exercise, where part appears as work done and part as heat. Thus, ATP is stored chemical energy that links the energy-yielding and the energy-requiring functions within all cells. The aim of this chapter is to fully explain ATP and how it is produced from carbohydrate, fat, and protein food sources.

Structurally, ATP is composed of a carbon-nitrogen base called adenine, a 5-carbon sugar called ribose, and three phosphates, symbolized by P_i (inorganic phosphate). Each phosphate group is linked by a high-energy bond. When one phosphate is removed, the remaining compound is *adenosine diphosphate* (ADP). When two phosphates are re-

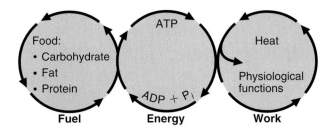

FIGURE 9.1

Generalized Scheme of Catabolic Energy Transformation in the Human Body

Energy is the capacity to do work. Energy exists in six forms: chemical, mechanical, heat, light, electrical, and nuclear. Movement of the human body (work) represents mechanical energy that is supported by the chemical energy derived from food fuels.

moved, the remaining compound is *adenosine monophosphate* (AMP).

The ATP energy reaction is reversible. When ATP is synthesized from ADP by adding P_i, energy is required. The addition of P_i is known as *phosphorylation.*

$$ADP + P_i + energy \rightarrow ATP$$

When ATP is broken down, energy is released. **Hydrolysis** is a chemical process in which a substance is split into simpler compounds by the addition of water. ATP is split by hydrolysis.

$$ATP \rightarrow ADP + P_i + energy \text{ for work} + heat$$

Note that the energy-requiring and energy-releasing reactions involving ATP are **coupled reactions,** which are linked chemical processes in which

Metabolism The total of all energy transformations that occur in the body.

Adenosine Triphosphate (ATP) Stored chemical energy that links the energy-yielding and energy-requiring functions within all cells.

Hydrolysis A chemical process in which a substance is split into simpler compounds by the addition of water.

Coupled Reactions Linked chemical processes in which a change in one substance is accompanied by a change in another.

a change in one substance is accompanied by a change in another. That is, one of these reactions does not occur without the other. As the chemical agent that links the energy-yielding and energy-requiring functions in the cell, ATP is also a universal agent, being the immediate source of energy for virtually all reactions requiring energy in all cells.

ATP is often referred to as cellular energy. Actually, ATP is a high-energy molecule. More specifically, it has a high-energy bond between the second and third phosphate group. When this phosphate is removed, energy is released. To better understand how the breakdown of ATP releases energy, consider an analogy. Think for a moment about a spring-loaded dart gun. The dart can be considered analogous to P_i. It takes a small amount of energy to "spring-load" the dart; this energy corresponds to the energy involved in the energy-requiring reaction:

$$ADP + P_i + energy \rightarrow ATP$$

Once the dart is loaded, the spring houses potential energy, which is released when the gun is fired. Firing corresponds to the energy-releasing reaction:

$$ATP \rightarrow ADP + P_i + energy$$

The energy available to do work in the intact cell is 12 kcal $\cdot$ mol^{-1} of ATP, although this energy may vary in different cells and under different conditions.[9]

ATP can be regenerated from ADP in three ways:

1. By interaction of ADP with CP (*creatine phosphate*, which is sometimes designated as PC, or *phosphocreatine*).
2. By anaerobic respiration in the cell cytoplasm.
3. By aerobic respiration in the cell mitochondria.

Cellular Respiration The process by which cells transfer energy from food to ATP in a stepwise series of reactions; relies heavily upon the use of oxygen.

Anaerobic In the absence of, not requiring, nor utilizing oxygen.

Aerobic In the presence of, requiring, or utilizing oxygen.

Substrate A substance acted upon by an enzyme.

Phosphocreatine is another high-energy compound stored in muscles. It transfers its phosphate—and, hence, its potential energy—to ADP to form ATP, leaving creatine:

$$ADP + PC \rightarrow C + ATP$$

PC stores are sacrificed to regenerate ATP and in a working muscle will be depleted in less than 15 sec. The rest of this chapter will concentrate on the more substantial production of ATP by the second and third techniques listed, namely, anaerobic and aerobic cellular respiration.

Cellular Respiration

The process by which cells transfer energy from food to ATP in a stepwise series of reactions is called **cellular respiration.** It is called cellular respiration because the cells rely heavily upon the oxygen that the respiratory system provides for them in order to produce energy. In addition, the by-product of energy production, carbon dioxide, is exhaled through the respiratory system. Cellular respiration can be either **anaerobic,** meaning it occurs in the absence of, does not require, nor uses oxygen, or **aerobic,** meaning it occurs in the presence of, requires, or uses oxygen. Brain cells cannot produce energy anaerobically, and cardiac muscle cells have only a minimal capacity for anaerobic energy production. Skeletal muscle cells, however, are able to produce energy aerobically and/or anaerobically as the situation demands it.

Figure 9.2 presents a basic outline of the products and processes of cellular respiration. A detailed discussion of these processes will follow. At this time, however, you need only note the following points.

1. All three major food nutrients, fats (FAT), carbohydrates (CHO), and proteins (PRO), can serve as fuel or **substrates**—the substances acted upon by enzymes—for the production of ATP.

2. The most important immediate forms of the substrates utilized are glucose (GLU), free fatty acids (FFA), and amino acids (AA). Both FFA and glycerol are derived from the breakdown of triglycerides. Some cells can use glycerol directly in glycolysis, but muscle cells cannot.

Fat   **Carbohydrate (CHO)**   **Protein (PRO)**

FIGURE 9.2

An Overview of Cellular Respiration

*Glycerol can enter glycolysis in liver or fat cells but not in muscle cells.

†Boxes represent the process; arrows show the direction of flow.

3. *Acetyl coenzyme A* (acetyl CoA) is the central converting substance (usually called the universal or common intermediate) in the metabolism of FAT, CHO, and PRO. Although the process of glycolysis will provide a small amount of ATP as well as acetyl CoA, both beta oxidation and oxidative deamination or transamination are simply preparatory steps by which FFA and AA are converted to acetyl CoA. That is, beta oxidation and oxidative deamination or transamination are simply processes for converting FFA and AA, respectively, to a common substrate that allows the metabolic pathway to continue. The end result is that the primary metabolic pathways of the Krebs cycle, electron transport system (ETS), and oxidative phosphorylation (OP) are the same no matter what the food precursor. This is certainly more efficient than having totally separate pathways for each food nutrient.

4. Each of the energy-producing processes (glycolysis, Krebs cycle, ETS/OP) consists of a series of steps. This is both good news and bad news for you

as a student. It is good news because it allows energy to be released gradually. If all of the energy contained in the food nutrients were released at one time, it would be predominantly released as heat and would destroy tissue. It is bad news because it is easy to be intimidated by or uninterested in so many steps, each with its own chemical structure, enzyme, and long, strange name. There is a logic to these steps, however, and it is on the logic and understanding (rather than the chemical structures) that this discussion will concentrate.

Carbohydrate Metabolism

The discussion of ATP production will begin with carbohydrate metabolism for several reasons. First, many of the energy requirements of the human body are met by carbohydrate metabolism. Second, carbohydrate is the only food nutrient that can be used to create energy anaerobically. Energy for both rest and exercise is provided primarily by aerobic metabolism. However, exercise can often require anaerobic energy production. In that situation carbohydrate is essential. Third, carbohydrate is the preferred fuel of the body because carbohydrate requires less oxygen in order to be metabolized than fat does. And finally, if you understand carbohydrate metabolism, it is relatively simple to understand how fats and proteins are metabolized.

Carbohydrates are composed of carbon, oxygen, and hydrogen. The complete metabolism of carbohydrate requires oxygen, which is supplied by pulmonary ventilation and external and internal respiration and is transported by the circulatory systems to the muscle cells. It produces carbon dioxide, which is removed via the circulatory and respiratory systems, and water.

The form of carbohydrate that is exclusively metabolized is *glucose,* a 6-carbon sugar arranged in a hexagonal formation and symbolized as $C_6H_{12}O_6$. Thus, all carbohydrate must be broken down into glucose before it can continue through the metabolic pathways. In its most simplistic form carbohydrate metabolism can be represented by the equation

$$C_6H_{12}O_6 + 6O_2 \rightarrow 6H_2O + 6CO_2 + \text{energy}$$

or glucose + oxygen → water + carbon dioxide
+ energy (as ATP)

When an excess of glucose is available to the cell, it can be stored as **glycogen,** which is a chain of glucose molecules chemically linked together, or converted to and stored as fat. The creation of glycogen from glucose is called *glycogenesis.* Glycogen is stored predominantly in the liver and muscle cells, as shown in the electron micrograph in Figure 9.3. When additional glucose is needed, stored glycogen is broken down (hydrolyzed) to provide glucose, a process called **glycogenolysis.** Since glycogen must first be broken down into glucose, the production of energy from glucose or glycogen is identical after that initial step. The complete breakdown of glucose and glycogen follows the

FIGURE 9.3

Glycogen Storage in Skeletal Muscle

In this electron micrograph of skeletal muscle (EM:25,000X), stored glycogen is visible as the small round black dots.

Source: Photo courtesy of Dian Molsen, Northern Illinois University Electron Microscope Laboratory.

Glycogen Stored form of carbohydrate composed of chains of glucose molecules chemically linked together.

Glycogenolysis The process by which stored glycogen is broken down (hydrolyzed) to provide glucose.

four-stage approach outlined in Figure 9.4 and detailed in later figures.

To keep the concepts *stages* and *steps* clear, think of the four stages as the four quarters of football game. Each quarter is composed of several series of plays in which the offensive team has four downs to make 10 yards and run more plays or score. In metabolism each stage is like a quarter. Each individ-

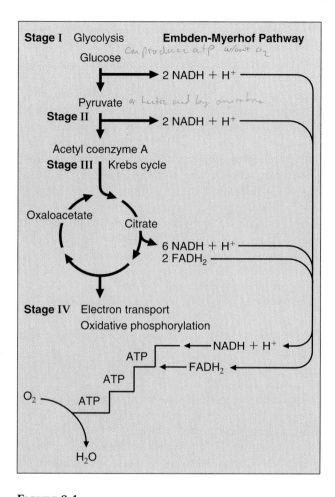

Stage I   Glycolysis   **Embden-Myerhof Pathway**
Glucose   *Can produce atp w/out O₂*

→ 2 NADH + H⁺

Pyruvate   *or lactic acid by anaerobic*
Stage II

→ 2 NADH + H⁺

Acetyl coenzyme A
Stage III   Krebs cycle

Oxaloacetate
Citrate

→ 6 NADH + H⁺
2 FADH₂

Stage IV   Electron transport
Oxidative phosphorylation

ATP   ← NADH + H⁺ ←
← FADH₂ ←
ATP
O₂   ATP

H₂O

FIGURE 9.4

**The Four Stages of Carbohydrate
Cellular Respiration**

however—the production of ATP energy—is a given, and the amount is precisely known for each fuel utilized.

Stage I: Glycolysis Overview

Much of the importance of glycolysis is simply that it prepares glucose to enter the next stage of metabolism (see Figure 9.4) by converting glucose to pyruvic acid. Also very important is that ATP can be produced during glycolysis. This process is the only way that we can produce ATP in the absence of oxygen (anaerobically).

Glycolysis, which literally means the breakdown or dissolution of sugar, is the energy pathway responsible for the initial catabolism of glucose in a 10- or 11-step process. Glycolysis begins with either glucose or glycogen and ends with the production of either pyruvate (pyruvic acid) by aerobic glycolysis or lactate (lactic acid) by anaerobic glycolysis.[5,9,12,13,17] (Note that names ending in *-ate* technically indicate the salts of their respective acids, that is, lactate is the salt of lactic acid. However, the salt and acid forms are often used interchangeably in descriptions of the metabolic pathways.)

Each step is catalyzed by a specific enzyme. An **enzyme** is a protein that accelerates the speed of a chemical reaction without itself being changed by the reaction. It does not cause a reaction that would not otherwise occur; it simply speeds up one that would occur anyway. Metabolic enzymes are easy to identify since their names end in the suffix *-ase*. Generally, their names are also related to the reaction they are catalyzing.

The activity of enzymes is affected by the concentrations of the substrate acted upon and of the enzyme itself, temperature, pH, and the presence or

ual step is analogous to a single football play. When steps are put together as in a series of plays in a drive, a **metabolic pathway** or sequence of enzyme-mediated chemical reactions resulting in a specific product is created. Although the quarters of a game and the stages of metabolism always follow the given numerical succession, there are two major differences. First, football plays should follow no particular order, or it wouldn't be much of a contest. Steps in a metabolic pathway, on the other hand, occur in an absolute, unvarying sequence. Second, one never knows exactly what the score of a football game will be, or even if there will be any scoring, until the game is over. The end result of metabolism,

Metabolic Pathway A sequence of enzyme-mediated chemical reactions resulting in a specified product.

Glycolysis The energy pathway responsible for the initial catabolism of glucose in a 10- or 11-step process that begins with glucose or glycogen and ends with the production of pyruvate (aerobic glycolysis) or lactate (anaerobic glycolysis).

Enzyme A protein that accelerates the speed of a chemical reaction without itself being changed by the reaction.

absence of poisons or medications. The discussions that follow assume that the enzymes are acting in a normal physiological environment. Only a few enzymes that are especially important in regulatory or rate-limiting roles will be named. *Regulatory* or *rate-limiting enzymes* are the enzymes that are most important in controlling the rate of energy production along a metabolic pathway—just as a traffic light regulates the flow of vehicles along a highway.

As a metabolic pathway, glycolysis begins with the absorption of glucose into the bloodstream from the small intestines or with the release of glucose into the bloodstream from the liver. These steps supply the fuel. Glucose must then be transported into the muscle cell. Transport occurs across the cell membrane via facilitated diffusion, utilizing a protein carrier and occurring down a concentration gradient. Transport is a passive process that does not require the expenditure of energy. The hormone insulin increases the activity of the glucose-transporting system, which involves the enzyme hexokinase.

Glycolysis takes place in the cytoplasm of the cell. The enzymes that catalyze each step are simply free floating in the cytoplasm. The transfer of the intermediary substances between enzymes takes place by *diffusion,* which is the tendency of molecules to move from a region of high concentration to one of low concentration. All of the intermediates (everything but glucose and the pyruvate or lactate) are *phosphorylated compounds*—that is, they contain phosphates. All of the phosphate intermediates, ADP, and ATP are unable to pass through the cell membrane. The cell membrane, however, is freely permeable to glucose and lactate.

Substrate-Level Phosphorylation The transfer of P_i directly from a phosphorylated intermediate or substrates to ADP without any oxidation occurring.

Oxidation A gain of oxygen, a loss of hydrogen, or the direct loss or electrons by an atom or substance.

Reduction A loss of oxygen, a gain of electrons, or a gain of hydrogen by an atom or substance.

Nicotinamide Adenine Dinucleotide (NAD) A hydrogen carrier in cellular respiration.

Flavin Adenine Dinucleotide (FAD) A hydrogen carrier in cellular respiration.

Glycolysis, as depicted in Figure 9.5, involves both the utilization and production of ATP. One ATP is used in the first step if the initial fuel is glucose. One ATP is used in step 3 whether the initial fuel is glucose or glycogen. Thus, 1 ATP is used for activation if the initial fuel is glycogen, but 2 ATP are used if the initial fuel is glucose. ATP is produced from ADP + P_i at steps 7 and 10 by a process known as substrate-level phosphorylation. **Substrate-level phosphorylation** is the transfer of P_i directly from the phosphorylated intermediates or substrates to ADP without any oxidation occurring. A net total of 3 ATP are gained if glycogen is the initial fuel, but only 2 ATP are gained if glucose is the initial fuel.

Exactly how glycolysis is accomplished is explained in the following step-by-step analysis. Clarification of the terms *oxidation* and *reduction* and a description of the role of nicotinamide adenine dinucleotide (NAD) and flavin adenine dinucleotide (FAD) are necessary before proceeding to these steps, however.

Oxidation-Reduction.   There are three kinds of **oxidation:** a gain of oxygen (hence the name), a loss of hydrogen, or the direct loss of electrons by an atom or substance.

The name of the process whereby an atom or substance gains electrons is called **reduction.** A good way to remember which is which is to put the two words with e's together: reduction = + e^-. Reduction can also mean a loss of oxygen or a gain of hydrogen by an atom or a substance.

When one substance is oxidized another is simultaneously reduced. The substance that is oxidized also loses energy; the substance that is reduced also gains energy.

Oxidation in the form of hydrogen removal occurs in several of the intermediary steps in catabolism. When hydrogen atoms are removed, they must be transported elsewhere. The two most important hydrogen carriers in cellular respiration are **nicotinamide adenine dinucleotide (NAD)** and **flavin adenine dinucleotide (FAD).** Both NAD and FAD can accept two electrons and two protons from two hydrogen atoms. Each does so in a slightly different manner, however. FAD (the oxidized form is FAD_{ox}) actually binds both protons and is written as $FADH_2$ (or FAD reduced, written FAD_{red}). NAD actually exists as NAD^+ (or NAD reduced, written NAD_{red}); when bonded to hydrogen, it is written as

Don't need to memorize

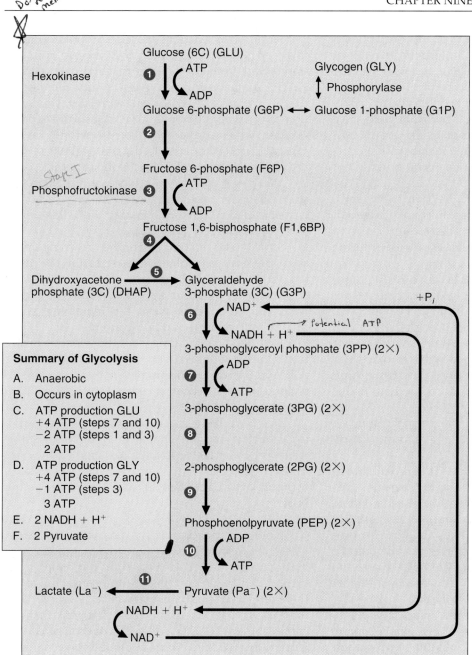

FIGURE 9.5

Stage I: Glycolysis

NADH + H⁺. The symbols NAD⁺ and FAD will be used to indicate the oxidized form, and NADH + H⁺ and FADH₂ will be used to indicate the reduced form of these carriers in this text, so it is clear where the hydrogen atoms are. NAD⁺ is by far the more important hydrogen carrier in human metabolism.

A helpful analogy of the roles of FAD and NAD is a taxi cab. The purpose of NAD and FAD is to transport (serve as taxis) for the hydrogen. NAD and FAD must pick up hydrogen passengers (be reduced) and they must drop them off (be oxidized) at another point without either the carrier (taxi) or the hydrogen (passengers) being permanently changed.

The Steps of Stage I.   Refer to Figure 9.5 as each step is explained in the text. [5,9,12,13,17]

Step 1. The glucose molecule is phosphorylated (has a phosphate attached) through the transfer of one phosphate group from ATP to the location of the sixth carbon on the glucose hexagon producing glucose 6-phosphate. This phosphorylation effectively traps the glucose in that particular cell, since the electrical charge of the phosphate group prohibits glucose from crossing the membrane, and the enzyme that can break this phosphate bond is not present in muscle cells.

The same is true for the glycogen in the cells. That is, it is trapped in the muscle where it is stored. On the other hand, the liver possesses enzymes to break down glycogen and release glucose into the bloodstream.

These facts are important because during high-intensity, long-term exercise glycogen stored in specific muscles must be used there. Furthermore, glycogen stored in muscles not used in that activity (that is, the upper body for a running event) cannot be removed as such from the inactive muscles and be transported to the active ones. Therefore, high levels of glycogen need to be stored in the muscles that will be used.

Step 2. The atoms that make up the glucose 6-phosphate are simply rearranged to form fructose 6-phosphate.

Step 3. Another molecule of ATP is broken down and the phosphate added at the first carbon. This addition places a phosphate group at each end of the molecule and results in the product fructose 1,6-di- or bisphosphate. The prefixes *di-* and *bis-* mean "two." In this case two phosphates are now part of the molecule. This step is catalyzed by the enzyme *phosphofructokinase* (PFK), which is the most important regulatory enzyme in glycolysis.

Step 4. This is the step from which glycolysis, meaning sugar breaking or splitting, gets its name, for here the 6-carbon sugar is split into two 3-carbon sugars. The two sugars are identical in terms of their component atoms but have different names (dihydroxyacetone phosphate, or DHAP, and glyceraldehyde 3-phosphate, or G3P) because the component atoms are arranged differently.

Step 5. The atoms of dihydroxyacetone phosphate are rearranged to form glyceraldehyde 3-phosphate, with the phosphate group at the third carbon. From this point on each step occurs twice (indicated by 2× in Figure 9.5), once for each of the three carbon subunits.

Step 6. Two reactions that are coupled occur in this step. In the first a pair of hydrogen atoms is transferred from the G3P to the hydrogen carrier NAD^+, reducing this to $NADH + H^+$. The fate of this $NADH + H^+$ will be dealt with later. This reaction releases enough energy to perform the second reaction, which adds a phosphate from the P_i always present in the cytoplasm to the first carbon, so that the product becomes 1,3-diphosphoglycerate.

Step 7. ATP is finally produced from ADP in this step when the phosphate from the first carbon is transferred to ADP, storing energy. Since this step is also doubled, 2 ATP are formed.

Step 8. This is simply another rearrangement step where the phosphate is moved from the number 3 to the number 2 carbon.

Step 9. A water molecule is removed, which weakens the bond between the remaining phosphate group and the rest of the atoms.

Step 10. The remaining phosphate is transferred from phosphoenolpyruvate (PEP) to ADP, forming ATP and pyruvate. The enzyme is pyruvate kinase. Again, since the reaction happens twice, 2 ATP are produced.

Step 11. If the hydrogen atoms carried by NAD^+ as $NADH + H^+$ are unable to enter the electron transport chain (as described in stage IV), they are transferred instead to pyruvic acid (pyruvate), forming lactic acid (lactate), which regenerates the NAD^+.

Note that the formula for the two pyruvic acid molecules formed is $2C_3H_4O_3$ while that of the original glucose was $C_6H_{12}O_6$. Both the number of carbon and oxygen atoms are the same, however, there are four hydrogens fewer in pyruvic acid than in glucose. These are the hydrogens that are carried by the NAD^+. If the endpoint of glycolysis is lactic acid ($2C_3H_6O_3$), all of the hydrogens are accounted for.

When the end product of glycolysis is pyruvic acid, the process is called aerobic glycolysis (or slow glycolysis). When glucose is converted to lactic acid, the process is called anaerobic glycolysis (or fast glycolysis). Glucose predominates as the fuel for slow glycolysis, and glycogen predominates as the fuel for fast glycolysis.

Mitochondria. Mitochondria (which is the plural form; the singular is *mitochondrion*) are subcellular organelles that are often called the power-houses of the cell. The formation of acetyl CoA, Krebs cycle, electron transport, and oxidative phosphorylation all take place in the mitochondria.

Figure 9.6 presents a diagram and an electron micrograph of a mitochondrion: a three-dimensional, discretely encapsulated, bean-shaped structure. In actual living tissue mitochondria exist in many different shapes—and, indeed, they constantly change shapes.

As shown in Figure 9.6, mitochondria have five distinct components. The first component is the outer membrane (labeled as 1 in the figure). As is usual, this membrane serves as a barrier and selectively permits the transfer of material into and out of the mitochondria. The second component (2) is an inner membrane. The inner membrane is parallel to the outer membrane in spots, but it also consists of a series of folds or convolutions called *crista* (3) (the plural is *cristae*). Protruding across and from the inner membrane is a series of protein-enzyme complexes called ball-and-stalk complexes (4) that have the appearance of a golf ball on a tee. Although the inner membrane has transport functions, the crista portion and especially the ball-and-stalk apparatus are specialized as the locations where ATP synthesis actually takes place.

The area between the two membranes is known simply as the intermembrane space (5). The center portion of the mitochondria is known as the *matrix* (6). The matrix is filled with a gellike substance composed of water and proteins. Metabolic enzymes and DNA (7) for organelle replication are stored here.

The fact that mitochondria contain their own DNA means that they are self-replicating. When a need for more ATP arises, mitochondria simply split in half and then grow to their former size. This property, discussed later, has specific implications for how an individual adapts to exercise training. It also explains why some cells have only a few mitochondria but others have thousands. Red blood cells are unique in that they contain no mitochondria.

Mitochondria tend to be located where they are needed. Within muscle cells they lie directly beneath the cell membrane (and are called *sarcolemmal mitochondria*) and among the contractile elements (which are called *interfibrillar mitochondria*).

Stage II: Formation of Acetyl Coenzyme A

Stage II (Figure 9.7) is a very short metabolic pathway consisting solely of the conversion of pyruvate to acetyl coenzyme A. [5,9,12,13,17] No ATP is either used or produced directly. However, a pair of hydrogen atoms (two, because all reactions still happen twice) are removed and picked up by NAD^+ to be transferred to the electron transport chain.

FIGURE 9.6

Mitochondrion

Mitochondria Cell organelles in which the Krebs cycle, electron transport, and oxidative phosphorylation take place.

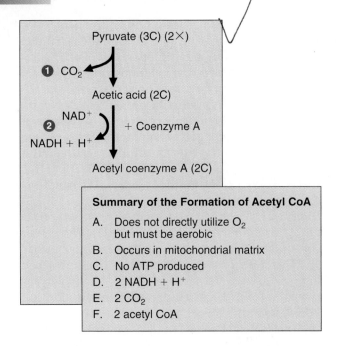

Summary of the Formation of Acetyl CoA

A. Does not directly utilize O_2 but must be aerobic

B. Occurs in mitochondrial matrix

C. No ATP produced

D. 2 NADH + H^+

E. 2 CO_2

F. 2 acetyl CoA

FIGURE 9.7

Stage II: The Formation of Acetyle Coenzyme A

The conversion of pyruvate to acetyl CoA takes place within the mitochondrial matrix (Figure 9.6). This conversion requires that the pyruvate be transported across the mitochondrial membranes via a specific carrier. No oxygen is used directly in this stage, but these steps will only occur in the presence of oxygen. As usual, enzymes catalyze each reaction.

The Steps of Stage II.   Refer to the diagram in Figure 9.7 for the two steps of stage II. [5,9,12,13,17]

Step 1. Pyruvate is converted to acetic acid. In the process one molecule of CO_2 is removed. This

Coenzyme A nonprotein substance derived from a vitamin that activates an enzyme.

Krebs Cycle A series of eight chemical reactions that begins and ends with the same substance; energy is liberated for direct substrate phosphorylation of ATP from ADP and P_i; carbon dioxide is formed and hydrogen atoms removed and carried by NAD and FAD to the electron transport system; does not directly utilize oxygen but requires its presence.

CO_2, as well as the CO_2 that will be formed in stage III, diffuses into the bloodstream and is ultimately exhaled via the lungs.

Step 2. Acetic acid is combined with coenzyme A to form acetyl coenzyme A (acetyl CoA). A **coenzyme** is a nonprotein substance derived from a vitamin that activates an enzyme. The conversion of pyruvate to acetyl CoA commits the pyruvate to stages III and IV since there is no biochemical means of reconverting acetyl CoA back to pyruvate.

Stage III: Krebs Cycle   What makes the **Krebs cycle** a cycle is that it both begins and ends with the same substance, called *oxaloacetate* (or oxaloacetic acid, which is abbreviated as OAA). The cycle is an eight-step process (see Figure 9.8) that actually comprises two metabolic pathways: one pathway for steps 1–3 and the second pathway for steps 5–8.

No ATP is used in the Krebs cycle, and only one step (5) results in the substrate-level phosphorylation production of ATP. However, four steps (3, 4, 6, and 8) result in the removal of hydrogen atoms, which are picked up by either NAD^+ or FAD. This result is critically important, because these are the hydrogen atoms that will provide the electrons for the electron transport system. Carbon dioxide is produced at steps 3 and 4. As with every step since the 6-carbon glucose molecule was split into two 3-carbon units in stage I (step 4, Figure 9.5), every reaction and product is doubled.

All of the enzymes and hence all of the reactions for the Krebs cycle occur within the mitochondrial matrix, with one exception. The exception is that the enzyme succinate dehydrogenase that catalyzes step 6 is located in the inner mitochondrial membrane.

The intermediate molecules as well as the preliminary molecules pyruvic acid and acetyl CoA are keto acids. Although no oxygen is used directly, this stage requires the presence of oxygen.

The Steps of Stage III.   The steps for the Krebs cycle [5,9,12,13,17] are presented in Figure 9.8, which you should refer to while reading the discussion.

Step 1. The 2-carbon acetyl CoA combines with the 4-carbon molecule oxaloacetate (OAA) to form citrate or citric acid. It is because of this first prod-

FIGURE 9.8

Stage III: The Krebs Cycle

Summary of Krebs Cycle

A. Does not directly utilize O_2 but must be aerobic
B. Occurs in mitochondrial matrix
C. 2 ATP (step 5)
D. 6 NADH + H^+ (steps 3, 4, and 8)
E. 2 $FADH_2$ (step 6) *4 ATP*
F. $4CO_2$

uct that the cycle is also known as the citric acid cycle. In the reaction the coenzyme A (CoA-SH) is removed from acetyl CoA and is free to convert more pyruvate to acetyl CoA or to be used later in the cycle.

Step 2. The atoms of citric acid (citrate) are re-arranged to become isocitrate.

Step 3. Two reactions occur. In the first hydrogen atoms are removed and accepted by the carrier NAD^+, forming NADH + H^+. In the second reaction a CO_2 is removed, leaving the 5-carbon α-ketoglutarate.

Step 4. Step 4 is basically a repetition of step 3 in that a pair of hydrogen atoms are removed and picked up by NAD^+ and a CO_2 is also removed. In addition, the remaining structure is attached to coenzyme A (CoA-SH). The resultant succinyl CoA

has only four carbons, which will remain intact throughout the rest of the cycle.

Step 5. In this step coenzyme A is displaced by a phosphate group, which, in turn, is transferred, via a substance called guanosine triphosphate (GTP), to ADP to form ATP. This is the only step in the Krebs cycle that produces and stores energy directly. As in glycolysis this ATP is produced by substrate-level phosphorylation.

Step 6. More hydrogen atoms are removed, but this time the carrier substance is FAD, forming $FADH_2$.

Step 7. Water is added, converting fumarate to malate.

Step 8. A pair of hydrogen atoms are removed and accepted by NAD^+. The remaining atoms once more make up oxaloacetate, and the cycle is ready to begin again.

The ATP produced in stages I and III can be used immediately to provide energy for the cell. The CO_2 diffuses into the bloodstream, is transported to the lungs, and is exhaled. Now we must determine what happens to all of the hydrogen atoms that are being carried as NADH + H$^+$ and FADH$_2$.

Stage IV: Electron Transport and Oxidative Phosphorylation

The **electron transport system (ETS)** or respiratory chain is the final metabolic pathway; it proceeds as a series of chemical reactions in the mitochondria that transfer electrons from the hydrogen atom carriers NAD and FAD to oxygen; water is formed as a by-product and the electrochemical energy released by the hydrogen ions is coupled to the formation of ATP from ADP and P$_i$.[5,9,12,13,17] The chain itself consists of a series of electron (e$^-$) and hydrogen ion (H$^+$) carriers im-

bedded in the inner membrane or cristae of the mitochondria. Most of these H$^+$ and e$^-$ carriers are proteins or a combination of metal ions and proteins. The major carriers are indicated in Figure 9.9. These carriers are flavoprotein 1 and 2, the coenzyme Q, and five cytochromes: b, c$_1$, c, a, and a$_3$. Coenzyme Q and cytochrome c are mobile and literally move the electrons between the other carriers.

The H$^+$ and e$^-$ come from the breakdown of the hydrogen atoms released in stages I, II, and III and transported by NAD$^+$ and FAD:

$$2H = 2H^+ + 2e^-$$

The H$^+$ are deposited in the fluid between the inner and outer mitochondrial membranes. The e$^-$ are shuttled along from one electron acceptor to the next (see Figure 9.9). The e$^-$ move along in a series of

FIGURE 9.9

Stage IV: Electron Transport and Oxidative Phosphorylation

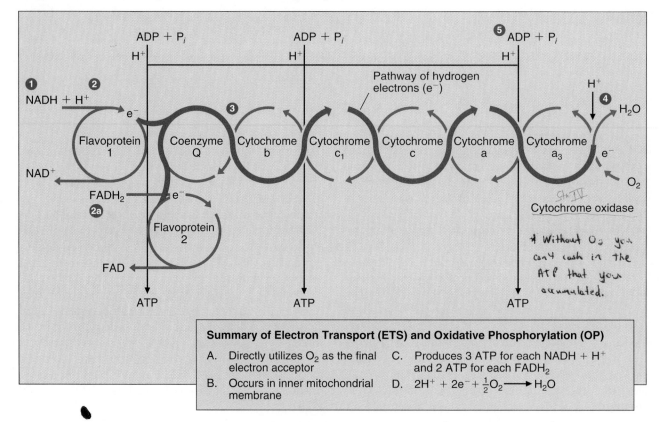

Summary of Electron Transport (ETS) and Oxidative Phosphorylation (OP)

A. Directly utilizes O_2 as the final electron acceptor

B. Occurs in inner mitochondrial membrane

C. Produces 3 ATP for each NADH + H$^+$ and 2 ATP for each FADH$_2$

D. $2H^+ + 2e^- + \frac{1}{2}O_2 \longrightarrow H_2O$

oxidation-reduction reactions, because each successive carrier has a greater affinity (force of chemical attraction) for them than the preceding one in the sequence. Oxygen has the greatest affinity of all for e^- and acts as the final e^- acceptor. The additional electrons on the oxygen give it a negative charge and attract the positively charged H^+, thus forming water.

The formation of ATP from ADP and P_i is coupled to the movement of H^+ and e^- along the electron transport chain. The movement of those ions releases energy that is used to phosphylate ADP to ATP. Because phosphate is added (phosphorylation) and the NADH + H^+ and $FADH_2$ are oxidized (electrons removed), the term **oxidative phosphorylation (OP)** is used to denote this formation of ATP. Thus oxidative phosphorylation is the process in which NADH + H^+ and $FADH_2$ are oxidized in the electron transport system and the energy released is used to synthesize ATP from ADP and P_i. Remember that the process of producing ATP directly in glycolysis and the Krebs cycle was called substrate-level phosphorylation because the P_i was transferred directly from phosphorylated intermediates to ADP without any oxidation occurring.

The Steps of Stage IV. Again, the series of steps [5,9,12,13,17] presented in Figure 9.9 are necessary so that the energy may be preserved and not released all at once and lost as heat, which would destroy tissue.

Step 1. NADH + H^+ arrives at flavoprotein 1 and transfers the electrons (e^-) and protons (H^+) from the hydrogen across the inner membrane.

Step 2. The H^+ are released and deposited into the intermembrane space.

Step 2a. This step is really a variation and not a sequential step. If the original hydrogen carrier was FAD instead of NAD^+, the transfer of electrons and protons occurs at flavoprotein 2 instead of flavoprotein 1.

Step 3. The electrons return to the inner membrane surface and pick up another pair of H^+ from the surrounding fluid, which they transport to the intermembrane space as before. This step is repeated three times for $6H^+$ if the carrier is NADH + H^+ and twice for $4H^+$ if the carrier is $FADH_2$. At the same time the electrons shuttle down the cytochromes, al-

ternately causing the cytochromes to gain (become oxidized) and lose (become reduced) the electrons.

Step 4. Oxygen accepts the electrons. This increase in negative charge attracts hydrogen ions and causes the formation of water. Figure 9.10 depicts this step graphically.

Step 5. The H^+ that have been transported into the intermembrane space create an electrochemical gradient. Since the drive is to equalize that gradient, the H^+ leak back into the mitochondrial matrix through special protein channels. The movement of H^+ creates an electrical current, and this electrical energy is somehow used to synthesize ATP from ADP + P_i, both of which are present in the matrix. One ATP molecule is produced for each pair of H^+. Therefore, each NADH + H^+ is responsible for producing 3 ATP, but each $FADH_2$ produces only 2 ATP.

Step 6. This final step is not shown in Figure 9.9 but is depicted in Figure 9.11. In this step the ATP diffuses out of the mitochondria in exchange for the inward movement of ADP needed for the continual production of energy.

Figure 9.11 summarizes the process of cellular respiration just discussed and shows the interrelationships in a cell. As you study the figure, refer to the individual stage explanations as needed.

ATP Production from Carbohydrate

The number of ATP produced directly by substrate-level phosphorylation and the number of hydrogen atoms being carried by NAD and FAD were pointed out for each stage. These numbers are summarized in Table 9.1 (p. 228). From this summary we can

---

Electron Transport System (ETS) The final metabolic pathway; it proceeds as a series of chemical reactions in the mitochondria that transfer electrons from the hydrogen atom carriers NAD and FAD to oxygen; water is formed as a by-product; the electrochemical energy released by the hydrogen ions is coupled to the formation of ATP from ADP and P_i.

Oxidative Phosphorylation (OP) The process in which NADH + H^+ and $FADH_2$ are oxidized in the electron transport system and the energy released is used to synthesize ATP from ADP and P_i.

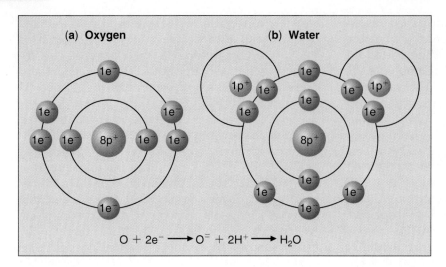

(a) Oxygen

(b) Water

$$O + 2e^- \longrightarrow O^= + 2H^+ \longrightarrow H_2O$$

FIGURE 9.10

Oxygen as the Final Electron Acceptor

(a) The outer shell of oxygen has room for eight electrons but contains only six. Thus it can accept two electrons at the end of electron transport. (b) When oxygen accepts these two electrons, it then has a double negative charge ($O^=$). Two hydrogen ions (H^+) are thus attracted, and water (H_2O) is formed.

compute the total yield of ATP from one molecule of glucose or glycogen.

Stage I (glycolysis) yields a gross production of 4 ATP but uses 2 ATP, yielding a net gain of 2 ATP from direct substrate-level phosphorylation, if the substrate is glucose. If the substrate is glycogen, only 1 ATP is used and the net gain is 3 ATP.

Two NADH + H^+ are also produced. These hydrogen atoms are transported from the cytoplasm, where glycolysis has taken place, into the mitochondria, if the level of pyruvate is not too high and if there is enough oxygen to accept the electrons at the end of the ETS. However, the mitochondrial membrane is impermeable to NADH + H^+, meaning that the membrane does not allow it to pass through. Therefore, a shuttle system must be employed.

Actually, two shuttle systems appear to operate—one for cardiac muscle and the other for skeletal muscle. The cardiac-muscle shuttle system is called the *malate-aspartate shuttle*. It operates by the NADH + H^+ in the cytoplasm giving up the hydrogens to malate, which carries them across the inner mitochondrial membrane. Here, mitochondrial NAD$^+$ picks up the H^+ and enters the ETS.[13]

The skeletal-muscle shuttle system is called the *glycerol-phosphate shuttle*. It operates by the NADH + H^+ in the cytoplasm giving up the hydrogens to glycerol phosphate, which carries them into the inner mitochondrial membrane. Here, FAD picks the H^+ up and enters the ETS. This shuttle predominates in skeletal muscle.[5,9,12,13,17] It is the carrier within the mitochondrion that determines how many ATP are produced.

Therefore, in heart muscle the yield from the glycolytic hydrogens is 6 ATP (2 NADH + H^+ × 3 = 6 ATP). That of skeletal muscle is only 4 ATP (2 FADH$_2$ × 2 = 4 ATP).

Stage II (the conversion of pyruvate to acetyl CoA) yields no substrate-level ATP, but it does produce 2 NADH + H^+. Since these molecules are already in the mitochondria, they directly enter the ETS: 2 NADH + H^+ × 3 = 6 ATP.

Stage III (the Krebs cycle) produces 2 ATP directly by substrate-level phosphorylation, NADH + H^+ at three steps, and FADH$_2$ at one step. Thus, (3 NADH + H^+ × 3 = 9 ATP) + (1 FADH$_2$ × 2 = 2 ATP). Since each step occurs twice for each 6-carbon glucose molecule, this yield must be doubled: 9 ATP + 2 ATP = 11 ATP × 2 = 22 ATP.

If we add all of these results for skeletal muscle when glucose is the fuel, we get:

2 ATP	(substrate-level phosphorylation, glycolysis)
4 ATP	(NADH + H^+ → FADH$_2$, glycolysis)
6 ATP	(NADH + H^+, Stage II)
2 ATP	(substrate-level phosphorylation, Krebs cycle)
22 ATP	(FADH$_2$ + NADH + H^+, Krebs cycle ETS/OP)

or   36 ATP for the aerobic oxidation of one molecule of glucose by skeletal muscle.

To make sure that you understand this calculation, determine the total ATP produced when the

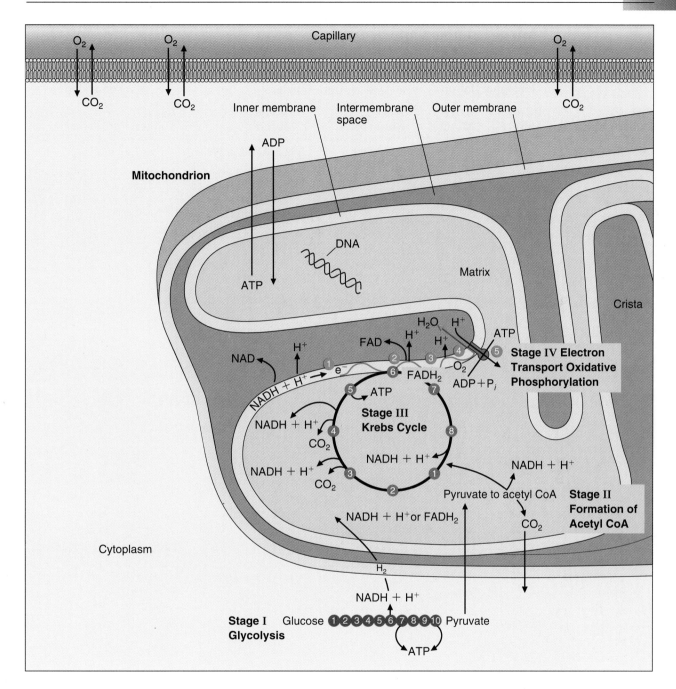

FIGURE 9.11

Cellular Respiration

aerobic oxidation takes place in heart muscle and the initial fuel is glucose. Check your answer against the value given in Table 9.1. Do the same computations assuming that glycogen, not glucose, is the energy substrate.

Fat Metabolism

Although the body may prefer to use carbohydrate as fuel from the standpoint of oxygen cost, the importance of fat as an energy source should not be

TABLE 9.1 ■ ATP Production from Carbohydrate

Metabolic Process Stage	ATP from Substrate-level Phosphorylation		Hydrogen Atoms and Carrier		ATP from Oxidative Phosphorylation	
	Heart Muscle	Skeletal Muscle	Heart Muscle	Skeletal Muscle	Heart Muscle	Skeletal Muscle
I. Glycolysis	+4 −2 2 (*3)	+4 −2 2 (*3)	2 NADH + H$^+$	†2 NADH + H$^+$		
II. Pyruvate → acetyl CoA	0	0	2 NADH + H$^+$	2 NADH + H$^+$		
III. Krebs cycle	2	2	6 NADH + H$^+$ 2 FADH$_2$	6 NADH + H$^+$ 2 FADH$_2$		
IV. ETS/OP: Hydrogen atoms from						
Stage I					6	4
Stage II					6	6
Stage III					22	22
Glucose:					2	2
					6	4
					6	6
					2	2
					22	22
Total					38	36
Glycogen:					3	3
					6	4
					6	6
					2	2
					22	22
Total					39	37

*If glycogen not glucose is fuel.

†Owing to shuttle differences in crossing into mitochondrial membrane, these hydrogen atoms are actually carried by FAD in the mitochondria, reducing the ATP production.

underestimated. Fat is found in many common foods. Fat, in the form of *triglyceride* (sometimes known as triacylglycerol), is the major storage form of energy in humans. Some triglyceride is stored within muscle cells (Figure 9.12), but the vast majority is deposited in adipose cells (Figure 9.13) and comprises approximately 10–15% of the body weight of young males and 20–25% of the body

FIGURE 9.12

Lipid Droplets in Skeletal Muscle

In this electron micrograph of skeletal muscle (EM: 27,200X) lipid droplets are visible in the light round circles, some of which have been labeled "L".

From: Cell and Tissue Ultrastructure by Cross and Mercer. Copyright © 1993 by W. H. Freeman and Company. Used with permission.

weight of young females.[11] Roughly half of this adipocyte storage occurs subcutaneously (under the skin). The remaining stores surround the major organs of the abdomino-thoracic cavity as support and protection. Triglycerides are turned over constantly in the body. In fact, your body fat is turned over completely about every 3–4 weeks, so you are definitely not carrying any of your "baby fat" with you today.[12]

Fat is an excellent storage fuel for several reasons. First, fat is an energy-dense fuel yielding 9.13 kcal per gram; both carbohydrate and protein yield slightly less than 4 kcal per gram. The reason for these figures is related to the chemical structure of the substrates—specifically, the amount of oxidizable carbon and hydrogen. It is easy to appreciate the difference by looking at the chemical composition of the free fatty acid palmitate, which is $C_{16}H_{32}O_2$. This fatty acid has almost three times the amount of C and H, but only a third the amount of O as glucose ($C_6H_{12}O_2$). Remember that it is H that donates the electrons used during oxidative phosphorylation.

Second, carbohydrate, in the form of glycogen, is stored in the muscles with a large amount of water: 2.7 g of water per gram of dried glycogen.

Triglyceride is stored dry. Thus, the energy content of fat is not diluted, and hard as it may be to believe, bulk is less than would otherwise be necessary. If humans had to store the comparable energy amount as carbohydrates, we would be at least twice as big![13]

FIGURE 9.13

Triglyceride Stored in Adipose Tissue

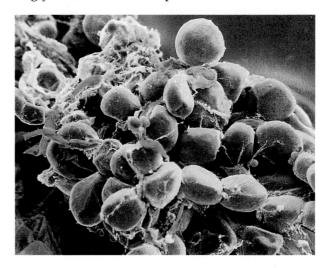

Third, glycogen stores are relatively small in comparison to fat stores. A person can deplete the stored glycogen in as little as 2 hr of heavy exercise or one day of bed rest, whereas fat supplies can last for weeks, even with moderate activity. Although many Americans often seem concerned about having too much body fat, this storage capacity is undoubtedly important for survival of the species when food is not readily available.

The triglycerides stored in adipose tissue must first be broken down into glycerol and free fatty acids before they can be used as fuel (Figure 9.2). One glycerol and three fatty acids make up a triglyceride. Seven fatty acids predominate in the body, but since three fatty acids combine with a glycerol to make up a triglyceride, there are 343 (7 × 7 × 7) different combinations possible.[15] Some common fatty acids are oleic acid, palmitic acid, stearic acid, linoleic acid, and palmitoleic acid.

Fatty acids may be saturated, unsaturated, or polyunsaturated. A saturated fatty acid has a chemical bonding arrangement that allows it to hold as many hydrogens as possible. Thus, *saturated* means "saturated with hydrogen." Unsaturated fatty acids have a chemical bonding arrangement with a reduced-hydrogen binding potential and therefore are unsaturated with respect to hydrogens. Polyunsaturated means several bonds are without hydrogens.

The breakdown of triglycerides into glycerol and fatty acids is catalyzed by the enzyme hormone-sensitive lipase. The glycerol is soluble in blood, but the free fatty acids (FFA) are not. Glycerol can enter glycolysis in the cytoplasm (as 3-phosphoglycerate, the product of step 7 in Figure 9.5), but it is not typically utilized by muscle cells in this fashion.[13,15] The direct role of glycerol as a fuel in the muscle cells during exercise is so minor that it need not be considered. However, glycerol can be converted to glucose by the liver.

FFA must be transported in the blood bound to albumin. Specific receptor sites on the muscle cell membrane receive the FFA into the cell. The FFA must then be translocated or transported from the cytoplasm into the mitochondria. Once in the mito-

chondrial matrix, the FFA undergoes the process of beta oxidation (Figure 9.14).

Beta Oxidation   **Beta oxidation** is a cyclic series of steps that breaks off successive pairs of carbon atoms from FFA, which are then used to form acetyl CoA. Remember that acetyl CoA is the common intermediate by which all foodstuffs enter the Krebs cycle and electron transport system. The number of cycles depends upon the number of carbons; most fatty acids have 14–24 carbons.

FIGURE 9.14

Beta Oxidation

Beta Oxidation A cyclic series of steps that breaks off successive pairs of carbon atoms from FFA, which are then used to form acetyl CoA.

When there is an adequate supply of oxaloacetate to combine with, the fat-derived acetyl CoA enters the Krebs cycle and proceeds through electron transport and oxidative phosphorylation. Figure 9.14 diagrams the steps of beta oxidation, which are explained next. As with glycolysis, ATP is used for activation; but unlike glycolysis, beta oxidation produces no ATP directly.

The Steps of Beta Oxidation

Step 1. The fatty acid molecule is activated by the breakdown of 1 ATP to AMP, releasing the energy equivalent of 2 ATP if broken down as it is normally to ADP. Concurrently, coenzyme A is added.

Step 2. FAD is reduced to $FADH_2$. The $FADH_2$ will enter the electron transport chain and produce 2 ATP.

Step 3. A molecule of water is added and NAD^+ is reduced to $NADH + H^+$. The $NADH + H^+$ will enter the electron transport chain and produce 3 ATP. Steps 2 and 3, with the removal of the hydrogen atoms, account for the oxidation portion of the name for this process.

Step 4. The bond between the alpha (α) carbon (C_2) and the beta (β) carbon (C_3) is broken, resulting in the removal of two carbons (C_1 and C_2), which are then used to form acetyl coenzyme A. The cleavage of carbons at the site of the beta carbon explains why the process is called beta oxidation.

Step 5. Steps 1–4 are repeated for each pair of carbons except the last, since the last unit formed is acetyl CoA itself. Therefore, the number of cycles that must be completed to oxidize the fat can be computed using the formula n/2 – 1 where n is the number of carbons. The acetyl CoA can enter the Krebs cycle and electron transport system (Figures 9.2, 9.8, and 9.9).

ATP Production from Fatty Acids   The number of ATP produced from the breakdown of fat depends on which fatty acid is utilized. The following example shows a calculation for palmitate.

■ EXAMPLE

Calculate the number of ATP produced from the breakdown of palmitate (palmitic acid).

The steps in the calculation follow

1. Palmitate is a 16-carbon fatty acid. Therefore, as noted in the previous step 5, it cycles through beta oxidation n/2 – 1 = 16/2 – 1 = 7 times.

2. Each cycle produces 1 $FADH_2$ and 1 $NADH + H^+$, as follows:

    $$FADH_2 \quad \rightarrow FAD \quad \quad 2\ ATP$$
    $$NADH + H^+ \quad \rightarrow NAD \quad \underline{+\ 3\ ATP}$$
    $$5\ ATP$$

    This reaction happens 7 times: $7 \times 5 = 35$ ATP.

3. Each cycle (7) plus the last step (1) produces acetyl CoA, for a total of 8. Each acetyl CoA yields 1 ATP, 3 $NADH + H^+$, and 1 $FADH_2$ in the Krebs cycle. The 3 $NADH + H^+$ will produce 9 ATP, and the $FADH_2$ will produce 2 ATP in the electron transport system. Thus, 12 ATP are produced for each acetyl CoA, for a total of 8 acetyl CoA $\times$ 12 ATP = 96 ATP.

4. Add the results of steps 2 and 3: 96 ATP + 35 ATP = 131 ATP. However, 1 ATP was utilized in step 1 of beta oxidation to activate the fatty acid. Furthermore, this ATP was broken down to AMP, not ADP; hence, the equivalent of 2 ATP were used. Subtracting this result from the total, we get 131 ATP – 2 ATP = 129 ATP from palmitate. ■

Recall that three acids plus one glycerol make up a triglyceride. These calculations apply to a single specific fatty acid. It has been estimated that for the mixture that comprises human adipose tissue the ATP yield is 138 molecules of ATP per molecule of fatty acid.

To determine whether you understand the ATP yield from fatty acids, calculate the ATP produced from an 18-carbon fatty acid such as stearate. Check your answer in the answer section at the end of the chapter.

Ketone Bodies and Ketosis   As mentioned earlier, in order for the acetyl CoA produced by beta oxidation to enter the Krebs cycle, a sufficient amount of oxaloacetate is necessary. When carbohydrate supplies are sufficient, this is no problem, and fat is said to burn in the flame of carbohydrate. However, when carbohydrates are inadequate (perhaps as a result of fasting, prolonged exercise, or diabetes mellitus), oxaloacetate is converted to glucose. The production of glucose from noncarbohydrate sources under these conditions is necessary, since some tissue, such as the brain and nervous system, rely predominantly on glucose as a fuel.[12]

When oxaloacetate is converted to glucose and is therefore not available to combine with acetyl CoA to form citrate, the liver converts the acetyl CoA derived from the fatty acids into metabolites called *ketones* or *ketone bodies*. Despite the similarity in the names, do not confuse these ketones with keto acids (pyruvic acid and the Krebs cycle intermediates) (Figure 9.8). There are three forms of ketones: acetoacetic acid, beta-hydroxybutyric acid, and acetone. All are strong acids. Acetone gives the breath a very characteristic fruity smell.

The ketone bodies can themselves be used as fuel by muscles, nerves, and the brain. If the ketones are not used but, instead, accumulate, a condition called *ketosis* occurs. The high acidity of ketosis can disrupt normal physiological functioning, especially acid-base balance. Ketosis is more likely to result from an inadequate diet (as in anorexia nervosa) or diabetes than from prolonged exercise, since the muscles will use the ketones as fuel. During exercise aerobically trained individuals can utilize ketones more effectively than untrained individuals.

Protein Metabolism

Proteins are found in many food sources. *Proteins are large molecules consisting of varying combinations of amino acids linked together.* Approximately 20 amino acids occur naturally.[8] Because there are so many ways these amino acids can combine, there is an almost infinite number of possible proteins. Like carbohydrates and fats, amino acids contain atoms of carbon, oxygen, and hydrogen. In addition, they may include sulfur, phosphorus, and iron. All amino acids have in common an amino group containing nitrogen (NH_2).

Proteins are extremely important in the structure and function of the body. Among other things they are components of hemoglobin, contractile elements of the muscle, hormones, fibrin for clotting,

Transamination The transfer of the NH_2 amino group from an amino acid to a keto acid.

Gluconeogenesis The creation of glucose in the liver from noncarbohydrate sources, particularly glycerol, lactate or pyruvate, and alanine.

tendons, ligaments, and portions of all cell membranes. Because proteins are so important in the body, the constituent amino acids are used predominantly as building blocks, not as a source of energy.

However, amino acids can be, and in certain instances are, used as a fuel source. When amino acids are used as a fuel source, muscles appear to preferentially, but not exclusively, utilize the group of amino acids known as branched-chain amino acids (BCAA): leucine, isoleucine, and valine. In this situation, as with carbohydrate and fat metabolism, the final common pathways of the Krebs cycle, electron transport, and oxidative phosphorylation are utilized. The site of entry into the metabolic pathways varies, as shown in Figure 9.2, with the amino acid.[17]

Six amino acids can enter metabolism at the level of pyruvic acid, 8 at acetyl CoA, 4 at alpha-ketoglutarate, 4 at succinate, 2 at fumarate, and 2 at oxaloacetate. All of these intermediates except acetyl CoA are, in turn, converted to pyruvate before being utilized to produce energy. The acetyl CoA is used directly in the Krebs cycle and electron transport, as previously described.

Transamination and Oxidative Deamination Before amino acids can be used as a fuel and enter the pathways at any place, the nitrogen-containing amino group (the NH_2) must be removed. Removal is accomplished by the process of transamination and sometimes oxidative deamination.[5,9,12,13,17] These processes are summarized in Table 9.2.

All but two amino acids appear to be able to undergo transamination. **Transamination** involves the transfer of the NH_2 amino group from an amino acid to a keto acid. Remember that keto acids include pyruvic acid, acetyl CoA, and the Krebs cycle intermediates. This process occurs in both the cytoplasm and the mitochondria, predominantly in muscle and liver cells. Transamination results in the formation of a new amino acid and a different keto acid. The most frequent keto acid acceptor of NH_2 is α-ketoglutarate, with glutamate being the amino acid formed.[12,17]

Two fates for glutamate are shown in Table 9.2. In the first glutamate is transaminated to alanine, another amino acid. Alanine, in turn, can be converted to glucose in a process called gluconeogenesis.[5,12] **Gluconeogenesis** is the creation of glucose in the liver from noncarbohydrate sources, particularly glycerol, lactate or pyruvate, and alanine.

TABLE 9.2 ■ Transamination and Oxidative Deamination

TRANSAMINATION	OXIDATIVE DEAMINATION
GENERALIZED	**GENERALIZED**
Amino acid (1) and keto acid (1) ⇌ amino acid (2) + keto acid (2).	Amino acid → keto acid + NH_3.
The NH2 group from amino acid (1) is transferred to keto acid (1), forming a different amino acid (2) and a different keto acid (2).	The NH_2 group is removed from an amino acid, forming a keto acid and ammonia.
	MOST COMMON
MOST COMMON	Glutamate + H_2O + NAD ⇌ NH_3 + α-ketoglutarate + NADH + H^+
Any one of 12 different amino acids + α-ketoglutarate ⇌ glutamate + keto acid	**FATE OF PRODUCTS**
	1. NADH + H^+ enters the electron transport system.
SPECIFIC EXAMPLE	2. α-ketoglutarate is a Krebs cycle intermediate.
Glutamate + pyruvate ⇌ alanine + α-ketoglutarate	3. NH_3 (ammonia) is removed in urine. The urea cycle is $2NH_3$ + CO_2 → $NH_2 CONH_2$ (urea) + H_2O.

In the second process glutamate undergoes oxidative deamination. In oxidative deamination the oxidized form of NAD is reduced, and the amino group (NH_2) is removed and becomes NH_3. NH_3 is ammonia, and high concentrations in the body are extremely toxic. The dominant pathway for NH_3 removal is by conversion to urea in the liver (via the urea cycle) and excretion in urine by the kidneys. Oxidative deamination is used much less frequently than transamination.

ATP Production from Amino Acids

Since the amino acid derivatives are ultimately utilized as pyruvate or acetyl CoA, the ATP production count from the amino acids is the same as for glucose from that point on, except that it is not doubled.[15] Refer to Figure 9.5 to remind yourself why the double count occurred and to Figure 9.2 to see amino acids entering the pathways denoted next.

Pyruvate → acetyl CoA =	NADH + H^+	3 ATP
Krebs cycle + ETS/OP		1 ATP
	3 NADH + H^+	9 ATP
	1 $FADH_2$	2 ATP
		15 ATP

Acetyl CoA would produce 12 ATP, since the NADH + H^+ production from pyruvate to acetyl CoA would be the only step missing.

The Regulation of Cellular Respiration and ATP Production

Intracellular

Intracellularly, the production of ATP—and, hence, the flow of substrates through the various metabolic pathways—is regulated predominantly by feedback mechanisms. As has been stated before, each step in each metabolic pathway is catalyzed by a specific enzyme. At least one of these enzymes in each pathway can be acted upon directly by other chemicals in the cell and, as a result, increases or decreases its activity. Such an enzyme is called a *rate-limiting enzyme*, and the other factors that influence it are called *modulators*. When the rate-limiting enzyme is inhibited, every step in the metabolic pathway beyond that point is also inhibited. When the rate-limiting enzyme is stimulated, every step in the metabolic pathway beyond that point is also stimulated.

The primary rate-limiting enzyme in glycolysis is phosphofructokinase (PFK), the enzyme that catalyzes step 3. PFK is stimulated, and subsequently the rate of glycolysis increased, by modulators such as ADP, AMP, P_i, and a rise in pH. ADP, AMP, and P_i modulators are the result of the breakdown of ATP. This is an example of a positive-feedback system in which the by-product of the utilization of a substance stimulates a greater production of that original substance. Conversely, PFK is inhibited, and subsequently the rate of glycolysis decreased, by the modulators ATP, CP, citrate (a Krebs cycle intermediate), FFA, and a drop in pH. Each of these modulators indicates that sufficient substances exist to supply ATP. This is an example of a negative-feedback system in which the formation of a product or other similarly acting product inhibits further production of the product.[13]

The primary rate-limiting enzyme in the Krebs cycle is isocitrate dehydrogenase (ICD), which catalyzes step 3. ICD is stimulated by ADP, P_i, and calcium (positive feedback) and is inhibited by ATP (negative feedback).[13]

Cytochrome oxidase—which catalyzes the transfer of electrons to molecular oxygen, resulting in the formation of water—is the rate-limiting enzyme for the electron transport system. It is stimulated by ADP and P_i (positive feedback) and is inhibited by ATP (negative feedback).[13]

A pattern in the modulators is readily evident, with ATP, ADP, and P_i being universally important. When ATP is present in sufficient amounts to satisfy the needs of the cell and to provide some reserve in storage, there is no need to increase its production. Thus, key enzymes in the metabolic pathways are inhibited. However, when muscle activity begins and ATP is broken down into ADP and P_i, these by-products stimulate all the metabolic pathways to produce more ATP so that the muscle contractions can continue.

Extracellular

During exercise the metabolic processes must not only provide ATP for energy but must also maintain blood glucose levels at near-resting values for the proper functioning of the entire organism. This is because the brain and nervous tissue must have glucose as a fuel. One of the ways of maintaining glucose levels is by the process of gluconeogenesis.

Gluconeogenesis   As defined earlier, gluconeogenesis is the creation (-*genesis*) of new (-*neo*) glucose (*gluco-*) in the liver from noncarbohydrate sources. The primary fuel sources for gluconeogenesis are glycerol, lactate or pyruvate, and alanine. Glycerol is released into the bloodstream when triglycerides are broken down (Figure 9.15).

Pyruvate is the end product of glycolysis (Figure 9.15). The majority of the pyruvate is converted to acetyl CoA and enters the Krebs cycle and electron transport system. However, a small portion diffuses out of the muscle cell and into the bloodstream.[15] Still another portion of the pyruvate (the actual amount depends on the intensity of the activity) is converted to lactate, which also diffuses into the bloodstream. About ten times as much lactate as pyruvate diffuses out of the muscle cells.

Alanine is formed by transamination when the amino group from one amino acid (preferentially, the BCAA or an amino acid derived from glutamate) is transferred to pyruvate (see Figure 9.15). Note that in the liver alanine is first reconverted to pyruvate (freeing the NH_3 to enter the urea cycle and be excreted) before being converted to glucose.

In all cases the conversion to glucose takes place in the liver. For each gram of glucose produced 1.02 g of glycerol, 1.43 g of pyruvate, 1.23 g of lactate, or 1.45 g of alanine is utilized.[15]

The glycerol-glucose cycle has no special name, but the pyruvate/lactate-glucose cycle is known as the *Cori cycle,* and the alanine-glucose cycle is called the *Felig cycle.* The Cori and Felig cycles help maintain normal blood glucose levels so that the brain, nerves, and kidneys as well as the muscles may draw from this supply.

Neurohormonal Coordination   The regulation of blood glucose levels, including gluconeogenesis, is governed jointly by the autonomic nervous system (particularly the sympathetic division) and the endocrine system, which function in a coordinated fashion. Figure 9.16 shows this integration of the two control systems for the regulation of energy production in responding to exercise.

When exercise begins, signals from the working muscles and motor centers in the central nervous system bring about a neurohormonal response mediated through the hypothalamus. The hypothalamus stimulates both the anterior pituitary and the sympathetic nervous system. The neurotransmitter norepinephrine is released directly from sympathetic nerve endings, and the hormones epinephrine and norepinephrine are released from the adrenal medulla. Epinephrine and norepinephrine both act directly on fuel sites and stimulate the anterior pituitary and pancreas. As a result of the dual stimulation of the anterior pituitary, hormones

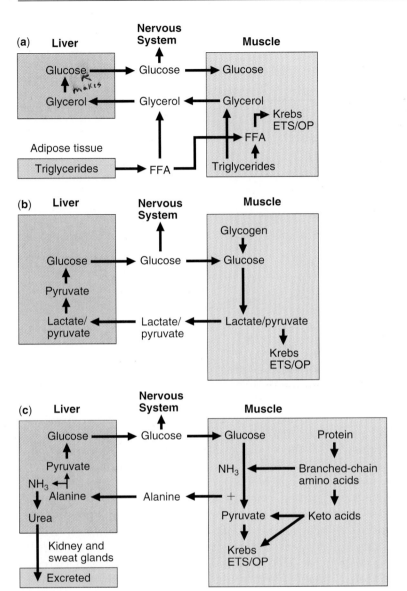

FIGURE 9.15

Gluconeogenesis

(a) Glycerol-glucose cycle, (b) Cori cycle, (c) Felig cycle.

are released—namely, growth hormone, cortisol, and thyroxine. The release of insulin is inhibited from the pancreas, but glucagon release is stimulated.[1,6] In general, the result is threefold (see also Table 9.3):

1. An increase in the mobilization and utilization of free fatty acid stores from extramuscular (adipose tissue) and intramuscular stores.

2. An increase in the breakdown of extramuscular (liver) and intramuscular stores of glycogen and the creation of glucose from noncarbohydrate sources (gluconeogenesis) in the liver.

3. A decrease in the uptake of glucose into the nonworking cells.

A two-tier system of hormonal involvement appears to operate on the basis of time of response. The catecholamines (epinephrine and norepinephrine) and glucagon react to an increase in muscular activity in a matter of seconds to minutes. Both assist in all three functions listed. However, epinephrine's influence on fat metabolism is relatively slow (approximately 20 min) and far greater than its affect on glucose metabolism.[7]

The actions of epinephrine, norepinephrine, and glucagon are backed up by growth hormone

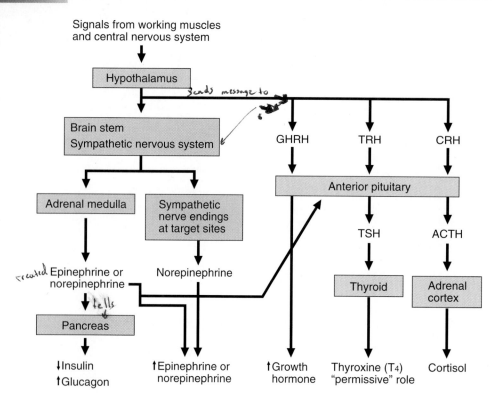

FIGURE 9.16 ✓

Extracellular Neurohormonal Regulation of Metabolism

Sources: Bunt,[1] Marieb,[2], Van de Graaff & Fox.[17]
Note: TRH is thyroid-releasing hormone; ACTH is adreno cortico-trophic hormone; GHRH is growth hormone releasing hormone; CRH is corticotrophic releasing hormone; TSH is thyroid stimulating hormone. ↓ decrease, ↑ increase.

and cortisol, respectively. The response of growth hormone and cortisol may take hours to become maximal. Thus, these latter two hormones are probably most important for carbohydrate conservation in long-duration activity. This result explains why they can bring about glycogen synthesis, which glucagon and the catecholamines do not.[7]

Insulin secretion is suppressed during exercise. This decrease in insulin and the increase in glucagon, growth hormone, and cortisol cause a decrease in the glucose uptake into cells other than the working muscles. The available glucose is thus spared for the working muscles and the nervous system.

During exercise the working muscles become highly permeable to glucose despite the lack of insulin. The reason for this change in permeability is unknown, but it is suspected that something in the muscle contractile process itself is responsible. The contractile process also helps to break down the intramuscular stores of glycogen and triglycerides.[6,7]

The increases in protein breakdown and in amino acid transport caused by growth hormone and cortisol (Table 9.3) are important in providing protein precursors for gluconeogenesis (Figure 9.15). The fact that these hormones are slow respon-ders also explains why protein is not used in significant amounts until long-duration activity.

Since the mobilization of free fatty acids involves the breakdown of triglycerides, glycerol is also released and made available for gluconeogenesis. Note that an accumulation of the other gluconeogenic precursor, lactate, will inhibit free fatty acid release from adipose tissue. Therefore, gluconeogenesis serves a dual purpose in helping to provide glucose and reducing the levels of lactate so that it does not interfere as much with fat utilization.

Thyroxine itself has a number of metabolic functions. However, its role in exercise metabolism appears to be one of potentiation or permissiveness. That is, it helps to create an environment in which the other metabolic hormones can function more effectively, rather than having any major effect itself.

The level of response and reaction to all of these hormones depends upon three things:

1. The type, duration, and intensity of the exercise; relative intensity appears to be more important than the absolute workload.

2. The nutritional, health, training status, and fiber type composition of the exerciser.

TABLE 9.3 ■ Hormonal Regulation of Metabolism During Exercise

		Hormone		
EFFECT	GLUCAGON	EPINEPHRINE AND NOREPINEPHRINE	GROWTH HORMONE*	CORTISOL
Glucose uptake and utilization	↓†		↓†	↓†
Glycogen breakdown (glycogenolysis)	↑	↑	↑	↑
Glycogen formation (glycogenesis)	↓	↓	↑	↑
Gluconeogenesis	↑	↑	↑	↑
FFA storage (lipogenesis)	↓		↓	↓
FFA mobilization (lipolysis)	↑	↑	↑	↑
Amino acid transport and uptake			↑	↑
Protein breakdown				↑

*Heavy exercise.   ↑ = Increases.
†Nonactive cells.   ↓ = Decreases.

3. The size of the fuel depots, the state of the hormone receptors, and the capacity of the involved enzymes.[6]

*F*uel Utilization at Rest and During Exercise

The preceding discussion explained how each of the major fuel sources—fats, carbohydrates, and proteins—produces ATP energy for the human body. At rest, it has been estimated that fats contribute from 41 to 67%, carbohydrates from 33 to 42%, and proteins from just a trace to 17% of the total daily energy requirements of the human body.[10]

During exercise various forms of each fuel are utilized to supply the working muscle with the additional ATP energy needed to sustain movement.

In order to understand which energy sources are used during exercise, it is first necessary to know approximately how much of each energy substrate is available for use. Table 9.4 shows the tissue fuel stores in an average adult male who weighs 65 kg and has 8.45 kg (13%) body fat and 30 kg of muscle. Protein stores have been omitted since the major tissue storage of protein is in the muscles and complete degradation (breakdown) of muscle to sustain energy metabolism is neither realistic nor desirable under normal circumstances.

Several important points should be noted from Table 9.4. First, triglycerides provide the greatest source of potential energy (77,150 kcal is enough energy to sustain life for approximately 47 days!). Second, comparatively, very little carbohydrate is actually stored. In fact, the human body's stores of carbohydrate are only enough to support life for 1¼ days if all three sources (muscle glycogen, liver glycogen, and circulating glucose) are added

TABLE 9.4 ■ Tissue Fuel Stores in Average Adult Males (body weight = 65 kg, percent body fat =13)

	Total Energy*			Estimated Period Fuel Would Supply Energy[†]		
TISSUE FUEL	g	kJ	Kcal	BASAL[‡] (DAYS)	WALK[‡] (DAYS)	RUN[‡] (MIN)
Triglycerides[§] (fatty acids)	8,450	322,789	77,150	47.46	11.25	5223
Liver glycogen[§]	80	1,275	305	0.19	0.05	20.7
Muscle glycogen (28.25 kg muscle[#])	425	7,384 **	1,743 **	1.07	0.25	118
Circulating glucose	20	319	76	0.05	0.01	5.2

*Conversion factors utilized: glucose, 3.81 kcal · g^{-1}; fatty acid, 9.13 kcal · g^{-1}; kcal × 4.184 = kJ.[2,15]

[†]Calculations assume that each fuel is the only fuel utilized. In reality, the fuels are utilized with mixtures that depend on the type, intensity, and duration of the activity and the training, fiber type proportions, and nutritional status of the exerciser.

[‡]Kilocalorie cost of exercise: basal 0.174 kcal · kg^{-1} · 10 min^{-1} walking at 3.5 mi · hr^{-1} = 0.733 kcal · kg^{-1} · 10 min^{-1}; running at 8.7 mi · hr^{-1} (6:54 mile) = 2.273 kcal · 10 min^{-1}.[3]

[§]65 kg body weight × 0.13 (fraction of body fat) = 8.45 kg fat.

$^{||}$Liver equals approximately 2.5% body weight. Normal glycogen content is 50 g · kg^{-1}.[15]

[#]Weight of the muscle is approximately equal to half the lean body mass.

**Muscle fatty acid values would equal this value since 1 kg of muscle contains approximately 13.5 g fatty acid and 1.5 g glycerol. The triglyceride value includes the muscle store.[15]

Sources: Based on Kapit, Macey, & Meisami;[8] Newsholme & Leech.[13]

together. Thus, carbohydrate replenishment on a regular basis is essential. Third, exercise has a major impact on how long each fuel can supply energy.

Table 9.4 assumes that each fuel is acting independently, which in fact never happens. Tables 9.5 and 9.6 provide more realistic views of what actually happens during exercise. Table 9.5 depicts the relative utilization of each substrate source as influenced by the type, intensity, and duration of the activity. Very short duration, very high intensity dynamic activity and static contractions are special cases that rely predominantly on energy substrates stored in the muscle fibers—that is, ATP-PC and glycogen (which can quickly be broken down into ATP to provide energy).

The other exercises listed in Table 9.5 are assumed to be predominantly dynamic and to a large extent aerobic (utilizing oxygen). In general, the lower the intensity, the more important fat is as a fuel; the higher the intensity, the more important carbohydrates are as fuel. Duration has a similar effect in that the shorter the duration, the more important carbohydrates are as a fuel, with fat being

utilized more and more as the duration lengthens. Fats come into play over the long term because the glycogen stores can and will be depleted. Indeed, long-duration activities often exhibit a three-part sequence in which muscle glycogen, bloodborne glucose (including glucose that has been broken down from liver glycogen and glucose that has been created by gluconeogenesis), and fatty acids successively predominate as the major fuel source. Protein may account for 5–15% of the total energy supply in activities lasting more than an hour.[4,10,14]

Table 9.6 provides an estimation of how fuel utilization varies by race distance [10 km (6.2 mi) and 42.2 km (26.2 mi), or marathon distance] and performance (a "fast" and a "slow" time for each distance). Compare the muscle glycogen utilization in the fast and the slow conditions. At the short distance (less than 1 hr) there is not much difference, but during the marathon almost six times as much muscle glycogen is used by the faster runner. Conversely, the greatest amount of fat is utilized by the slow marathoner. Circulating glucose use is much higher in marathoners because the longer duration and lower intensity permit the liver to generate

TABLE 9.5 ■ Relative Degree of Fuel Utilization in Muscle for Various Types of Exercise

		Exercise Condition				
FUEL	REST	VERY HIGH INTENSITY, VERY SHORT DURATION (< 3 MIN), AND STATIC CONTRACTIONS	HIGH-INTENSITY (80–85% MAX), SHORT-DURATION (< 40 MIN)	HIGH-INTENSITY (70–80% MAX), MODERATE-DURATION (40–150 MIN)	MODERATE-INTENSITY (60–70% MAX), LONG-DURATION (> 150 MIN)	LOW-INTENSITY (< 50% MAX), LONG-DURATION (> 150 MIN)
Muscle glycogen	Negligible	High	High	High	Moderate	Low
Liver glycogen and bloodborne glucose	Moderate	Negligible	High	High	Moderate	Moderate
Free fatty acid (FFA)	Moderate	Negligible	Low	Moderate	High	High
Amino acid	Low	Negligible	Negligible	Low	Low	Low

Sources: Based on Felig & Wahren,[14] Pernow & Saltin,[14] Saltin.[16]

* The greater intensity the more glycogen one would use.
+ The lesser intensity the more fatty acids will be burned as a fuel.

(by gluconeogenesis) and release glucose into the bloodstream. The 10-km runner has sufficient muscle glycogen stores and does not need to rely on external glucose production. Very little protein (BCAA) is used by either of the 10-km runners, but a small amount provides some energy for the marathoners.

A complex interaction exists between exercise energy needs and the fuel sources that provide this energy within the human organism.

TABLE 9.6 ■ Fuel Utilization by 70-kg Male Runner at Different Distances and Levels of Performance

	10 km		42.2 km	
	FAST	SLOW	FAST	SLOW
Performance	0:30:00	1:00:00	2:21:00	5:12:00
Circulating glucose (g)	9.7	13.4	120.5	217.8
Muscle glycogen (g)	149.0	134.0	403.0	69.0
Liver glycogen (g)	20.1	10.9	73.7	103.9
Fatty acids (g)	7.0	12.0	104.0	229.0
Branched-chain amino acids (g) (BCAA)	0.7	0.9	15.7	48.5

Source: Péronnet et al.[15]

SUMMARY

1. The process by which ATP is formed from food is called cellular respiration.

2. Carbohydrate metabolism consists of four stages that convert glucose or glycogen into carbon dioxide, water, and ATP energy.

3. Stage I of carbohydrate metabolism is known as glycolysis. Glycolysis consists of a series of 10 or 11 steps; it occurs in the cytoplasm of cells and is anaerobic. It begins with glucose or glycogen and ends with pyruvate (pyruvic acid) or lactate (lactic acid). In the process a net gain of 2 ATP is achieved by substrate-level phosphorylation if the fuel was glucose and 3 ATP if the fuel was glycogen. A pair of $NADH + H^+$ also result.

4. Stage II of carbohydrate metabolism has no identifying name, but it results in the formation of acetyl coenzyme A from pyruvate. These two steps occur in the mitochondrial matrix; although no oxygen is used directly, the process must be aerobic. No ATP is produced, but two pairs of hydrogen atoms are released and picked up by NAD^+, forming $NADH + H^+$.

5. Stage III of carbohydrate metabolism is the Krebs cycle (sometimes known as the citric acid cycle). This stage consists of eight steps and also occurs in the mitochondrial matrix; again, no oxygen is used directly, but it also must be aerobic. Two ATP are produced by substrate-level phosphorylation and pairs of hydrogen atoms are removed at four separate steps. In three cases the hydrogens are picked up by NAD^+ and in the fourth by FAD.

6. Stage IV of carbohydrate metabolism is known as electron transport and oxidative phosphorylation. Electron transport takes place in the inner mitochondrial membrane and, as the name implies, consists of relaying electrons from the hydrogen atoms from one protein carrier to another and transporting the remaining hydrogen ions into the intermembrane space. In the process an electrical current is created. This electrical energy is then used to synthesize ATP from ADP by the addition of a phosphate. For each hydrogen carried to the electron transport system by NAD^+, 3 ATP are formed. For each hydrogen carried by FAD to the electron transport chain, 2 ATP are formed.

7. A total of 36 ATP are produced if the fuel subtrate is glucose and the muscle is skeletal. A total of 37 ATP are produced if the fuel substrate is glycogen and the muscle is skeletal. A total of 38 ATP are produced if the fuel substrate is glucose and the muscle is cardiac. A total of 39 ATP are produced if the fuel substrate is glycogen and the muscle is cardiac.

8. Triglycerides stored in adipose cells or stored intramuscularly are the major storage form of energy in humans. Triglycerides are composed of fatty acids and glycerol. Muscle cells can only use fatty acids as a fuel.

9. Fatty acid can only be utilized as a fuel source aerobically within the mitochondria. Fatty acids must undergo the process of beta oxidation—which involves the removal of hydrogen atoms (oxidation) and the removal of pairs of carbons (at the beta carbon location) to form acetyl coenzyme A—before entering the Krebs cycle and electron transport.

10. The ATP produced from each fatty acid depends upon the number of carbon pairs. For the mixture that comprises human adipose tissue the ATP yield is 138 molecules of ATP per molecule of fatty acids.

11. When glucose supplies are inadequate and oxaloacetate must be converted to glucose, the acetyl coenzyme A derived from fatty acids is converted into three forms of ketones: acetoacetic acid, beta-hydroxybutyric acid, and acetone. Acetone gives the breath a characteristic fruity smell.

12. Amino acids are used primarily in anabolic processes in human cells, building proteins such as hemoglobin and the contractile elements of muscle. However, amino acids—and especially the branched-chain amino acids (valine, leucine, and isoleucine)—can be used as a fuel source and may contribute as much as 5–15% of the energy supply in long term, dynamic endurance activity.

13. All amino acids contain an amino group (NH_2). Before an amino acid can be used as a fuel, this amino group must be removed. Removal of the amino group is accomplished by two processes: oxidative deamination or transamination (most common). Entry into the Krebs cycle and electron transport then occurs at several locations, but ultimately all of the intermediates except acetyl CoA are converted to pyruvate before being used to produce energy.

14. Fifteen ATP are derived from each of the amino acid derivatives utilized as pyruvate, and 12 ATP are produced from each derivative utilized as acetyl CoA.

15. ATP energy production has both intracellular and extracellular regulation. Intracellular regulation operates primarily by the feedback stimulation (by ADP, AMP, P_i, and a rise in pH) or inhibition (by ATP, CP, citrate, and a drop in pH) of the rate-limiting enzyme. Extracellular regulation is achieved by the coordinated action of the sympathetic nervous system (via norepinephrine) and the hormonal system (norepinephrine, epinephrine, glucagon, cortisol, growth hormone, and cortisol).

16. The goal of metabolism during exercise is threefold:

(a) To increase the mobilization and utilization of free fatty acid from adipose tissue and intramuscular stores.

(b) To decrease the uptake of glucose into nonworking muscle cells while at the same time providing glucose for nerve and brain cells.

(c) To increase the breakdown of liver and muscle stores of glycogen and create glucose from non-carbohydrate sources in the liver.

17. The creation of glucose from noncarbohydrate sources is called gluconeogenesis. The primary fuel sources for gluconeogenesis are glycerol, lactate or pyruvate, and alanine.

18. Fatty acids comprise the largest fuel supply. Other fuels, in descending order, are total muscle glycogen, liver glycogen, and circulating glucose.

19. Which energy substrate is utilized and in what amounts depends upon the complex interaction of the type, duration, and intensity of exercise; the proportion of muscle fiber types involved; and the training status, long-term nutritional state, and short-term dietary status of the exerciser.

20. In general, very short duration, high-intensity dynamic activity and static contractions are special cases that rely predominantly on the ATP-PC and glycogen stored in the muscle fibers.

21. In dynamic aerobic activity the higher the intensity, the more important carbohydrates (glucose and glycogen) are as a fuel; the lower the intensity, the more important fats are as a fuel. Likewise, the shorter the duration, the more important carbohydrates are as a fuel; the longer the duration, the more that fat is utilized. In activities lasting more than an hour. protein makes a small but important contribution to the energy supply.

Answer

The number of ATP produced from the 18-carbon fatty acid stearate.

1. $n/2 - 1 = 18/2 - 1 = 8$ cycles of beta oxidation
2. $FADH_2 = 8 \times 2$ ATP $= 16$ ATP
   $NADH_2 = 8 \times \underline{3 \text{ ATP}} = \underline{24 \text{ ATP}}$
   $ 8 \times 5$ ATP $= 40$ ATP
3. Acetyl CoA = 9:
   $ 9 \times 12$ ATP $= 108$ ATP
4. Activation energy $= -2$ ATP
5. Total: 108 ATP
   $\underline{+ 40 \text{ ATP}}$
   148 ATP
   $\underline{-2 \text{ ATP}}$
   146 ATP

REVIEW QUESTIONS

1. Distinguish between anabolism and catabolism. Is cellular respiration anabolic or catabolic?

2. Name and briefly summarize the four steps of carbohydrate metabolism.

3. Explain how a count of 36 ATP is achieved by cellular respiration if the fuel substrate is glucose in skeletal muscle. Why is the ATP count from carbohydrate sometimes 37, 38, or 39 instead of 36?

4. Why is beta oxidation necessary before fat can be used as an energy substrate? Describe what occurs during beta oxidation.

5. State how the calculation is completed to determine the number of ATP produced from fatty acids. Complete an example using a fat having 24 carbons.

6. Name and describe the process that amino acids must undergo before being used as a fuel substrate. Why is this process necessary?

7. Identify the locations in the metabolic pathways where amino acids may enter. How does the ATP count differ between these locations?

8. Why is acetyl coenzyme A called the universal common intermediate?

9. Why would the breath of someone suffering from anorexia nervosa smell sweet?

10. Describe the role of enzymes in the metabolic pathways. Identify the rate-limiting enzymes in stages I, III, and IV of carbohydrate metabolism. How are enzymes regulated?

11. What are the goals of metabolic regulation during exercise? How are these goals achieved by the interaction of the sympathetic nervous system and the hormonal system?

12. Compare the relative availability and use of carbohydrate, fat, and protein fuel substrates on the basis of intensity and duration of exercise.

REFERENCES

1. Bunt, J. C.: Hormonal alterations due to exercise. *Sports Medicine.* 3(5):331–345 (1986).
2. Bursztein, S., D. H. Elwyn, J. Askanazi, & J. M. Kinney: *Energy Metabolism, Indirect Calorimetry and Nutrition.* Baltimore: Williams & Wilkins (1989).
3. Consolazio, C. F., R. E. Johnson, & L. J. Pecora: *Physiological Measurements of Metabolic Functions in Man.* New York: McGraw-Hill (1963).
4. Felig, P., & J. Wahren: Fuel homeostasis in exercise. *New England Journal of Medicine.* 293(4):1078–1084 (1975).
5. Frisell, W. R.: *Human Biochemistry.* New York: Macmillan (1982).
6. Galbo, H.: *Hormonal and Metabolic Adaptation to Exercise.* New York: Thieme-Stratton (1983).

7. Guyton, A. C.: *Textbook of Medical Physiology* (7th edition). Philadelphia: Saunders (1986).

8. Kapit, W., R. I. Macey, & E. Meisami: *The Physiology Coloring Book.* New York: Harper & Row (1987).

9. Lehninger, A. L.: *Bioenergetics* (2nd edition). Menlo Park, CA: Benjamin (1971).

10. Lemon, P. W. R., & F. J. Nagel: Effects of exercise on protein and amino acid metabolism. *Medicine and Science in Sports and Exercise.* 13(3):141–149 (1981).

11. Malina, R. M., & C. Bouchard: *Growth, Maturation and Physical Activity.* Champaign, IL: Human Kinetics Publishers (1991).

12. Marieb, E. N.: *Human Anatomy and Physiology.* Redwood City, CA: Benjamin/Cummings (1989).

13. Newsholme, E. A., & A. R. Leech: *Biochemistry for the Medical Sciences.* New York: John Wiley (1983).

14. Pernow, B., & B. Saltin (eds.): *Muscle Metabolism During Exercise.* New York: Plenum (1971).

15. Péronnet, F. G. Thibault, M. Ledoux, & G. Brisson: *Performance in Endurance Events: Energy Balance, Nutrition, and Temperature Regulation in Distance Running.* London, Ontario, Canada: Spodym (1987).

16. Saltin, B.: Metabolic fundamental in exercise. *Medicine and Science in Sports.* 5(3):137–146 (1973).

17. Van de Graaff, K. M., & S. I. Fox: *Concepts of Human Anatomy and Physiology* (2nd edition). Dubuque, IA: Brown (1989).

10

Anaerobic Metabolism During Exercise

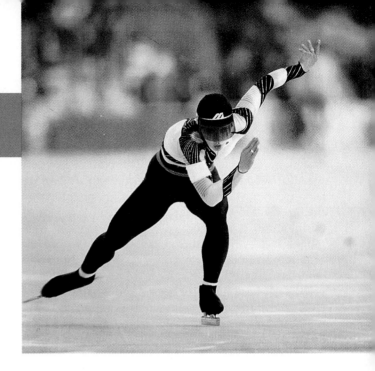

After studying the chapter, you should be able to:

- Describe the energy continuum as it relates to varying durations of maximal maintainable exercise.

- Provide examples of sports or events within sports in which the ATP-PC, lactic, or oxygen system predominates.

- List the major variables that are typically measured to describe the anaerobic response to exercise and, where appropriate, the actual exercise test itself.

- Explain the physiological reasons why lactate may accumulate in the blood.

- Distinguish between the power and the capacity of the ATP-PC, lactic, and oxygen systems.

- Identify the oxygen deficit and excess postexercise oxygen consumption, and explain the causes of each.

- Describe the changes in ATP and PC that occur during constant-load, heavy exercise lasting 3 min or less.

- Describe the changes in lactate accumulation that occur during constant-load, heavy exercise lasting 3 min or less and during incremental exercise to maximum.

- Differentiate between the terms *anaerobic threshold*, *ventilatory threshold*, and *lactate threshold*; and explain why *anaerobic threshold* is a misnomer.

- Discuss why the accumulation of lactate is a physiological problem.

- Explain the fate of lactate during exercise and recovery.

- Compare anaerobic metabolism during exercise for males versus females; children and adolescents versus young and middle-aged adults; and the elderly versus young and middle-aged adults.

- Identify the impact of genetics on anaerobic characteristics.

The Energy Continuum

The previous chapter explained how ATP, the ultimate energy source for all human work, is produced by cellular respiration. The emphasis there was on the energy substrate (carbohydrate, fat, or protein) that was utilized as a fuel. This chapter and the next will look at ATP production and utilization on the basis of the need for oxygen. Anaerobic metabolism does not require oxygen to produce ATP, but aerobic metabolism does. Critical to understanding anaerobic and aerobic exercise metabolism is the fact that these processes are not mutually exclusive. That is, anaerobic metabolism and aerobic metabolism are not either/or situations in terms of how ATP is provided. Both systems can and usually do work concurrently. When describing whether muscular exercise is aerobic or anaerobic, the concern is with which system predominates.

Figure 10.1 reviews the three sources of ATP introduced in Chapter 9. Figure 10.1a describes *alactic anaerobic metabolism*, sometimes called the *phosphagen* or *ATP-PC system*. Once ATP has been created, it is stored in the muscle. This amount is relatively small and can provide energy for only 1–2 sec of maximal effort. However, another high-energy compound, phosphocreatine (PC), also known as creatine phosphate (CP), can be used to resynthesize ATP from ADP instantaneously. The amount of PC in muscle is about three times that of ATP.[34] Any time the energy demand is increased—whether the activity is simply turning a page of this book, coming out of the blocks for a sprint, or starting out on a long bicycle ride—at least part of the immediate need for energy is supplied by these stored forms, which must ultimately be replenished. These sources are also used preferentially in high-intensity, very short duration activity. Together, the ATP-PC supply can support slightly less than 10 sec of maximal activity. This ATP-PC system neither uses oxygen nor produces lactic acid and is thus said to be alactic anaerobic.

Figure 10.1b represents *anaerobic glycolysis*, also called the *lactic acid (LA) system*. When the demands for ATP exceed the capacity of the phosphagen system and the aerobic system (either at the initiation of any activity or during high-intensity, short-duration exercise), anaerobic glycolysis is utilized. This is rather like calling in the reserves, for glycolysis can provide the supplemental energy quickly. This

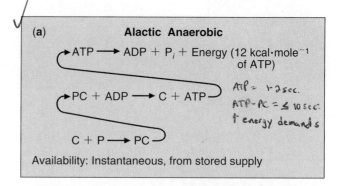

(a)   **Alactic Anaerobic**

ATP ⟶ ADP + P_i + Energy (12 kcal·mole^{-1} of ATP)

PC + ADP ⟶ C + ATP

C + P ⟶ PC

ATP = 1-2 sec.
ATP-PC = ≤ 10 sec.
↑ energy demands

Availability: Instantaneous, from stored supply

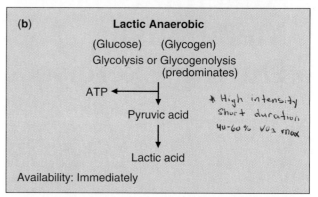

(b)   **Lactic Anaerobic**

(Glucose)   (Glycogen)
Glycolysis or Glycogenolysis
(predominates)

ATP ⟵

Pyruvic acid

Lactic acid

✻ High intensity
Short duration
40-60 % VO₂ max

Availability: Immediately

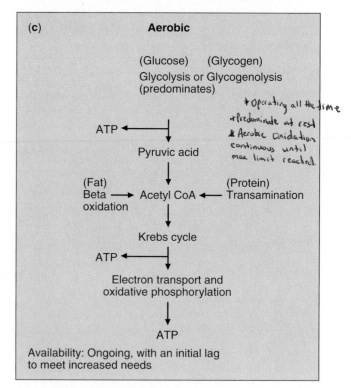

(c)   **Aerobic**

(Glucose)   (Glycogen)
Glycolysis or Glycogenolysis
(predominates)

ATP ⟵

Pyruvic acid

(Fat)   (Protein)
Beta ⟶ Acetyl CoA ⟵ Transamination
oxidation

Krebs cycle

ATP ⟵

Electron transport and
oxidative phosphorylation

ATP

✻ Operating all the time
✻ Predominate at rest
✻ Aerobic oxidation continuous until max limit reached.

Availability: Ongoing, with an initial lag to meet increased needs

FIGURE 10.1

Anaerobic and Aerobic Sources of ATP

system makes things like a 1500-m speed skating event possible. That is the benefit. The cost is that the production of lactic acid often exceeds clearance, and lactate accumulates. Since this system does not involve the utilization of oxygen but does result in the production of lactic acid, it is said to be lactic anaerobic.

Figure 10.1c shows *aerobic oxidation,* also termed the O_2 *system.* The generation of ATP from aerobic glycolysis, the Krebs cycle, and electron transport–oxidative phosphorylation is constantly in operation at some level. Under resting conditions this system provides basically all of the energy needed. When activity begins or occurs at moderate levels of intensity, oxidation increases quickly and proceeds at a rate that supplies the needed ATP. If the workload is continuously incremented, aerobic oxidation proceeds at a correspondingly higher rate until its maximal limit is reached. The highest amount of oxygen the body can consume during heavy dynamic exercise for the aerobic production of ATP is called *maximal oxygen uptake,* or $\dot{V}O_2$max. Because $\dot{V}O_2$max is primarily an index of cardiorespiratory capacity, it is discussed in depth in that unit. However, because $\dot{V}O_2$max reflects the amount of oxygen available for the aerobic production of ATP, it is also an important metabolic measure. Both aerobic and anaerobic exercises are often described in terms of a given percentage of $\dot{V}O_2$max (either less than or greater than 100% $\dot{V}O_2$max). Anaerobic metabolic processes are important at the onset of all aerobic exercise, contribute significantly at submaximal levels, and increase their contribution as the exercise intensity gets progressively higher. Depending on an individual's fitness level, lactic anaerobic metabolism begins to make a significant contribution to dynamic activity at approximately 40–60% $\dot{V}O_2$max. However, even then the ability to process oxygen is most important. Since the aerobic system does involve the use of oxygen and proceeds completely to oxidative phosphorylation, it is said to be aerobic or oxidative (O_2).

These three sources of ATP—the phosphagen system (ATP-PC), the glycolytic system (LA), and the oxidative system (O_2)—are recruited in a specific sequence called the *time-energy system continuum.* This continuum assumes that the individual is working at a maximal maintainable intensity for a continuous duration. This means that it is assumed that an individual can go all out for 5 min or less or

can work at 100% $\dot{V}O_2$max for 10 min, at 95% $\dot{V}O_2$max for 30 min, at 85% $\dot{V}O_2$max for 60 min, and at 80% $\dot{V}O_2$max for 120 min. Of course, there are individual differences, but these assumptions are reasonable in general.

Figure 10.2 indicates the relative contributions of each of the energy systems to the total energy requirement under these conditions. These values are estimates that sometimes overlap but that do provide general trends as well as some specific values.[5, 33] For example, during an all-out event that lasts 30 sec the dominant metabolism is anaerobic (80%), with approximately 33% being provided by the ATP-PC system and 47% by the LA system. Which system predominates during an event which takes 5 min and what are the percentages? If you take time to analyze the graph, you should discover that the breakdown at 5 min is a mirror image of what occurs at 30 sec. Now 80% of the energy is provided by aerobic oxidative metabolism and only 20% by anaerobic metabolism, split 3% ATP-PC and 17% LA.

Four basic patterns can be discerned from this continuum. These patterns will be helpful later for determination of training programs.

1. All three energy systems (ATP-PC, LA, O_2) are involved in providing energy for all durations of exercise.

2. The ATP-PC system predominates in activities lasting 10 sec or less and still contributes at least 8% of the energy supply for maximal activities up to 2 min in length. Since the ATP-PC system is involved primarily at the onset of longer activities, it becomes a smaller portion of the total energy supply as the duration gets longer.

3. Anaerobic metabolism (ATP-PC + LA) predominates in supplying energy for exercises lasting less than 2 min. However, even exercises lasting as long as 10 min utilize at least 15% anaerobic sources. Within the anaerobic component the longer the duration, the greater the relative importance of the lactic acid system is in comparison to the phosphagen system.

4. By 5 min of exercise the O_2 system is clearly the dominant system. The longer the duration, the more important it becomes.

The rest of this chapter will concentrate on the anaerobic contribution to energy metabolism.

FIGURE 10.2

Time-Energy System Continuum

Approximate relative contributions of aerobic and anaerobic energy production at maximal maintainable intensity for varying durations.

Source: Åstrand & Rodahl,[5] Gollnick & Hermansen.[33]

Note: The graphs assume 100% $\dot{V}O_2$max at 10 min; 95% $\dot{V}O_2$max at 30 min; 85% $\dot{V}O_2$max at 60 min; and 80% $\dot{V}O_2$ max at 120 min. ATP-PC $\leq$ 10 s.

Chapter 11 will concentrate on the aerobic contribution to energy metabolism, although again it must be emphasized that the two systems work together, with one or the other predominating based primarily on the duration of the activity.

*M*easurement of Anaerobic Metabolism

Laboratory Procedures

Unfortunately, there is no generally accepted means by which to directly measure the anaerobic energy contribution to exercise. There are, however, two general approaches to describing the anaerobic exercise response. One approach describes changes in the chemical substances either used in alactic anaerobic metabolism (specifically, ATP and PC levels) or produced as a result of lactic anaerobic metabolism (lactic acid or lactate). The second approach quantifies the amount of work performed or the power generated during short-duration, high-intensity activity. The assumption is that such activity could not be done without anaerobic energy; therefore, mea-

suring such work or power indirectly measures anaerobic energy utilization.

ATP-PC and Lactate   The measurement of ATP, PC, and lactate can be done by chemical analysis of muscle biopsy specimens. Lactate is the most frequently measured variable, in part because it can also be measured from blood samples. The blood sample may be obtained either by venipuncture or finger prick, both of which are less invasive than a muscle biopsy. Another reason for the popularity of lactate analysis is the user-friendly, fast, accurate, and relatively inexpensive analyzers that are available. Figure 10.3 shows an analyzer that requires a minimal blood sample (a 25-μL capillary tube obtained by a finger prick), is portable, and takes less than 5 min for each sample analysis.

Lactic acid is produced in muscle cells when the NADH + H$^+$ formed in glycolysis (step 6) is oxidized to NAD$^+$ by a transfer of the hydrogen atom to pyruvic acid, which forms lactic acid.[19, 62] In muscle tissue lactic acid is produced in amounts that are in equilibrium with pyruvic acid under normal resting conditions. In addition, lactic acid is always produced by red blood cells, portions of the kidneys,

(a)

(b)

FIGURE 10.3

Lactate Analysis

A small sample of blood is obtained by a finger prick (a) and injected into a lactate
analyzer (b) for determination of lactate concentration [La].

and certain tissues within the eye. At normal pH
levels lactic acid will almost completely dissociate
into hydrogen ions (H) and lactate ($C_3H_5O_3^-$, designated as La$^-$). Thus, technically, lactic acid is
formed, but lactate is what is measured in the
bloodstream. Despite this distinction, the terms *lactic acid* and *lactate* are often used synonymously.[19]

Both resting and exercise values depend upon
the balance between lactic acid production and removal or clearance. This balance of production and
removal is called *turnover*. When production exceeds removal, lactate is said to accumulate. High-
intensity–short-duration or near-maximal exercise
is the most common cause of lactate accumulation.
Under these circumstances glycolysis proceeds at a
rate that produces larger quantities of NADH   H
than the mitochondria has oxygen to accept. In this
case "something" still has be done with the hydrogen atoms so that the NAD can be regenerated.
What happens is that the NADH   H is oxidized
to NAD by a transfer of the hydrogen atoms to
pyruvic acid, which forms lactic acid. Lactic acid
then dissociates into hydrogen ions and lactate.

Lactate is a small molecule that moves easily
from the muscles to the blood and most other fluid
compartments. However, it takes time to reach an
equilibrium between muscle and blood, especially if
large amounts are being created, as can happen during high-intensity exercise. This equilibrium and the

achievement of peak blood values may take as long
as 5–10 min. Until equilibrium occurs, muscle lactate values will be higher than blood lactate values.
This also means that the highest blood lactate values
are typically seen after several minutes of recovery,
not during high-intensity work.[33]

Lactate levels are reported using a variety of
units. The two most common are millimoles per liter
(mmol L^{-1} sometimes designated as mM) or milligrams per 100 milliliters of blood (mg 100 mL^{-1} sometimes designated as mg% or mg dL^{-1}). One mmol L^{-1}
is equal to 9 mg 100 mL^{-1}. Resting levels of lactate of
1–2 mmol L^{-1} or 9–18 mg 100 mL^{-1} are typical. A
value of 8 mmol L^{-1} or 72 mg 100 mL^{-1} is usually
taken to indicate that an individual has worked
maximally.[5] Peak values as high as 32 mmol L^{-1} or
288 mg 100 mL^{-1} have been reported.

Lactic acid is a by-product of anaerobic metabolism. However, anaerobiosis (lack of oxygen) is not
the only situation in which lactic acid is produced.
The following four circumstances also lead to lactic
acid production and possible accumulation.

1. The enzyme that catalyzes the conversion of
pyruvic acid to lactic acid (lactate dehydrogenase) is
much more active than the enzymes that provide
alternate pathways for pyruvate metabolism, including the rate-limiting enzymes in the Krebs
cycle (one of which is isocitrate dehydrogenase).

Therefore, lactic acid production is an inevitable consequence of glycolysis.[20, 30]

2. During heavy exercise, activity of the sympathetic nervous system stimulates the release of epinephrine and glucagon (see Figure 9.19). Both of these hormones bring about the breakdown of glycogen, leading ultimately to high levels of glucose-6-phosphate (G6P). (Refresh your memory by referring to Figure 9.5, if necessary, to locate G6P in glycolysis.) High levels of G6P increase the rate of glycolysis and, hence, the production of pyruvic acid. As noted previously, high levels of pyruvic acid lead to the production of lactate.[20]

3. During exercise, muscle contraction stimulates glycogenolysis in order to use glycogen as a fuel in glycolysis. Therefore, increased lactic acid production occurs whether or not oxygen levels are sufficient.[28]

4. During high-intensity, short-duration activities muscle fibers, which are predominantly glycolytic, are preferentially recruited. These fast-contracting glycolytic fibers produce lactic acid when they contract whether or not oxygen is present in sufficient amounts. This response appears to be a function of the specific lactic dehydrogenase enzyme found in these fibers.[35] Thus, although lactic acid is associated with high-intensity, short-duration work, it does not absolutely indicate a lack of oxygen. It does reflect the use of the anaerobic glycolytic pathway and the balance between glycolytic and mitochondrial activity.

Tests of Anaerobic Power and Capacity

Energy system capacity is defined as the total amount of energy that can be produced by an energy system. **Energy system power** is defined as the maximal amount of energy that can be produced per unit of time. Table 10.1 clearly shows that the phosphagen (ATP-PC) system is predominantly a power system with very little capacity. The lactic anaerobic glycolytic system has almost equal power and capacity, just slightly favoring capacity. The information on the aerobic (O_2) system is included here just to show how truly high in power and low in capacity the anaerobic systems are.

Although the ATP-PC system can put out energy at the rate of 72 kcal · min^{-1}, it can only sustain that value by working maximally for 9–10 sec, for a total output of only 11 kcal (72 kcal · min^{-1} ÷ 60 sec · min^{-1} = 1.2 kcal · sec; 11 total kcal ÷ 1.2 kcal · sec = 9.17 sec). The LA system has a lower power (36 kcal · min^{-1}) but can sustain it for almost 1 min and 20 sec (48 kcal ÷ 36 kcal · min^{-1} = 1.33 min = 1:19.8). By comparison, if the O_2 system worked at a power output of 9 kcal · min^{-1}, exercise could be sustained for more than 2 hr (1268 kcal ÷ 9 kcal · min^{-1} = 141 min = 2:21) just using carbohydrate fuel sources. In fact, when all fuel supplies are included, the capacity of the aerobic system is, for all intents and purposes, unlimited.

When measuring the anaerobic systems, one would ideally have a test that could distinctly evaluate alactic anaerobic power, alactic anaerobic capacity, lactic anaerobic power, and lactic anaerobic capacity. Because no such tests exist, attempts have been made to get this information indirectly by measuring (1) the total mechanical power generated during high-intensity, short-duration work; (2) the amount of mechanical work done in a specific

TABLE 10.1 ■ Estimated Maximal Power and Capacity in Untrained Males

ENERGY SYSTEM	Power		Capacity	
	Kcal · min^{-1}	kJ · min^{-1}	Kcal	kJ
ATP-PC (phosphagen)	72	300	11	45
LA (anaerobic glycolysis)	36	150	48	200
O_2 (aerobic glycolysis + Krebs cycle + ETS-OP; fuel = CHO)	7.2–19.1	30–80	359–1268	1500–5300

Sources: Bouchard, Taylor, & Dulac;[16] Bouchard et al.[17]

period of time; or (3) the time required to perform a given amount of presumably anaerobic work.[36] Two such tests are commonly used in laboratory settings, the Wingate Anaerobic Test (WAT) and the Maragaria-Kalamen Stair Climb.[17]

The Wingate Anaerobic Test.   The Wingate Anaerobic Test depicted in Figure 10.4 is probably the most well known of several bicycle ergometer tests used to measure anaerobic power and capacity. The test is an all-out ride for 30 sec against a resistance based on body weight. Resistance values of 0.075 kg · kg⁻¹ body weight for children, 0.086 kg · kg⁻¹ body weight for adult females, and 0.095 kg · kg⁻¹ body weight for adult males appear to be optimal. Athletes may need values as high as 0.10 kg · kg⁻¹ of body weight, but the most common value used (as in the example that follows) is 0.075 kg · kg⁻¹ body weight.[78] The revolutions (rev) of the flywheel are counted per second during the test, and from the available information three variables are determined.

Computer-generated results from a typical test are given in Table 10.2. The subject was a 129-lb

FIGURE 10.4

Wingate Anaerobic Test

This subject is ready to perform the Wingate Anaerobic Test. Once he is pedaling as fast as he can, the tester will release the weight held in her hand, providing a resistance based upon the subject's body weight. The subject will then continue to pedal as quickly as possible for 30 seconds. Data from sensors attached to the flywheel are relayed to the computer for calculation of peak power, mean power, and fatigue index.

female physical education major, but not an athlete. Note that these results are for a leg test; an arm version is also available. Calculations for the resistance she used (4.4 kg) are shown on Table 10.2. The data contained in the table will be used to calculate three variables: peak power, mean power, and fatigue index. **Peak power** (PP) is defined as the maximal power (force times distance divided by time) exerted during very short (5 sec or less) duration work. **Mean power** (MP) is defined as the average power (force times distance divided by time) exerted during short (typically 30 sec) duration work. The **fatigue index** (FI) is the percentage of peak power drop-off during high-intensity, short-duration work. Each of these variables requires the use of different time periods in the calculations.

The first variable computed is *peak power* (PP), the maximum power exerted during the highest 5 sec period. This usually occurs early in the activity and, in the example given, is the time between 2 and 6 sec where 10.25 rev were completed. Peak power can be expressed in absolute terms as kgm · 5 sec⁻¹ or prorated to a full minute as kgm · min⁻¹ or watts (W). Peak power can also be expressed relative to body weight as kgm · 5 sec⁻¹ · kg⁻¹, kgm · min⁻¹ · kg⁻¹, or W · kg⁻¹. The formula for peak power is

(10.1)   peak power (kgm · 5 sec⁻¹) = maximal revolutions in 5 sec × distance that the flywheel travels per revolution (m) × force setting (kg)

or   PP = rev(max) in 5 sec × D · rev⁻¹ × F

Energy System Capacity The total amount of energy that can be produced by an energy system.

Energy System Power The maximal amount of energy that can be produced per unit of time.

Peak Power (PP) The maximum power (force times distance divided by time) exerted during very short (5 sec or less) duration work.

Mean Power (MP) The average power (force times distance divided by time) exerted during short- (typically 30 sec) duration work.

Fatigue Index (FI) Percentage of peak power drop-off during high-intensity, short-duration work.

TABLE 10.2 ■ Results for the Wingate Leg Test

Weight is 129 lb = 58.50 kg; resistance for legs is 58.50 kg × 0.075 kg · kg^{-1} body weight = 4.4 kg.

SECONDS	REVOLUTIONS PER SECOND	INCLUSIVE TIME (SEC)	5-SEC TOTAL REVOLUTIONS	kgm · min^{-1}· kg^{-1}	W · kg^{-1}
1	8				
2	9				
3	8				
4	8				
5	7	1–5	10.00	54.15	8.85
6	9	2–6	10.25	55.50	9.07
7	7	3–7	9.75	52.80	8.63
8	7	4–8	9.50	51.44	8.41
9	7	5–9	9.25	50.09	8.18
10	6	6–10	9.00	48.74	7.96
11	6	7–11	8.25	44.67	7.30
12	6	8–12	8.00	43.32	7.08
13	6	9–13	7.75	41.97	6.86
14	6	10–14	7.50	40.61	6.64
15	6	11–15	7.50	40.61	6.64
16	6	12–16	7.50	40.61	6.64
17	5	13–17	7.25	39.26	6.41
18	6	14–18	7.25	39.26	6.41
19	5	15–19	7.00	37.91	6.19
20	6	16–20	7.00	37.91	6.19
21	5	17–21	6.75	36.55	5.97
22	5	18–22	6.75	36.55	5.97
23	5	19–23	6.50	35.20	5.75
24	5	20–24	6.50	35.20	5.75
25	5	21–25	6.25	33.84	5.53
26	5	22–26	6.25	33.84	5.53
27	4	23–27	6.00	32.49	5.31
28	5	24–28	6.00	32.49	5.31
29	4	25–29	5.75	31.14	5.09
30	4	26–30	5.50	29.78	4.87

Total pedal revolutions = 45.25.
Highest 5-sec absolute peak power = 3247.20 kgm · min^{-1}.
Highest 5-sec relative peak power = 55.50 kgm · min^{-1}· kg^{-1}
= 9.07 W · kg^{-1}

Mean absolute power = 2389.20 kgm · min^{-1}.
Mean relative power = 40.84 kgm · min^{-1}· kg^{-1} = 6.67 W · kg^{-1}
Fatigue index = 100 – (lowest 5 sec divided by highest 5 sec) × 100 = 46.34%.

■ EXAMPLE

Thus for this example the calculation is

$$PP = 10.25 \text{ rev} \times 6 \text{ m} \cdot \text{rev}^{-1} \times 4.4 \text{ kg}$$
$$= 270.6 \text{ kgm} \cdot 5 \text{ sec}^{-1}$$

Prorated to a full minute, PP is

$$PP = 270.6 \text{ kgm} \cdot 5 \text{ sec}^{-1} \times 12 \quad (60 \text{ sec} \cdot \text{min}^{-1} \div 5 \text{ sec} = 12)$$
$$= 3247.2 \text{ kgm} \cdot \text{min}^{-1}$$

Relative to body weight PP is

$$PP = 3247.2 \text{ kgm} \cdot \text{min}^{-1} \div 58.5 \text{ kg}$$
$$= 55.50 \text{ kgm} \cdot \text{min}^{-1} \cdot \text{kg}^{-1}$$

When converted to watts ($1 \text{ W} = 6.12 \text{ kgm} \cdot \text{min}^{-1}$), the relative value is

$$PP = 55.5 \text{ kgm} \cdot \text{min}^{-1} \div 6.12 \text{ kgm} \cdot \text{min}^{-1} \cdot \text{W}^{-1}$$
$$= 9.07 \text{ W} \cdot \text{kg}^{-1} \quad \blacksquare$$

Originally, peak power was thought to reflect only alactic processes—alactic anaerobic capacity, in particular. However, subsequent research has shown that muscle lactate levels rise to high values as early as 10 sec into such high-intensity work. This result indicates that glycolytic processes are occurring almost immediately along with ATP-CP breakdown. Therefore, peak power cannot be interpreted as being only alactic.[10]

The second variable calculated is *mean power,* and it can also be expressed in both absolute and relative units. Mean power (MP) is the average power sustained throughout the 30-second ride. The formula for mean power is

(10.2) mean power (kgm · 30 sec^{-1} = total number of revolutions in 30 sec × distance that the flywheel travels per revolution (m) × force setting (kg)

or $MP = \text{rev(total) in 30 sec} \times D \cdot \text{rev}^{-1} \times F$

■ EXAMPLE

Thus, for this example the calculation is

$$MP = 45.25 \text{ rev} \times 6 \text{ m} \cdot \text{rev}^{-1} \times 4.4 \text{ kg}$$
$$= 1194.6 \text{ kgm} \cdot 30 \text{ sec}$$

Prorated to a full minute, MP is

$$MP = 1194.6 \text{ kgm} \times 2 \quad (60 \text{ sec} \cdot \text{min}^{-1} \div 30 \text{ sec} = 2)$$
$$= 2389.2 \text{ kgm} \cdot \text{min}^{-1}$$

Related to body weight MP is

$$MP = 2389.2 \text{ kgm} \cdot \text{min}^{-1} \div 58.5 \text{ kg} = 40.84 \text{ kgm} \cdot \text{min}^{-1} \cdot \text{kg}^{-1}$$

When converted to watts MP is

$$MP = 40.84 \text{ kgm} \cdot \text{min}^{-1} \cdot \text{kg}^{-1} \div 6.12 \text{ kgm} \cdot \text{min}^{-1} \cdot \text{W}^{-1}$$
$$= 6.67 \text{ W} \cdot \text{kg}^{-1} \quad \blacksquare$$

Mean power is sometimes said to represent lactic anaerobic capacity, although this has not been substantiated.[10]

The third variable that can be computed is the *fatigue index* (FI), or the percentage of peak power drop-off during high-intensity, short-duration work. It is calculated using the highest 5-sec power (PP) and the lowest 5-sec power (LP). Little is known about the relationship of the fatigue index to anaerobic fitness.[10]

(10.3) fatigue index (%) = 100 − [(lowest power kgm · 5 sec^{-1}) ÷ (peak power kgm · 5 sec^{-1})] × 100

or $$FI = 100 - \left(\frac{PP}{LP}\right) \times 100$$

■ EXAMPLE

In our example the highest 5-sec power is 270.6 kgm. Using the peak power formula of Equation 10.1 but with the lowest 5-sec total, we get

$$LP = 5.50 \text{ rev} \times 6 \text{ m} \cdot \text{rev}^{-1} \times 4.4 \text{ kg}$$
$$= 145.2 \text{ kg} \cdot 5 \text{ sec}^{-1}$$
$$100 - (145.2 \text{ kg} \cdot 5 \text{ sec}^{-1} \div 270.6 \text{ kg} \cdot 5 \text{ sec}^{-1}) \times 100$$
$$= 46.34\% \quad \blacksquare$$

Although the WAT is not a purely anaerobic test (the aerobic component has been measured at between 13 and 29%), it is predominantly anaerobic. It compares well (with correlations generally above 0.75) with other tests of anaerobic power and capacity and is widely used.[10, 63]

The Margaria-Kalamen Stair Climb. To perform the Margaria-Kalamen test, an individual runs for 6 m on the level and then climbs a staircase, taking three steps at a time. Power in kgm · sec^{-1} is calculated by using, respectively, the weight of the subject, the vertical height between the third and ninth steps, and the time between the third and ninth steps.[17, 78] The use of electronic switch mats or photoelectric cells is essential for accuracy. This test is considered to be a test of alactic anaerobic power because of the short time involved—usually less than 5 sec for the entire test and close to 1 sec for the measured time between the third and ninth steps.

Field Tests. There are no field tests available to estimate the ATP-PC used or the lactate produced during exercise. However, performance in high-intensity, short-duration activity can give an indication of anaerobic power and capacity. Two types of activities are commonly used: vertical jump tests and sprints or middle-distance runs.

In vertical jump tests several different protocols are utilized, including variations in the starting posture, the use or nonuse of arms, and what body part displacement is measured. The one commonality is the end value measured: the height jumped. When the jump is performed on a force platform, actual power values can be calculated, and the test is considered to be a laboratory test. When the jump is performed as a field test on a normal surface, work (force times distance), not power, is estimated. The height of the vertical jump and peak power as determined from force plate data have been shown to be highly correlated ($r = 0.92$). For these reasons, vertical jump height is seen as an acceptable indicator of anaerobic alactic power.[78]

For sprints and middle-distance runs, the involvement of the various energy systems is related to the time of the all-out activity, as shown in Figure 10.2. Therefore, runs whose distance can be covered in a distinct time range (depending somewhat on age, sex, and training status) can be utilized as field tests of anaerobic metabolism.[21] For example, dashes of 40, 50, or 60 yd or m will take approximately 4–15 sec and can be used as an indication of alactic anaerobic power and/or capacity. Longer runs, probably between 200 and 800 m (or 220 and 880 yd) and lasting 40–120 sec, can be used as an indication of lactic anaerobic power and capacity. Faster speeds in covering a given distance would indicate increased anaerobic power and/or capacity.

The Anaerobic Exercise Response

Oxygen Deficit and Excess Postexercise Oxygen Consumption

When exercise begins, no matter how light or heavy it is, there is an immediate need for additional energy. Thus, the most obvious exercise response is an increase in metabolism. All three energy systems will be involved in this response, with their relative contributions being proportional to the intensity and duration of the activity.

FIGURE 10.5

Oxygen Deficit and Excess Postexercise Oxygen Consumption (EPOC) during Submaximal Exercise (a) and Supramaximal Exercise (b)

(a) During light to moderate submaximal exercise, both the oxygen deficit, indicated by the convex curve at the start of exercise, and the excess postexercise oxygen consumption, indicated by the concave curve during the recovery time period, are small. (b) During heavy or supramaximal exercise both the O_2 deficit and the EPOC are large. Under both conditions energy is supplied during the O_2 deficit period by using stored ATP-PC, anaerobic glycolysis, and oxygen stores in capillary blood and on myoglobin. The heavier the exercise the more the reliance on anaerobic glycolysis. The EPOC is a result of the restoration of ATP-PC, removal of lactate, restoration of O_2 stores, elevated cardiovascular and respiratory function, elevated hormonal levels, and especially, the elevated body temperature.

Figure 10.5 shows two scenarios for going from rest to different intensities of exercise. In Figure 10.5a the activity is a moderate submaximal bout. The oxygen requirement for this particular exercise is 1.4 L · min⁻¹. The individual has a V̇O₂max of

2.5 L · min^{-1}. Therefore, this individual is working at 56% $\dot{V}O_2$max. The area under the smoothed curve during both exercise and recovery represents oxygen used. Notice, however, that there is an initial lag during which the oxygen supplied and utilized is below the oxygen requirement for providing energy. This difference between the oxygen required during exercise and the oxygen supplied and utilized is called the **oxygen deficit.** Because of this supply and demand discrepancy anaerobic sources must be involved in providing energy at the onset of all activity.

The O_2 deficit has traditionally been explained as the inability of the circulatory and respiratory systems to respond quickly enough to the increased energy demands. Evidence, however, now indicates that the O_2 deficit is probably due to limited cellular utilization of O_2 as a result of metabolic adjustments.[70] That is, the increasing levels of ADP, P_i, and NADH + H$^+$, brought about by the suddenly elevated energy demands, stimulate both aerobic and anaerobic energy processes, not just one or the other. Thus, it is not that the aerobic system cannot supply all of the needed energy but that the regulatory system does not allow it to. Therefore, during the transition from rest to work, energy is supplied by:

1. O_2 transport and utilization.
2. Utilization of O_2 stores in capillary blood and on myoglobin.
3. The splitting of stored ATP-PC.
4. Anaerobic glycolysis, with the concomitant production of lactic acid.[71]

Eventually, if the exercise intensity is low enough (as in the example in Figure 10.5a), the aerobic system will predominate and the oxygen supply will equal the oxygen demand. This condition is called steady-state, steady-rate, or steady-level exercise.

Figure 10.5b shows a smoothed plot of O_2 consumption at rest and during and after an exercise bout in which the O_2 requirement is greater than $\dot{V}O_2$max, sometimes called supramaximal exercise. The initial period of lag between O_2 supply and demand is once again evident and, as in the first example, the added energy is provided by stored ATP-PC, anaerobic glycolysis, and stored O_2. However, in this case, when the O_2 consumption

plateaus or levels off, it is at $\dot{V}O_2$max, and more energy is still needed if exercise is to continue.

This plateau is not considered to be a steady state because the energy demands are not being totally met aerobically. The supplemental energy is provided by anaerobic glycolysis. Exactly what the energy demand is in this situation is difficult to determine precisely, since, as stated before, lactic acid levels do not reflect production alone. However, without the anaerobic energy contribution this activity could not continue. The maximal ability to tolerate lactic acid accumulation will determine to a large extent how long the activity can continue.

The recovery from exercise exemplified by the concave curves following the cessation of exercise in both Figures 10.5a and 10.5b shows that oxygen consumption drops quickly (a fast component lasting 2–3 min) and then tapers off (a slow component lasting 3–60 min). The magnitude and duration of this elevated oxygen consumption will depend primarily on the intensity of the preceding exercise. In the case of light submaximal work (Figure 10.5a) recovery takes place quickly; after heavy exercise (Figure 10.5b) recovery takes much longer.

Historically, this period of elevated metabolism after exercise has been called the O_2 debt, the assumption being that the "extra" O_2 consumed during the "debt" period was being utilized to "pay back" the deficit incurred in the early part of exercise.[6, 77] More recently, the terms O_2 recovery or **excess postexercise oxygen consumption (EPOC)** have come into favor. EPOC is defined as the oxygen consumption during recovery that is above normal resting values.

A critical question is what causes this elevated metabolism in recovery. Although there is, at this time, no complete explanation of EPOC, six factors have been suggested.

1. *Restoration of ATP-PC stores:* About 10% of the EPOC is utilized to rephosphorylate creatine

---

Oxygen Deficit The difference between the oxygen required during exercise and the oxygen supplied and utilized. Occurs at the onset of all activity.

Excess Postexercise Oxygen Consumption (EPOC) Oxygen consumption during recovery that is above normal resting values.

and ADP to PC and ATP, respectively, thus restoring these substances to resting levels.[6,30] Approximately 50% of the ATP-PC is restored in 30 sec.[59] This time is called the *half-life* of ATP-PC. Full recovery requires slightly over 2 min.[28] Figure 10.6 shows the breakdown of ATP and PC during heavy exercise. It also shows the restoration of ATP from energy substrate sources and then PC restoration from the regenerated ATP until both the PC and ATP resting levels are regained.

2. Restoration of O_2 stores: Although the amount of O_2 stored in the blood (bound to hemoglobin) and muscle (bound to myoglobin) is not large, it does need to be replenished at the cessation of exercise. Replenishment probably occurs completely within 2–3 min.[6,77]

3. Elevated cardiovascular-respiratory function: Both the respiratory system and the cardiovascular system remain elevated postexercise. That

FIGURE 10.6

Use and Regeneration of ATP-PC

ATP → ADP + P_i + energy for muscle contraction (large inner circle). During heavy exercise the ADP is regenerated to ATP by the breakdown of CP (CP + ADP → C + ATP) (small inner circle). Only in recovery will the nearly depleted CP stores be restored from the breakdown of ATP resulting from aerobic metabolic production (large outside oval).

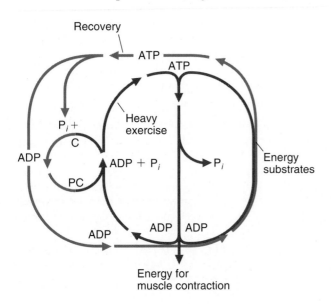

is, neither the breathing rate and depth nor heart rate recover instantaneously. Although this circumstance enables the extra amounts of oxygen to be processed, the actual energy cost of these cardiovascular-respiratory processes probably accounts for only 1–2% of the excess oxygen.[6,77]

4. Elevated hormonal levels: During exercise the circulating levels of the catecholamines (epinephrine and norepinephrine), thyroxine, and cortisol are all increased (Figure 9.16 and Table 9.3). In addition to their fuel mobilization and utilization effects, these hormones increase Na^+–K^+ pump activity in muscles and nerves by changing cell membrane permeability to Na^+ and K^+. As an active transport process, the Na^+–K^+ pump requires ATP. The increased need for ATP means an increased need for O_2. Until the hormones are cleared from the bloodstream, the additional O_2 and ATP use is a significant contributor to the EPOC.[6,30]

5. Elevated body temperature: When ATP is broken down to supply the energy for chemical, electrical, or mechanical work, heat is produced as a by-product. During exercise, heat production may exceed heat dissipation, causing a rise in body core temperature. For each degree Celsius that body temperature rises, the metabolic rate increases approximately 13–15%.[50] Thus, in recovery, although the need for high levels of energy to support the exercise has ceased, the influence of the elevated temperature has not, since cooling takes some time to occur. This temperature effect is by far the most important reason for EPOC, accounting for as much as 60–70% of the slow component after exercise at 50–80% $\dot{V}O_2$max.[6,30]

6. Lactate removal: The lactate that has accumulated must be removed. Historically, it was thought that the majority of this lactate was converted to glycogen and that this conversion was the primary cause of the slow component of EPOC. The fate of lactic acid is now seen as more complex and its contribution as a causative factor for EPOC as minimal.[30,77] This idea will be discussed in more detail later in this chapter.

ATP-PC Changes

Figure 10.7 indicates what happens to ATP and PC levels in both muscle and blood during constant-

FIGURE 10.7

Time Course for the Depletion of CP and ATP and the Accumulation of Lactate in Muscle and Veins Muscle levels of ATP are maintained relatively constant during high-intensity, short-duration exercise at the expense of CP. Muscle lactate levels rise sooner and higher than venous levels owing to the diffusion time lag and dilution.

(105 - 110 % VO2 Max ≤ 3')

Source: Modified from P. D. Gollnick & L. Hermansen. Biochemical adaptation to exercise: Anaerobic metabolism. In J. H. Wilmore (ed.), *Exercise and Sport Sciences Reviews.* New York: Academic Press (1973). Reprinted by permission of Williams & Wilkins.

• 60-70% of resting ATP still Present(at the expense of PC)(Help from glycolysis, ↑LA)
• La⁻ depend on intensity
• Lag for diffusion time (Venous Lactate)
• > 90% of VO2 max - typical La⁻ response

load, heavy exercise (105–110% V̇O₂max) lasting 3 min or less. As shown in the figure, the ATP level in the muscle decreases only slightly. In fact, the maximum ATP depletion observed in skeletal muscle after heavy exercise is only about 30–40% in both males and females. Thus, even after exhaustive work 60–70% of the resting amount of ATP is still present.[21, 34]

Conversely, the level of PC changes dramatically such that it is nearly depleted. The greatest depletion of PC occurs in the initial 20 sec of exercise, with the result that ATP is almost maintained at resting levels during that time span. From 20 to 180 sec the decline in PC and ATP is both gradual and parallel.[33] Obviously, the ATP level is maintained at the expense of the PC. However, some ATP is also being provided from glycolysis, as indicated by the rise in lactate. Compare the theoretical basis of the Wingate Anaerobic Test with these data.

Lactate Changes

Lactate levels in response to exercise primarily depend on the intensity of the exercise. Only short-duration, high-intensity exercise and incremental exercise to maximal work will be considered here.

Figure 10.7 includes both muscle and blood lactate response to high-intensity, short-duration (3 min or less), constant-load exercise. As the figure shows, muscle lactate levels rise immediately with the onset of such hard work (105–110% V̇O₂max) and continue to rise throughout the length of the task. The blood lactate values show a similar pattern, if the lag for diffusion time is taken into account.[33] This lactate response (a rapid and consistent accumulation) is representative of what occurs when the exercise bout is greater than 90% V̇O₂max.[33]

Figure 10.8 shows the lactate response to incremental exercise on a cycle ergometer. The oxygen consumption (Figure 10.8a) increases in a linear pattern to meet the increasing demands for energy, but blood lactate (Figure 10.8b) shows very little initial change and then increases continuously in a curvilinear fashion.[43,44] These particular results are below the 8 mmol · L⁻¹ generally considered to indicate a maximal test, however.

The Lactate Threshold(s)   Since the early 1970s a great deal of attention has been paid to a concept that has been labeled variously as the *anaerobic threshold*, the *ventilatory threshold(s)*, or the **lactate threshold(s).** The original concept of an anaerobic threshold is based upon the lactate response to incremental exercise, as depicted in Figure 10.9, and the relationship of the lactate response to minute ventilation (the volume of air breathed each minute).

As espoused by Wasserman and his colleagues,[83] the *anaerobic threshold* is defined as the exercise intensity, usually described as a percentage of V̇O₂max or workload, above which blood lactate levels rise and minute ventilation increases dispro-

> **Lactate Thresholds** Points on the linear-curvilinear continuum of lactate accumulation that appear to indicate sharp rises, often labeled as the first (LT1) and second (LT2) lactate threshold.

Figure 10.8

Changes in Oxygen Consumption and Blood Lactate as a Function of Work Rate

The rise in O_2 consumption is directly proportional to the increase in workload. Blood lactate levels show very little change at low work rates and then increase continuously in a curvilinear pattern.

Source: Modified from E. F. Hughes, S. C. Turner, & G. A. Brooks. Effects of glycogen depletion and pedaling speed on anaerobic threshold. *Journal of Applied Physiology.* 52(6): 1598–1607 (1982). Reprinted by permission of the American Physiological Society.

portionately in relation to oxygen consumption. The onset of anaerobic metabolism (or anaerobiosis), which is assumed to lead to the lactate accumulation, is attributed to the failure of the cardiovascular system to supply the oxygen required to the muscle tissue. The disproportionate rise in ventilation is attributed to excess carbon dioxide resulting from the buffering of the lactic acid.[48,82]

Theoretically, these interactions can occur as follows: Lactic acid is a strong acid, and as noted before in this chapter, it readily dissociates into hydrogen ions (H^+) and lactate (La^-). Because an excess of hydrogen ions would change the pH (or acid-base balance) of the muscles and blood, the body attempts to bind these hydrogen ions to a chemical buffer. For example, sodium bicarbonate (a weak base) may be used as a buffer in the reaction:

$$NaHCO_3 + HLa \leftrightarrow NaLa + H_2CO_3$$

sodium bicarbonate + lactic acid ↔ sodium lactate + carbonic acid

Carbonic acid is a much weaker acid than lactic acid and can be further dissociated into water and carbon dioxide:

$$H_2CO_3 \leftrightarrow H_2O + CO_2$$

Carbon dioxide is a potent stimulant for respiration and can easily be removed from the body through respiration, thereby assisting in the maintenance of pH.[64] The carbon dioxide thus formed is said to be nonmetabolic carbon dioxide, since it does not result from the immediate breakdown of an energy substrate (carbohydrate, fat, or protein).

Figure 10.9 clearly shows that there are distinct breaks from linearity in respiration (Figure 10.9c) despite a continuous rectilinear rise in heart rate (Figure 10.9a) and oxygen consumption (Figure 10.9b) during incremental work to maximum. These breakpoints (Figure 10.9c) have been labeled as VT1 (the first ventilatory threshold) and VT2 (the second ventilatory threshold). They were originally thought to result from corresponding lactate thresholds (labeled in Figure 10.9d as LT1 and LT2, the first lactate threshold and the second lactate threshold) as a result of the buffering of lactic acid. The original work by Wasserman and others postulated only one anaerobic threshold (which would have been VT1 in Figure 10.9c), but later work identified at least two thresholds, which were given various names.[47,66,75] The designations VT1 and VT2 and LT1 and LT2 are used here for simplicity and because no causal mechanism is implied.

The idea that the point of lactate accumulation can be determined noninvasively by respiratory values typically measured during laboratory exercise testing of oxygen consumption is appealing, since few people truly enjoy having multiple blood samples taken. However, the terminology, determi-

Incremental work expressed as workload or % $\dot{V}O_2$max

FIGURE 10.9

Ventilatory and Lactate Thresholds during Incremental Work to Maximum

Both heart rate (a) and O_2 consumption (b) increase in direct rectilinear patterns during an incremental work task whether the work is expressed in terms of absolute workload or percentage of $\dot{V}O_2$max. In contrast, both ventilation (c) and lactate (d) appear to exhibit two distinct breakpoints as they rise. The circumstance of VT1 occurring at the same time as LT1 and VT2 occurring at the same time as LT2 is coincidental.

nation, and mechanistic explanations are not without controversy.[81]

The primary concern is that the presence of lactate does not automatically mean that the oxygen supply is inadequate.[43] This fact was discussed at length earlier in this chapter. To quickly review, blood lactate levels are a result of (1) the muscle fibers recruited to do the work; (2) the rate of lactate production by working muscles; (3) the oxidation of pyruvate in the mitochondria; (4) the rate of efflux of lactate from the contracting muscles; and (5) the rate of lactate removal from the bloodstream by nonworking muscles, the kidneys, and the liver. Lactate accumulation does not occur at the time of increased production; rather, it occurs when the turnover rate (or balance between production and removal) cannot keep up.

Figure 10.10a shows this concept graphically. That is, as the exercise and oxygen consumption increases, the rate of lactate appearance (R_a) in the muscle does also (Figure 10.10b). At low-intensity exercise the rate of lactate disappearance (R_d) does not differ much from R_a. However, as the intensity increases, the gap between R_a and R_d grows progressively wider. The result is the blood lactate concentration [La⁻] depicted in Figure 10.10a. Thus, it is incorrect to label the appearance of elevated levels of lactic acid in the blood as representing an anaerobic threshold.

A second concern is exactly how to interpret the lactate response to incremental work. Look closely at the lactate patterns in Figures 10.8 and 10.9. Basically, the circles representing individual data points are the same. However, in Figure 10.9 lines are imposed on the data points that clearly indicate two breaks in the linearity, or two thresholds.[75] The same data points are described as being a continuous and exponential curve in Figure 10.8.[44] Recent experimental evidence and mathematical models[44] support the curvilinear interpretation, not the breakpoint one. Nevertheless, the term *lactate threshold* continues to be used to indicate marked increases in the accumulation of lactate.

A third concern involves carbon dioxide. Carbon dioxide is involved in the control of respiration (see Chapter 2). An excess of hydrogen ions from a source such as lactic acid can cause an increase in the amount of carbon dioxide through the bicarbonate buffering system just described. However, the presence of lactic acid is not the only mechanism

FIGURE 10.10

**The Rate of Appearance (R_a), the Rate
of Disappearance (R_d), and the Resultant
Accumulation of Lactate as a Consequence
of Incremental Exercise**

The measured change in lactate concentration [La$^-$]
(a) is a result of a growing imbalance between the
rate of appearance (R_a) and the rate of disappearance
(R_d) (b) as exercise intensity increases.

Source: G. A. Brooks. Anaerobic threshold: Review of the concept and directions for future research. *Medicine and Science in Sports and Exercise.* 17(1): 22–31 (1985). Reprinted by permission.

that can account for an increase in carbon dioxide or
the concomitant increase in minute ventilation.[46]
Evidence is particularly strong in McArdle's syndrome patients. McArdle's syndrome patients are
deficient in the enzyme phosphorylase, which is
necessary to convert glycogen to lactic acid. Thus,
no matter how hard these patients exercise, their
lactic acid values remain negligible. On the other
hand, their minute ventilation values have the same

distinctive breakpoints shown by anyone not deficient in phosphorylase.[39] Thus, something other
than the accumulation of lactic acid must be operating to explain the ventilatory response.

Fourth, the lactate thresholds and the ventilatory thresholds do not change to the same extent in
the same individuals as a result of training, glycogen depletion, and/or varying pedaling rates.[43,65] If
they were causally linked, they should change together.

Current theory, therefore, says that although
lactic acid increases and ventilatory breaks or
thresholds often occur simultaneously, these responses are due to coincidence, not cause and effect.[19,81] Exactly what these various thresholds mean
is still unknown.

Despite a lack of complete understanding of the
lactate threshold, the amount of work an athlete can
do before accumulating large amounts of lactate has
a definite bearing on performance. Distance running performance, for example, depends to a large
extent on some combination of $\dot{V}O_2$max, the oxygen
cost of running at a given submaximal speed (called
economy), and the ability to run at a high percentage of $\dot{V}O_2$max without a large accumulation of lactic acid.[23,27,52] An indication of the running speed
that represents the optimal percentage of $\dot{V}O_2$max
can be achieved by determining the lactate thresholds. The first lactate threshold (LT1) generally occurs between 40 and 60% of $\dot{V}O_2$max; the second
(LT2) is generally over 80% of $\dot{V}O_2$max and possibly
as high as 95% of $\dot{V}O_2$max. LT1 is sometimes
equated with a lactate concentration of 2 mmol · L^{-1}
and LT2 with a lactate concentration of 4 mmol · L^{-1}.
This 4 mmol · L^{-1} level, called the *onset of blood lactate accumulation* (OBLA), is frequently used to decide both training loads and racing strategies.[40,47]
Running at a pace that results in a continual accumulation of lactate has a detrimental effect on endurance time that is directly related to changes
brought about by the lactate.

Table 10.3 summarizes the anaerobic metabolic
exercise responses discussed in this section.

Why Is Lactic Acid a Problem? It is the
hydrogen ions (H$^+$) that dissociate from lactic acid,
rather than undissociated lactic acid or lactate (La$^-$),
that present the primary problems to the body. This
distinction is important, because at normal pH levels lactic acid is almost completely dissociated im-

TABLE 10.3 ■ Anaerobic Exercise Responses

VARIABLE	HIGH CONSTANT INTENSITY, 3-MIN DURATION OR LESS	INCREMENTAL WORK TO MAXIMUM
ATP	↓ 30–40%	
PC	↓ 60–70%	
La⁻	↑ From 2 to 12 mmol·L⁻¹	Minimal rise until approximately 40–60% $\dot{V}O_2$max; then continuous curvilinear rise to 8 mmol·L⁻¹ or more

↑ increases ↓ decreases

mediately to H^+ and La^- ($C_3H_5O_3^-$).[19] As long as the amount of free H^+ does not exceed the ability of the chemical and physiological mechanisms to buffer them and maintain the pH at a relatively stable level, there are few problems. Most problems arise when the amount of lactic acid—and hence H^+—exceeds the body's immediate buffering capacity and pH decreases. The blood has become more acidic. At that point pain is perceived and performance suffers. The mechanisms of these results are described in the following subsections.

Pain.   Anyone who has raced or run the 400-m distance all out understands the pain caused by lactic acid. Such an event takes between approximately 45 sec and 3 min (depending on the ability of the runner) and relies heavily on the ATP-PC and LA systems to supply the needed energy. The resultant hydrogen ions accumulate and stimulate pain nerve endings located in the muscle.[37]

Performance Decrement.   The decrement in performance associated with lactic acid is brought about by fatigue that is both metabolic and muscular in origin.

1. Metabolic fatigue is a result of a reduced production of ATP linked to enzyme changes, changes in membrane transport mechanisms, and changes in substrate availability.

Enzymes—in particular, the rate-limiting enzymes in the metabolic pathways—can be inactivated by high hydrogen ion concentrations (low pH). The hydrogen ion attaches to these enzyme molecules and in so doing changes their size, shape, and hence ability to function. Phosphofructokinase (PFK) is thought to be particularly sensitive, although oxidative enzymes can also be affected.[45]

At the same time, changes occur in membrane transport mechanisms (either to the carriers in the membrane or to the permeability channels). These changes affect the movement of molecules across the cell membrane and between the cytoplasm and organelles such as the mitochondria.[45]

Energy substrate availability can be inhibited by a high concentration of hydrogen ions. Glycogen breakdown is slowed by the inactivation of the enzyme glycogen phosphorylase. Fatty acid utilization is decreased because lactic acid inhibits mobilization. Thus, a double-jeopardy situation is evident. With fatty acid availability low a greater reliance is placed on carbohydrate sources at the time when glycogen breakdown is inhibited. At the same time, phosphocreatine (PC) breakdown is accelerated, leading to a faster depletion of substrate for ATP regeneration.[5,25, 45]

Thus, both the inactivation of enzymes and the decrement in substrate availability will lead to a reduction in the production of ATP and, ultimately, a decrement in performance.

2. Muscular fatigue is evidenced by reduced force and velocity of muscle contraction. The contraction of skeletal muscle and the influence of lactic acid on muscular fatigue are explained in depth in Chapters 17 and 18, respectively. Suffice it to say here that a lowered pH can have two major effects on muscle contraction. The first is an inhibition of actomyosin

ATPase, the enzyme responsible for the breakdown of ATP to provide the immediate energy for muscle contraction. The second is an interference of H^+ with the actions and uptake of calcium (Ca^{2+}) that is necessary for the excitation-contraction coupling and relaxation of the protein cross-bridges within the muscle fiber. High levels of lactate ions (La^-) may also interfere with cross-bridging. [42] The result of these actions is a decrease in both the force a muscle can exert and the velocity of muscle contraction.

The Fate of Lactate Carbon and hydrogen tracer studies have shown that lactate has two major fates during exercise and in recovery: (1) to serve as a fuel source and (2) to serve as a source of carbon atoms for a number of other substances (see Table 10.4).[20, 30] Remember that lactic acid is composed of carbon, hydrogen, and oxygen ($C_3H_6O_3$).

Both the heart and active skeletal muscle tissue utilize lactate as a fuel. Muscle fiber types are fully described in Chapter 17, but briefly, fibers that produce energy predominantly by anaerobic glycolysis are called glycolytic; those that produce energy predominantly aerobically are called oxidative. Lactate formed in glycolytic muscle fibers (Type II B, FG) can diffuse into the venous system and be recirculated to more oxidative skeletal fibers (Type I, SO and Type II A, FOG) and the heart. Or it can diffuse directly into adjacent oxidative muscle fibers (SO) where it is utilized to produce energy. In either case, lactate becomes a fuel source by being converted back to pyruvate. This pyruvate then follows the normal pathways through acetyl-CoA, the Krebs cycle, and electron transport. In the process it is oxidized to ATP, CO_2, and H_2O. This process accounts for approximately 55–70% of the lactate removal.[20]

In addition, as described earlier, the carbon structure of lactate can be converted to other structures through gluconeogenic or transamination processes forming glucose, glycogen, keto acids (Krebs cycle intermediates) (20% or less), or amino acids (5–10%). In turn, the amino acids serve as components for other body proteins. A very small amount (less than 2%) remains as lactate.[20]

Lactate Removal Postexercise Lactate is removed from the bloodstream relatively rapidly following exercise.[32] However, removal does not occur at a constant rate. If it did, then higher levels of lactate would take proportionately longer to dissipate than lower levels. For example, if you could do one push-up in 2 sec and you couldn't change that rate or speed, then 10 push-ups would take twice as long to do as 5 push-ups (20 versus 10 sec). On the other hand, if you could change that rate, you might be able to do 10 in the same time as you did 5 (in 10 sec). Many chemical reactions have this ability to change the rate or speed at which they occur. That is, the rate is proportional to the amount of substrate and product present. The more substrate available and the less product, the faster the reaction proceeds, and vice versa. This characteristic is called the *mass action effect*. Lactate appears to be one of those substrates whose utilization and conversion is linked with the amount of substrate present.[15]

Thus, despite wide interindividual differences (which may be related to muscle fiber type), in a resting recovery situation approximately half of the lactate is removed in about 15–20 min no matter what the starting level is. This time is called the half-life of lactate. Near-resting levels are achieved in about 30–60 min, regardless of the starting level.

TABLE 10.4 ▪ The Fate of Lactate During Recovery from Heavy Exercise[20]

FATE	PERCENTAGE
Is converted to pyruvic acid and oxidized to ATP, CO_2, and H_2O	55–70%
Is reconverted to muscle and liver glycogen	20% or less
Provides carbons for amino acids and other proteins	5–10%
Remains as lactate	2% or less

Source: Brooks.[20]

Handwritten note at top: Law of Mass Action: more LA present during exercise the faster the rate of removal.

Handwritten note: Complete Removal = 30-60 minutes

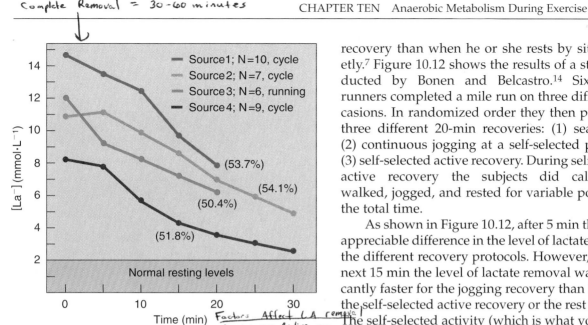

FIGURE 10.11

The Time Course of Lactate Removal During Resting Recovery from Exercise

During resting recovery from exercise, lactate exhibits a half-life of 15–25 minutes.

Sources: (1) Bonen et al.;[15] (2) Belcastro & Bonen;[11] (3) Bonen & Belcastro;[14] (4) McGrail, Bonen, & Belcastro.[61]

Handwritten note below Figure 10.11: Factors Affect LA removal: 1. Passive or Active recovery 2. Modality during recovery 3. Is Recovery continuous or Intermittent.

Thus, the initial postexercise concentration of lactate is the first factor that influences the rate of removal. The higher the concentration, the faster the rate of removal is.[15,41,42]

Figure 10.11 shows typical resting recovery curves from cycling and running studies. Note that in each case the value close to 50% (shown in parentheses) of the initial postexercise lactate levels occurs between 15 and 25 min of recovery.

The second factor that determines the rate of lactate removal is whether the individual follows a rest (passive) recovery or an exercise (active) recovery regimen. Third, if an exercise recovery is employed, the intensity of the exercise (expressed as a percentage of $\dot{V}O_2$max) will make a difference. Fourth, the modality of the exercise employed in the recovery phase may influence the optimal percentage of $\dot{V}O_2$max at which removal occurs. And finally, whether the recovery exercise is continuous or intermittent seems to make a difference.

Evidence suggests that lactate removal occurs more quickly when an individual exercises during recovery than when he or she rests by sitting quietly.[7] Figure 10.12 shows the results of a study conducted by Bonen and Belcastro.[14] Six trained runners completed a mile run on three different occasions. In randomized order they then performed three different 20-min recoveries: (1) seated rest, (2) continuous jogging at a self-selected pace, and (3) self-selected active recovery. During self-selected active recovery the subjects did calisthenics, walked, jogged, and rested for variable portions of the total time.

As shown in Figure 10.12, after 5 min there is no appreciable difference in the level of lactate between the different recovery protocols. However, over the next 15 min the level of lactate removal was significantly faster for the jogging recovery than for either the self-selected active recovery or the rest recovery. The self-selected activity (which is what you would typically see athletes doing at a track meet), although not as good as continuous jogging (in part

FIGURE 10.12

Lactate Removal in Active Versus Passive Recovery

Lactate removal is faster under active than passive conditions, although the magnitude of the benefit of active recovery depends on the type and intensity of the activity. In this study, continuous jogging at 61.4% $\dot{V}O_2$max was more effective than a mixture of walking, jogging, and calisthenics.

Source: Bonen & Belcastro.[14]

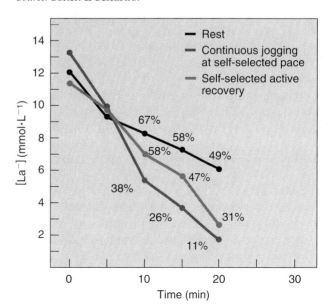

because it was intermittent), was still significantly better than resting recovery.

After 20 min of jogging recovery, the lactate that remained was well within the normal resting levels of 1–2 mmol · L⁻¹. The self-selected active recovery had removed 70% of the lactate, but the resting recovery had only removed 50% of the lactate. Thus, full recovery was, and generalizing is, delayed if a seated rest is employed. Since athletes who run the distances from 400 to 1500 m (or the English equivalents of 440 yd to 1 mi) often double at track meets, such a delay could impair their performances in the second event. On the basis of these results, an athlete competing or training at distances that are likely to cause large accumulations of lactic acid should cool down with an active continuous recovery.

Why does activity increase the rate of lactate removal? The rate of lactate removal by the liver appears to be the same whether an individual is resting or exercising. However, during exercise blood flow is increased, as is the oxidation of lactate by skeletal muscles.[7,11,33,42,61] These changes appear to be primarily responsible for the beneficial effects of an active recovery.

At what intensity should an active recovery be performed? Studies that have attempted to answer this question have found an inverted U-shaped response.[11,42] That is, up to a point, a higher intensity of exercise (as measured by percentage of $\dot{V}O_2$max) during recovery is better. But after that point, as the intensity continues to rise, the removal rate decreases. This pattern is exemplified in Figure 10.13, where the curve is both U-shaped and skewed toward the lower $\dot{V}O_2$max percentage values, with the optimal rate being between 29 and 45% of $\dot{V}O_2$max. These data were collected after cycle ergometer rides. Data collected for track and treadmill exercises show the same type of U-shaped curve response, but in the 55–70% $\dot{V}O_2$max range.[11,42] This difference in optimal intensity may be a function of the modality (there is a higher static component for the cycle ergometer than for running) or of the training status of the subjects tested.

The actual value of these optimal percentages should not be surprising. The lactate threshold has been shown to occur between 40 and 60% of $\dot{V}O_2$max and may be higher in trained individuals. Thus, it appears that the optimal intensity for recovery would be just below an individual's lactate threshold, where lactate production is minimal but clearance is maximized.

FIGURE 10.13

Lactate Removal Rate as a Function of the Percentage of $\dot{V}O_2$max in Recovery Exercise for Cycling

Source: A. N. Belcastro & A. Bonen. Lactic acid removal rates during controlled and uncontrolled recovery exercise. *Journal of Applied Physiology.* 39(6): 932–936 (1975). Modified and reprinted by permission of the American Physiological Association.

One word of caution: Although an active recovery is best for lactate removal, it can delay glycogen resynthesis by further depleting glycogen stores.[22] This has more relevance for an individual attempting to recover from a hard interval-training session than for someone just completing a middle-distance race and preparing for another. Glycogen depletion is likely to be more severe in the former case, and getting rid of the lactate quickly is more of an immediate concern in the latter case. For athletes recovering from an interval training session or competing in heats on successive days the best procedure may be to combine an initial dynamic active recovery (just to the point of regaining a near-resting heart rate) with stretching and then engage in a passive recovery during which carbohydrates are consumed.

*M*ale Versus Female Anaerobic Characteristics

The anaerobic characteristics of females are in general lower than those of males during the young and middle-aged adult years. Much of the difference is undoubtedly related to the smaller overall muscle mass of the average female compared with that of the average male.[84]

The Availability and Utilization of ATP-PC

Neither the local resting stores of ATP per kilogram of muscle nor the utilization of ATP-PC during exercise varies between the sexes.[20, 32] However, in terms of total energy available from these phosphagen sources, males will exceed females due to muscle mass differences.

The Accumulation of Lactate

Resting levels of lactate are the same for males and females. Lactate thresholds, when expressed as a percentage of $\dot{V}O_2$max, are also the same for both sexes, although the absolute workload at which the lactate thresholds occur will be higher for males than for females. Thus, at any given absolute workload that is still submaximal but above LT1 or LT2, females will have a higher lactate value than males. Consequently, the workload is more stressful for fe-

males and requires a greater anaerobic contribution. However, at a given relative workload or percentage of $\dot{V}O_2$max above the lactate thresholds, lactate concentrations are equal for both sexes.[84]

Lactate values at maximal exercise from ages 16 through 50 are higher by approximately 0.5–2.0 mmol $\cdot$ L^{-1} for males than for females (see Figure 10.14). Once again, females are generally doing less in terms of an absolute workload than males at maximum.

The accumulation of lactate during maximal exercise presents a special dilemma for nursing mothers. A portion of the lactate present in blood diffuses into breast milk and remains present for at least 90 min.[79,80] Infants have fully developed taste buds at birth and can detect sour tastes such as that produced by lactic acid. In fact, some infants will reject postexercise milk if it contains lactic acid.[79] If a nursing mother finds that her infant fusses or refuses to nurse after she has exercised, she can try one of several things. The first option is to feed the baby just prior to exercising or collect the milk at that time and store it for later feeding. The second possibility is to experiment with lower-intensity workouts that will not lead to a substantial lactate accumulation.

FIGURE 10.14

Lactate Values After Maximal Exercise as a Function of Age and Sex

Sources: Compiled from computed mean values data for 4–20-year-old subjects, Cumming,[24] Saris,[69] Åstrand,[4] and Eriksson[26]. Computed mean values data for 20–60-year-old subjects, Bouhuys et al.,[18] Sidney & Shepard,[73] I. Åstrand,[1] Robinson,[68] and P. Åstrand.[2]

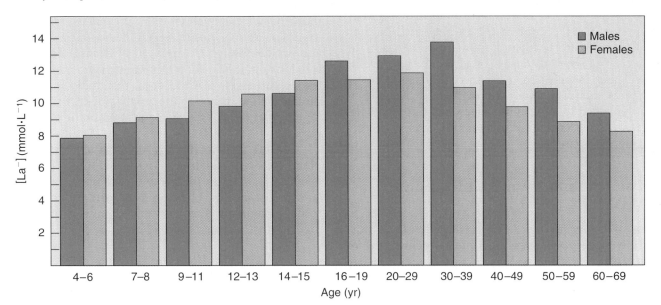

Finally, postexercise milk may have to be discarded and supplemental feeding implemented.

Mechanical Power and Capacity

As previously mentioned, on average males produce higher absolute work output than females. Data available from the Wingate Anaerobic Test show that values for peak power for women are approximately 65% of values for men if expressed in watts, improve to 83% if expressed in watts per kilogram of body weight, and come close to being equal at 94% when expressed in watts per kilogram of lean body mass. The corresponding comparisons for mean power are 68%, 87%, and 98%, respectively. The peak power of women (in watts per kilogram of body weight) is very similar to the mean power of men. The fatigue index does not show a significant sex difference, indicating that both sexes tire at the same rate.[58]

Anaerobic Exercise Characteristics of Children

The anaerobic characteristics of children are not as well-developed as those of adults. Furthermore, children do not tend to be the metabolic specialists that adults are. For example, one would not expect Leroy Burrell (1994 world record holder in the 100-m dash, with a time of 9.85) to do well at the marathon distance, nor Joan Benoit Samuelson (first women's Olympic marathon winner in 1984) to be successful at the sprint distances. Yet watch children at play (Figure 10.15) and, more often than not, the fastest at short distances or strength-type events will also do well at long distances or in aerobic-type games such as soccer. Although much research is still needed to explain the anaerobic differences between children and adults, some patterns are becoming apparent.[8]

The Availability and Utilization of ATP-PC

Local resting stores of ATP per kilogram of wet muscle weight appear to be the same for a child and for an adult. Levels of resting PC per kilogram of wet muscle weight have been reported as slightly lower

FIGURE 10.15

Children tend not to be metabolic specialists in their play, but can perform anaerobic short-distance or strength-type activities (as show here) as well as aerobic long-distance type activities.

in children[8, 72] or no different from adult levels.[26, 72] There is agreement that the rate of utilization of these reserves during exercise does not differ. However, since children are smaller in stature than adults, the total amount of energy that can be generated from this source is lower.

The Accumulation of Lactate

On the average, blood lactate values obtained during submaximal exercise and after maximal exercise are lower in children than in adults.[69,72] Furthermore, peak lactate values after maximal exercise exhibit a relatively positive rectilinear increase with age until adulthood. Figure 10.14 exemplifies this relationship. It also shows that there is no meaningful sex difference in children in the ability to accumulate lactate, although the girls' values are slightly higher than the boys' values throughout the growth period.

Several theories have been postulated to explain children's inability to sustain high lactate levels. All of these ideas are based upon two assumptions: that the children tested did indeed put forth a maximal effort, and that there is a physiological cause for the observed differences.

The Muscle Enzyme Theory   Eriksson[26] and others have shown that phosphofructokinase

(PFK) activity in 11–13-yr-old boys is 2.5–3 times lower than in trained or sedentary adult men. Since PFK is a rate-limiting enzyme of glycolysis, this lowered activity may be indicative of a decreased ability to produce lactic acid. In addition, the availability and the utilization of glycogen as a substrate are both lower in children than in adults. However, other glycolytic enzymes, such as lactic dehydrogenase (the enzyme involved in the conversion of pyruvic acid to lactic acid), show just the opposite response. That is, the highest level of activity has been seen in 12–14-yr-old boys.[13] Therefore, no definitive conclusion can be made about the role of the glycolytic enzymes.

In general, the oxidative enzymes show higher activity in young children than in older individuals.[13,85] This result, along with higher mitochondrial density and intracellular lipids, means that there is an improved lipid utilization in the child. Thus, it may be that children have a finer balance between aerobic and anaerobic metabolism than adults. Additional evidence for this observation comes from the fact that children show a lower oxygen deficit and reach a steady state faster than adults.[2,67,72]

Sexual Maturation Theory There is limited evidence that suggests that the increase in glycolytic capacity (and hence the production of lactate) in children is related to the hormonal changes that occur to bring about sexual maturation.[85] In particular, testosterone is thought to have a role. If so, the levels would have to be small enough to allow for the differences in girls as well as in boys.

Neurohormonal Regulation Theory It has been shown that sympathetic nervous system activity is significantly lower in children than in adults at maximal exercise. One of the results of sympathetic stimulation during exercise is hepatic vasoconstriction. The liver plays a major role in the clearance of lactate. If blood flow to the liver is reduced, not as much lactate is cleared. Thus, since the child maintains a higher liver blood flow, more lactate can be cleared. This implies that children are not deficient in the production of lactate but are, instead, better able to remove or reconvert it than adults.[12,57,69]

Which of these theories, or which combination of them, is correct remains to be shown.

The Lactate Threshold(s)

The phenomenon of ventilatory breakpoints and lactate accumulation is seen in children as well as in adults.[31] Because children do not utilize anaerobic metabolism as early in work as adults do, the work level of children at the fixed lactate levels of 4 mmol · L^{-1} will be relatively higher than that of adults.[49,67] Williams et al.[85] report a value of almost 92% of $\dot{V}O_2$max for 4 mmol · L^{-1} of lactate in 11–13-yr-old boys and girls. Values for adults tend to be about 15% below this value. Thus, the child is working relatively harder (at a higher %$\dot{V}O_2$max) than the adult at the same lactate level. Consequently, the assessment of exercise capacity and the monitoring of training by a 4-mmol · L^{-1} value is inappropriate in prepubertal children.

Mechanical Power and Capacity

Peak power and peak power per kilogram of body weight have consistently been shown to be lower in prepubertal boys and girls than in adolescents or young adults when evaluated by the Margaria-Kalamen Stair Climb test. The results are similar to those for the Wingate Anaerobic Test, although there is a lack of information on females of all ages. In boys peak power increases consistently from age 10 to young adulthood. Mean power follows the same pattern. This is true whether the values are expressed in absolute terms (watts) or are corrected for body weight (watts per kilogram). The absolute differences between children and adults, however, are much greater (that is, the child can achieve only about 30% of the adult values) than the relative differences, (that is, the child can achieve about 60–85% of the adult values). Peak values seem to occur in the late thirties for the legs and the late twenties for the arms.[9,44] Figure 10.16 shows these results graphically.

*A*naerobic Exercise Characteristics of Older Adults

Evidence detailing anaerobic characteristics in the elderly is scarce. The reason is undoubtedly a combination of caution on the part of researchers and uncertain motivation on the part of subjects when faced with the necessarily high intensity

FIGURE 10.16

The Effect of Age on Anaerobic Performance

Cross-sectional data on 306 males who performed both an arm and a leg Wingate Anaerobic Test. The pattern of increase in values from childhood to young adulthood is similar for leg (a & c) and arm (b & d) cycling whether the unit of measurement is absolute (a & b) or relative (c & d).

Source: O. Inbar & O. Bar-Or. Anaerobic characteristics in male children and adolescents. *Medicine and Science in Sports and Exercise.* 18(3): 264–269 (1986). Reprinted by permission.

exercise. What data are available indicate that anaerobic variables show a common aging pattern. That is, there is typically a peak in the second or third decade and then a gradual decline into the sixth decade. Despite this the elderly can still participate successfully in basically anaerobic activities (Figure 10.17). One must always remember when interpreting aging results, however, that no one knows how much of the reduction is a direct result of aging, how much is the result of detraining that accompanies the reduced activity level of the elderly, and how much is the result of disease.

The Availability and Utilization of ATP-PC

Local resting stores of ATP-PC are reduced and levels of creatine and ADP are elevated in muscles of the elderly.[49, 74] Results from the Margaria-Kalamen Stair Climb test have shown a reduction in ATP-PC power of as much as 45% and a reduction in ATP-PC capacity of 32% from youth to old age.[72] This means that ATP-PC stores are both reduced and unable to be used as quickly. The result is a decrease in alactic anaerobic power.

The Accumulation of Lactate

On the average, resting levels of blood lactate are remarkably consistent across the entire age span, varying only from 1 to 2 mmol · L⁻¹.

Lactate values during the same absolute submaximal work show a tendency to be higher for individuals over the age of 50 yr.[1,2,3,68] However, this generalization is confounded by the fact that at any given absolute load of work the older individual is working at a higher percentage of his or her maximal aerobic power, which would be expected to involve anaerobic metabolism more.[73] When younger and older individuals work at the same relative workload (% $\dot{V}O_2$max), lactate concentrations are lower in older persons than in the young, probably

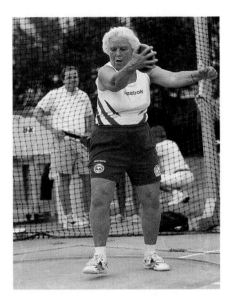

FIGURE 10.17

Anaerobic metabolic processes function less effectively in the elderly than in younger adults, but participation in anaerobic sports such as throwing the discus can still be enjoyed.

because the elderly are using less muscle mass to do less work.[54] Data are unavailable on the lactate thresholds in the elderly.

Maximal lactate levels reach a peak between 16 and 39 yr of age and then show a gradual decline (see Figure 10.14). Both males and females exhibit the same pattern, with the absolute values of females being considerably lower than those of males.

Physiological factors appear to contribute to the decline in maximal lactate values with age.[72,76] First, activity of the enzyme lactate dehydrogenase (which catalyzes the conversion of pyruvic acid to lactic acid) decreases in all muscle fiber types. This decrease effectively slows glycolysis. The reduction in glycolysis may also be related to reduced amounts of glycogen stored in the skeletal muscles of the elderly.

Second, the elderly possess a smaller ratio of muscle mass to blood volume, a smaller ratio of capillary to muscle fiber, and a concomitant slower diffusion of lactic acid out of the active muscle fibers and into the bloodstream.[72] Thus, it may not be that the elderly have a large deficiency in anaerobic ca-

pacity at the cellular level; rather, it may simply be that measurements from blood samples are underestimations. Of course, a combination of the first and second factors may also be operating.

Mechanical Power and Capacity

The average peak power value obtained on the Margaria-Kalamen Stair Climb test (Figure 10.18a) declines precipitously over the 20–70-yr age range.[17] Published results are unavailable for the Wingate Anaerobic Test for individuals over the age of 40 and for females except in the 18–28-yr range.[60] However, Makrides et al.[58] have presented data on 50 male and 50 female subjects from 15 to 70 yr of age on a test similar to the WAT (Figure 10.18b). In this case peak power represents an instantaneous value rather than a 5-sec value. Mean power is still the average of 30 sec of pedaling but at a controlled rate of 60 rev · min⁻¹. The results from this study show a decline of approximately 6% for each decade of age for sedentary individuals of both sexes. However, the absolute values for the females are consistently lower than those for the males. Indeed, in the Makrides study the peak power of the females coincides with the mean power of the males. For both sexes lean thigh volume was found to be closely related to peak power and mean power, but it did not account for all the variation in the values or in the decline with age.

*H*eritability of Anaerobic Characteristics

There is an old saying that "sprinters are born and distance runners are made." Is this statement scientifically defensible? The answer is both yes and no. Since sprinters are the anaerobic athletes, only sprinters will be dealt with here. Very little research has been done on the genetic contribution to differences in alactic and lactic anaerobic power and capacity, which form the basis for successful sprint performances. However, because there is so much interindividual variation in anaerobic values and abilities, genetics is likely to play an important role. Heritability studies ideally compare measures of a given trait for pairs of monozygous (MZ), or identical, twins and dizygous (DZ), or fraternal, twins.

FIGURE 10.18

Mechanical Power Changes with Age in Males and Females

(a) Average peak power ratings determined from the Margaria-Kalamen Stair Climb are higher for males than females across the age span from adolescence to middle adulthood. Males and females show steady and parallel declines in peak power during the adult years. (b) Instantaneous peak power and mean power measured during a 30-sec cycle ergometer test are higher for males (MW_I and MW_M, respectively) than for females (FW_I and FW_M, respectively) across the age span from late adolescence to older adulthood. Female instantaneous peak power (FW_I) is equal to male mean power (MW_M).Instantaneous peak power and mean power show rectilinear and parallel declines with age in males and females. Each line was calculated from the experimentally determined equation associated with that line on the graph.

Sources: (a) Data from Bouchard et al.[17] (b) Data from Makrides et al.[58]

The expectation is that the MZ twins will show less variability (that is, be more similar in the trait) than the DZ twins. The studies detailed here comprise what is known at this time.

Klissouras[53] compared the lactate response to incremental treadmill running in 10 pairs of male DZ and 15 pairs of males MZ twins from 7 to 13 yr of age. The young age of the subjects was thought to be helpful in controlling for the effect of environment. The lactate responses were more similar for the more closely genetically related MZ twins than for the DZ twins (Table 10.5). The study concluded that the genetic determination for lactate accumulation was 81.4%.

Komi and colleagues provided data on 15 pairs of male and 14 pairs of female twins between the ages of 10 and 14 yr[56] and 20 pairs of male and 11 pairs of female twins between the ages of 15 and 24 yr.[55] The variability in maximal mechanical power as measured by the Margaria-Kalamen Stair Climb was found to be 99.2% genetically determined in the preadolescent boys and 97.8% in the older men. The variability could not be computed for the girls and women.

Simoneau et al.[74] studied the alactic anaerobic capacity in four groups with increasing genetic communality—that is, adopted siblings, biological siblings, dizygotic twins, and monozygotic twins.

TABLE 10.5 ■ Intrapair Correlations of Heritability for Anaerobic Characteristics

		ATP-PC System		
SOURCE	PAIRS	J · kg⁻¹	J · kg⁻¹ · FFW⁻¹*	LA SYSTEM (mmol · L⁻¹)
Klissouras[53]	DZ twins (N = 15)			0.76
	MZ twins (N = 10)			0.93
Simoneau et al.[74]	Adopted siblings (N = 19)	−0.01	0.06	
	Biological siblings (N = 55)	0.46	0.38	
	DZ twins (N = 31)	0.58	0.44	
	MZ twins (N = 49)	0.80	0.77	

*FFW = fat free body weight.

Both sexes were included, and the ages ranged from 9 to 33 yr. Alactic anaerobic capacity was determined by the total work output (in joules) on a bicycle ergometer in 10 sec. Table 10.5 shows that the correlations between the work output of the pairs of siblings or twins got steadily higher as the shared genetics increased between the groups. As expected, there was not much difference between the separate-birth biological siblings and dizygotic twins when expressed in joules per kilogram of body weight or joules per kilogram of fat free body weight weight (FFW). The total genetic effect was estimated to be between 44 and 76%.

On the basis of these data it can only be concluded that there is some degree of genetic influence on anaerobic characteristics but the exact amount is unknown. It can therefore be said that, at least to a certain extent, sprinters are born. On the other hand, as discussed in Chapter 11, so probably are distance runners.

SUMMARY

1. Anaerobic metabolism does not require oxygen to produce ATP, but aerobic metabolism does.

2. Anaerobic and aerobic metabolism work together to provide ATP and, hence, energy for exercise. Depending on the duration and intensity of the activity, one or the other predominates.

3. The ATP-PC system predominates in high-intensity exercise that lasts 30 sec or less. The LA system predominates in high-intensity exercise lasting between 30 sec and 1½ min. The aerobic system predominates in exercise lasting from 3–5 min to hours. This sequence is called the time-energy system continuum.

4. There is no generally accepted way to directly measure the anaerobic energy contribution to exercise. One indirect approach is to describe the changes in ATP, PC, and lactate levels. Another is to quantify the amount of work performed or power generated during short-duration, high-intensity activity.

5. The onset of all exercise is characterized by a discrepancy between oxygen demand and oxygen utilization known as the oxygen deficit. This deficit is due not to the cardiovascular-respiratory system's inability to respond but to limited cellular utilization of oxygen as a result of metabolic adjustments. That is, when ATP is broken down into ADP + P_i and elevated levels of NADH + H⁺ are present, both aerobic and anaerobic metabolic pathways are stimulated to produce more ATP.

6. During the transition from rest to exercise, energy is supplied by:
   (a) Oxygen transport and utilization.
   (b) The use of oxygen stores in venous blood and on myoglobin.
   (c) The splitting of stored ATP-PC.
   (d) Anaerobic glycolysis with the concomitant production of lactic acid.

7. During exercise the balance between aerobic and anaerobic metabolism depends on the intensity of the activity in relation to the individual's maximal ability to produce energy using oxygen ($\dot{V}O_2$max).

8. During recovery from exercise oxygen consumption remains elevated. The term *excess postexercise oxygen consumpyion* (EPOC) is used to refer to this phenomenon. The following factors appear to be ongoing during recovery.

(a) Restoration of ATP-PC stores
(b) Restoration of oxygen stores
(c) Elevated cardiorespiratory function
(d) Elevated hormonal levels
(e) Elevated body temperature
(f) Lactate removal

9. During high-intensity, short-duration (3 min or less) anaerobic exercise ATP levels decrease 30–40%, PC levels decrease 60–70%, and lactate accumulation can increase well over 1000%.

10. During incremental work to maximum lactate accumulates slowly until approximately 40–60% $\dot{V}O_2$max when the continual accumulation is exponentially curvilinear. The term *lactate threshold* (LT) is commonly (although not absolutely accurately) used to describe the point where large increases in lactate accumulation occur.

11. LT1 is typically found between 40 and 60% $\dot{V}O_2$max, and LT2 is found between 80 and 95% $\dot{V}O_2$max. An absolute value of 4 mmol · L^{-1} is termed the OBLA and is often used as a training and racing guideline.

12. The relationship between the lactate thresholds and ventilatory thresholds appears to be primarily coincidental.

13. The term *anaerobic threshold* is a misnomer and should not be used because the presence of lactate does not automatically mean that the oxygen supply is inadequate. Blood lactate levels are determined by five things:

(a) The muscle fibers recruited to do the work.
(b) The rate of lactate produced by working muscles.
(c) The rate of oxidation of pyruvate in the mitochondria.
(d) The rate of removal of lactate from the working muscles.
(e) The rate of lactate removal from the bloodstream by nonworking muscles, the liver, and the kidneys.

14. Lactic acid dissociates into hydrogen ions (H^+) and lactate (La^-). If the amount of hydrogen ions exceeds the ability of the chemical and respiratory mechanisms to buffer them, pH decreases and the blood becomes more acidic.

15. Performance decrements occur with high concentrations of H^+ because of:

(a) Pain.
(b) Reduced production of ATP through inactivation of enzymes or changes in membrane transport.

(c) Inhibition of energy substrate availability because glycogen breakdown is slowed or because fatty acid mobilization is slowed.
(d) Reduced force and velocity of muscle contraction.

16. During recovery from heavy exercise lactate is cleared five ways.

(a) It is oxidized to ATP, CO_2, and H_2O.
(b) It is reconverted to muscle and liver glycogen via gluconeogenesis.
(c) It is converted to amino acids and Krebs cycle intermediates.
(d) It provides carbons for proteins.
(e) It remains as lactate.

17. Lactate removal from the bloodstream after exercise follows the law of mass action: The more lactate present, the faster the rate of removal. The half-life of lactate is approximately 15–20 min, with full removal achieved between 30 and 60 min.

18. The time required for lactate removal can be decreased by doing an active recovery at an intensity of approximately 30–45% $\dot{V}O_2$max for cycling and 55–70% $\dot{V}O_2$max for running.

19. The anaerobic characteristics of children are not well developed in comparison with those of adults. The lower amount of ATP-PC available is related to children's small body size.

20. Peak lactate values after incremental exercise to maximum are lower in children than adults and vary directly with age throughout the growth years. There is no meaningful male-female difference in the ability to accumulate lactate during childhood.

21. Mechanical power and capacity are lower for children and adolescents than for adults, whether expressed in absolute terms or corrected for body weight.

22. During the adult years males accumulate higher levels of blood lactate as a result of maximal work than do females, and males exhibit higher mechanical power and capacity even when they are adjusted for body weight.

23. Anaerobic metabolic processes decline from young and middle-aged to older adults. The decline includes lower resting levels of ATP-PC.

24. Peak lactate values after incremental exercise to maximum decline after approximately 40 yr of age. Females exhibit considerably lower peak values than males.

25. The mechanical power and capacity of the elderly decline steadily. The decline is greater in females than in males.

26. The exact degree of genetic influence on anaerobic characteristics is unknown, although estimates range from 44–99%.

REVIEW QUESTIONS

1. Describe the energy continuum. For each of the following sports or events, determine the percentage contribution from the ATP-PC, LA, and O_2 systems.

    (a) 100-m dash

    (b) 800-m run

    (c) soccer (not goalie)

    (d) triathlon

    (e) volleyball spike

    (f) 100-m swim

    (g) mile run

    (h) stealing a base

    (i) wrestling period

2. List the major variables that are typically measured to describe the anaerobic response to exercise. Where possible, provide an example of an exercise test from which the variable could be determined.

3. Explain the five physiological reasons for the production of lactic acid. What determines whether or not lactate accumulates in the blood?

4. Arrange the ATP-PC, LA, and O_2 systems from highest to lowest in terms of (a) power and (b) capacity. What is the difference between power and capacity?

5. Diagram the oxygen deficit and excess postexercise oxygen consumption for an activity that requires 110% $\dot{V}O_2$max in an individual whose $\dot{V}O_2$max equals $4 \text{ L} \cdot \text{min}^{-1}$ and whose resting oxygen is $0.25 \text{ L} \cdot \text{min}^{-1}$. Explain how energy is provided during the oxygen deficit time period and why oxygen remains elevated during recovery.

6. Diagram and explain the changes that take place in ATP, PC, and $[\text{La}^-]$ during constant-load, heavy exercise lasting 3 min or less.

7. Diagram the lactate response to incremental work to maximum. The ventilatory and lactate thresholds often occur at approximately the same time. Debate whether this is a result of cause and effect or coincidence. Can either the lactate thresholds or the ventilatory thresholds be accurately described as anaerobic thresholds? Why or why not?

8. What are the physiological effects of lactate accumulation?

9. What happens to lactate during exercise and recovery? What is the best way to clear lactate quickly during recovery?

10. What are the effects of sex and age on anaerobic metabolism during exercise?

11. Approximately how much of an individual's anaerobic ability is due to genetic factors? Are sprinters made or born?

REFERENCES

1. Åstrand, I.: Aerobic work capacity in men and women with special reference to age. *Acta Physiologica Scandinavica* (Suppl.). 169: 1–92 (1960).

2. Åstrand, P.-O.: *Experimental Studies of Physical Working Capacity in Relation to Sex and Age.* Copenhagen: Munksgaard (1952).

3. Åstrand, P.-O.: Human physical fitness with special reference to sex and age. *Physiological Reviews.* 36(3):307–335 (1956).

4. Åstrand, P.-O., L. Engstrom, B. O. Eriksson, P. Karlberg, I. Nylander, B. Saltin, & C. Thoren: Girl swimmers: With special reference to respiratory and circulatory adaption and gynecological and psychiatric aspects. *Acta Paediatrica* (Suppl.). 147:1–73 (1963).

5. Åstrand, P.-O., & K. Rodahl: *Textbook of Work Physiology: Physiological Bases of Exercise.* New York: McGraw-Hill (1977).

6. Bahr, R.: Excess postexercise oxygen consumption—Magnitude, mechanisms and practical implications. *Acta Physiologica Scandinavica* (Suppl.). 605:9–70 (1992).

7. Bangsbo, J., T. Graham, L. Johansen, & B. Saltin: Muscle lactate metabolism in recovery from intense exhaustive exercise: Impact of light exercise. *Journal of Applied Physiology.* 77(4):1890–1895 (1994).

8. Bar-Or, O.: *Pediatric Sports Medicine for the Practitioner: From Physiological Principles to Clinical Applications.* New York: Springer-Verlag, 1–65 (1983).

9. Bar-Or, O.: The prepubescent female. In M. M. Shangold & G. Mirkin (eds.), *Women and Exercise: Physiology and Sports Medicine.* Philadelphia: Davis, 109–119 (1988).

10. Bar-Or, O.: The Wingate Anaerobic Test: An update on methodology, reliability and validity. *Sports Medicine.* 4:381–394 (1987).

11. Belcastro, A. N., & A. Bonen: Lactic acid removal rates during controlled and uncontrolled recovery exercise. *Journal of Applied Physiology.* 39(6):932–936 (1975).

12. Berg, A., & J. Keul: Biochemical changes during exercise in children. In R. M. Malina (ed.), *Young Athletes: Biological, Psychological, and Educational Perspectives.* Champaign, IL: Human Kinetics Publishers (1988).

13. Berg, A., S. S. Kim, & J. Keul: Skeletal muscle enzyme activities in healthy young subjects. *International Journal of Sports Medicine.* 7:236–239 (1986).

14. Bonen, A., & A. N. Belcastro: Comparison of self-selected recovery methods on lactic acid removal rates. *Medicine and Science in Sports.* 8(3):176–178 (1976).

15. Bonen, A., C. J. Campbell, R. L. Kirby, & A. N. Belcastro: A multiple regression model for blood lactate removal in man. *Pflügers Archives.* 380:205–210 (1979).

16. Bouchard, C., A. W. Taylor, & S. Dulac: Testing maximal anaerobic power and capacity. In J. D. MacDougall, H. W. Wenger, & H. J. Green (eds.), *Physiological Testing of the High-Performance Athlete* (2nd edition). Champaign, IL: Human Kinetics Publishers, 175–221 (1991).

17. Bouchard, C., A. W. Taylor, J. A., Simoneau, & S. Dulac: Testing anaerobic power and capacity. In J. D. MacDougall, H. A. Wenger, & H. J. Green (eds.), *Physiological Testing of the Elite Athlete* (1st edition). Hamilton, Ontario: Canadian Association of Sport Sciences Mutual Press Limited, 61–73 (1982).

18. Bouhuys, A., J. Pool, R. A. Binkhorst, & P. van Leeuwen: Metabolic acidosis of exercise in healthy males. *Journal of Applied Physiology.* 21(3):1040–1046 (1966).

19. Brooks, G. A.: Anaerobic threshold: Review of the concept and directions for future research. *Medicine and Science in Sports and Exercise.* 17(1):22–31 (1985).

20. Brooks, G. A.: The lactate shuttle during exercise and recovery. *Medicine and Science in Sports and Exercise.* 18(3):360–368 (1986).

21. Cheetham, M. E., L. H. Boobis, S. Brooks, & C. Williams: Human muscle metabolism during sprint running. *Journal of Applied Physiology.* 61(1):54–60 (1986).

22. Choi, D., K. J. Cole, B. H. Goodpaster, W. J. Fink, & D. L. Costill: Effect of passive and active recovery on the resynthesis of muscle glycogen. *Medicine and Science in Sports and Exercise.* 26(8):992–996 (1994).

23. Costill, D. L., H. Thomason, & E. Roberts: Fractional utilization of the aerobic capacity during distance running. *Medicine and Science in Sports.* 5(4):248–252 (1973).

24. Cumming, G. R., L. Hastman, & J. McCort: Treadmill endurance times, blood lactate, and exercise blood pressures in normal children. In R. A. Binkhorst, H. C. G. Kemper, & W. H. M. Saris (eds.), *Children and Exercise XI.* Champaign, IL: Human Kinetics Publishers 140–150 (1985).

25. Davis, J. A.: Response to Brooks' manuscript. *Medicine and Science in Sports and Exercise.* 17(1):32–34 (1985).

26. Eriksson, B. O.: Physical training, oxygen supply and muscle metabolism in 11–13 year old boys. *Acta Physiologica Scandinavica* (Suppl.). 384:1–48 (1972).

27. Farrell, P. A., J. H. Wilmore, E. F. Coyle, J. E. Billing, & D. L. Costill: Plasma lactate accumulation and distance running performance. *Medicine and Science in Sports and Exercise.* 11:338–344 (1979).

28. Fox, E. L.: Measurement of the maximal lactic (phosphagen) capacity in man. *Medicine and Science in Sports* (abstract). 5:66 (1973).

29. Freund, H., S. Oyono-Enguéllé, A. Heitz, C. Ott, J. Marbach, M. Gartner, & A. Pape: Comparative lactate kinetics after short and prolonged submaximal exercise. *International Journal of Sports Medicine.* 11(4):284–288 (1990).

30. Gaesser, G. A., & G. A. Brooks: Muscular efficiency during steady-rate exercise: Effects of speed and work rate. *Journal of Applied Physiology.* 38(6):1132–1139 (1975).

31. Gaisl, G., & J. Buchberger: Determination of the aerobic and anaerobic thresholds of 10–11 year old boys using blood-gas analysis. In K. Berg & B. O. Eriksson (eds.), *Children and Exercise IX.* Baltimore: University Park Press, International Series of Sport Sciences (1979).

32. Gollnick, P. D., W. M. Bayly, & D. R. Hodgson: Exercise intensity, training, diet, and lactate concentration in muscle and blood. *Medicine and Science in Sports and Exercise.* 18(3):334–340 (1986).

33. Gollnick, P. D., & L. Hermansen: Biochemical adaptations to exercise: Anaerobic metabolism. In J. H. Wilmore (ed.), *Exercise and Sport Sciences Reviews.* New York: Academic Press (1973).

34. Gollnick, P. D., & D. W. King: Energy release in the muscle cell. *Medicine and Science in Sports.* 1(1):23–31 (1969).

35. Green, H. J.: Muscle power: Fiber type recruitment, metabolism and fatigue. In N. L. Jones, M. McCartney, & A. J. McComas (eds.), *Human Muscle Power.* Champaign, IL: Human Kinetics Publishers (1986).

36. Green, S.: Measurement of anaerobic work capacities in humans. *Sports Medicine.* 19(1):32–42 (1995).

37. Guyton, A. C.: *Textbook of Medical Physiology* (7th edition). Philadelphia: Saunders (1986).

38. Hagberg, J. M., E. F. Coyle, J. E. Carroll, J. M. Miller, W. H. Martin, & M. H. Brooke: Exercise hyperventilation in patients with McArdle's disease. *Journal of Applied Physiology.* 52:991–994 (1982).

39. Heck, H., A. Mader, G. Hess, S. Mücke, R. Müller, & W. Hollmann: Justification of the 4-mmol/L lactate threshold. *International Journal of Sports Medicine.* 6:117–130 (1985).

40. Hermansen, L., S. Maehlum, E. D. R. Pruett, O. Vaage, H. Waldum, & T. Wessel-Aas: Lactate removal at rest and during exercise. In H. Howald & J. R. Poortmans (eds.), *Metabolic Adaptation to Prolonged Exercise.* Basel: Birkhäuser, 101–105 (1975).

41. Hermansen, L., & I. Stensvold: Production and removal of lactate during exercise in man. *Acta Physiologica Scandinavica.* 86:191–201 (1972).

42. Hogan, M. C., L. B. Gladden, S. S. Kurdak, & D. C. Poole: Increased [lactate] in working dog muscle reduces tension development independent of pH. *Medicine and Science in Sports and Exercise* 27(3):371–377, 1995.

43. Hughes, E. F., S. C. Tuner, & G. A. Brooks: Effect of glycogen depletion and pedaling speed on anaerobic threshold. *Journal of Applied Physiology.* 52(6):1598–1607 (1982).

44. Hughson, R. L., K. H. Weisiger, & G. D. Swanson: Blood lactate concentration increases as a continuous function in progressive exercise. *Journal of Applied Physiology.* 62(5):1975–1981 (1987).

45. Hultman, E., & K. Sahlin: Acid-base balance during exercise. In R. S. Hutton & D. I. Miller (eds.), *Exercise and Sport Sciences Reviews.* 8:41–128 (1980).

46. Inbar, O., & O. Bar-Or: Anaerobic characteristics in male children and adolescents. *Medicine and Science in Sports and Exercise.* 18(3):264–269 (1986).

47. Jacobs, I. Blood lactate: Implications for training and sports performance. *Sports Medicine.* 3:10–25 (1986).

48. Jones, N. L., & R. E. Ehrsam: The anaerobic threshold. In R. L. Terjung (ed.), *Exercise and Sport Sciences Reviews.* 10:49–83 (1982).

49. Kanaley, J. A., & R. A. Bioleau: The onset of the anaerobic threshold at three stages of physical maturity. *Journal of Sports Medicine and Physical Fitness.* 28(4):367–374 (1988).

50. Kapit, W., R. I. Macey, & E. Meisami: *The Physiology Coloring Book.* New York: Harper & Row (1987).

51. Kenney, R. A. *Physiology of Aging: A Synopsis.* Chicago: Year Book Medical (1982).

52. Kinderman, W., G. Simon, J. Keul: The significance of the aerobic-anaerobic transition for the determination of workload intensities during endurance training. *European Journal of Applied Physiology.* 42:25–34 (1979).

53. Klissouras, V.: Heritability of adaptive variation. *Journal of Applied Physiology.* 31(3):338–344 (1971).

54. Kohrt, W. M., R. J. Spina, A. A. Ehsani, P. E. Cryer, & J. O. Holloszy: Effects of age, adiposity, and fitness level on plasma catecholamine responses to standing and exercise. *Journal of Applied Physiology.* 75(4):1828–1835 (1993).

55. Komi, P. V., & J. Karlsson: Physical performance, skeletal muscle enzyme activities, and fibre types in monozygous and dizygous twins of both sexes. *Acta Physiologica Scandinavica* (Suppl.). 462:5–28 (1979).

56. Komi, P. V., V. Klissouras, & E. Karvinen: Genetic variation in neuromuscular performance. *Internationale Zeitschrift fur Angewandte Physiologie.* 31:289–304 (1973).

57. Mácek, M., & J. Vávra: Anaerobic threshold in children. In R. A. Binkhorst, H. C. G. Kemper, & W. H. M. Saris (eds.), *Children and Exercise XI.* Champaign, IL: Human Kinetics Publishers, 110–113 (1985).

58. Makrides, L., G. J. F. Heigenhauser, N. McCartney, & N. L. Jones: Maximal short term exercise capacity in healthy subjects aged 15–70 years. *Clinical Science.* 69:197–205 (1985).

59. Margaria, R., M. T. Edwards, & D. B. Dill: The possible mechanisms of contracting and paying the oxygen debt and the role of lactic acid in muscular contraction. *American Journal of Physiology.* 106:689–715 (1933).

60. Maud, P. J., & B. B. Shultz: Norms for the Wingate Anaerobic Test with comparison to another similar test. *Research Quarterly for Exercise and Sport.* 60(2):144–151 (1989).

61. McGrail, J. C., A. Bonen, & A. N. Belcastro: Dependence of lactate removal on muscle metabolism in man. *European Journal of Applied Physiology.* 39:87–97 (1978).

62. Newsholme, E. A., & A. R. Leech: *Biochemistry for the Medical Sciences.* New York: Wiley (1983).

63. Patton, J. F., & A. Duggan: An evaluation of tests of anaerobic power. *Aviation and Space Environmental Medicine.* 58:237–242 (1987).

64. Pitts, R. F.: *Physiology of the Kidney and Body Fluids* (3rd edition). Chicago: Year Book Medical (1974).

65. Poole, D. C., & G. A. Gaesser: Response of ventilatory and lactate threshold to continuous and interval training. *Journal of Applied Physiology.* 58(4):1115–1121 (1985).

66. Reinhard, V., P. H. Muller, & R. M. Schmulling: Determination of anaerobic threshold by the ventilation equivalent in normal individuals. *Respiration.* 38:36–42 (1979).

67. Reybrouck, T. M.: The use of the anaerobic threshold in pediatric exercise testing. In O. Bar-Or (ed.), *Advances in Pediatric Sport Sciences.* Champaign, IL: Human Kinetics Publishers (1989).

68. Robinson, S.: Experimental studies of physical fitness in relation to age. *Arbeitsphysiologie.* 10:251–323 (1938).

69. Rowland, T. W.: *Exercise and Children's Health.* Champaign, IL: Human Kinetics Publishers (1990).

70. Sahlin, K., J. M. Ren, & S. Broberg: Oxygen deficit at the onset of submaximal exercise is not due to a delayed oxygen transport. *Acta Physiologica Scandinavica.* 134:175–180 (1988).

71. Saris, W. H. M., A. M. Noordeloos, B. E. M. Ringnalda, M. A. Van't Hof, & R. A. Binkhorst: Reference values for aerobic power of healthy 4 to 18 year old Dutch children: Preliminary results. In R. A. Binkhorst, H. C. G. Kemper, & W. H. M. Saris (eds.), *Children and Exercise XI.* Champaign, IL: Human Kinetics Publishers, 151–160 (1985).

72. Shephard, R. J.: *Physical Activity and Growth.* Chicago: Year Book Medical (1982).

73. Sidney, K. H., & R. J. Shephard: Maximum and submaximum exercise tests in men and women in the seventh, eighth, and ninth decade of life. *Journal of Applied Physiology: Respiratory, Environmental and Exercise Physiology.* 43(2) 280–287 (1977).

74. Simoneau, J. A., G. Lortie, C. Leblanc, & C. Bouchard: Anaerobic alactacid work capacity in adopted and biological siblings. In R. M. Malina & C. Bouchard (eds.), *Sport and Human Genetics.* Champaign, IL: Human Kinetics Publishers, 165–171 (1986).

75. Skinner, J. S., & T. H. McLellan: The transition from aerobic to anaerobic metabolism. *Research Quarterly for Exercise and Sport.* 51(1):234–248 (1980).

76. Smith, E. L., & R. C. Serfass (eds.): *Exercise and Aging: The Scientific Basis.* Hillside, NJ: Enslow Publishers (1981).

77. Stainsby, W. N., & J. K. Barclay: Exercise metabolism: O_2 deficit, steady level O_2 uptake and O_2 uptake for recovery. *Medicine and Science in Sports.* 2(4):177–181 (1970).

78. Vandewalle, H., G. Pérès, & H. Monod: Standard anaerobic exercise tests. *Sports Medicine.* 4:268–289 (1987).

79. Wallace, J. P., G. Inbar, & K. Ernsthausen: Infant acceptance of postexercise breast milk. *Pediatrics.* 89(6): 1245–1247 (1992).

80. Wallace, J. P., & J. Rabin: The concentration of lactic acid in breast milk following maximal exercise. *International Journal of Sports Medicine.* 12(3):328–331 (1991).

81. Walsh, M. L., & E. W. Banister: Possible mechanisms of the anaerobic threshold: A review. *Sports Medicine.* 5:269–302 (1988).

82. Wasserman, K., & M. B. McIlroy: Detecting the threshold of anaerobic metabolism in cardiac patients during exercise. *American Journal of Cardiology.* 14:844–852 (1964).

83. Wasserman, K., B. J. Whipp, S. N. Koyal, & W. L. Beaver: Anaerobic threshold and respiratory gas exchange during exercise. *Journal of Applied Physiology.* 35:236–243 (1973).

84. Wells, C. L.: *Women, Sport and Performance: A Physiological Perspective* (2nd edition). Champaign, IL: Human Kinetics Publishers (1991).

85. Williams, J. R., N. Armstrong, & B. J. Kirby: The 4mM blood lactate level as an index of exercise performance in 11–13 year old children. *Journal of Sport Sciences.* 8:139–147 (1990).

11

Aerobic Metabolism During Exercise

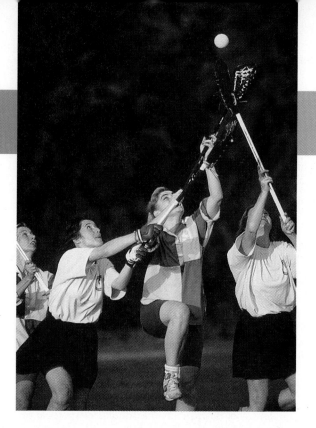

After studying the chapter, you should be able to:

- List and explain the major variables used to describe the aerobic metabolic response to exercise.

- Explain the laboratory and field assessment techniques used to obtain information on aerobic metabolism during exercise.

- Compare and contrast oxygen consumption during dynamic aerobic (a) short-term, light- to moderate-intensity exercise; (b) prolonged, moderate to heavy submaximal exercise; and (c) incremental exercise to maximum.

- Describe how the oxygen cost of breathing changes during exercise.

- Calculate the respiratory exchange ratio and interpret what it means in terms of energy substrate utilization.

- Compare and contrast lactate accumulation during short-term, light- to moderate-intensity exercise

and prolonged, moderate to heavy dynamic aerobic exercise.

- Calculate the metabolic cost of activity in both kilocalories and metabolic equivalents, and explain how each can be applied.

- Differentiate between gross efficiency, net efficiency, delta efficiency; differentiate between the efficiency and the economy of movement.

- List the ways in which an exercising individual can increase his or her efficiency.

- Compare the walking and running economy between children and young or middle-aged adults, and discuss the possible reasons for the differences.

- Explain why efficiency and economy are important to exercise performance.

- State the impact of genetics on aerobic metabolism during exercise.

Introduction

The previous chapter concentrated on anaerobic exercise responses. That is, it examined situations in which energy was provided predominately by the stored ATP-PC or by the production of ATP through anaerobic glycolysis. The chapter emphasized that during high-intensity, short-duration activity, carbohydrate was the only fuel used, lactate accumulated as a by-product, and no oxygen was required.

The preceding chapter also described the metabolic response to incremental work to maximum. In this situation the workload begins at low levels of intensity and progresses at regular intervals to the highest load possible. Incremental work to maximum typically lasts between 5 and 30 min, depending on the size of the increments and the fitness level of the exerciser. As the chapter pointed out, low workloads are primarily aerobic. But at some point, as the workload is raised, anaerobic metabolism becomes important, contributes significantly to the energy production in a way that, unfortunately, cannot be routinely measured, and results in a significant accumulation of lactate.

This chapter will concentrate on the aerobic portion of incremental work to maximum and on short- and long-duration submaximal work. Keep in mind throughout this chapter that aerobic metabolism predominates in activity lasting 3–5 min or longer but that the onset of all activity involves some amount of anaerobic metabolism during the oxygen deficit period. Excess postexercise oxygen consumption (EPOC) occurs following submaximal as well as maximal exercise.

Laboratory Measurement of Aerobic Metabolism

The primary goal of measuring aerobic metabolism is to quantify how much energy is necessary to complete a given activity. There are a couple of ways to approach this goal. To understand these approaches, consider two known aspects of aerobic metabolism: First, it requires oxygen; and second, it produces heat as a by-product. Therefore, aerobic metabolism can be assessed by measuring oxygen consumption or heat production. Oxygen consumption is measured by indirect open-circuit spirome-

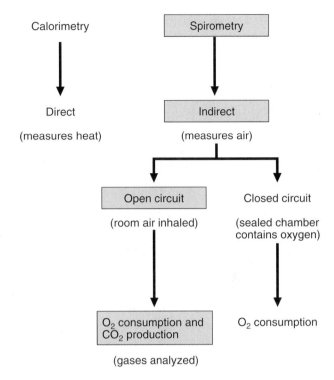

FIGURE 11.1

Measurement of Aerobic Metabolism

Aerobic metabolism can be measured by direct calorimetry or indirect spirometry. In exercise physiology open-circuit indirect spirometry, in which expired gases are analyzed for O_2 consumed and CO_2 produced, are typically used.

Note: Boxes indicate processes typically utilized in exercise physiology.

try, and heat production is measured by calorimetry, as summarized in Figure 11.1.

Calorimetry

The term *calorimetry* is derived from the word *calories*, the basic unit of heat energy. **Calorimetry** is the measurement of heat energy liberated or absorbed in metabolic processes. *Direct calorimetry* actually measures heat production. This measurement re-

---

Calorimetry The measurement of heat energy liberated or absorbed in metabolic processes.

quires the use of specially constructed chambers in which the heat produced by a subject increases the temperature of the air or water surrounding the walls and is thereby measured.

Accurate exercise data are difficult to obtain since exercise equipment, even if it fits into the usually small quarters, can also emit heat. In addition, the body may store heat (as evidenced by a rise in body temperature) and/or sweat (which must be accounted for). Despite these drawbacks, the direct measurement of heat is the most precise use of the term *calorimetry*.

Spirometry

Spirometry is an indirect calorimetry method for estimating heat production in which expired air is measured and analyzed for the amount of oxygen consumed and carbon dioxide produced. This method is based upon the fact that oxygen consumption at rest or during submaximal exercise, when expressed as calories, is equal to the heat produced by the body as measured by direct calorimetry. However, since heat is not measured directly, spirometry is an indirect measure. The oxygen consumption is also directly proportional to the aerobic production of ATP. The measurement of oxygen consumed is based upon the amount of air breathed. Spirometry is the measurement of air breathed.

In a *closed system* the subject breathes from a sealed container filled with gas of a designated composition (often 99.9% O_2). Expired CO_2 is usually absorbed by a chemical such as soda lime. The rate of utilization of the available O_2 is then determined. This system has a large error and is rarely used. It is mentioned here so that the terminology of an open circuit can be understood.

In *open-circuit spirometry* the subject inhales room or outdoor air from his or her surroundings and exhales into the same surroundings. The oxygen content of the inhaled air is normally 20.93%; the carbon dioxide does not need to be absorbed but

> **Spirometry** An indirect calorimetry method for estimating heat production or calorimetry in which expired air is measured and analyzed for the amount of oxygen consumed and carbon dioxide produced.

is simply exhaled into the surrounding atmosphere. A sample of the expired air is analyzed for oxygen and carbon dioxide content.

Putting these factors together results in the descriptor *open-circuit indirect spirometry*. The term *open-circuit indirect calorimetry* should be reserved for use when calories are calculated from oxygen consumption, but in fact it is often used interchangeably with *open-circuit indirect spirometry*.

Measuring O_2 consumption by open-circuit indirect spirometry is a valid way to assess aerobic metabolism during resting and steady-state submaximal exercise, conditions when the relationship between O_2 consumption and ATP production remains linear. However, in situations when anaerobic energy production is also involved, the actual energy cost of the exercise will be underestimated, because the linear relationship no longer exists and there is no way to account for the anaerobic portion.

Open-circuit indirect spirometry can be used to measure oxygen consumption during any physical activity. However, the size, sensitivity, and lack of portability of the equipment have limited its use to modalities that can be performed in a laboratory or a special swimming pool setup. By far the most popular exercise-testing modalities in the laboratory are the motor-driven treadmill and the cycle ergometer. Measurement can be done at rest, during submaximal exercise, or at maximal levels of exertion. The following section will describe in detail how this measurement is accomplished and, in so doing, will discuss the aerobic response to varying patterns of exercise.

*A*erobic Exercise Responses

Figure 11.2 shows an individual attached to an analysis system for open-circuit indirect spirometry. The individual interacts with the system through the breathing valve, which permits air to flow in only one direction at a time—in from room air and out toward the sampling chamber. The use of the noseclip ensures that all breathing is done through the mouth.

Oxygen Consumption and Carbon Dioxide Production

Figure 11.3 shows schematic configurations of an open-circuit system in which either the volume of

FIGURE 11.2

Subject Undergoing Assessment of Aerobic Metabolism During Exercise

inspired air (Figure 11.3a) or expired air (Figure 11.3b) is measured and the expired air is analyzed for the percentage of oxygen and carbon dioxide. Although oxygen consumption is the variable of primary interest, because of its direct relationship with ATP, determining the amount of carbon dioxide produced is also important, since that measure will enable us to determine information about fuel utilization and caloric expenditure.

Oxygen consumption ($\dot{V}O_2$) is the amount of oxygen taken up, transported, and used at the cellular level. It equals the amount of oxygen inspired minus the amount of oxygen expired. **Carbon dioxide produced ($\dot{V}CO_2$)** is the amount of carbon dioxide generated during metabolism, primarily from aerobic cellular respiration. It equals the amount of carbon dioxide expired minus the amount of carbon dioxide inspired. The amount of a gas equals the volume of air (either inhaled or exhaled) times the percentage of the gas. Therefore, to determine these amounts, we need to measure the volume of air either inhaled or exhaled and the percentages of oxygen and carbon dioxide in exhaled air. The percentages of oxygen and carbon dioxide in inhaled air are known to be 20.93% and 0.03%, respectively.

The mathematical relationships just described can be formulated as follows:

(11.1) oxygen consumption (L · min^{-1}) = [volume of air inspired (L · min^{-1}) × percentage of oxygen in inspired air] – [volume of air expired (L · min^{-1}) × percentage of oxygen in expired air]

or $\dot{V}O_2$ cons = $\dot{V}_I$ × % O_2 insp – $\dot{V}_E$ × % O_2 expir

(11.2) carbon dioxide produced (L · min^{-1}) = [volume of air expired (L · min^{-1}) × percentage of carbon dioxide in expired air] – [volume of air inspired × percentage of carbon dioxide in inspired air]

or $\dot{V}CO_2$ prod = $\dot{V}_E$ × % CO_2 expir – $\dot{V}_I$ × % CO_2 insp

Since the volume of air inhaled does not usually equal the volume of air exhaled, knowing either the value of air inhaled or exhaled and the gas percentages allows us to calculate the other air volume. These calculations are fully described in Appendix B.

Most laboratories use a computer programmed with software to solve Eqs. 11.1 and 11.2. Appendix B explains what is involved and how to do the computations manually. Table 11.1 gives the results of such a computer program for a metabolic test. The first 3 min represent resting values. The next 8 min were determined during treadmill walking at 3.5 mi · hr^{-1} (94 m · min^{-1}, or 5.6 km · hr^{-1}) at 7% grade. Ignore for the time being minutes 33 through 37 as well as the missing minutes. Locate in Figure 11.3, the pieces of equipment referred to as you follow the discussion of these variables. The dot above the volume symbol ($\dot{V}$) indicates per unit of time, which is usually 1 min.

The volume of air inspired ($\dot{V}_I$) or expired ($\dot{V}_E$) is measured by a pneumoscan or flowmeter (labeled as the dry-gas meter in Figure 11.3). Typically, all ventilation values are reported as expired values

Oxygen Consumption ($\dot{V}O_2$) The amount of oxygen taken up, transported, and used at the cellular level.

Carbon Dioxide Produced ($\dot{V}CO_2$) The amount of carbon dioxide generated during metabolism.

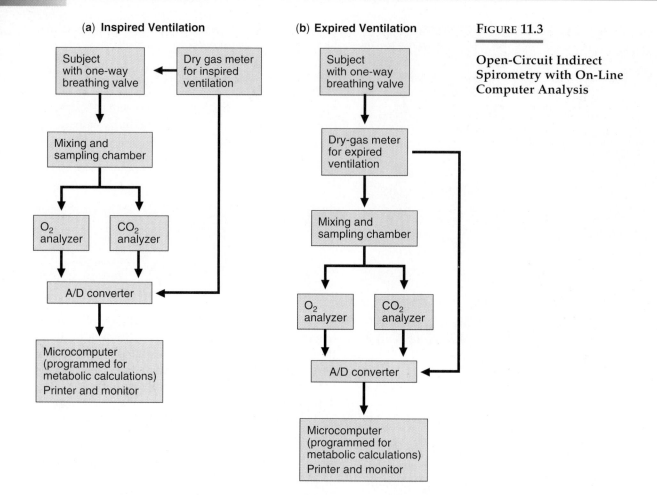

(a) Inspired Ventilation

(b) Expired Ventilation

FIGURE 11.3

Open-Circuit Indirect Spirometry with On-Line Computer Analysis

that have been adjusted to standard temperature (0°C), standard pressure (760 mmHg), and dry (without water vapor) conditions, known as STPD. The process and rationale for standardizing ventilatory volumes were discussed fully in Chapter 2. Standardization permits comparisons between data collected under different conditions. Two things should be noted about the $\dot{V}_E$ STPD values. First, the values for exercise (Ex) are higher than those at rest (R) ($\overline{X}R = 7.93$ L·min^{-1} $\overline{X}Ex = 25.41$). Second, within each condition the values are very stable.

The air the subject exhales is sampled from a mixing chamber and analyzed by electronic gas analyzers that have been previously calibrated by gases of known composition. Information regarding the percentage of expired oxygen ($O_2\%$ in Table 11.1) and CO_2 ($CO_2\%$ in Table 11.1) is relayed from the gas analyzers along with the ventilation values through an analog-to-digital (A/D) converter,

which gets the electronic signals in proper form to a microcomputer.

Remember that room air is composed of 20.93% O_2, 0.03% CO_2, and 79.4% N_2 and other trace elements such as argon and krypton. The N_2 component is considered to be inert in human metabolism. However, as we have seen in the metabolic pathways, O_2 is consumed when ATP is created aerobically and CO_2 is produced. Therefore, in general, the $O_2\%$ will decrease from values in ambient air and range somewhere around 15–16% during moderate exercise. The CO_2 values will be greater than those in room air, increasing to somewhere around 4–6% during moderate exercise. Note these values in Table 11.1. During rest not much oxygen is used, so the percentage exhaled is relatively high ($\overline{X}R = 17.09\%$). The accompanying $CO_2\%$ is, as would be expected, relatively low ($\overline{X}R = 3.28\%$). During the exercise portion more O_2 is being used to produce

TABLE 11.1 ■ Aerobic Metabolic Responses at Rest and During Submaximal Exercise

Sex = Female   Ambient Temperature = 18°C;

Age = 22 yr   Barometric Pressure = 752 mmHg;

Weight = 53.4 kg   Relative Humidity = 5%.

TIME (min)	$\dot{V}_E$ STPD (L·min^{-1})	$O_2\%$	$CO_2\%$	$\dot{V}O_2$ (L·min^{-1})	$\dot{V}CO_2$ (L·min^{-1})	$\dot{V}O_2$ (mL·kg^{-1}·min^{-1})	RER	HR (b·min^{-1})
REST (STANDING)								
1	7.57	17.11	3.26	0.3	0.23	5.61	0.81	75
2	7.58	17.21	3.2	0.29	0.23	5.43	0.82	75
3	8.64	16.95	3.37	0.34	0.28	6.55	0.8	75
$\overline{X}$	7.93	17.09	3.28	0.31	0.25	5.86	0.81	75
3.5 mi·hr^{-1} WALKING (STEADY STATE); 7% GRADE								
1	21.96	15.85	4.34	1.14	0.93	21.53	0.81	120
2	24.20	15.85	4.60	1.25	1.10	23.59	0.87	136
3	23.46	15.73	4.76	1.25	1.10	23.40	0.88	136
4	26.07	16.02	4.66	1.29	1.20	24.15	0.93	136
5	25.71	15.95	4.73	1.29	1.20	24.34	0.92	136
6	27.53	16.03	4.68	1.35	1.27	25.46	0.93	136
7	25.71	15.91	4.79	1.29	1.22	24.34	0.93	136
8	28.64	16.06	4.68	1.39	1.33	26.21	0.94	136
$\overline{X}$	25.41	15.93	4.66	1.28	1.17	24.13	0.90	136
3.5 mi·hr^{-1} WALKING (OXYGEN DRIFT); 7% GRADE								
33	28.64	16.26	4.56	1.33	1.29	25.09	0.96	140
34	31.21	16.33	4.55	1.43	1.41	26.96	0.98	144
35	31.21	16.32	4.54	1.43	1.39	26.96	0.97	144
36	30.84	16.16	4.67	1.47	1.43	27.71	0.96	146
37	32.31	16.19	4.68	1.52	1.50	28.65	0.97	150

This individual had a $\dot{V}O_2$max of 47.64 mL·kg^{-1}·min^{-1}, or 2.42 L·min^{-1}.

energy; therefore, there is a lower percentage of O_2 exhaled ($\overline{X}E$ = 15.93%). The use of more O_2 to create more energy also results in the production of more CO_2 ($\overline{X}Ex$ = 4.66%).

The computer uses a software program of metabolic formulas to correct ventilation for temperature (room temperature if V_I is measured; expired air temperature if V_E is measured), relative humidity (if V_I is measured), and barometric pressure. Then using the expired percentage values of O_2 and CO_2, it calculates values for the volume of O_2 consumed

($\dot{V}O_2$ L·min^{-1} and $\dot{V}O_2$ in mL·kg^{-1}·min^{-1}), CO_2 produced ($\dot{V}CO_2$ in L·min^{-1}), and the ratio of the volume of CO_2 produced divided by the volume of O_2 consumed, known as the respiratory exchange ratio (RER). Sometimes this relationship is designated simply as R but we will use RER throughout this text. The VO_2 and VCO_2 values are actual volumes of the gases that are used and produced by the body, respectively. The L·min^{-1} unit represents the absolute amount of gas on a per-minute basis. The mL·kg^{-1}·min^{-1} unit takes into account body size [the body weight (BW) is given at the top of the table], and hence is considered to be a relative value; that is, it describes how many milliliters of gas are consumed (or produced) for each kilogram of body weight each minute.

The absolute unit is highly influenced by body size, with large individuals showing the highest values. Therefore, it is most useful when comparing an individual to himself or herself under different conditions, such as before and after a training program, to determine if an improvement in fitness has occurred. Use of the absolute unit is particularly important if individuals have lost weight, because the $mL \cdot kg^{-1} \cdot min^{-1}$ value will go up as the weight goes down whether or not actual fitness has improved. The $mL \cdot kg^{-1} \cdot min^{-1}$ value, to an extent, equates individuals by factoring out the influence of body size. It is typically used for comparisons between individuals.

Another unit that can be used to express O_2 consumed and CO_2 produced on a relative basis is $mL \cdot kg \, FFB^{-1} \cdot min^{-1}$ or $mL \cdot kg \, LBM^{-1} \cdot min^{-1}$, where FFB stands for fat-free body and LBM stands for lean body mass. To calculate these units, percent body fat must be known and used to determine what portion of the total body weight is fat-free or lean. This unit is often used in comparisons between the sexes. However, it is not a very practical measure since no one has yet figured how to avoid carrying one's fat during exercise.

At rest the subject in the example in Table 11.1 is using about $0.31 \, L \cdot min^{-1}$, or $310 \, mL \cdot min^{-1}$, of oxygen and producing about $0.25 \, L \cdot min^{-1}$ of carbon dioxide. During exercise she is using $1.28 \, L \cdot min^{-1}$ of oxygen and producing $1.17 \, L \cdot min^{-1}$ of carbon dioxide.

Short-Term, Light- to Moderate-Intensity Submaximal Exercise

Look at minutes 1–8 in Table 11.1. During this light exercise there is very little minute-to-minute variation in any of the variables after the first minute of adjustment. A comparison of the mean oxygen cost of these 8 min ($24.13 \, mL \cdot kg^{-1} \cdot min^{-1}$) with her $\dot{V}O_2max$ ($47.64 \, mL \cdot kg^{-1} \cdot min^{-1}$) shows that the subject is working at approximately 50% $\dot{V}O_2max$. When the exercise performed is at less than 70% $\dot{V}O_2max$ and the duration is from 5 to 10 min, the oxygen consumption should level off and remain relatively constant for the duration of the work (Figure 11.4a). This condition is known as steady state or steady-rate exercise. The time to achieve steady state varies from 1 to 3 min in youths and young adults at low and moderate levels of intensity, but it will increase with higher-intensity exercise.[55] The time to achieve steady state increases in the elderly.

Prolonged, Moderate to Heavy Submaximal Exercise

Now look carefully at minutes 33 through 37 in Table 11.1. Pay particular attention to the $\dot{V}O_2 \, L \cdot min^{-1}$ and $mL \cdot kg^{-1} \cdot min^{-1}$ values. Despite the fact that the workload has not changed, a gradual increase is seen in these variables. When exercise is performed at a level greater than 70% $\dot{V}O_2max$; or when exercise is performed at a lower percentage of $\dot{V}O_2max$, as in this case, but for a long duration; or if the conditions are hot and humid, a phenomenon known as **oxygen drift** occurs. In oxygen drift the oxygen consumption increases despite the fact that the oxygen requirement of the activity has not changed. A schematic representation of oxygen drift is presented in Figure 11.4b.

The oxygen consumption increases (drifts upward) because of rising blood levels of catecholamines (epinephrine and norepinephrine), lactate accumulation (if the % $\dot{V}O_2$ is high enough), shifting substrate utilization (to greater carbohydrate), increased cost of ventilation, and increased body temperature. Thus, although any given level of exercise typically requires a specific amount of oxygen, this amount will show some individual and circumstantial variation.[32]

Incremental Exercise to Maximum

Table 11.2 provides the results of a computer program for an incremental treadmill test to maximum. In this case the subject was a very fit male senior exercise science major who regularly and successfully competed in long-distance running, cycling, and duathlon events. In an incremental exercise test such as this the subject is asked to continue to the

---

Oxygen Drift A situation that occurs in submaximal activity of long duration, or above 70% $\dot{V}O_2max$, or in hot and humid conditions where the oxygen consumption increases, despite the fact that the oxygen requirement of the activity has not changed.

FIGURE 11.4

Oxygen Consumption Responses to Various Exercises

(a) Short-duration, light to moderate, steady-state dynamic aerobic exercise. (b) Long-duration, moderate to heavy, submaximal dynamic aerobic exercise. (c) Incremental dynamic aerobic exercise to maximum.

point of volitional fatigue—that is, until he is too tired to go on any longer. Throughout the test the speed and/or grade is systematically raised so that the exercise becomes progressively harder. The protocol used for this particular test is called the modi-

fied Balke. For this test the speed is kept constant at 3.5 mi·hr⁻¹ (94 m·min⁻¹). The grade is 0% for the first minute and 2% for the second minute; it increases 1% per minute thereafter. Because the increments are small, the individual should be able to adjust to the load in just 1 min for most of the submaximal portion. This subject was able to continue for 28 min.

Because the work is different, the ventilation, $\dot{V}O_2$, and $\dot{V}CO_2$ responses are also different from those of the submaximal steady-state exercise in Table 11.1. In the incremental task ventilation, $\dot{V}O_2$, and $\dot{V}CO_2$ values all increase as a result of the increasing demands for and production of energy. For this particular subject the volume of expired air ($\dot{V}_E$ STPD) rose from 25.21 L·min⁻¹ at minute 2 to 139.04 L·min⁻¹ at minute 28. This result demonstrates the reserve capacity in the ventilatory system. Oxygen consumption increased from slightly over 1 L·min⁻¹ (or almost 17 mL·kg⁻¹·min⁻¹) to just over 5 L·min⁻¹ at maximum. At this point the subject was producing as much ATP as he could aerobically. The highest amount of oxygen an individual can take in, transport, and utilize to produce ATP aerobically while breathing air during heavy exercise is **maximal oxygen consumption ($\dot{V}O_2$max).**

The exercise tester has to decide whether any given test truly is a maximal effort before labeling the highest $\dot{V}O_2$ value as maximal. Several criteria can be used to decide if test results represent a maximal test. One was mentioned in the previous chapter: a lactate value greater than 8 mmol·L⁻¹.[7,8] Here you do not have that information. A second is really a cardiovascular criterion: a HR ± 12–15 b·min⁻¹ of predicted maximal heart rate (220 – age). A third is whether a plateau occurred in the oxygen values. Such a plateau is defined as a rise of 2.1 mL·kg⁻¹·min⁻¹ or less, or a rise of 0.15 L·min⁻¹ or less, in oxygen consumption ($\dot{V}O_2$) with an increase in workload.[75] Did this subject meet the HR and $\dot{V}O_2$ criteria for a true maximal test? Check the answers at the end of the chapter to see if you are correct (number 1).

Maximal Oxygen Consumption ($\dot{V}O_2$max) The highest amount of oxygen an individual can take in and utilize to produce ATP aerobically while breathing air during heavy exercise.

TABLE 11.2 ▪ **Aerobic Metabolic Responses During an Incremental Treadmill Test (Modified Balke Protocol)**

Sex = Male   Ambient Temperature = 23°C

Age = 22 yr   Barometric Pressure = 739 mmHg

Weight = 66 kg   Relative Humidity = 13%

TIME (min)	$\dot{V}_E$ STPD	$O_2\%$	$CO_2\%$	$\dot{V}O_2$ (L·min^{-1})	$\dot{V}O_2$ (mL·kg^{-1}·min^{-1})	$\dot{V}CO_2$ (L·min^{-1})	RER	HR (b·min^{-1})
2	25.21	16.47	4.45	1.12	16.96	1.10	0.99	82
3	27.31	16.36	4.54	1.25	18.93	1.22	0.98	84
4	29.06	16.30	4.62	1.33	20.30	1.30	0.98	100
5	29.75	16.18	4.71	1.41	21.36	1.39	0.98	98
6	33.62	16.09	4.84	1.62	24.54	1.60	0.99	108
7	30.17	16.08	4.99	1.45	21.96	1.49	1.03	105
8	34.37	15.99	5.03	1.68	25.45	1.72	1.01	120
9	37.92	16.09	5.03	1.81	27.42	1.89	1.04	117
10	37.17	16.07	4.96	1.79	27.12	1.83	1.02	115
11	38.84	15.89	5.00	1.95	29.69	1.93	0.98	123
12	39.56	15.82	5.10	2.01	30.60	2.00	0.99	122
13	39.84	15.57	5.23	2.15	32.57	2.07	0.96	124
14	43.37	15.51	5.30	2.36	35.75	2.28	0.96	132
15	46.64	15.62	5.41	2.45	37.27	2.50	1.01	144
16	47.37	15.68	5.42	2.45	37.27	2.54	1.03	138
17	50.87	15.85	5.21	2.55	38.78	2.62	1.02	143
18	51.53	15.52	5.48	2.78	42.12	2.80	1.01	146
19	55.12	15.73	5.38	2.83	42.87	2.95	1.03	155
20	56.84	15.74	5.32	2.91	44.24	3.00	1.02	158
21	58.54	15.63	5.38	3.08	46.81	3.12	1.01	162
22	59.95	15.58	5.43	3.19	48.33	3.23	1.01	167
23	68.06	15.59	5.47	3.61	54.69	3.70	1.02	180
24	78.06	15.69	5.55	4.01	60.90	4.30	1.07	181
25	85.18	15.70	5.62	4.36	66.21	4.75	1.08	188
26	94.24	15.78	5.75	4.68	71.06	5.39	1.14	192
27	112.96	16.29	5.51	4.98	75.45	6.18	1.24	196
28	139.04	16.97	4.94	5.11	77.52	6.83	1.34	200

The rectilinear increase in $\dot{V}O_2$ can be generalized to all healthy individuals whether they are male or female, young or old, high or low in terms of fitness. This pattern is schematically represented in Figure 11.4c. However, the plateau is not always evident in children and the elderly. In these cases the term *peak oxygen consumption* ($\dot{V}O_2$peak) to describe the highest value attained is more accurate than the term *maximal oxygen consumption* ($\dot{V}O_2$max).

As a result of the increasing ATP production, the amount of CO_2 produced also increases. Note in Table 11.2 that the amount of CO_2 produced ($\dot{V}CO_2$) is generally not equal to the amount of O_2 consumed ($\dot{V}O_2$). Note also that despite the incremental nature of this test, the $O_2\%$ and $CO_2\%$ do not vary much. There is a slight decline in $O_2\%$ and a parallel rise in $CO_2\%$ after the first 10 min and then relatively steady values until the last 2 min, when the $O_2\%$ goes back up and the $CO_2\%$ goes back down just a little. Frequently, as a subject nears maximal exertion, the $O_2\%$ may rise to 17% and the $CO_2\%$ may drop to 3%. These small percentage changes, especially when they occur in the last couple of minutes, are compensated for by the increasingly larger volumes of air being ventilated.

Static and Dynamic-Resistance Exercise

Physiological responses to static exercise are generally described in relation to the percentage of maximal voluntary contraction (MVC) at which they take place. Depending on the muscle group involved, static contractions below 15–25% MVC do not fully occlude blood flow, and so oxygen can be delivered to working muscles. At such loads, however, little extra energy above resting level is required, and oxygen consumption increases minimally, perhaps as little as 50 mL · min⁻¹, but for as long as half an hour.[5,71]

The higher the % MVC of the static contraction, the greater the intramuscular pressure is, the more likely it is that the blood flow will be completely arrested or occluded, and the shorter the time that the contraction can be maintained. If, despite an MVC of 30% or greater, occlusion of blood flow is not complete, an increase in oxygen consumption occurs. This increased oxygen consumption is higher than the amount at lower percentages of MVC but still far below the rise in values that occurs during the aerobic endurance exercises previously described.

In addition to a lower oxygen consumption, there is one other major difference between static and dynamic endurance exercise. At the cessation of static exercise, when blood flow is fully restored, a sudden increase in oxygen consumption is seen (Figure 11.5) before the slow, gradual decline of the typical EPOC curve begins.[5,71]

The primary source of energy for dynamic-resistance activity such as weight lifting or wrestling is anaerobic.[37,38] In part, anaerobic energy is used because dynamic-resistance exercise has a static component to it. In part, anaerobic energy is used due to the high intensity and short duration of the exercise. Despite the predominance of anaerobic energy sources, there is an aerobic component to dynamic-resistance activity as well. As mentioned

in the previous chapter, even the most widely used anaerobic test, the Wingate Anaerobic Test, has an aerobic energy contribution of almost 30%.[11] The more the repetitions and the longer the duration of the sets in a weight-lifting workout, the greater will be the aerobic contribution. Actual values are not available for different routines because such activities are intended for anaerobic, not aerobic, benefits. Undoubtedly, however, the oxygen costs of weight-lifting routines are less than the oxygen costs of most aerobic endurance activities but higher than the cost of purely static exercise.

The Oxygen Cost of Breathing

Part of the oxygen used both at rest and during exercise goes to support the respiratory muscles. This value does not remain constant but varies with the intensity of activity. During rest the respiratory system uses about 1–2% of the total body oxygen consumption, or 2.5 mL · min⁻¹ of oxygen. The oxygen cost of ventilation is higher in children than in adults and the elderly.[10,60]

During light to moderate submaximal dynamic aerobic exercise, where $\dot{V}_E$ is less than 60 L · min⁻¹, the respiratory oxygen cost changes minimally to, at most, about 25–100 mL · min⁻¹. At heavy submaximal exercise, where $\dot{V}_E$ is anywhere from 60 to 120 L · min⁻¹, respiratory oxygen use may rise from 50 to 400 mL · min⁻¹. During incremental exercise to maximum, the initial $\dot{V}_E$ during the lower exercise stages shows a very gradual curvilinear rise, reflecting the submaximal changes described previously. At workloads above those requiring a $\dot{V}_E$ greater than 120 L · min⁻¹, a dramatic exponential curve occurs. In this curve, by the time a $\dot{V}_E$ of 180 L · min⁻¹ is achieved in a very fit individual, 1000–1300 mL · min⁻¹ of oxygen is used simply to support respiration.[60]

There may be a theoretical maximal level of ventilation above which any further increase in oxygen consumption would be used entirely by the ventilatory musculature.[23,58,60] Precisely where this critical level of ventilation occurs is unknown. However, even if there is no such thing as a critical ventilation level, respiration does utilize a significant portion, 3–13%, of the $\dot{V}O_2$ during heavy exercise.[23,70] Smoking increases the oxygen cost of respiration during exercise. However, even an abstinence of just one day can substantially reduce this effect of cigarette smoking.[65,71] In old age the oxygen cost of breathing

FIGURE 11.5

Respiratory and Metabolic Responses to Heavy Static Exercise

Heavy static exercise causes small respiratory (a-vO$_2$ diff and $\dot{V}_E$) and metabolic ($\dot{V}O_2$ and RER) responses during the actual contraction. However, each of these variables exhibits an increased rebound effect immediately upon cessation of the exercise before slowly returning to pre-exercise values.

Source: E. Asmussen. Similarities and dissimilarities between static and dynamic exercise. *Circulation Research* (Suppl.). 48(6): I-3–I-10 (1981). Copyright 1981 by the American Heart Association. Reprinted by permission.

may be a significant factor in limiting exercise performance.[71]

Respiratory Quotient/Respiratory Exchange Ratio

Once the $\dot{V}O_2$ consumed and $\dot{V}CO_2$ produced during exercise are known, a great deal of useful information can be derived. One such derived variable is given in both Table 11.1 and Table 11.2: RER, or respiratory exchange ratio.

> **Respiratory Quotient (RQ)** The ratio of the amount of carbon dioxide produced divided by the amount of oxygen consumed at the cellular level.

The RER reflects on a total body level what is happening at the cellular level. The ratio of the amount of carbon dioxide (CO_2) produced to the amount of oxygen consumed (O_2) at the cellular level is termed the **respiratory quotient (RQ).** The formula is

(11.3) respiratory quotient = carbon dioxide produced (molecules) ÷ oxygen consumed (molecules)

or
$$RQ = \frac{CO_2}{O_2}$$

This formula may also be computed using liters per gram in place of molecules.

The values of carbon dioxide produced and oxygen consumed are known for the oxidation of carbohydrate, fat, and protein, both on a chemical or molecular level and in absolute amounts ($L \cdot g^{-1}$). The latter values are presented in Table 11.3. The amount of oxygen consumed and the amount of carbon dioxide produced vary between the major fuel sources because of differences in the chemical composition of the fuels. The examples that follow compute the cellular level RQ for each major fuel source both per mole of a specific substrate (the carbohydrate, glucose, $C_6H_{12}O_6$; the fat, palmitic acid, $C_{16}H_{32}O_2$; and the protein, albumin, $C_{72}H_{112}N_2O_{22}S$), and per gram of carbohydrate (glucose), fat (fatty acid) as well as total protein and branched chain amino acids. In each case the oxygen used (left side of the equation) and carbon dioxide produced (right side of the equation) is inserted into Eq. 11.3 to determine RQ.

■ EXAMPLE

For carbohydrates:
Glucose (per mole)

$$C_6H_{12}O_6 + 6O_2 \rightarrow 6CO_2 + 6H_2O + \text{energy}$$

$$RQ = \frac{6CO_2}{6O_2} = 1.0$$

Glucose (per gram, from Table 11.3):

$$1 \text{ g glucose} + 0.75 \text{ L O}_2 \rightarrow 0.75 \text{ L CO}_2$$
$$+ H_2O + 3.75 \text{ kcal}$$

$$RQ = \frac{0.75 \text{ L CO}_2}{0.75 \text{ L O}_2} = 1.0$$

For fat:
Palmitic acid (per mole)

$$C_{16}H_{32}O_2 + 23O_2 \rightarrow 16CO_2 + 15H_2O + \text{energy}$$

$$RQ = \frac{16 \text{ CO}_2}{23 \text{ O}_2} = 0.7$$

Fatty acids (per gram, from Table 11.3)

$$1 \text{ g fatty acid} + 2.02 \text{ L O}_2 \rightarrow 1.43 \text{ L CO}_2$$
$$+ H_2O + 9.3 \text{ kcal}$$

$$RQ = \frac{1.43 \text{ L CO}_2}{2.02 \text{ L O}_2} = 0.71$$

TABLE 11.3 ■ Energy Production from Carbohydrate, Fats, and Protein

	CARBOHYDRATE		PROTEIN		FAT
Primary utilization in exercise	High-intensity, short-duration exercise		Ultradistance exercise and glucose precursor		Low-intensity, long-duration exercise and glucose precursor
Form in which utilized by muscles	Glucose	Glycogen	*	Branched-chain amino acids	Fatty acids
Oxygen needed to utilize per gram ($L \cdot g^{-1}$)	$0.75 \text{ L} \cdot g^{-1}$	$0.83 \text{ L} \cdot g^{-1}$	$0.965 \text{ L} \cdot g^{-1}$	$1.24 \text{ L} \cdot g^{-1}$	$2.02 \text{ L} \cdot g^{-1}$
Energy produced per gram ($kcal \cdot g^{-1}$)	$3.75 \text{ kcal} \cdot g^{-1}$ $15.68 \text{ kJ} \cdot g^{-1}$	$4.17 \text{ kcal} \cdot g^{-1}$ $17.43 \text{ kJ} \cdot g^{-1}$	$4.3 \text{ kcal} \cdot g^{-1}$ $17.97 \text{ kJ} \cdot g^{-1}$	$3.76 \text{ kcal} \cdot g^{-1}$ $18.09 \text{ kJ} \cdot g^{-1}$	$9.3 \text{ kcal} \cdot g^{-1}$ $38.87 \text{ kJ} \cdot g^{-1}$
Energy produced per liter of oxygen ($kcal \cdot L\,O_2^{-1}$)	$5.03 \text{ kcal} \cdot L\,O_2^{-1}$ $21.03 \text{ kJ} \cdot L\,O_2^{-1}$	$5.03 \text{ kcal} \cdot L\,O_2^{-1}$ $21.03 \text{ kJ} \cdot L\,O_2^{-1}$	$4.46 \text{ kcal} \cdot L\,O_2^{-1}$ $18.64 \text{ kJ} \cdot L\,O_2^{-1}$	$3.03 \text{ kcal} \cdot L\,O_2^{-1}$ $12.67 \text{ kJ} \cdot L\,O_2^{-1}$	$4.61 \text{ kcal} \cdot L\,O_2^{-1}$ $19.27 \text{ kJ} \cdot L\,O_2^{-1}$
Carbon dioxide produced ($L \cdot g^{-1}$)	$0.75 \text{ L} \cdot g^{-1}$	$0.83 \text{ L} \cdot g^{-1}$	$0.781 \text{ L} \cdot g^{-1}$	$0.92 \text{ L} \cdot g^{-1}$	$1.43 \text{ L} \cdot g^{-1}$

*Values for protein are given. However, the BCAA values are more realistic for muscle activity per 1 g PRO = 1.17 g AA.[55, 62]

For protein:
Albumin (per mole)

$$C_{72}H_{112}N_2O_{22}S + 77O_2 \rightarrow 63CO_2 + 38H_2O$$
$$+ SO_3 + 9CO(NH_2) \text{ (urea)}$$

$$RQ = \frac{63CO_2}{77O_2} = 0.82$$

Protein (per gram, from Table 11.3)

$$1 \text{ g protein} + 0.965 \text{ L O}_2 \rightarrow 0.781 \text{ L CO}_2$$
$$+ H_2O + 4.3 \text{ kcal}$$

$$RQ = \frac{0.781 \text{ L CO}_2}{0.965 \text{ L O}_2} = 0.81$$

Note that if the branched-chain amino acids are used, the RQ would be lower:

$$1 \text{ g BCAA} + 1.24 \text{ L O}_2 \rightarrow 0.92 \text{ L CO}_2$$
$$+ H_2O + 3.76 \text{ kcal}$$

$$RQ = \frac{0.92 \text{ L CO}_2}{1.24 \text{ L O}_2} = 0.74$$

The values of 1.0 for carbohydrate, 0.7 for fat, and 0.81 for protein are the classic accepted values for RQ. ∎

Since these values for RQ have been derived from the cellular oxidation of specific foodstuffs, knowing the RQ allows one to estimate the fuels utilized. However, individuals do not often use only one fuel; thus, the "classic values" are rarely seen. Therefore, in a resting individual an RQ of 0.93 indicates a high reliance on carbohydrate, and an RQ of 0.75 indicates a high reliance on fat. An RQ of 0.82 indicates either a fasting individual burning protein (usually from muscle mass, if in a starvation situation) or more likely, an individual using a normal mixed diet of all three fuels. Remember that protein is not normally used as a major fuel source, especially at rest.

Although these interpretations are acceptable in the resting individual, there are several difficulties with the RQ and its meaning during exercise. In the first place, the O_2 and CO_2 values measured in open-circuit indirect spirometry are ventilatory measures that are indicative of total body gas exchange and not just working muscle. Second, anything that causes hyperventilation will cause an excess of CO_2 to be exhaled, thus falsely elevating the ratio. This result is often seen in stress situations in anticipation of an exercise test or in early recovery from maximal work. Third, if exercise is of a high enough intensity to involve anaerobic metabolism, causing an increase in acidity (a decrease in pH) and a concomitant rise in nonmetabolic CO_2 release, RQ no longer represents just fuel utilization. Values during exercise, especially as an individual approaches maximal effort, usually exceed 1.0. In this case the assumption is that the fuel source is carbohydrate and the excess CO_2 is a result of anaerobic metabolism. Conversely, after an initial increase during recovery, CO_2 is retained, causing low values.[56] For these reasons the term **respiratory exchange ratio (RER)** is a more accurate one than RQ to describe the ratio of $\dot{V}CO_2$ produced to $\dot{V}O_2$ consumed when determined by open-circuit spirometry.

This involvement of anaerobic metabolism that results in RER values greater than 1.0 allows us to use RER as an additional criterion to determine whether an exercise test was truly maximal. The criterion for a true maximal test is an RER greater than 1.1 or at least 1.0.[50]

Although changing the name from RQ to RER is a more accurate description, RER values still do not enable us to distinguish between different forms of a fuel, such as glucose, glycogen, fatty acids, or ketone bodies. Also, when only ventilatory CO_2 and O_2 are measured, there is no indication of protein utilization. In order to measure protein utilization, we must measure the amount of nitrogen excreted (in urine and sweat). This task is, at best, a cumbersome one and, at worst, almost impossible to do in exercise situations.[22, 27] Thus, the RER that is measured by the $\dot{V}CO_2 \text{ L} \cdot \text{min}^{-1} \div \dot{V}O_2 \cdot \text{L} \cdot \text{min}^{-1}$ during exercise is a nonprotein RER. Again, since protein is not thought to be utilized as a fuel until long-duration activity is in progress, this simplification is not deemed to materially affect the relative percentage of carbohydrate and fat utilization in most situations.

Table 11.4 presents the relative percentages of calories used from carbohydrate and fat for all RER values between 0.7 and 1.0.[24] Referring to Table 11.1,

Respiratory Exchange Ratio (RER) The ratio of the volume of CO_2 produced divided by the volume of O_2 consumed.

TABLE 11.4 ■ **Percentage of Calories from Carbohydrate (CHO) and Fat and the Caloric Equivalents for Nonprotein RER Values for Each Liter of Oxygen Used**

RER	CHO%	FAT%	CALORIC EQUIVALENT (kcal · L O_2^{-1})	RER	CHO%	FAT%	CALORIC EQUIVALENT (kcal · L O_2^{-1})
0.70	0.0	100.0	4.686	0.86	52.4	47.6	4.875
0.71	1.4	98.6	4.690	0.87	55.8	44.2	4.887
0.72	4.8	95.2	4.702	0.88	59.2	40.8	4.899
0.73	8.2	91.8	4.714	0.89	62.6	37.4	4.911
0.74	11.6	88.4	4.727	0.90	66.0	34.0	4.924
0.75	15.0	85.0	4.739	0.91	69.4	30.6	4.936
0.76	18.4	81.6	4.751	0.92	72.8	27.2	4.948
0.77	21.8	78.2	4.764	0.93	76.2	23.8	4.961
0.78	25.2	74.8	4.776	0.94	79.6	20.4	4.973
0.79	28.6	71.4	4.788	0.95	83.0	17.0	4.985
0.80	32.0	68.0	4.801	0.96	86.4	13.6	4.998
0.81	35.4	64.6	4.813	0.97	89.8	10.2	5.010
0.82	38.8	61.2	4.825	0.98	93.2	6.8	5.022
0.83	42.2	57.8	4.838	0.99	96.6	3.4	5.035
0.84	45.6	54.4	4.850	1.00	100.0	0.0	5.047
0.85	49.0	51.0	4.862				

Source: Modified from T. M. Carpenter. *Tables, Factors, and Formulas for Computing Respiratory Exchange and Biological Transformations of Energy* (4th ed.). Washington, D.C.: Carnegie Institution of Washington, Publication 303C (1964). Reprinted by permission.

we see that during rest the individual in the example had an RER of 0.81. From Table 11.4 this value means that 35.4% of her fuel was carbohydrate and 64.6% fat at that time. During her 8 min of steady-state work the RER averaged 0.90, indicating a major shift in fuel supply. At that RER 66% of the fuel was carbohydrate and 34% fat.

During the last 5-min interval (minutes 33–37 in Table 11.1), we see an even greater reliance on carbohydrate with almost 90% of the energy used being supplied by carbohydrate sources. If submaximal exercise were to continue for another 2 hr or more, the RER values would drop back down, indicating a depletion of available carbohydrate fuel stores. How low the RER values would go depends on the amount of carbohydrate originally stored, as well as the exact intensity and duration of the activity. For this reason, athletes often try to carbohydrate load prior to endurance events so that carbohydrate stores are initially high and will last

longer. Carbohydrate loading is fully discussed in Chapter 13.

Now look at Table 11.2. Determine the approximate percentages of carbohydrate and fat used at minutes 2, 14, and 28. Check your answer (number 2 at the end of the chapter) to see if you are correct. These early minute RER values are higher than expected for the workload, probably from hyperventilation in anticipation of the maximal effort to come in the exercise test. The last three RER values are greater than 1.1 and indicate the involvement of anaerobic metabolism.

Lactate Changes

Lactate levels in response to exercise depend primarily on the intensity of the exercise. Figure 11.6 depicts what occurs in both short-term and long-term low-intensity submaximal dynamic aerobic activity. During the first 3 min of such steady-state work the lactate (La⁻) level rises (Figure 11.6a). This increase reflects the lactate accumulated during the oxygen deficit.[42] When a very similar workload is continued for 60 min, the lactate level remains unchanged after the initial rise (Figure 11.6b). As explained in the previous chapter, the reason for this result lies in the balance between lactate production (the rate of lactate appearance) and lactate clearance (the rate of lactate disappearance).

Figure 11.7 shows the results from a study that directly measured the rate of lactate appearance (R_a) and the rate of lactate disappearance (R_d) by radioactive tracers as well as the blood levels of lactate concentration ([La⁻]).[19] In the transition from rest to steady-state submaximal exercise the rate of both lactate appearance and lactate disappearance increased. During the next 30 min of exercise the turnover rate was higher than at rest. The result was an initial increase in [La⁻], which declined after 5

FIGURE 11.7

The Impact of the Rates of Lactate Appearance and Disappearance on Lactate Accumulation during Light and Heavy Submaximal Aerobic Exercise

During light (700 kgm · min⁻¹ submaximal aerobic exercise, the rate of lactate disappearance (R_d) (left Y axis) lags behind the rate of lactate appearance (R_a) (left Y axis) to a small extent, but then catches up so that the 30-min lactate concentration [La⁻] value (right Y axis) approximates rest. During heavy submaximal exercise (minutes 30–45) the R_d lags behind R_a and [La⁻] increases.

Source: G. A. Brooks. Anaerobic threshold: Review of the concept and directions for further research. *Medicine and Science in Sports and Exercise.* 17(1): 22–31 (1985). Reprinted by permission.

FIGURE 11.6

Lactate Accumulation during Short- and Long-Term Dynamic Aerobic Constant Submaximal Work

After an initial rise in accumulation during the oxygen deficit period (a), lactate levels off and remains relatively constant during long duration submaximal aerobic work (b).

Source: Based on data from Freund et al.[39]

min of activity to almost resting levels by 30 min. When the workload was increased, the rate of clearance (R_d) was no longer able to keep up with the rate of production (R_a), and the lactate concentration in the blood [La⁻] showed a sharp increase.

Figure 11.8 shows how lactate level varies with competitive distance in highly trained male runners. At the shorter distances the predominant energy source is anaerobic, and the anticipated high lactate values are seen. As the distance increases and more of the energy is supplied aerobically, the intensity that can be maintained decreases. As a result, lactate also decreases, doing so in a negative exponential curvilinear pattern. By approximately 30 km (18 mi) the lactate levels are no different than they are at rest.

The importance of the intensity of exercise, even at the marathon distance, is illustrated in Figure

FIGURE 11.8

Lactate Accumulation Resulting from Increasing Distances of Competitive Running Races

Blood lactate accumulation shows an inverse curvilinear relationship with distance in running races.

Source: D. L. Costill. Metabolic responses during distance running. *Journal of Applied Physiology.* 28(3): 251–255 (1970). Reprinted by permission of the American Physiological Society.

11.9. Two groups of runners were equated according to their $\dot{V}O_2$max. One group ran a simulated marathon on the treadmill at 73.3% $\dot{V}O_2$max (in 2 hr 45 min or less); the other group ran the same distance but at 64.5% $\dot{V}O_2$max (in 3 hr 45 min or slightly less). Within the slow group blood lactate values remained relatively stable and at a level considered to be within normal resting amounts. The blood lactate levels in the fast group were significantly higher throughout the marathon than those of the slow group. As absolutes, however, both sets of values were barely above normal resting levels.

In general, during light to moderate work (that is, less than 50–60% of $\dot{V}O_2$max), the blood lactate level is likely to rise slightly at first. Then it either will remain the same or will decrease slightly, even if the exercise lasts 30–60 min.

At moderate to heavy intensities between 50 and 85% $\dot{V}O_2$max (depending on the genetic characteristics and training status of the individual), lactate levels will elevate rapidly during the first 5–10 min of exercise. If the workload continues for more than 10 min, the lactate level may continue to rise,

FIGURE 11.9

Blood Lactate Accumulation during the Marathon

Blood lactate accumulation during a fast marathon (2 hr and 45 min or less) was greater than the accumulation during a slow marathon (3 hr and 45 min or less). The lactate levels for the slow marathoners never exceeded normal resting levels and the lactate levels for the fast marathoners barely exceeded normal resting levels.

Source: M. J. O'Brien, C. A. Viguie, R. S. Mazzeo, & G. A. Brooks. Carbohydrate dependence during marathon running. *Medicine and Science in Sports Exercise.* 25 (9): 1009–1017 (1993). Reprinted by permission.

may stabilize, or may decline, depending on the individual and other conditions.

Table 11.5 summarizes the oxygen consumption, RER energy substrate, and lactate responses to dynamic aerobic endurance exercise.

Estimation of Caloric Intake and Expenditure

Table 11.3 not only shows the oxygen consumed and carbon dioxide produced when each of the energy substrates is utilized, but it also indicates the potential energy in terms of kilocalories per gram (kcal · g^{-1}) or kilocalories per liter of oxygen (kcal · L O$_2$$^{-1}$) for each substrate. The kcal · L O$_2$$^{-1}$ figures show that carbohydrates are most efficient in the use of oxygen to provide energy, followed by fat,

TABLE 11.5 ■ **Aerobic Exercise Responses**

EXERCISE	O$_2$ CONSUMPTION	RER	LACTATE
Short-term (5–10 min), light-to-moderate intensity submaximal exercise	Increases until energy needs are met and then levels off	Increases over rest	Slight increase at onset of any exercise, barely above resting levels
Long-term (5–10 min to hours) or high-intensity (greater than 70% VO$_2$max) submaximal exercise	Increases until energy needs are met and then levels off at least temporarily; oxygen drift usually occurs	Increases over rest; the higher the intensity, the higher the RER; if duration is long enough, RER will decrease as CHO supplies are depleted	May rise slightly, stay the same, or decrease slightly; close to resting values
Incremental exercise to maximum	Increases in a rectilinear pattern proportional to the workload; plateaus at maximum	Increases in general rectilinear fashion; maximal values should be greater than 1.0	Curvilinear accumulation to high levels greater than 8 mmol · min^{-1}

and finally by protein. However, there really is not a great deal of variation among the substrates.

The potential energy for carbohydrate and for protein depends on whether the form is glucose (3.75 kcal · g^{-1}) or glycogen (4.17 kcal · g^{-1}), all amino acids (4.3 kcal · g^{-1}) or just the branched-chain amino acids (3.76 kcal · g^{-1}). When food is ingested, these distinctions cannot be made; and the net average energy values are rounded to the whole numbers of 4 kcal · g^{-1} for carbohydrate and protein and 9 kcal · g^{-1} for fat. These values are called *Atwater factors* and are used to represent the energy potential of food. From the known values of VO$_2$ L · min^{-1} and RER it is possible to compute the kilocalorie (or kilojoule) energy expenditure.

Table 11.4 presents the **caloric equivalent**—the number of kilocalories produced per liter of oxygen consumed—for all values of RER between 0.7 and 1.0. The kilocalories produced per liter of oxygen

(kcal · LO$_2^{-1}$) varies from 4.686 at an RER of 0.7 to 5.047 at an RER of 1.0. If the amount of oxygen consumed and the caloric equivalent are known, the caloric cost of an activity can be computed.

To compute the kcal · min^{-1} cost, one must first find the caloric equivalent for the RER in Table 11.4. The rest of the computation is simply a matter of multiplying the oxygen cost by the caloric equivalent. The formula is

(11.4) caloric cost of an activity (kcal · min^{-1}) = oxygen consumed (L · min^{-1}) × caloric equivalent (kcal · LO$_2^{-1}$)

■ EXAMPLE

Assume that an individual had an RER of 0.91 during exercise that used 2.15 LO$_2$ · min^{-1}. The caloric equivalent for an RER of 0.91 is 4.936 kcal · LO$_2^{-1}$ so the calculation becomes

$$2.15 \, O_2 \, L \cdot min^{-1} \times 4.936 \, kcal \cdot LO_2^{-1}$$
$$= 10.61 \, kcal \cdot min^{-1}$$ ■

This **caloric cost** represents the energy expenditure of the activity. It may be expressed as calories or joules per minute (kcal · min^{-1} or kJ · min^{-1}) or relative to body weight (kcal · kg^{-1} · min^{-1} or kJ · kg^{-1} · min^{-1}) or as total calories if the calories per

Caloric Equivalent The number of kilocalories produced per liter of oxygen consumed.

Caloric Cost Energy expenditure of an activity performed for a specified period of time. It may be expressed as total calories (kcal), calories or kjoules per minute (kcal · min^{-1} or kJ · min^{-1}) or relative to body weight (kcal · kg^{-1} · min^{-1} or kJ · kg^{-1} · min^{-1}).

minute is multiplied by the total number of minutes of participation.

If you know the oxygen consumed during any activity, but you do not know the RER, you can estimate the caloric value of that activity by multiplying by 5.0 kcal $\cdot$ LO$_2^{-1}$. The 5 kcal $\cdot$ LO$_2^{-1}$ value is very close to the average caloric equivalent and is easy to remember. Since one kilocalorie equals 4.18 kilojoules, to convert kcal $\cdot$ min^{-1} to kJ $\cdot$ min^{-1}, multiply by 4.18. For the example we are discussing, we get

$$10.61 \text{ kcal} \cdot \text{min}^{-1} \times 4.18 \text{ kJ} \cdot \text{kcal}^{-1} = 44.36 \text{ kJ} \cdot \text{min}^{-1}$$

Determine the caloric cost (in kilocalories and kilojoules) for minute 14 of Table 11.2. Check your answer (number 3, at the end of the chapter). Remember that this caloric cost is an estimate of the aerobic portion only. If we attempt to calculate the caloric cost of all 28 min of the incremental task, the resulting number will be an underestimation, because we cannot calculate the anaerobic energy expenditure. Furthermore, these values include what an individual would expend if he or she were resting quietly. The term used when resting energy expenditure is included is *gross energy expenditure*. If resting energy expenditure is subtracted from gross energy expenditure, net energy expenditure—or the energy expended to do the exercise itself—is the result. Knowledge of the caloric cost of an activity is helpful in prescribing exercise.

Do the calculations requested in Box 11.1.

The Metabolic Equivalent (MET)

Although most people are used to seeing energy cost expressed as kilocalories, exercise physiologists and physicians often use MET values. MET is an acronym derived from the term *Metabolic EquivalenT*. One MET represents the average, seated, resting energy cost of an adult and is set at 3.5 mL $\cdot$ kg^{-1} $\cdot$ min of oxygen, or 1 kcal $\cdot$ kg^{-1} $\cdot$ hr^{-1}.

In reality, resting metabolic rate varies among individuals. If an individual's resting, seated energy expenditure is known, this value can be substituted for the 3.5 mL $\cdot$ kg^{-1} $\cdot$ min^{-1} average, but in practice, variations from the average value are not considered to be substantial enough to invalidate its use. Multiples of the 1-MET resting baseline represent the **MET** level or multiples of the resting rate of oxygen consumption of any given activity. Thus, an activity performed at the level of 5 METs would require five times as much energy as is expended at rest.

To calculate MET levels, divide the amount of oxygen utilized (in mL $\cdot$ kg^{-1} $\cdot$ min^{-1}) by 3.5. Hence, if an individual expends 29 mL $\cdot$ kg^{-1} $\cdot$ min^{-1} of O$_2$ on a task, the MET level is 29 mL $\cdot$ kg^{-1} $\cdot$ min^{-1} ÷ 3.5 mL $\cdot$ kg^{-1} $\cdot$ min^{-1} = 8.3 METs.

To convert from MET to kcal $\cdot$ min^{-1}, it is necessary to know the individual's body weight and use the relationship 1 kcal $\cdot$ kg^{-1} $\cdot$ hr^{-1} = 1 MET.[3] For example, if the 8.3-MET activity was done by a female of average weight (68 kg), the calculation is

$$8.3 \text{ METs} = \frac{(8.3 \text{ kcal} \times 68 \text{ kg})}{60 \text{ min} \cdot \text{hr}^{-1}} = 9.4 \text{ kcal} \cdot \text{min}^{-1}$$

How many METs is the subject in Table 11.2 exercising at in minute 14? The answer is at the end of the chapter (number 4).

Table 11.6 presents a list of common activities in both METs and kcal $\cdot$ kg^{-1} $\cdot$ min^{-1} for adults. These values can be used for exercise prescriptions. Table 11.7 provides a classification of work intensities for sedentary individuals based on oxygen consumption (mL $\cdot$ kg^{-1} $\cdot$ min^{-1} or L $\cdot$ min^{-1}) and caloric cost (kcal $\cdot$ min^{-1} and kcal $\cdot$ kg^{-1} $\cdot$ min^{-1}). These values can be used as a rough guide for determining how long work can be sustained at each intensity. For example, hiking at a level of 0.05–0.12 kcal $\cdot$ kg^{-1} $\cdot$ min^{-1} (from

Box 11.1 A Question of Understanding

A reasonable and beneficial level of exercise for fat loss is 300 kcal per session.[4] The oxygen cost of riding a bicycle ergometer at 2 Kp (600 kgm $\cdot$ min^{-1}, or 100 W) at 60 rev $\cdot$ min^{-1} is 1200 mL O$_2$ $\cdot$ min^{-1} above resting metabolism. At this rate, how long should an individual ride in order to burn an excess of 300 kcal? Ignore the cost involved in a warm-up or cool-down. Check your answer at the end of the chapter.

MET A unit that represents the metabolic equivalent in multiples of the resting rate of oxygen consumption of any given activity.

TABLE 11.6 ■ **MET and Caloric Values for Various Physical Activities**

PHYSICAL ACTIVITY	MET RANGE	kcal · kg^{-1} · min^{-1}	PHYSICAL ACTIVITY	MET RANGE	kcal · kg^{-1} · min^{-1}
Archery	3–4	0.05–0.07	Rope jumping	8–12	0.13–0.20
Backpacking	5–11	0.08–0.18	Running		
Badminton	4–9	0.07–0.15	12 min · mi^{-1}	8.7	0.15
Basketball			11 min · mi^{-1}	9.4	0.16
Nongame	3–9	0.05–0.15	10 min · mi^{-1}	10.2	0.17
Game play	7–12	0.12–0.20	9 min · mi^{-1}	11.2	0.19
Bed exercise	1–2	0.02–0.03	8 min · mi^{-1}	12.5	0.21
(cardiac)			7 min · mi^{-1}	14.1	0.24
Bicycling,	7	0.12	6 min · mi^{-1}	16.3	0.27
10 mph			Sailing	2–5	0.03–0.08
Bowling	2–4	0.03–0.07	Scuba diving	5–10	0.08–0.17
Calisthenics	3–8	0.05–0.13	Skating, ice and	5–8	0.08–0.13
Canoeing,	3–8	0.05–0.13	roller		
rowing,			Skiing,		
kayaking			Downhill	5–8	0.08–0.13
Dancing			Cross-country	6–12	0.10–0.20
Social	3–7	0.05–0.12	Water	5–7	0.08–0.12
and square			Soccer	5–12	0.08–0.20
Aerobic	6–9	0.10–0.15	Squash	8–12	0.13–0.20
Football (touch)	6–10	0.10–0.17	Stair climbing	4–8	0.07–0.13
Golf			Swimming	4–8	0.07–0.13
Power cart	2–3	0.03–0.05	Table tennis	3–5	0.05–0.08
Walking,	4–7	0.07–0.12	Tennis	4–9	0.07–0.15
carrying bag			Volleyball	3–6	0.05–0.10
Handball	8–12	0.13–0.20	Walking		
Hiking, cross-	3–7	0.05–0.12	1.7 mi · hr^{-1}	2.3	0.04
country			2.0 mi · hr^{-1}	2.4	0.04
Horseback riding	3–8	0.05–0.13	2.5 mi · hr^{-1}	2.9	0.05
Paddleball,	8–12	0.13–0.20	3.0 mi · hr^{-1}	3.3	0.06
racquetball			3.4 mi · hr^{-1}	3.6	0.06

Source: Modified from American College of Sports Medicine.[3]

Note: 1 MET = 1 kcal · kg^{-1} · hr^{-1}; 1 kcal · kg · hr ÷ 60 = 1 kcal · kg^{-1} · min^{-1}.

Table 11.6) can be sustained at least 8 hr a day for several weeks (from Table 11.7), as many individuals who have traveled the length of the Appalachian Trail from Georgia to Maine will attest. Conversely, running at 6 min · mi^{-1} (10 mph) is such heavy work (0.27 kcal · kg^{-1} · min^{-1} from Table 11.6) that it would easily exhaust the untrained individual in just a few minutes (Table 11.7). Trained individuals would be able to sustain heavy levels of work for longer periods of time.

*F*ield Estimates of Energy Expenditure During Exercise

Metabolic Calculations Based on Mechanical Work or Standard Energy Use

In situations where an accurate assessment of mechanical work is possible, energy expenditure,

TABLE 11.7 ■ Work Classifications Based on Metabolic Cost of Sedentary Individuals

CLASSIFICATION	$\dot{V}O_2$ (L · min⁻¹)	kcal · min⁻¹	kcal · kg⁻¹ · min⁻¹*	TIME WORK CAN BE SUSTAINED
LIGHT				
Mild	< 0.75	< 4	< 0.06	Indefinitely
Moderate	0.76–1.50	4.1–7.5	0.07–0.11	8 hr daily
HEAVY				
Optimal	1.51–2.00	7.6–10	0.12–0.15	8 hr daily for a few weeks only
Strenuous	2.01–2.50	10.1–12.5	0.16–0.18	4 hr 2–3 times per week for a few weeks consecutively
SEVERE				
Maximal	2.51–3.00	12.51–15.00	0.19–0.22	1–2 hr occasionally
Exhausting	> 3.00	> 15.0	> 0.22	Few minutes, rarely

Source: Modified from Wells, Balke, & Van Fossan.[76]

*Assume 150 lb or 68 kg, which is the average American weight for a 64.5-in. female. The actual values will vary for different body weights.

expressed as oxygen consumption (mL · min⁻¹, mL · kg⁻¹ · min⁻¹, or METs) can be estimated by a series of calculations. The equations used for the calculations are based on known oxygen costs for steady state horizontal walking (0.1 mL · kg⁻¹ · min⁻¹ for each m · min⁻¹), horizontal running (0.2 mL · kg⁻¹ · min⁻¹ for each m · min⁻¹), vertical rise (1.8 mL · kg⁻¹ · min⁻¹ for each m · min⁻¹), leg work against resistance (2 mL · kgm⁻¹) and arm work against resistance (3 mL · kgm⁻¹).[3] These values do not include the resting metabolic rate of 1 MET or 3.5 mL · kg⁻¹ · min⁻¹.

■ EXAMPLE

If an individual were walking on a track at a 20 min · mi⁻¹ pace (3 mi · hr⁻¹), which is a velocity of 80.4 m · min⁻¹ (3 mi · hr⁻¹ × 26.8 m · min⁻¹ · mi · hr⁻¹), the calculation would be as follows:

$$\text{walking oxygen consumption} = 80.4 \text{ m·min}^{-1} \times \left(\frac{0.1 \text{ mL · kg}^{-1} \cdot \text{min}^{-1}}{\text{m · min}^{-1}} \right)$$

$$+ 3.5 \text{ mL·kg}^{-1} \cdot \text{min}^{-1} = 11.54 \text{ mL·kg}^{-1} \cdot \text{min}^{-1}$$

This value can easily be converted to METs as previously described by dividing by 3.5 mL · kg⁻¹ · min⁻¹. At the 20 min · mi⁻¹ pace, this is 3.3. METs. If you check Table 11.6, you will see that 3.3 is the MET value given for walking at 3 mi · hr⁻¹. ■

In addition to this equation for horizontal walking, other equations are available and are presented in Appendix B for uphill walking, horizontal and uphill running, bench stepping, leg cycle ergometry, and arm cycle ergometry.[3]

These equations are useful for exercise prescription purposes in a school, health club or clinical setting where it is not possible to directly measure energy expenditure. Physicians, as mentioned before, often prescribe exercise by MET level and assume that the exercise leader will be able to determine the proper pace for walking or running, resistance on a cycle ergometer, or height and rate for step aerobics. The equations enable the exercise leader to do just that. However, it must always be remembered that the resultant values are just estimates for any given individual in any specific setting. Therefore, workloads should be fine-tuned by using heart rate or rate of perceived exertion (RPE) responses as described in Chapter 5.

Motion Sensors and Accelerometers

Attempts have been made to determine energy cost in the field by measuring movement, assuming that more movement means that more calories have been expended. Probably the most familiar type of motion sensor is the pedometer. After it is set with an individual's stride length, a *pedometer* can be used to record the distance an individual travels by foot. Thus, it is an indication of the quantity of movement. Electronic motion sensors that measure both frequency (or quantity) of movement and intensity of movement are called *accelerometers*.[48] The most popular accelerometer is the Caltrac. Figure 11.10 shows an individual wearing a Caltrac while walking. Both activity counts and estimated caloric values are displayed directly by Caltrac and require no additional calculations by the user. However, the accuracy of Caltrac for individual assessment of caloric cost has not been definitively determined.[18,44,45,51,59]

Activity Recalls and Questionnaires

The least complex system for estimating energy expenditure, at least from the standpoint of technology, is some form of self- or observer activity report.[48] To determine the caloric cost of a particular exercise session, we must first know the activity that was performed and its intensity and duration. Then the caloric cost of that activity is determined from a chart like the one presented in Table 11.6. Finally, we must know the body weight of the individual exercising. The information is then substituted into the following formula:

> **(11.5)**   total caloric cost of the activity (kcal) = caloric cost per kilogram of body weight per minute ($kcal \cdot kg^{-1} \cdot min^{-1}$) × body weight (kg) × exercise time (min)

■ EXAMPLE

If a 65-yr-old, 84-kg female walks 3 mi in 1:15, how many kilocalories does she expend?

In order to use Table 11.6, we must first convert 3 mi in 1 hr and 15 min to mi per hour.

$$3 \text{ mi} \div \left(\frac{75 \text{ min}}{60 \text{ min}} \right) = 2.4 \text{ mph}$$

Looking at Table 11.6, we see that 2.5 mph is the closest we can get. Thus, an individual walking at 2.5 mph expends $0.05 \text{ kcal} \cdot kg^{-1} \cdot min^{-1}$. Substituting into this formula, we get

$$0.05 \text{ kcal} \cdot kg^{-1} \cdot min^{-1} \times 84 \text{ kg} \times 75 \text{ min} = 315 \text{ kcal}$$

Therefore, this individual has expended 315 kcal in her walk, which is a good fitness workout.   ■

If an assessment of total daily energy expenditure or even weekly average expenditure is desired, the process becomes more tedious and, as a result, is probably less exact. Even the most willing individuals have only so much time to spend writing down everything they do; and if it is recorded after the fact, some things will be forgotten. Nevertheless, keeping a diary both of approximate energy expended and ingested can provide valuable information for individuals.

FIGURE 11.10

A Caltrac Accelerometer

This woman is wearing a Caltrac accelerometer that senses the frequency of her movement as she walks. The results provide an estimate of energy expended.

*E*fficiency and Economy

Efficiency

Walk into an appliance store to buy a furnace, hot water heater, washer, dryer, air conditioner, or refrigerator and each of the choices will have a label proclaiming its efficiency rating. Brand X uses only such and such an amount of electricity (for just pennies a day!) to heat 40 gallons of water, wash a load of clothes, and so on. Down the street the car dealer is shouting the praises of the latest midsized economy car. Plenty of leg room, holds five adults comfortably, and gets 35 mi per gallon of gas! In each case the concept is the same. We want to get the most output (in heating, cooling, or miles) for the least input and expense (electrical power, gas, or money). The same holds true when we consider physical labor or exercise output: We want to get the most output (work) for the least input (ATP, kilocalories, or fuel used).

The human body conforms to the first law of thermodynamics, which is also called the law of conservation of energy. Simply put, this law states that energy can neither be created nor destroyed but can only be changed in form. When an individual exercises or performs other external work, the actual work achieved represents only a portion of the total energy utilized. The rest of the energy appears as heat, which must be dissipated or the body temperature will rise. The percentage of energy input that appears as useful external work is called the **mechanical efficiency,** or simply the efficiency of that task.

Efficiency can be calculated in at least three ways. The simplest calculation of efficiency is as *gross efficiency.*

(11.6)

$$\text{gross efficiency} = \frac{\text{work output}}{\text{energy expended}} \times 100$$

■ EXAMPLE

Calculate the gross efficiency for a 22-yr-old female whose body weight (BW) is 65.5 kg. She has ridden a Monark cycle ergometer (flywheel distance = 6 meters) at 50 rev $\cdot$ min^{-1} with a load of 2.5 kp for 15 min.

The external output is calculated as work equals force times distance (W = F × D).

$$W = 2.5 \text{ kp} \times (50 \text{ rev} \cdot \text{min}^{-1} \times 6 \text{ m} \times 15 \text{ min})$$
$$= 11250 \text{ kgm}$$

It takes 426.8 kgm of work to equal one kilocalorie. Therefore, 11250 kgm ÷ 426.8 kcal $\cdot$ kgm^{-1} = 26.36 kcal of work output.

The amount of energy expended is calculated by using Eq. 11.4 and multiplying by the total time of the exercise. The average oxygen consumption for the ride was 1.73 L $\cdot$ min^{-1} and the RER was 0.91. At an RER of 0.91 the caloric equivalent (Table 11.4) is 4.936 kcal $\cdot$ L O$_2$$^{-1}$. Substituting into Eq. 11.4 we get

$$1.73 \text{ L O}_2 \cdot \text{min}^{-1} \times 4.936 \text{ kcal} \cdot \text{L O}_2^{-1}$$
$$= 29.95 \text{ kcal} \cdot \text{min}^{-1} \times 15 \text{ min} = 128.09 \text{ kcal}$$

of energy expended.

Eq. 11.6 can now be used to determine gross efficiency.

$$\text{gross efficiency} = \frac{26.36 \text{ kcal}}{128.09 \text{ kcal}} \times 100 = 20.58\% \blacksquare$$

A slightly more complex method uses *net efficiency.* In net efficiency the energy expended is corrected for resting metabolic rate.

(11.7)

$$\text{net efficiency} = \frac{\text{work output}}{\substack{\text{energy expended} - \text{resting} \\ \text{metabolic rate for the same} \\ \text{time period}}} \times 100$$

■ EXAMPLE

This means in the example used for gross efficiency that the individual's resting metabolic rate (measured to be 1.11 kcal $\cdot$ min^{-1} or 16.6 kcal for the 15 min) must be subtracted from the total energy expenditure of 128.09 kcal before computing for efficiency. Thus, substituting in Eq. 11.7 we get

$$\text{net efficiency} = \frac{26.36 \text{ kcal}}{128.09 \text{ kcal} - 16.6 \text{ kcal}} \times 100 = 23.64\% \blacksquare$$

The third technique for reporting efficiency requires the use of at least two workloads and is based on the difference between the two loads. It is called *delta efficiency.*

(11.8)

$$\text{delta efficiency} = \frac{\text{difference in work output between two loads}}{\substack{\text{difference in energy expenditure between} \\ \text{the same two loads}}} \times 100$$

Mechanical Efficiency The percentage of energy input that appears as useful external work.

■ EXAMPLE

Calculate the delta efficiency for the 22-yr-old female in the last two examples whose body weight is 65.5 kg. This time she has performed two exercise stages on a treadmill, the first at 0% grade and the second at 10% grade. The speed was a constant 94 m·min^{-1} (3.5 mi·hr^{-1}). The difference in work output is therefore primarily determined by the difference in percent grade, in this case a 10% difference. Treadmill delta efficiency calculations are usually done on a per minute basis. Therefore, instead of calculating the change in work (W = F × D) as in the first two examples, the change in work rate or power (P), which is work divided by time, is used.

$$\Delta P \, kgm \cdot min^{-1} = BW \, (kg) \times speed \, (m \cdot min^{-1})$$
$$\times (\% \, slope/100)^{1,40}$$

Substituting, we get

$$\Delta P = 65.5 \, kg \times 94 \, m \cdot min^{-1} \times (10/100)$$
$$= 615.7 \, kgm \cdot min^{-1}$$

Using the conversion of 426.8 kgm of work is equal to 1 kcal, we then divide 615.7 kgm · min^{-1} by 426.8 kgm for a difference in work output of 1.44 kcal · min^{-1}.

As before, energy expenditure is calculated by using Eq. 11.4. The average oxygen consumption at 0% grade is 0.91 L·min^{-1} with an RER of 0.73. The caloric equivalent (Table 11.4) of the 0.73 RER is 4.714 kcal · LO$_2$$^{-1}$. Substituting into Eq. 11.4 this becomes

$$0.91 \, LO_2 \cdot min^{-1} \times 4.714 \, kcal \cdot LO_2^{-1} = 4.29 \, kcal \cdot min^{-1}$$

The average oxygen consumption at 10% grade was 1.75 LO$_2$$^{-1}$ and the RER was 0.86. The caloric equivalent of an RER of 0.86 is 4.875 kcal · LO$_2$$^{-1}$. Substituting these values into Eq. 11.4 we have

$$1.75 \, LO_2 \cdot min^{-1} \times 4.875 \, kcal \cdot LO_2^{-1} = 8.53 \, kcal \cdot min^{-1}$$

To obtain the difference in energy expended at the two workloads, we simply subtract

$$8.53 \, kcal \cdot min^{-1} - 4.29 \, kcal \cdot min^{-1} = 4.24 \, kcal \cdot min^{-1}$$

Eq. 11.8 can now be used to solve for delta efficiency:

$$delta \, efficiency = \frac{1.44 \, kcal \cdot min^{-1}}{4.25 \, kcal \cdot min^{-1}} \times 100 = 33.9\% \quad ■$$

When used on the same exercise modality, the different methods of calculating efficiency will yield very different results. For example, Gaesser and Brooks[40] calculated gross efficiencies of 7.5–20.4%, net efficiencies of 9.8–24.1%, and delta efficiencies of 24.4–34% on the bicycle ergometer under the same controlled experimental conditions. Despite these differences, each technique is best suited for particular uses.

Gross efficiency is most useful when values for specific workloads, speeds, or the like, are of interest. For example, it answers the question: What is the efficiency of cycling into a 15-mph (24-kph) head wind, and how might that change with body position? Gross efficiency is also important for applications in nutritional studies where gross energy expenditure is a matter of concern for adequate replenishment, such as during the Tour de France, when replacement is essential if a cyclist is to continue hard riding day after day. Gross efficiency also is the measure that has been reported most frequently, and so it is important for comparison purposes.[36]

Since the energy expended during rest really is not used to do external work, net efficiency is actually a better indication of the efficiency of work per se. At the same time, it is not a particularly realistic value, since an individual performing any external work is still expending resting energy.

The most accurate means for determining the effect of speed or work rate on efficiency is the use of delta efficiency. It gives an indication of the relative energy cost of performing an additional increment of work. Delta efficiency is also the technique of choice when calculating efficiency on a treadmill. Its use is necessary because technically no work (calculated as force times distance) is done when the treadmill is horizontal (0% grade), despite the fact that energy is used.

All efficiency calculations assume a submaximal steady-state or steady-rate condition and require that both work output and energy expenditure be expressed in the same units, typically kilocalories. The calculations may be done for the total time, as in the 15-min bicycle ergometer ride used in the example for gross efficiency, or per unit of time, as in the per-minute calculations for the treadmill of delta efficiency. However, time can be a factor, since efficiency is generally high when a large amount of work is performed in a short period of time and low when a small amount of work is performed over a long period of time.[73]

Because the same amount of physical work in the same or a different exercise modality does not cause the same metabolic effect, it is the energy cost ($\dot{V}O_2$ consumption) that is the deciding factor in determining efficiency.[73] Figure 11.11 shows this basic relationship. As the energy cost ($\dot{V}O_2$ mL·kg^{-1}·min^{-1} on the left y-axis) increases, efficiency (% efficiency on the right y-axis) decreases, and vice versa.

Certain factors have been shown to change efficiency and thus can be manipulated by an individual in order to optimize efficiency. For example, the optimal seat height on a bicycle at any given power output has been found to be approximately 109% of leg length. Optimal pedaling frequency at any given power output has been shown to be between 40 and 60 rev·min^{-1} for trained and untrained individuals, despite the fact that trained cyclists self-select a rate closer to 90 rev·min^{-1}. The higher revolutions per minute used by the trained cyclist may optimize muscular forces and lower limb stresses but not metabolic efficiency.[77] When the revolutions per minute are kept constant on a bicycle ergometer, efficiency tends to increase from low to high work-

loads.[26,43,73] The optimal speed for walking when distance is held constant is between 60 and 100 m·min^{-1} (about 2.25 and 3.75 mph, or 16–27 min·mi). The optimal grade when speed is held constant is approximately 5% downhill (–5%). The optimal stride length when speed is held constant varies considerably among individuals. Most runners, however, intuitively select a stride length that is very close to optimal for themselves. Therefore, coaches who attempt to alter stride length may be harming efficiency.

Exercise efficiency values are most frequently reported in the 20–25% range. These values may be slightly higher (20–45%) if they are calculated as delta efficiencies and slightly lower (5–20%) if the activity involves air or wind resistance. Overcoming air resistance requires additional energy at all speeds of running and velocities of wind (including no wind). Hence, in a running or cycling race participants often draft off (or tuck in behind) the front runner. The first athlete must work harder than the athlete tucked behind, who does less work, hoping to save sufficient energy to put on a surge at the end and pass the more fatigued front runner.

The extra energy cost due to air resistance is proportional to the velocity at which the runner is moving raised to the second power, or m·sec^2. This amounts to approximately 2% extra energy expenditure for the marathon distance, 4–8% for middle-distance events, and 8–16% for sprints at world-class speeds. Although these percentages may not sound like much, they can be the equivalent of 5 min for the marathoner. At high levels of competition this is a tremendous amount of time and would make a considerable difference in the results.[6,35,36,40,61,63]

Although a head wind can require additional energy, and thus decrease efficiency, the reverse is not true. A tailwind never assists the runner by decreasing the energy cost proportionally.

The mechanical efficiency of cycling, whether calculated as net efficiency or delta efficiency, appears to be similar in prepubertal children, postpubertal adolescents, and adults.[46,66] It may be slightly reduced in the elderly. These similarities are true whether the calculations are based on relative (% $\dot{V}O_2$max) or on absolute (kgm·min^{-1} or W) workloads. The similarities also hold for males and females alike.[9,41,72,74] Because of the constancy of efficiency, cycling is a good family activity.

FIGURE 11.11

Optimizing Efficiency

Source: Cavanaugh and Kram.[25]

Note: Optimization means minimizing energy expenditure and maximizing work output.

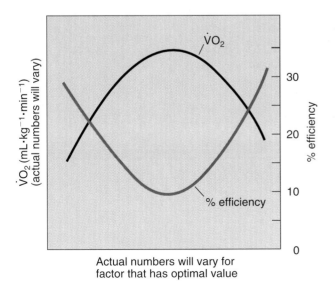

Actual numbers will vary for factor that has optimal value

Economy of Walking and Running

As has been shown, the calculation of efficiency is a ratio of work output to energy expenditure output. However, measuring external work output may be impossible in many activities such as horizontal walking and running during which the reciprocal movements of the arms and legs cancel each other and no vertical gain is attained. Consequently, the energy expended or oxygen cost is often used alone for walking and running as a measure of economy, not efficiency.

Economy is the oxygen cost of walking or running at varying speeds. The most basic generalization about economy is that, over a wide range of velocities, the energy cost (in $mL \cdot kg^{-1} \cdot min^{-1}$ of O_2) is rectilinearly related to the speed (in $m \cdot min^{-1}$). This generalization is true at least at 0% grade on a treadmill when the speed can be accomplished at a submaximal steady-state level.[28] Figure 11.12 shows this fundamental relationship. The black lines were computed from the equations recommended by the American College of Sports Medicine[3] and presented in Appendix B.[3] These equations in turn were based on a compilation of research. Note that the relationship between speed and oxygen consumption is not a continuous straight line encompassing both walking (Figure 11.12a) and running (Figure 11.12b). For walking speeds between approximately 50 and 100 $m \cdot min^{-1}$ each $m \cdot min^{-1}$

FIGURE 11.12

The Economy of Walking and Running for Children Versus Adults

The oxygen cost (expressed as $\dot{V}O_2$ $mL \cdot kg^{-1}$ min^{-1}) of walking (a) and running (b) increases rectilinearly as velocity increases. However, the slope of the two lines is different, and they do not form a continuous line from slow walking to fast running. Prepubertal males and prepubertal females are less economical than adult males and females as indicated by the higher oxygen cost at each and every velocity.

Sources: American College of Sports Medicine[3]; Rowland et al.,[68] and Rowland and Green.[67]

adds $0.1 \text{ mL} \cdot \text{kg}^{-1} \cdot \text{min}^{-1}$ above resting to the cost of the walk; for running speeds above $134 \text{ m} \cdot \text{min}^{-1}$ the increment is $0.2 \text{ mL} \cdot \text{kg}^{-1} \cdot \text{min}^{-1}$. Speeds between 100 and $134 \text{ m} \cdot \text{min}^{-1}$ represent an awkward area for most people; where it is too fast to walk but too slow to run. Additionally, outdoor running over ground is probably more demanding in terms of oxygen cost than indoor running on the treadmill at any given velocity.[32,54]

For any given individual, running economy appears to be relatively stable if environmental, equipment, and testing factors (such as body temperature, air resistance, footwear, time of day, and training status) are controlled.[55] Day-to-day variations between 1.6 and 11% have been reported in the literature for well-trained and elite male runners. On the other hand, differences among individuals in terms of running economy are often extensive, ranging from 20 to 30%, in subjects of equal training and performance status. The reason for these observations has not been determined.[24,32]

The Influence of Sex on Economy

The influence of sex on the interindividual variation in economy is unclear. Studies report that males expend more energy (Figure 11.12, green lines), less energy, or the same amount of energy in walking and running as do females (Figure 11.12, gold lines) when values are expressed relative to body mass (per kilogram of body weight). What is clear is that even if the oxygen cost is equal at any given speed, the female, who typically has a lower $\dot{V}O_2max$, will be working at a higher % $\dot{V}O_2max$ than the male.[7,12,17,20,31,32,55] This fact has implications for the pace at which long distance events can be run.

The Influence of Age on Economy

Age has a clear-cut effect on economy. Ample evidence exists to show that children and adolescents are less economical than adults when running over a wide range of speeds. There is scant evidence to indicate that the elderly may be less economical than young and middle-aged adults. Further research is needed in this area.[2,5,32,41,49,55,64,67,68,69]

Figures 11.12a and 11.12b show the results of two studies conducted in the same laboratory in which male prepubertal children (9–13 yr) were compared with adult males (23–33 yr)[68] and female prepubertal children (8–12 yr) were compared with

adult females (22–35 yr)[67] and how the four groups compared to the theoretical computed oxygen consumption values. In both sexes the energy cost at all speeds of running was higher for the children than the adults when expressed relative to body mass. No values for walking were available for the males, but at $80 \text{ m} \cdot \text{min}^{-1}$ there was no apparent age difference for the females. The differences at the running speeds held true whether expressed as an absolute load $(\text{m} \cdot \text{min}^{-1})$ or relative load (% $\dot{V}O_2max$). The adult values were much closer to the calculated values than the children's, indicating that the equations should not be used for children.

Figures 11.13a and 11.13b show that not only do children and adolescents differ from adults in terms of economy of running but they also differ from each other.[6] Indeed, there is a progressive decline in oxygen cost (progressive increase in economy) from the youngest (4–6 yr) to the oldest (16–17 yr) age groups in both the boys and girls. A compilation of studies shows the decline in oxygen cost to be about 2% per year from 8 to 18 yr when the same work is performed.[55] Similar data are available for walking at $80-100 \text{ m} \cdot \text{min}^{-1}$ at increasing grades for both boys and girls. These changes are evident from cross-sectional studies in which different individuals are tested at each age, and in longitudinal studies of the same individuals at different ages.[10,28,34]

Much speculation has surrounded the cause of this low economy in children. Five factors are known to be affected by growth and may offer at least a partial explanation.

1. ***High basal metabolic rate.*** The basal metabolic rate (BMR) is the minimum level of energy required to sustain the body's vital functions in the waking state as measured by oxygen consumption. BMR is highest in young children and progressively declines to adulthood, where it stabilizes until it again declines in old age.[66] (See Figures 11.14 and 15.2.) Hence, gross exercise oxygen consumption values may be higher in children than in adults because resting metabolic rates are higher. Bar-Or[10] has pointed out that this difference in resting metabolism is only $1-2 \text{ mL} \cdot \text{kg}^{-1} \cdot \text{min}^{-1}$ and, although

---

Economy   The oxygen cost of walking or running at varying speeds.

Figure 11.13

Running Economy of Children and Adolescents

Running economy improves as both male (a) and female (b) children age. This can be seen by the almost parallel and successively lower $\dot{V}O_2$ $mL \cdot kg^{-1} \cdot min^{-1}$ values across the tested velocities of running.

Source: P.-O. Åstrand. *Experimental Studies of Physical Working Capacity in Relation to Sex and Age.* Copenhagen: Munksgaard (1952). Modified and printed by permission.

this value represents a 25–35% greater BMR in children than in adults, it is unlikely to account for all of the difference in submaximal exercise values. Indeed, when Åstrand[5] utilized net oxygen values instead of gross (by subtracting the BMRs), the differences between the age groups was reduced but not eliminated.

2. *Large surface area/mass ratio.* A phenomenon exists in the animal kingdom in which smaller animals (such as mice, squirrels, rabbits, or the young of any species) exhibit higher resting metabolic rates per unit of body mass than larger animals (dogs, horses, elephants, or the adults of any species). However, when the unit of comparison is not body mass (that is, per kilogram) but body surface area (that is, per square meter), metabolic rates are similar. This is called the surface law. The surface law appears to be important in the maintenance of normal core temperatures. Body heat loss is directly related to surface area. The larger the surface area, the greater the heat loss is. Relatively speaking, small and/or young adults have greater surface areas per unit of mass than large and/or adult animals. Hence, a higher resting metabolic rate is necessary to maintain body temperature. This phenomenon may be the reason for the elevated BMR in the young.[66,67,68] When Rowland and his colleagues[67,88] changed the unit of comparison from $mL \cdot kg^{-1} \cdot min^{-1}$ to $mL \cdot m^2 \cdot min^{-1}$, the differences between the prepubertal and adult subjects of both sexes were no longer significant and were almost eliminated.

3. *Immature running mechanics.* Anyone watching a young child and an adult run together can easily see the differences in motor skill.[66,68] The young child appears to take numerous small, choppy steps involving lots of extraneous move-

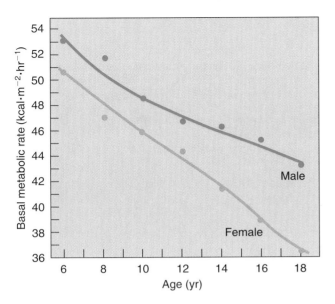

FIGURE 11.14

Changes in Basal Metabolic Rate with Age

Source: From *Exercise and Children's Health* (pp. 56, 57) by Thomas W. Rowland, Champaign, IL: Human Kinetics Publisher. Copyright 1990 by Thomas Rowland. Reprinted by permission.

ments. Technically, the child has a higher stride frequency; a shorter stride length (although it is proportional to his or her height); a greater vertical displacement; increased ankle, knee, and hip extension at takeoff; a longer nonsupport phase; and a shorter placement of the support foot in front of the center of gravity. The only one of these variables that seems to have any direct affect on the oxygen cost of running is stride frequency. Each stride requires energy to accelerate and brake the body's mass. When only one stride is considered, the oxygen cost does not differ between children and adults. However, at any given pace the child has a greater frequency of strides simply because he or she is anatomically smaller. Thus, more oxygen is utilized to provide the greater energy need.[68]

Support for the importance of stride frequency is also evident from cycling. Cycling is independent of both weight (the body weight is supported by the seat) and pedaling frequency (analogous to stride frequency), since the latter is controlled by setting the revolutions per minute if an ergometer is used. In this situation, as stated previously, no difference in efficiency is apparent between children and adults.

Remember that each individual intuitively selects the most economical combination of stride frequency and length for running . It is best not to attempt to "make" children more economical by training them to lengthen their strides. Stride frequency decreases and stride length increases naturally as the child grows.

4. *Less efficient ventilation.* The volume of air breathed in order to consume 1 L of oxygen is called the *ventilatory equivalent* (VE). Children have a higher VE than adults. The processing of this additional air requires an added expenditure of energy. This increased metabolic cost of respiration may account for part of the increased oxygen costs at submaximal work in children, although not all research evidence is in agreement.[66,67,68,69]

5. *Decreased anaerobic capacity.* As discussed in the preceding chapter, children are less able to generate ATP anaerobically than adults. The measurement of economy by oxygen consumption evaluates only the aerobic energy contribution. It is possible that at higher, but still submaximal, workloads, adults provide a greater amount of the required energy anaerobically and thus exhibit an artificially low oxygen cost value.[66,68] Evidence from RER values supports this contention. Children typically show lower RERs during submaximal exercise than do adults. Direct measurement of free fatty acid and glycerol levels show, however, that the lower RERs are not the result of an increased utilization of fat as a fuel as might be expected. Instead, it is postulated that the lower RERs result from lower amounts of nonmetabolic "excess CO_2," that is, the CO_2 generated from the buffering of lactic acid.

Why Do Economy and Efficiency Matter?

Economy or efficiency probably matter little in high-intensity, short-term activities such as maximal weight lifts and sprints or in skilled movements such as golf. However economy or efficiency is extremely important in endurance events. Among those factors critical for success in endurance performances are a high $\dot{V}O_2$max, the ability to work at a high % $\dot{V}O_2$max aerobically, and a high economy

Box 11.2 A Question of Understanding

The Fitt family plans to run the Cornfest 10-km (6.2 miles) race together. Dr. Phyllis Fitt (the mother) is an exercise physiologist and recently tested every-one in her lab. Given the following information, what is the fastest time they can run with a reasonable chance of everyone finishing in good shape together?

	Daughter	Son	Mother	Father	Grandmother
Age (yr)	12	8	37	45	57
$\dot{V}O_2$max (mL·kg^{-1}·min^{-1})	48	50	50	52	40
$\dot{V}O_2$ (mL·kg^{-1}·min^{-1})					
10 min·mi^{-1}	37	39	30	32	33
9 min·mi^{-1}	40	43	32	34	36
8 min·mi^{-1}	45	48	38	41	40
7 min·mi^{-1}	48	50	43	46	

Hint: Competitive runners typically average 80–90% $\dot{V}O_2$max during distance races of 5–10 mi; fun run-ners might be expected to be at the lower end of this value.

---

measured as a low submaximal oxygen cost at high velocities.[26,28,30,31,55]

Although a high $\dot{V}O_2$max is considered to be a prerequisite for success in distance or endurance events, it generally does not determine performance if participants are relatively homogeneous in that trait. For example, Costill[28] presents data from two runners (Ted Corbitt and Jim McDonagh) who had similar $\dot{V}O_2$max values (64 and 65 mL·kg^{-1}·min^{-1}). Over a period of two years they competed against each other in 15 major races and the same runner (McDonagh) won each and every time! Obviously, the physiological explanation did not lie in $\dot{V}O_2$max.

The importance of % $\dot{V}O_2$max that can be sustained for long periods is exemplified by the success of such runners as Grete Waitz, Frank Shorter, and Derek Clayton.[28] These world-class runners were estimated to use between 85 and 90% $\dot{V}O_2$max when they competed in marathons, whereas less successful marathoners average about 75 to 80% $\dot{V}O_2$max. Typically, such a high percentage (85–90%) could only be maintained for the shorter (10 mi or less) distance. By being able to continue at that rate for over twice as long as normal, these individuals gained a competitive edge.

Velocity at $\dot{V}O_2$max The speed at which an individual can run when working at his or her maximal oxygen consumption; based both on submaximal running economy and $\dot{V}O_2$max.

Additionally, if two runners of widely varying $\dot{V}O_2$max (runner A = 65 mL·kg^{-1}·min^{-1}; runner B = 50 mL·kg^{-1}·min^{-1}) but similar economy attempt to train together, say at an 8-min pace ($\dot{V}O_2$ cost = 40 mL·kg^{-1}·min^{-1}), runner B will be working much harder (80% $\dot{V}O_2$max) than runner A (62% $\dot{V}O_2$max). This variation in effort often occurs when females (average lower $\dot{V}O_2$max, equal economy) run with males.

Differences in economy have a similar effect on performance. If, for example, runner A and runner B had the same $\dot{V}O_2$max (65 mL·kg^{-1}·min^{-1}) but widely varying economies at an 8-min pace (runner A = 55 mL·kg^{-1}·min^{-1}; runner B = 40 mL·kg^{-1}·min^{-1}), then runner A would be working much harder (85% $\dot{V}O_2$max) than runner B (62% $\dot{V}O_2$max). This difference is probably why McDonagh (mentioned earlier) continually beat Corbitt in their races. At all velocities faster than 8 min·mi^{-1} Corbitt used significantly more oxygen than Mc-Donagh.[28] He had to be able to make up this difference by running at a higher % $\dot{V}O_2$max or he would lose. Obviously, it was the latter which occurred.

This scenario also occurs when a child (on average equal in $\dot{V}O_2$max to an adult but lower in economy) runs with an adult. At any given speed the child (unless there is a great disparity in his or her favor for $\dot{V}O_2$max) will be working harder than the adult. Although it is important for parents and teachers to encourage children to be active and for adults to do activities with children, the fact that the child will be working proportionally harder at any

TABLE 11.8 ■ **Information for Predicted Velocity at $\dot{V}O_2$max for Subjects A and B (Figure 11.15)**

	$\dot{V}O_2$ mL·kg⁻¹·min⁻¹ at indicated speed (m·min⁻¹)					$\dot{V}O_2$max (mL·kg⁻¹·min⁻¹)	v$\dot{V}O_2$max (m·min⁻¹)	10-km RUN TIME	% v$\dot{V}O_2$max FOR 10 km
SUBJECT	196	215	230	248	268				
A	38.03	40.58	44.30	45.10	—	54.68	304.56	38:21	83.2
B	—	46.13	48.28	50.54	54.88	60.88	306.50	38:09	83.1

Source: Based on Bird.[13]

given running pace must be taken into account. The parent or teacher should match the pace of the child or encourage just a slightly faster pace—not make the child keep up with what feels comfortable to the adult. As a consequence, the adult will have to do his or her hard training without the child along, but the child will enjoy the experience much more. Since there appears to be no difference in efficiency in cycling as a function of either sex or age, as long as the wheel sizes (and hence revolutions per minute) are equal, cycling may be a better family activity than running. See Box 11.2 and work through it now.

What may matter most to a competitive runner is a combination of economy and $\dot{V}O_2$max known as velocity at $\dot{V}O_2$max (v$\dot{V}O_2$max). The **velocity at $\dot{V}O_2$max** is the speed at which an individual can run when working at his or her maximal oxygen consumption based both on submaximal running economy and $\dot{V}O_2$max. Table 11.8 and Figure 11.15 show how this value is calculated and what it means. To calculate v$\dot{V}O_2$max, $\dot{V}O_2$ values (Y axis) are plotted at several submaximal speeds (X axis) for each individual, and a regression line—a line that best fits the $\dot{V}O_2$ values—is established. The line is extended to include the individual's measured $\dot{V}O_2$max. The speed (or velocity) at which the $\dot{V}O_2$max occurs is then determined by dropping a perpendicular line from the extended line to the X axis. This velocity is taken as the velocity at $\dot{V}O_2$max (v$\dot{V}O_2$max). As the figure shows, it is possible to achieve the same v$\dot{V}O_2$max with a high economy (that is, a low energy cost at submaximal speeds) and a low $\dot{V}O_2$max (subject A) or with a low economy (that is, a high energy cost at submaximal speeds) and a high $\dot{V}O_2$max (subject B). Individuals such as these two with a similar v$\dot{V}O_2$max would be expected to have similar

performances in endurance running events.[13,54] All other factors (such as % $\dot{V}O_2$max) being relatively equal, an individual with a high v$\dot{V}O_2$max would be expected to perform better than an individual with a low v$\dot{V}O_2$max.

The low economy of children may be important in explaining another phenomenon. Typically, endurance performance as measured by treadmill time to fatigue, 12-min-run distance, mile-run time, and so on, improves in children with age despite a constant $\dot{V}O_2$max (see Figure 11.16). Furthermore, although young athletes generally exhibit $\dot{V}O_2$max values that are higher than those of nonathletes, when training programs are followed, endurance

FIGURE 11.15

Predicted Velocity at $\dot{V}O_2$max

Source: Based on Bird.[13]

performance often improves exclusively—or at least more than does $\dot{V}O_2$max. It is possible that improvements in submaximal running economy (through improved skill in the short term) and age improvements in qualitative changes in oxygen delivery (not indicated by $\dot{V}O_2$max) and/or the improvement of anaerobic strength and speed components in the long term account for the enhanced endurance performances regardless of what occurs with $\dot{V}O_2$max. Indeed, submaximal running economy has been found to be statistically related to and to account for a considerable portion of the variance in endurance performance in children and adolescents in most (but not all) studies on this topic. Since $\dot{V}O_2$max remains relatively stable and the O_2 cost of any given speed decreases, the child is progressively working at a lower % $\dot{V}O_2$max as he or she ages. Hence, the individual would be expected to be able to perform (endure) at the same speed for a longer period of time, cover more ground in the same time span, and/or increase the speed at which any given distance is covered.[10,21,33,34,47,52,53,66,69]

Finally, for all the reasons cited in the discussion so far, one cannot use adult prediction equations based on $\dot{V}O_2$/speed relationships to predict $\dot{V}O_2$max in children.

Heritability of Aerobic Characteristics

Very little information is available on the impact of genetics on submaximal aerobic metabolism or its determinant characteristics. Bouchard et al.[16] studied the energy cost of incremental, submaximal, bicycle ergometer work on 22 pairs of sedentary male dizygous (DZ) twins and 31 pairs of sedentary male monozygous (MZ) twins (16–29 yr old). As anticipated, the MZ twins were more similar in oxygen utilization than the DZ twins. However, the heritability estimate (degree of genetic influence) declined from 90% when exercise was performed at 50 W, to 78% when exercise was performed at 75 W, to 46% when exercise was performed at 100 W. Variability due to heritability was nonsignificant at workloads of 125 and 150 W. Thus, a significant genetic effect was suggested for low work intensities but not for high ones. Energy substrate utiliza-

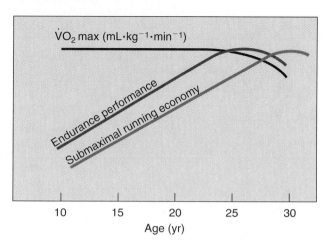

FIGURE 11.16

The Relationship Between Maximal Oxygen Consumption, Endurance Performance, and Submaximal Running Economy from Childhood to Early Adulthood

As children age endurance performance typically improves often despite no improvement in $\dot{V}O_2$ $mL \cdot kg^{-1} \cdot min^{-1}$. One possible explanation is the parallel improvement in submaximal running economy. In early adulthood all three measures begin to decline.

Source: From *Exercise and Children's Health* (pp. 56, 57) by Thomas W. Rowland, Champaign, IL: Human Kinetics Publisher. Copyright 1990 by Thomas Rowland. Reprinted by permission.

tion (as determined by RER) did not exhibit a consistently greater similarity in the MZ twins than in the DZ twins. These results do little to clarify the possibility of a genetic influence on aerobic characteristics.

Endurance performance—defined as maximal aerobic capacity and measured as total work output in 90 min of pedaling on a bicycle ergometer—was found to be more highly correlated in MZ twins than in DZ twins but had a heritability estimate of only 32%.[14] On the subcellular level no gene-associated variation has been found in mitochondrial density or metabolic enzyme activity.[14,15]

Despite these meager results, a strong genetic potential is deemed important for successful performance and absolutely essential for elite-level competition.

SUMMARY

1. Aerobic metabolism can be measured directly by calorimetry (the measurement of heat production) or indirectly by spirometry (the measurement of air breathed and the analysis of oxygen and carbon dioxide gases). Typically, open-circuit indirect calorimetry is used.

2. During aerobic exercise the amount of oxygen consumed and carbon dioxide produced increases. If the exercise is a short-term submaximal activity, the metabolic costs level off where the energy requirements are met. This activity is called steady-state or steady-rate submaximal exercise.

3. If a submaximal exercise lasts for a long time, is above approximately 70% $\dot{V}O_2$max, or takes place under hot and humid conditions, oxygen drift occurs. The oxygen consumption drifts upward owing to rising levels of catecholamines, lactate, and body temperature as well as an increasing cost of ventilation and a shift in substrate utilization.

4. During incremental exercise to maximum the oxygen consumed rises in a rectilinear pattern proportional to the workload increments until the individual can increase oxygen utilization no more and a plateau occurs. The highest amount of oxygen an individual can take in, transport, and utilize during heavy exercise is called maximal oxygen consumption ($\dot{V}O_2$max).

5. On the cellular level the ratio of carbon dioxide produced to oxygen consumed is termed the respiratory quotient (RQ); as analyzed from expired air, it is termed the respiratory exchange ratio (RER). Nonprotein RER is used most frequently in determining energy substrate utilization, with 0.7 being interpreted as fat, 1.0 as carbohydrate, and 0.85 as an approximate 50–50 mixture of both.

6. During exercise the higher the intensity, the higher the RER value is. During long-duration submaximal exercise RER may decrease as the carbohydrate stores are depleted. During incremental exercise to maximum RER may increase above 1.0, reflecting carbon dioxide increases from nonmetabolic sources.

7. During short-term submaximal exercise lactate accumulation will increase slightly, depending on the actual exercise intensity. If the submaximal exercise continues for a long duration, the lactate accumulation may rise slightly, stay the same, or even decrease slightly. The absolute values are not much different from resting levels. The lactate response to incremental work, as described in the previous chapter, is a curvilinear accumulation to high values.

8. Knowledge of the amount of oxygen consumed, the RER during the same time span, and the caloric equivalent permit the calculation of caloric expenditure (kcal · min⁻¹) and metabolic equivalents (METs).

9. Estimates of energy expenditure in nonlaboratory (field) settings can be done by using a series of metabolic formulas, by using motion sensors, or by using activity recall questionnaires and previously established caloric cost charts.

10. Mechanical efficiency, either gross, net, or delta, is some ratio of work output to energy expended. Economy is simply a measure of the energy expended (oxygen consumed); it is used when measuring the work output is difficult. Because the energy cost of walking and running is rectilinear over a wide range of speed, it is possible to estimate oxygen cost or MET values when the speed is known.

11. Individual variation in running economy is high between individuals but is low within the same individual. No clear-cut distinction in running economy has been shown between females and males. Children and adolescents are less economical than adults when running over a wide range of speeds. The elderly may also be less economical than young and middle-aged adults.

12. The exact reason why children are less economical than adults is unknown. However, the following factors have been considered possibilities:

(a) A high basal metabolic rate

(b) A large surface area/mass ratio

(c) Immature running mechanics

(d) Less efficient ventilation

(e) Decreased anaerobic capacity

13. A high economy (that is, a low oxygen cost) at any given velocity of running is beneficial to performance, especially if it is combined with a high $\dot{V}O_2$max and the ability to work consistently at a high % $\dot{V}O_2$max. The higher the velocity at $\dot{V}O_2$max and the greater percentage of $v\dot{V}O_2$max an individual can maintain, the better his or her performance will be. The improvement in running economy may explain why, as they grow and/or train, children typically improve in endurance run performance (such as the mile run) but do not show any significant improvement in $\dot{V}O_2$max.

14. The genetic influence on aerobic metabolic components is unclear. A heritability estimate of about 32% has been found for endurance performance.

Answers

1. Yes, this is a true max. RER = 1.34 (greater than 1.0 criterion level); HR = 200 b · min⁻¹ (predicted 220 – 22 = 198 ± 15 = 183 – 213); $\dot{V}O_2$ mL · kg⁻¹ · min⁻¹ difference minutes 27 – 28 = 2.07 (less than 2.1); $\dot{V}O_2$ reaches a plateau.

Answers (cont.)

2. Minute   2: RER = 0.99; CHO = 96.6%;
          FAT = 3.4%
   Minute 14: RER = 0.96; CHO = 86.4%;
          FAT = 13.6%
   Minute 28: RER = 1.34; CHO = 100%

3. RER = 0.96
   $\dot{V}O_2$ L $\cdot$ min^{-1} = 2.36
   kcal $\cdot$ L O_2^{-1} = 4.998 (from Table 11.4)
   4.998 kcal $\cdot$ L O_2^{-1} $\times$ 2.36 L O_2 $\cdot$ min^{-1}
   = 11.79 kcal $\cdot$ min^{-1}
   11.79 kcal $\cdot$ min^{-1} $\times$ 4.18 kJ $\cdot$ kcal^{-1}
   = 49.28 kJ $\cdot$ min^{-1}

4. $\dfrac{35.75 \text{ mL} \cdot \text{kg}^{-1} \cdot \text{min}^{-1}}{3.5 \text{ mL} \cdot \text{kg}^{-1} \cdot \text{min}^{-1}}$ = 10.21 METs

Box 11.1 Answers

1200 mL $\cdot$ min^{-1} O_2 = 1.2 L $\cdot$ min O_2

1.2 L $\cdot$ min^{-1} $\times$ 5 kcal $\cdot$ L^{-1} = 6 kcal $\cdot$ min^{-1}

300 kcal $\div$ 6 kcal $\cdot$ min^{-1} = 50 min

Box 11.2 Answers

Computing the % $\dot{V}O_2$max values for the given oxygen costs of each individual at each speed, we get:

Oxygen Cost	Daughter	Son	Mother	Father	Grand-mother
10 min $\cdot$ mi^{-1}	77	78	60	62	83
9 min $\cdot$ mi^{-1}	83	86	64	65	90
8 min $\cdot$ mi^{-1}	94	98	76	79	100
7 min $\cdot$ mi^{-1}	100	100	86	88	—

Therefore, the family could probably stay together easily at a 10 min $\cdot$ mi^{-1} pace, a little less easily due to grandmother at a 9 min $\cdot$ mi^{-1} pace. Perhaps grandmother and the kids should run together somewhere between 9 min $\cdot$ mi^{-1} and 10 min $\cdot$ mi^{-1} and let mom and dad go faster.

REVIEW QUESTIONS

1. List the variables used to describe the aerobic metabolic response to exercise. Describe how each one is obtained from laboratory or field tests. Explain what each variable means.

2. Diagram the oxygen consumption response during (a) short term, light-to-moderate-intensity dynamic exercise; (b) prolonged, moderate to heavy submaximal dynamic exercise; and (c) incremental aerobic exercise to maximum.

3. Describe the relationship between the oxygen cost of breathing and exercise intensity.

4. Explain the respiratory quotient and the respiratory exchange ratio. Relate them to the determination of energy substrate utilization, theoretically and numerically.

5. Compare lactate accumulation during (a) short-term, light-to-moderate-intensity dynamic aerobic exercise and (b) prolonged, moderate to heavy dynamic aerobic exercise. Contrast these responses to the short-term, high-intensity dynamic anaerobic exercise and incremental dynamic aerobic exercise to maximum detailed in the previous chapter.

6. Explain the similarities and differences in describing activity by kilocalories and MET levels. How can both be practically applied?

7. Differentiate, in terms of definition, calculation, and application, between gross efficiency, net efficiency, and delta efficiency. How can a cyclist maximize his or her efficiency?

8. Compare running economy by sex and age. Discuss possible reasons for any observed differences. Give three situations where any observed differences could have significant practical meaning.

9. Show how efficiency or economy can have an impact an exercise performance.

10. Describe the impact of genetics on aerobic metabolism during exercise.

REFERENCES

1. Adams, g. M.: *Exercise Physiology Laboratory Manual.* Dubuque, IA: Brown (1990).

2. Adams, W. C., M. M. McHenry, & E. M. Bernauer: Multistage treadmill walking performance and associated cardiorespiratory responses of middle-aged men. *Clinical Science.* 42:355–370 (1972).

3. American College of Sports Medicine: *Guidelines for Exercise Testing and Prescription* (5th edition). Philadelphia: Lea & Febiger (1995).

4. American College of Sports Medicine: The recommended quantity and quality of exercise for developing and maintaining cardiorespiratory and muscular fitness in healthy adults. *Medicine and Science in Sports and Exercise.* 22(2):265–274 (1990).

5. Asmussen, E.: Similarities and dissimilarities between static and dynamic exercise. *Circulation Research* (Suppl. I). 48(6):I-3–I-10 (1981).

6. Åstrand, P.-O.: *Experimental Studies of Physical Working Capacity in Relation to Sex and Age.* Copenhagen: Munksgaard (1952).

7. Åstrand, P.-O.: Human physical fitness with special reference to sex and age. *Physiological Reviews.* 36(3):307–335 (1956).

8. Åstrand, P.-O., & K. Rodahl: *Textbook of Work Physiology: Physiological Bases of Exercise.* New York: McGraw-Hill (1977).

9. Bal, M. E., E. M. Thompson, E. M. McIntosh, C. M. Taylor, & C. MacLeod: Mechanical efficiency in cycling of girls six to fourteen years of age. *Journal of Applied Physiology.* 6:185–188 (1953).

10. Bar-Or, O.: *Pediatric Sports Medicine for the Practitioner: From Physiological Principles to Clinical Applications.* New York: Springer-Verlag, 1–65 (1983).

11. Bar-Or, O.: The Wingate Anaerobic Test: An update on methodology, reliability and validity. *Sports Medicine.* 4:381–394 (1987).

12. Bhambhani, Y., & M. Singh: Metabolic and cinematographic analysis of walking and running in men and women. *Medicine and Science in Sports and Exercise.* 17(1):131–137 (1985).

13. Bird, J.: The contribution of selected physiological variables to 10 kilometer run time in trained, heterogeneous adult male runners. Unpublished master's thesis, 31 (1991).

14. Bouchard, C.: Genetics of aerobic power and capacity. In R. M. Malina & C. Bouchard (eds.), *Sports and Human Genetics.* Champaign, IL: Human Kinetics Publishers, 59–88 (1986).

15. Bouchard, C., & B. Lortie: Heredity and endurance performance. *Sports Medicine.* 1(1):38–64 (1984).

16. Bouchard, C., A. Tremblay, A. Nadeau, J. P. Despres, G. Thériault, M. R. Boulay, G. Lortie, C. Leblanc, & G. Fournier: Genetic effect in resting and exercise metabolic rates. *Metabolism.* 38(4):364–370 (1989).

17. Bransford, D. R., & E. T. Howley: Oxygen costs of running in trained and untrained men and women. *Medicine and Science in Sports.* 9(1):41–44 (1977).

18. Bray, M. S., J. R. Morrow, J. M. Pivarnik, & J. T. Bricker: Caltrac validity for estimating caloric expenditure with children. *Pediatric Exercise Science.* 4:166–179 (1992).

19. Brooks, G. A.: Anaerobic threshold: Review of the concept and directions for future research. *Medicine and Science in Sports and Exercise.* 17(1):22–31 (1985).

20. Bunc, V., & J. Heller: Energy cost of running in similarly trained men and women. *European Journal of Applied Physiology.* 59:178–183 (1989).

21. Burkett, L. N., B. Fernhall, & S. C. Walter: Physiological effects of distance run training on teenage females. *Research Quarterly for Exercise and Sport.* 56(3):215–220 (1985).

22. Bursztein, S., D. H. Elwyn, J. Askanzi, & J. M. Kinney: *Energy Metabolism, Indirect Calorimetry and Nutrition.* Baltimore: Williams & Wilkins (1989).

23. Bye, P. T. P., G. A. Farkas, & C. Roussos: Respiratory factors limiting exercise. *Annual Review of Physiology.* 45:439–451 (1983).

24. Carpenter, T. M.: *Tables, Factors, and Formulas for Computing Respiratory Exchange and Biological Transformations of Energy* (4th edition). Washington, D.C.: Carnegie Institution of Washington, Publication 303C (1964).

25. Cavanagh, P. R., & R. Kram: Mechanical and muscular factors affecting the efficiency of human movement. *Medicine and Science in Sports and Exercise.* 17(3):326–331 (1985).

26. Conley, D. L., & G. S. Krahenbuhl: Running economy and distance running performance of highly trained athletes. *Medicine and Science in Sports and Exercise.* 12(5):357–360 (1980).

27. Consolazio, C. F., R. E. Johnson, & L. J. Pecora: *Physiological Measurements of Metabolic Functions in Man.* New York: McGraw-Hill (1963).

28. Costill, D. L.: *Inside Running: Basics of Sport Physiology.* Indianapolis: Benchmark Press (1986).

29. Costill, D. L.: Metabolic responses during distance running. *Journal of Applied Physiology.* 28(3):251–255 (1970).

30. Costill, D. L., H. Thomason, & E. Roberts: Fractional utilization of the aerobic capacity during distance running. *Medicine and Science in Sports.* 5(4):248–252 (1973).

31. Cunningham, L. N.: Relationship of running economy, ventilatory threshold, and maximal oxygen consumption to running performance in high school females. *Research Quarterly for Exercise and Sport.* 61(4):369–374 (1990).

32. Daniels, J. T.: A physiologist's view of running economy. *Medicine and Science in Sports and Exercise.* 17(3):332–338 (1985).

33. Daniels, J., & N. Oldridge: Changes in oxygen consumption of young boys during growth and running training. *Medicine and Science in Sports.* 3(4):161–165 (1971).

34. Daniels, J., N. Oldridge, F. Nagle, & B. White: Differences and changes in VO_2 among young runners 10 to 18 years of age. *Medicine and Science in Sports and Exercise.* 10(3):200–203 (1978).

35. Davies, C. T. M.: Effects of wind assistance and resistance on the forward motion of a runner. *Journal of Applied Physiology: Respiratory, Environmental and Exercise Physiology.* 48(4):702–709 (1980).

36. Donavan, C. M., & G. A. Brooks: I. Muscular efficiency during steady-rate exercise. II. Effects of walking speed and work rate. *Journal of Applied Physiology: Respiratory, Environmental and Exercise Physiology.* 43(3):431–439 (1977).

37. Fleck, S. J., & W. J. Kraemer: *Designing Resistance Training Programs.* Champaign, IL: Human Kinetics Publishers (1987).

38. Fox, E. L., & D. K. Mathews: *Interval Training: Conditioning for Sports and General Fitness.* Philadelphia: Saunders (1974).

39. Freund, H., S. Oyono-Enguéllé, A. Heitz, C. Ott, J. Marbach, M. Gartner, & A. Pape: Comparative lactate kinetics after short and prolonged submaximal exercise. *International Journal of Sports Medicine.* 11(4):284–288 (1990).

40. Gaesser, G. A., & G. A. Brooks: Muscular efficiency during steady-rate exercise: Effects of speed and work rate. *Journal of Applied Physiology.* 38(6):1132–1139 (1975).

41. Girandola, R. N., R. A. Wiswell, F. Frisch, & K. Wood: Metabolic differences during exercise in pre- and postpubescent girls. *Medicine and Science in Sports and Exercise* (abstract). 13(2):110 (1981).

42. Gollnick, P. D., & L. Hermansen: Biochemical adaptations to exercise: Anaerobic metabolism. In J. H. Wilmore (ed.), *Exercise and Sport Sciences Reviews.* New York: Academic Press (1973).

43. Hagberg, J. M., Mullin, M. D. Giese, & E. Spitznagel: Effect of pedaling rate on submaximal exercise responses of competitive cyclists. *Journal of Applied Physiology: Respiratory, Environmental and Exercise Physiology.* 51(2):447–451 (1981).

44. Haskell, W. L., M. C. Yee, A. Evans, & P. J. Irby: Simultaneous measurement of heart rate and body motion to quantitate physical activity. *Medicine and Science in Sports and Exercise.* 25(1):109–115 (1993).

45. Haymes, E. M., & W. C. Byrnes: Walking and running energy expenditure estimated by Caltrac and indirect calorimetry. *Medicine and Science in Sports and Exercise.* 25(12):1365–1369 (1993).

46. Klausen, K., B. Rasmussen, L. K. Glensgaard, & O.V. Jensen: Work efficiency of children during submaximal bicycle exercise. In R. A. Binkhorst, H. C. G. Kemper, & M. Saris (eds.), *Children and Exercise XI*. Champaign, IL: Human Kinetics Publishers, 210–217 (1985).

47. Krahenbuhl, G. S., D. W. Morgan, & R. P. Pangrazi: Longitudinal changes in distance-running performance of young males. *International Journal of Sports Medicine*. 10(2): 92–96 (1989).

48. Laporte, R. E., H. J. Montoye, & C. J. Caspersen: Assessment of physical activity in epidemiologic research: Problems and prospects. *Public Health Reports*. 100(2):131–146 (1985).

49. Larish, D. D., P. E. Martin, & M. Mungiole: Characteristic patterns of gait in the healthy old. *Annals of the New York Academy of Sciences*. 515:18–32 (1987).

50. MacDougall, J. D., H. A. Wenger, & H. J. Green (eds.): *Physiological Testing of the Elite Athlete* (first edition). Hamilton, Ontario Canadian Association of Sport Sciences: Mutual Press Limited (1982).

51. Maliszewski, A. F., P. S. Freedson, C. J. Ebbeling, J. Crussemeyer, & K. B. Kastango: Validity of the Caltrac accelerometer in estimating energy expenditure and activity in children and adults. *Pediatric Exercise Science*. 3(2):141–151 (1991).

52. Mayers, N., & B. Gutin: Physiological characteristics of elite prepubertal cross-country runners. *Medicine and Science in Sports*. 11(2):172–176 (1979).

53. McCormack, W. P., K. J. Cureton, T. A. Bullock, & P. G. Weyand: Metabolic determinants of 1-mile run/walk performance in children. *Medicine and Science in Sports and Exercise*. 23(5):611–617 (1991).

54. Morgan, D., F. Baldini, P. Martin, & W. Kohrt: Ten km performance and predicted velocity of VO$_2$max among well-trained male runners. *Medicine and Science in Sports and Exercise*. 21:78–83 (1989).

55. Morgan, D. W., P. E. Martin, & G. S. Krahenbuhl: Factors affecting running economy. *Sports Medicine*. 7:310–330 (1989).

56. Newsholme, E. A., & A. R. Leech: *Biochemistry for the Medical Sciences*. New York: Wiley (1983).

57. O'Brien, M. J., C. A. Viguie, R. S. Mazzeo, & G. A.Brooks: Carbohydrate dependence during marathon running. *Medicine and Science in Sports and Exercise*. 25(9): 1009–1017 (1993).

58. Otis, A. B.: The work of breathing. *Physiological Reviews*. 34:449–458 (1954).

59. Pambianco, G., R. R. Wing, & R. Robertson: Accuracy and reliability of the Caltrac accelerometer for estimating energy expenditure. *Medicine and Science in Sports and Exercise*. 22(6):858–862 (1990).

60. Pardy, R. L., S. N. A. Hussain, & P. T. Macklem: The ventilatory pump in exercise. *Clinics in Chest Medicine*. 5(1): 35–49 (1984).

61. Pendergast, D. R., P. E. de Prampero, A. B. Craig, D. R.Wilson, & D. W. Rennie: Quantitative analysis of the front crawl in men and women. *Journal of Applied Physiology: Respiratory, Environmental and Exercise Physiology*. 43(3): 475–479 (1977).

62. Péronnet, F., G. Thibault, M. Ledoux, & G. Brisson: *Performance in Endurance Events: Energy Balance, Nutrition, and Temperature Regulation in Distance Running*. London, Ontario: Spodym (1987).

63. Pugh, L. G. C. E.: Oxygen intake in track and treadmill running with observations on the effect of air resistance. *Journal of Physiology*. 207:823–835 (1970).

64. Robinson, S., D. B. Dill, R. D. Robinson, S. P. Tzankoff, & J. A. Wagner: Physiological aging of champion runners. *Journal of Applied Physiology*. 41(1):46–51 (1976).

65. Rode, A., & R. J. Shepard: The influence of cigarette smoking upon the oxygen cost of breathing in near-maximal exercise. *Medicine and Science in Sports*. 3(2):51–55 (1971).

66. Rowland, T. W.: *Exercise and Children's Health*. Champaign, IL: Human Kinetics Publishers (1990).

67. Rowland, T. W., & G. M. Green: Physiological responses to treadmill exercise in females: Adult-child differences. *Medicine and Science in Sports and Exercise*. 20(5):474–478 (1988).

68. Rowland, T. W., J. A. Achinachie, T. J. Keenan, & G. M. Green: Physiologic responses to treadmill running in adult and prepubertal males. *International Journal of Sports Medicine*. 8(4):292–297 (1987).

69. Rowland, T. W., J. A. Auchinachie, T. J. Keenan, & G. M. Green: Submaximal aerobic running economy and treadmill performance in prepubertal boys. *International Journal of Sports Medicine*. 9(3):201–204 (1988).

70. Shepard, R. J.: The oxygen cost of breathing during vigorous exercise. *Quarterly Journal of Experimental Physiology*. 51:336–350 (1966).

71. Shepard J. T., C. G. Blomquist, A. R. Lind, J. H. Mitchell, & B. Saltin: Static (isometric) exercise: Retrospection and introspection. *Circulation Research* (Suppl. I). 48(6):I-179–I-188 (1981).

72. Sidney, K. H., & R. J. Shepard: Maximum and submaximum exercise tests in men and women in the seventh, eighth, and ninth decade of life. *Journal of Applied Physiology: Respiratory, Environmental and Exercise Physiology*. 43(2): 280–287 (1977).

73. Stegeman, J.: *Exercise Physiology: Physiological Bases of Work and Sport*. Chicago: Year Book Medical Publishers (1981).

74. Taylor, C. M., M. E. Bal, M. W. Lamb, & G. MacLeod: Mechanical efficiency in cycling of boys seven to fifteen years of age. *Journal of Applied Physiology*, 2:563–570 (1950).

75. Taylor, H. L., E. Buskirk, & A. Henschel: Maximal oxygen intake as an objective measure of cardiorespiratory performance. *Journal of Applied Physiology*. 8:73–80 (1955).

76. Wells, J. G., B. Balke, & D. D. VanFossan: Lactic acid accumulation during work. A suggested standardization of work classification. *Journal of Applied Physiology*. 10(1):51–55 (1957).

77. Widrick, J. J., P. S. Freedson, & J. Hamill: Effect of internal work on the calculation of optimal pedaling rates. *Medicine and Science in Sports and Exercise*. 24(3):376–382 (1992).

12

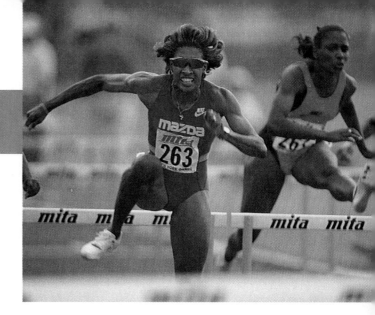

Metabolic Training Principles and Adaptations

After studying the chapter, you should be able to:

- Name and apply the training principles for metabolic enhancement.

- Describe and explain the metabolic adaptations that normally occur as a result of a well-designed and carefully followed training program.

- Discuss the impact of genetics on metabolic trainability, and derive a practical application from that discussion.

*I*ntroduction

In order to provide a training program that meets the metabolic goals of the individual it is necessary to systematically apply the training principles. The way in which these principles are applied will determine the extent to which the aerobic and/or anaerobic systems of energy production are emphasized, which, in turn, will determine the training adaptations that occur.

*A*pplication of the Training Principles for Metabolic Enhancement

A general description of the training principles was included in Chapter 1. Each training principle has a special meaning in relation to the metabolic production of energy to support exercise.

Specificity

Any training program must begin with a determination of the goal.[30, 55] For example, a 50-yr-old male enrolled in a fitness program who wants to break 60 min at a local 10-km race will have a very different training program than a 16-yr-old high school student competing at the 400- and 800-m distances.

Once the goal is established, it is possible to determine an estimate of the relative contributions of the major energy systems by use of a graph such as the one shown in Figure 10.2. For the 50-yr-old male just mentioned approximately 98% of the energy for his 60-min, 10-km run is derived from the O_2 system, with the remaining 2% coming from the ATP-PC and LA systems. These percentages vary little even if an individual's time is considerably slower or even somewhat faster than 60 min. Thus, the O_2 system should be emphasized in this individual's training regimen.

The high school middle-distance runner is a different story. To plan her training program, it is necessary to know her typical times at those distances. In general, she would be expected to be in the 1:00–3:00 range for both distances. (The American National 1989–1990 record for a 15–16-yr-old female was 0:53.74 for the 400-m run and 2:11.34 for the 800-m run.[4]) Events in this range stress all three energy systems with a heavier reliance on the ATP-PC and LA anaerobic systems as her performance speed increases. Since a faster time is the goal, she should emphasize and work on the anaerobic systems.

In general, only by stressing the primary energy system (or systems) used during the performance of the activity can improvement be expected. The one exception to this rule appears to be the development of an *aerobic base* through long-distance endurance work in the off-season for athletes in just about any sport (see Figure 1.5). This base can be viewed as preparation for more intense and specific training for anaerobic sports. The most specific training for metabolic improvement should occur in the preseason phase (see Figure 1.5).[55] Do Box 12.1 now to refresh your knowledge of time, distance, and energy systems.

For those sports where time is not the measuring stick for performance (such as basketball, football, softball, tennis, and volleyball), it is important to carefully analyze the separate components of the sport and determine which energy system supports each. For example, many people don't realize (until they think about it) that the average football play lasts between 4 and 7 sec and that the total action in a 60-min game, although spread over 3 hr, may be only 12 min. Thus, football training must emphasize the ATP-PC system (the 4–7-sec range), not the O_2 system (the 60-min time). Drills or circuits can be devised that stress the energy systems determined by the sport analysis to be the most important.

Specificity also applies to the major muscle groups and exercise modality involved. Most of the

---

Box 12.1 A Question of Understanding

The American National records in the 1500-m metric mile for girls progress from 7:39 (under 10 yr), to 7:04 (age 11–12 yr), to 4:37.32 (age 13–14 yr), to 4:25.57 (age 15–16 yr).[4] How does the energy system contribution vary with these times? Explain this variation on the basis of what you know about the development of the aerobic and anaerobic systems as a child matures. Compare your answer with the answer at the end of the summary.

biochemical training adaptations that occur do so only in the muscles that have been trained repeatedly in the way in which they will be used. Thus, the would-be triathlete who emphasizes bicycling and running in his or her program and spends little time on swimming should be more successful (in terms of individual potential) if he or she competed in duathlons instead.

Overload

Overload of the metabolic systems is typically achieved in one of two ways: first, by manipulating time and distance; and second, by monitoring lactic acid levels. Maximal oxygen uptake, although a measure of aerobic power and a means of quantifying training load, is more a cardiovascular than a metabolic variable. Factors contributing to the improvement of $\dot{V}O_2$max and the use of % $\dot{V}O_2$max as an overload technique are therefore primarily discussed in the section on application of the training principles in the cardiovascular unit (see Chapter 6).

The Time or Distance Technique   The *time or distance technique* involves some version of continuous and/or interval training. As the name implies, *continuous training* occurs when an individual selects a distance or a time to be active and continues uninterrupted to the end. Typically, a steady pace is maintained throughout the duration of the activity. Thus, the runner who completes an 8-mi training run at a 7:30-min · mi⁻¹ pace has done a continuous workout. Sometimes, if such a continuous steady-state aerobic training session is maintained for an extended period of time or distance, it is called a **long slow distance (LSD)** workout. If several periods of increased speed are randomly interspersed into a continuous aerobic workout, the term *fartlek* is used. Thus, a **fartlek** workout, named from the Swedish word meaning "speed play," combines the aerobic demands of a continuous run with the anaerobic demands of sporadic speed intervals. The distance, pace, and frequency of the speed intervals can vary depending upon what the individual wishes to accomplish that day.

Interval training is an aerobic and/or anaerobic workout that consists of three elements: a selected work interval (usually a distance), a target time for that distance, and a predetermined recovery or relief period before the next repetition of the work interval.[30] The energy system stressed is determined on the basis of the length of time of the work interval. Thus, a work time of less than 30 sec stresses the ATP-PC system; one between 30 sec and 3 min stresses the LA system. Anything over 3–5 min emphasizes the O_2 system. The target time is based on each individual's ability at the selected distance. The length and type of recovery period employed depends upon the energy system stressed; but the length is typically between 30 sec and 6 min, and the type may be rest or light or moderate activity.

ATP-PC System.   The amount of time required to restore half of the ATP-PC that has been used—that is, the half-life restoration period for ATP-PC—is approximately 30 sec, with full restoration occurring by 2 min.[30] Thus, if an individual has run for 10 sec and recovers for 30 sec, approximately half of the ATP-PC has been restored. A run of 30 sec with a recovery of 90 sec restores almost all of the ATP-PC.

During the same recovery time myoglobin O_2 replenishment is also taking place. The amounts replenished and restored are influenced by the activity of the participant during the recovery phase, with the greatest restoration occurring with rest or light activity such as stretching and walking.

Because the ATP-PC stores recover so quickly, they can be called upon repeatedly to provide energy. Repeatedly stimulating the ATP-PC system should bring about an increase in the capacity of that system. Any major involvement of the LA system is avoided by keeping the work intervals short so that little lactate accumulation occurs.

Long Slow Distance (LSD) Workout   A continuous aerobic training session performed at a steady-state pace for an extended period of time or distance.

Fartlek Workout   A type of training session, named from the Swedish word meaning "speed play," that combines the aerobic demands of a continuous run with the anaerobic demands of sporadic speed intervals.

Interval Training   An aerobic and/or anaerobic workout that consists of three elements: a selected work interval (usually a distance), a target time for that distance, and a predetermined recovery period before the next repetition of the work interval.

LA System.   To stress the lactic acid system re-quires work durations of 30 sec to 3 min. Lactic acid is produced in excess of clearance amounts during heavy work of this duration, resulting in an accu-mulation of lactate in the blood. Since lactate has a half-life of 15–25 min, with full clearance taking al-most an hour, it is neither practical nor beneficial to allow for even half-life clearance of lactate between repetitions.

Tolerance to lactic acid is increased by incom-plete recovery periods of 1 min 30 sec to 3 min. This amount of rest allows for the replenishment of ATP-PC and myoglobin O_2, and it allows the high-intensity work in the next work interval to be par-tially supplied by the ATP-PC energy system before stressing the LA system again.[31] It is inten-sity (from among the three overload factors of fre-quency, intensity, and duration) that is most important in improving the capacity of the LA sys-tem. Work-relief recovery is typically utilized at these work times, since active recovery does speed up lactate clearance.

O_2 System.   Long work bouts, which are still only a portion of the competitive event (that is, 0.5–1-mi [800 m to 1600 m] repeats for a 10-km run-ner), can be done to stress the O_2 system. The pace is typically close to average pace during competi-tion and may exceed it. The smaller the proportion of the distance, the faster the pace is and the more repetitions there are. However, the intent is that the intervals be done aerobically. For example, if a 10-km runner finishes in 1 hr 2 min, each mile (1.6 km) was run in 10 min. Mile (1.6 km) repeats should be run in training at a slightly faster pace—perhaps 9:40 or 9:45. Since this pace is already relatively low intensity work, a rest or walking recovery is best.

The distance for an interval workout (excluding warm-up and cool-down) should rarely exceed 2–5 mi (3.2–8 km) with a frequency of 1–3 days per week.[21] High-intensity interval training taxes the muscles and joints and care must be taken to avoid injury or overtraining. Refer to Chapter 1 for a re-view of the signs and symptoms of overtraining, if necessary. Continuous work at lower intensities al-lows for greater frequency and longer durations, both of which lead to a greater volume of training. A higher training volume is particularly important to endurance athletes.

The Lactate Monitoring Technique   As-sessing blood lactate concentration ([La⁻]) is the sec-ond common technique for monitoring overload. Ideally, this technique involves the direct measure-ment of blood lactate levels resulting from a given workout. When such facilities are available, the fol-lowing gradation of difficulty for individual exer-cise workouts has been suggested.[43, 50, 65, 74]

Easy recovery workouts	<2 mmol $\cdot$ L⁻¹ [La⁻]
LSD endurance workouts	≈ 2 mmol $\cdot$ L⁻¹ [La⁻]
Hard, intense endurance workouts	3–4 mmol $\cdot$ L⁻¹ [La⁻]
High-intensity interval workouts	>4 mmol $\cdot$ L⁻¹ [La⁻]

The optimal [La⁻] range for training endurance capacity appears to be close to 4 mmol $\cdot$ L⁻¹. Values above that stress the LA system more. The [La⁻] can be as high as 13–19 mmol $\cdot$ L⁻¹ during high-intensity interval work. Recall that the 2 mmol $\cdot$ L⁻¹-level is often labeled LT1 (the first lactate threshold) and the 4 mmol $\cdot$ L⁻¹-level is labeled LT2 (the second lactate threshold) or OBLA (see Chapter 10). Direct mea-surement of La⁻ during training is not very practi-cal, however, because of the necessity for special equipment and the necessity of taking multiple blood samples.

An alternative method, if an individual has ac-cess to laboratory testing facilities, is to determine the relationship between [La⁻] and HR values. Then HR can be used to estimate the [La⁻] level during training sessions and the intensity modified accord-ingly.[26, 37] For example, suppose an [La⁻] level of 2 mmol $\cdot$ L⁻¹ coincides with an HR of 120 b $\cdot$ min⁻¹ and 4 mmol $\cdot$ L⁻¹ with 160 b $\cdot$ min⁻¹. Then the LSD activities should be done at an HR of 120 b $\cdot$ min⁻¹; the recovery work at an HR lower than 120 b $\cdot$ min⁻¹; intense continuous work should be per-formed at a HR of approximately 160 b $\cdot$ min⁻¹; and hard interval work should be performed at a HR between 160 and 180 b $\cdot$ min⁻¹.

If no equipment is available for measuring [La⁻], an attempt can be made to use a field test de-signed by Conconi.[19] In this test the athlete per-forms repeats of an appropriate distance, usually between 200 and 800 m for runners. Each repeat is increased in speed by no more than $0.5 \text{ km} \cdot \text{hr}^{-1}$, and heart rate is monitored for each repeat. The point of deflection from rectilinearity of the heart rate at gradually increased speeds over the same distance may give an estimate of the $4 \text{ mmol} \cdot \text{L}^{-1}$ level in some individuals. Unfortunately, not all individuals show this response pattern with a deflection. If such a deflection does occur, the corresponding heart rate can then be used to judge that level of intensity during workouts. The difficulty lies in the fact that heart rate primarily reflects the functioning of the cardiovascular system, but lactate levels reflect the metabolic energy system. Fox, Bowers, and Foss[29] estimate that to ensure that 100% of the individuals are working at or above their "anaerobic threshold," heart rate would have to be greater than 90% of the maximal heart rate or equal to or greater than 85% of the heart rate reserve.

Whichever system is used to prescribe an individual's training session, it is important to provide a mixture of workout types to maximize the possibility for improvement and prevent boredom.

Adaptation

Adaptation is evident when a given distance or workload can be covered in a faster time with an equal or lower perception of fatigue or exertion and/or in the same time span with less physiological disruption (lower HR or [La$^-$] values) and faster recovery. The key to adaption for energy production in muscles appears to be allowing for sufficient recovery time between hard-intensity workouts. Cyclic training programs that alternately stress the desired specific energy system (hard day) and allow it to recover (easy day) induce optimal adaptation.[55, 71] Too many successive hard days working the same muscles and same energy system can lead to a lack of adaptation because of overtraining, and too many successive easy days can lead to a lack of adaptation because of undertraining.

Progression

Once adaptation occurs, the workload should be progressed if further improvement is desired. Progression can be done by increasing the distance or workload, decreasing the time, increasing the number of repetitions or sessions, decreasing the length of the relief interval, or changing the frequency of the various types of workouts per week. The key to successful progression is an increase in intensity and total training volume. The progression should be gradual. A general rule of thumb is that the increment in **training volume**—which is the total amount of work done, usually expressed as mileage or load—should not exceed more than 10% per week. For example, if an individual is currently cycling 60 mi per week, the distance should not be increased by more than 6 mi the following week.

Often in fitness work the challenge is to prevent an individual from doing too much too soon. The 50-yr-old man remembers when he was a high school star athlete and wants to regain that feeling and physique *now!* The fitness leader must gently be more realistic and err, if at all, on the side of caution in exercise prescription and progression.

The limit of metabolic adaptation appears to be achieved in approximately 10 days to 3 weeks if training is not progressed.[44] The ultimate limit may be set by genetics.

Individualization

The first step in individualizing training is, as mentioned earlier, to match the sport, event, or fitness goal of the participant with the specific mix of energy system demands. The second step is to evaluate each individual. The third step is to develop a periodization sequence for off-season, preseason, early and late in-season, and active rest phases. The fourth step is to develop a format, that is, the number of days devoted per week for each type of training or energy system stressed. The fifth step is to determine the training load (distance, workload, repetitions, or the like) on the basis of the individual's evaluation and modified by how he or she responds and adapts to the program. Interpreting and adjusting to an individual's response is the art of being a coach or fitness leader.

Training Volume The total amount of work done, usually expressed as mileage or load.

Maintenance

Once a specific level of endurance adaptation has been achieved, it appears that this level can be maintained by the same or by a reduced volume of work. However, the way that the volume is reduced is critical. If the training intensity is maintained, reductions of one-third to two-thirds in frequency and duration have been shown to maintain aerobic power ($\dot{V}O_2max$), endurance performance (at a given absolute or relative submaximal workload), and lactate accumulation levels at submaximal loads. This maintenance may last for at least several months. One day per week may be sufficient for short periods of time (say during a one-week vacation) if intensity is maintained.[17, 57, 70] Conversely, a reduction in intensity brings about a reduction in training adaptation.

It also seems to be important that the mode of exercise is consistent or closely simulated, since, as mentioned previously, many of the training adaptations that occur are specific to the muscles involved. Thus, *cross training*—the utilization of different modalities to reduce localized stress but increase overall training volume—is likely to be more beneficial for the cardiovascular system than for the metabolic system.

The level of maintenance training necessary for the anaerobic energy systems to operate at maximal levels is unknown. However, sprint performances deteriorate less quickly in response to a decrease in training than do endurance performances.[73]

Many fitness participants are primarily in a maintenance mode after the initial several months or first year of participation. The appropriate level for maintenance should be determined by individual goals. Maintenance should occur primarily during the in-season training cycle of an athlete.

A special kind of maintenance called tapering is often used by athletes in individual sports such as swimming, cycling, and running. A **training taper** is a reduction in training volume prior to important

---

Training Taper A reduction in training prior to important competitions that is intended to allow the athlete to recover from previous hard training, maintain physiological conditioning, and improve performance.

---

competitions that is intended to allow the athlete to recover from previous hard training, maintain physiological conditioning, and improve performance. Athletes often fear that if they taper for more than just a few days, their competitive fitness and performance will suffer. However, studies consistently show that if intensity is maintained while training volume is reduced, physiological adaptations are retained and performance is either equaled or improved after a taper of 7 to 21 days.[22, 49, 51, 64]

The one group of individuals who probably do not respond to these maintenance and taper guidelines with joy are those who are injured. Maintaining a high level of intensity in the training modality is one of the most difficult tasks for an injured individual. Research continues in an attempt to solve this problem, such as trying to determine whether work in the water can be substituted for land-based work. In the meantime, the injured individual who cannot continue to train at his or her preinjury level should probably accept the fact that he or she will experience a loss of adaptation.

Retrogression/Plateau/Reversibility

The training principle of retrogression, plateau, and reversibility is not one that a coach or fitness leader applies as much as anticipates and reacts to. At one or more points in the process of training, an individual will fail to improve with progression and will either stay at the same level (*plateau*) or show a performance or physiological decrement (*retrogression*). When a pattern of nonimprovement occurs, it is important to check for other signs of overtraining. A shift in training emphasis or the inclusion of more easy days may be warranted. Remember that a reduction in training does not necessarily lead to detraining. Of course, not all plateaus can be explained as overtraining; sometimes there is no explanation.

If an individual ceases training completely, for whatever reason, detraining will occur. This *reversibility* of training adaptations in skeletal and metabolic potential occurs within days to weeks after training ceases. A reduction in both maximal and submaximal performance ultimately follows. It should come as no surprise that those metabolic factors that show the greatest improvement with training—that is, those involved with aerobic energy production (see training adaptations later in this chapter)—also show the greatest reversal. Within three to six weeks after the cessation of activity, pre-training levels are typically reached again, especially if the training program was of short duration. Individuals with a long and established training history, however, tend to show an initial rapid decline in some aerobic variables but then level off at higher-than-pretraining levels. Anaerobic metabolic variables show less incremental increase with training and less loss with detraining. This fact may explain why sprint performance is more resistant to inactivity than endurance performance. Complete bed rest or immobilization accelerates detraining.[23, 57, 59, 73]

Retraining does not occur as rapidly as detraining and is not easier or more rapid than initial training.[73] Although direct experimental evidence is scanty, the consequences of detraining and retraining appear to be similar for adults, children, and adolescents.[6]

Warm-Up and Cool-Down

The information about warm-up is sparse in relation to the effects on metabolic function, but several generalizations seem to be warranted. An elevated body temperature—and more specifically, an elevated muscle temperature—increases the rate at which the metabolic processes in the cells can proceed. This rate increase occurs in large part because enzyme activity is temperature-dependent, exhibiting a steady rise from $0°C$ to approximately $40°C$ before plateauing and ultimately declining. At the same time, oxygen is more readily released from red blood cells and transported into the mitochondria at elevated temperatures.[68] One consequence of increased body temperature is a decreased oxygen deficit at the initiation of exercise.[40] Another consequence is a greater availability of oxygen to the muscles during work. When more oxygen is available sooner, less reliance is placed on anaerobic metabolism, and less lactate accumulates at any given heavy workload. At lighter endurance workloads a greater utilization of fats for the production of energy is possible earlier in the activity. This early use of fats serves to spare carbohydrate and extend the time a given high-intensity effort can be continued. These beneficial metabolic effects of a warm-up appear to exist for children and adolescents as well as adults.[6]

In devising a warm-up to achieve these metabolic benefits, several considerations need to be taken into account.[32]

1. The activity should involve large muscle groups that will elevate the body temperature from $37°$ to $38°$ or $39°C$. This temperature elevation generally occurs simultaneously with the onset of sweating.

2. The activity should last approximately 5–20 min and end no longer than 15 min before the hard phase of the workout or competitive performance. The harder the planned workout, the longer the warm-up phase should be. The less time elapsing between the warm-up and the performance, the better it is for an athlete.

3. The intensity of the warm-up should be such that it does not fatigue the participant. Highly fit individuals can utilize longer, more intense warm-ups than low fit individuals. Generally speaking, the warm-up for endurance activities can occur at a lower intensity (25–30% $\dot{V}O_2$max or less than 35% HRmax) than for sprinting or anaerobic activities (45–50% $\dot{V}O_2$max or 50–60% HRmax). Higher values in the 60–80% $\dot{V}O_2$max (70–85% HRmax) may be needed by highly conditioned athletes to elevate core temperature. In any case, it is probably best to stay below the lactate threshold.

4. The warm-up may be built into an endurance workout if the participant begins at a low intensity and progresses nonstop into higher levels of work.

5. Identical warm-ups of explosive tasks (such as long or high jumping) at full speed should be used sparingly. The action can be patterned at lower levels.

6. An intermittent or interval type warm-up has been found to be more beneficial for children than a continuous warm-up.[6]

The primary metabolic value of a cool-down lies in the fact that La$^-$ is dissipated faster during an active recovery. As described in Chapter 10, the lactate removal rate is maximized if the cool-down activity is of moderate intensity (a little higher than the individual tends to self-select) and continues for approximately 20 min.

In general, all of the training principles appear to apply to both sexes and, except where noted, to all ages. At the very least, there is insufficient evidence for modifying any of the general concepts on the basis of age or sex, although individual differences should always be kept in mind.

Metabolic Adaptations to Exercise Training

When the training principles just discussed are systematically applied and rigorously followed, a number of adaptations occur relative to the production and utilization of energy. The extent to which the adaptations occur depends upon the initial fitness level of the individual and his or her genetic potential. Figure 12.1 is an expanded version of Figure 9.4 showing the metabolic pathways you studied earlier. Numbers have been inserted following the naming of some factors to indicate sites where these adaptations occur. The following discussion will follow that numerical sequence. Refer to Figure 12.1 as you read.

FIGURE 12.1

Metabolic Training Adaptations

The circled numbers indicate sites where training changes occur. The boxes indicate processes.

Substrate or Fuel Supply

Regulatory Hormones   Primary among the metabolic adaptations to a training program are changes that occur in the hormones responsible for the regulation of metabolism (see Chapter 9, Figure 9.16 and Table 9.3). Although little is known about the impact of training on the hypothalamic-releasing factors and adrenocorticotrophic hormone (ACTH), a definite pattern is seen for the five hormones directly involved in substrate regulation. That pattern is one of a blunted response in which the amount of hormone secreted during submaximal activity is reduced. This pattern occurs whether the load is absolute or relative and in both the fast-responding and slow-responding hormones. Thus, the rise in glucagon is lower and the suppression of insulin less; the rise in norepinephrine and epinephrine is less; the rise in growth hormone is less; and the rise in cortisol is less during submaximal exercise in trained individuals than in untrained individuals.[35] Because of these smaller disruptions at submaximal levels, more work can be done before maximum is reached.

Carbohydrate   Both endurance and sprint training bring about an increase of muscle and liver glycogen reserves (Figure 12.1, site 1). In addition, at the same absolute submaximal workload (that is, the same rate of oxygen consumption) muscle and liver glycogen depletion occurs at a slower rate in the trained individual than in the untrained individual.[1, 38, 45, 46, 52] Thus, the trained individual uses less carbohydrate in his or her fuel mixture. This change is seen in lower RER values. Since glycogen is the primary source of fuel for high-intensity work, a larger supply of glycogen used less quickly enables an individual to participate in fairly intense activities at submaximal levels for longer periods of time before fatigue occurs. On the other hand, sprint training can also increase the rate of glycogenolysis at higher levels of work, giving the exerciser a fast supply of energy when needed for short bursts of maximal or supramaximal activity.

Fat   The trained individual is able to use his or her carbohydrate stores more slowly than the untrained individual because of the changes that occur in fat metabolism (Figure 12.1, site 2). Both trained and untrained individuals have more than adequate stores of fat. However, the rate of free fatty acid oxidation is determined not by the storage amount but by the concentration of free fatty acids in the bloodstream and the capacity of the tissues to oxidize the fat. Training brings about several adaptations in fat metabolism, including the following:

1. An increased mobilization or release of free fatty acids from the adipose tissue.

2. An increased level of plasma free fatty acids during submaximal exercise.

3. An increase in fat storage adjacent to the mitochondria within the muscles.

4. An increased capacity to utilize fat at any given plasma concentration.

The increased reliance on fat as a fuel is said to have a *glycogen-sparing effect* and is responsible for lowered RER values at the same absolute and same relative (% $\dot{V}O_2$max) work intensities. Because glycogen supplies last longer, there is a delay in fatigue and greater endurance at submaximal work levels. Both endurance and sprint training have glycogen-sparing effects.[1, 38, 45, 46]

Protein   Despite the fact that proteins are the least important energy substrate, changes do occur as a result of endurance training, which enhance their role (Figure 12.1, site 3). Adaptations in protein metabolism include an increased ability to utilize the branched chain amino acid leucine and an increased capacity to form alanine and release it from muscle cells. This increased production of alanine is accompanied by decreased levels in the plasma, probably indicating an accelerated removal for gluconeogenesis. In ultraendurance events this increased gluconeogenesis effect would be beneficial in maintaining blood glucose levels.[1, 46, 47]

Enzyme Activity

The key to increasing the production of ATP is enzyme activity. Since every step in each metabolic pathway is catalyzed by a separate enzyme, the potential for this training adaptation to influence energy production is great. However, it appears that not all enzymes respond to the same training stimulus nor change to the same extent.

Glycolytic Enzymes   The results of studies investigating the activity of the glycolytic enzymes have been contradictory, with most showing little (if any) change but some showing increased activity. Glycolysis (Figure 12.1, site 4) is involved in both the aerobic and anaerobic production of energy, and it may be that high-intensity training is required for some glycolytic enzymes to adapt but that others respond better to endurance training. Four key enzymes have shown significant training changes: hexokinase, phosphorylase, phosphofructokinase, and lactic dehydrogenase.

Hexokinase.   Hexokinase facilitates the entry of glucose from the bloodstream into the glycolytic pathway and its activity increases with endurance training. This increased activity is beneficial in endurance events when the liver is supplying glucose to the bloodstream.

Phosphorylase.   Phosphorylase catalyzes the breakdown of glycogen stored in the muscle cells so that glycogen may be used as fuel in glycolysis. An increase in phosphorylase activity has been found with high-intensity sprint training. The ability to break down glycogen quickly is important in near-maximal, maximal, and supramaximal exercise.

Phosphofructokinase (PFK).   PFK is the main rate-limiting enzyme of glycolysis. Results from both endurance and sprint training studies are inconsistent but tend to suggest an increase in activity with adequate levels of training. Increased PFK activity leads to a faster and greater quantity of ATP being produced glycolytically.

Lactic Dehydrogenase (LDH).   LDH catalyzes the conversion of pyruvate into lactate. It exists in several discrete forms, including a cardiac muscle form that has a low affinity for pyruvate (thus making the formation of lactate less likely) and a skeletal muscle form that has a high affinity for pyruvate (thus making the formation of lactic acid more likely). Endurance training tends to have two effects on LDH. It lowers the overall activity of LDH, and it causes a shift from the skeletal muscle to the cardiac muscle form. Thus, lactate is less likely to be produced in skeletal muscle and pyruvate is more likely to enter the mitochondria for use as an aerobic fuel. Both of these changes are beneficial to endurance performance.[1, 39, 46, 65]

Shuttles   You will recall that the hydrogen ions removed in glycolysis must be transported across the mitochondrial membrane by a shuttle since that membrane is impermeable to $NADH + H^+$ (Figure 12.1, site 5). No training changes have been found to occur in the glycerol-phosphate shuttle enzymes that predominate in skeletal muscle. Conversely, large increases in the enzymes of the cardiac muscle's malate-aspartate shuttle both in the cytoplasm and mitochondria have been found. This increase enhances aerobic metabolism in the heart.[46]

Mitochondrial Enzymes   Changes in the mitochondrial enzymes of the Krebs cycle, electron transport, and oxidative phosphorylation are coupled with changes in the mitochondria themselves (Figure 12.1, site 6). Both the size and the number of the mitochondria increase with training. Thus, mitochondria occupy a proportionally larger share of the muscle fiber space. The sarcolemmal mitochondria are affected to a greater degree than the interfibrillar mitochondria. The stimulus for these increases appears to be contractile activity itself, rather than any external stimulus such as hormonal changes, since only those muscles directly involved in the exercise training show these changes. For example, a runner would exhibit an increase in mitochondrial size and number only in the legs, whereas a cross country skier would show mitochondrial increases in both arms and legs.

Within limits, the extent of the augmentation in the mitochondria seems to be a function of the total amount of contractile activity. That is, the more contractions there are, the greater is the change in the mitochondria. It does not seem to matter whether the increase in contractile activity is achieved by completing more contractions per unit of time (speed work) or by keeping the rate of contractions steady but increasing the duration (endurance training). Resistance training does not appear to enhance mitochondria.

With larger mitochondria more transport sites are available for the movement of pyruvate into the mitochondria. The enzymatic activity per unit of mitochondria appears to be the same for trained and untrained individuals; however, the greater mitochondrial protein content means an overall greater enzyme activity to utilize the pyruvate. Interestingly, although most mitochondrial enzymes increase in activity, not all do; nor is the rate of change the same for all. The overall effect of the increased enzyme activity and the increased availability of pyruvate is an enhanced capacity to generate ATP by oxidative phosphorylation. This augmented capacity is more important in supplying energy for submaximal exercise than for maximal exercise.[1, 38, 45, 46]

Oxygen Utilization

Maximal Oxygen Uptake   Maximal oxygen uptake ($\dot{V}O_2$max) increases with training. Even though this is a measure of the amount of oxygen utilized at the muscle level (Figure 12.1, site 7), $\dot{V}O_2$max is determined more by the cardiovascular system's ability to deliver oxygen than by the muscle's ability to use it. Evidence for the subsidiary role of muscle in determining $\dot{V}O_2$max includes the fact that individuals can have essentially the same mitochondrial content but very different $\dot{V}O_2$max values. Conversely, individuals with equivalent $\dot{V}O_2$max values can have quite different mitochondrial enzyme levels. Additionally, small training changes can occur in one (mitochondrial activity or $\dot{V}O_2$max) without concomitant changes in the other—although, typically, both will increase. These differences probably explain why some runners are more economical (use less oxygen at a given pace than others do) and others possess a greater aerobic power (have a higher $\dot{V}O_2$max).[46]

Submaximal Oxygen Cost   The oxygen cost ($\dot{V}O_2$ in mL · min^{-1} or mL · kg^{-1} · min^{-1}) (Figure 12.1, site 7) of any given absolute submaximal workload is the same before and after training, assuming that no skill is involved where efficiency would change.[38,46] For example, if an individual has a smooth, coordinated front crawl stroke but has not participated in lap swimming, the oxygen cost of covering any given distance at a set pace will remain the same as this person trains. However, for an individual who is just learning the front crawl stroke, the oxygen cost would actually go down. It would decrease not because of a change in the exercise oxygen requirements but because extraneous inefficient movements that add to the oxygen cost are eliminated as skill is improved.[24, 27, 36]

Running economy depends both on the energy needed to move at a particular speed (*external energy*) and on the energy used to produce that energy (*internal energy*). Specifically, internal energy is associated with oxygen delivery (ventilation and heart rate in particular), thermoregulation, and substrate metabolism (remember that it takes more oxygen to utilize fat as a fuel than to burn carbohydrate). Theoretically, internal energy demand can be lowered by decreasing ventilation and heart rate costs and by increasing the percentage of carbohydrate. The first two changes do typically occur with training, but the last one does not. Indeed, the trained individual utilizes a higher percentage of fat at any given submaximal load than does an untrained individual. The primary possibility for improving external energy demand is stride length. However, studies have shown that experienced runners freely select the optimal stride length, so additional improvements in training status do little to change stride length. High-intensity interval training has produced improvements in running economy, but the evidence is not strong.[5,20,65] Decreased efficiency or economy, on the other hand, can occur. If so, it should be interpreted as a symptom of overtraining.[33]

If an individual increases his or her $\dot{V}O_2$max and yet the oxygen cost of any given (absolute) workload remains the same, then the % $\dot{V}O_2$max at which that individual is doing the given workload will go down. The task will be relatively easier for the individual, and endurance performance will be greatly enhanced. This improvement is a consequence of the biochemical adaptations in the muscle rather than changes in oxygen delivery.

The myoglobin concentration in muscles increases with endurance training in the muscles directly involved in the activity. As a consequence, the rate of oxygen diffusion through the cytoplasm into the mitochondria increases, making more oxygen available quickly.

Oxygen Deficit and Drift   The oxygen deficit at the onset of activity is smaller, but is not eliminated, in a trained individual. The primary reason for this reduction is that oxidative phosphorylation is activated sooner owing to the increased number of mitochondria that are sensitive to low levels of ADP and P_i. This result is advantageous to the exerciser, because less lactic acid will be produced and less creatine phosphate will be depleted.[45, 46]

The magnitude of oxygen drift will also be less after training. This change may be caused by concomitant reductions in epinephrine, norepinephrine, lactate, and body temperature rise during any given submaximal workload.[16, 41]

Lactate Accumulation

Lactic acid is produced when the hydrogen atoms carried on NADH + H$^+$ are transferred to pyruvic acid in a reaction catalyzed by lactic dehydrogenase (Figure 12.1, site 8). Lactate accumulates when the rate of production exceeds the rate of clearance. It is a matter of some debate whether the rate of production decreases or the rate of clearance increases more as a result of training. All of the substances involved in the production reaction, however, are influenced by adaptations that would favor a decreased production.

Pyruvate is the end product of carbohydrate metabolism (glycolysis). Less carbohydrate is utilized at an absolute submaximal workload after training; therefore, less pyruvate is available for conversion into lactate. More hydrogen atoms are transported into the mitochondria in cardiac cells owing to increased activity of the malate-aspartate shuttle, thereby decreasing the number of hydrogen atoms in the cytoplasm. And the LDH enzyme shifts from the skeletal muscle form, which favors lactic acid production, to the cardiac muscle form, which has a lower affinity for pyruvate. In addition, glycolysis is inhibited following training by several factors, two of which are related to the increased utilization of fat during submaximal exercise. The first is a high concentration of free fatty acid in the cytoplasm, and the second is a high level of citrate (the first product in the Krebs cycle). Both factors cause the rate-limiting enzyme PFK to slow down glycolysis and, hence, decrease the possible production of lactic acid. Finally, a smaller increase in the concentration of epinephrine and norepinephrine has been found at the same absolute and relative workloads in trained individuals. This decreased sympathetic stimulation may also decrease the activation of glycogenolysis and the potential production of lactic acid.[38, 46]

At the same time, lactate clearance is higher in trained than untrained individuals due to an enhanced blood flow to the liver, which aids in lactate removal. In addition, there is an overall uptake of lactate by the muscles. The enhanced uptake of lactate by active and inactive muscles means that the change in the rate of clearance probably is more important than the change in the rate of production.[15,25,54] The result is a decreased concentration of lactate in the muscles and blood at the same relative workload (% $\dot{V}O_2$max) after training.

As a consequence of the change in the ratio of lactate clearance to production, a higher workload (both in absolute and relative terms) is required to achieve lactate levels in the 2-to-4-mmol · L^{-1} range. This means that an individual can improve performance by exercising at a higher relative intensity for a given period of time and yet delay the onset of fatigue since the so-called lactate thresholds have been raised.[3, 43, 46, 66, 72, 74]

At maximal work the level of lactic acid accumulation is higher as a result of training. The higher level probably results from the greater glycogen stores and increased activity of some of the glycolytic enzymes other than LDH.[1, 38] It may also be a result that is more psychological than physiological, in that the trained individual is more motivated and is better able to tolerate the pain caused by lactic acid.[35]

ATP Production, Storage, and Turnover

ATP-PC   Although exercise training increases the potential for the production of larger quantities of ATP by oxidative phosphorylation (Figure 12.1, site 9), it does not change the efficiency of converting fuel to ATP or ATP to work. Thirty-six ATP are still produced from glucose in skeletal muscle, and the potential energy per mole of ATP is still between 7 and 12 kcal.[1, 38, 39, 45, 52, 66]

However, the amount of ATP and PC stored in the resting muscle is higher in the trained than in the untrained individual, especially if muscle mass increases. Whether this amount is large enough to markedly increase anaerobic capacity is questionable. At the same absolute workload there is less depletion of the PC and ATP levels after training. At the same relative workload PC depletion and ATP degradation does not change with training. However, the

TABLE 12.1 ■ **Estimated Maximal Power and Capacity for Untrained (UT) and Trained (TR) Males**

	Power				Capacity			
	kcal · min⁻¹		kJ · min⁻¹		kcal · min⁻¹		kJ · min⁻¹	
SYSTEM	UT	TR	UT	TR	UT	TR	UT	TR
Phosphagens (ATP-PC)	72	96	300	400	11	13	45	55
Anaerobic glycolysis (LA)	36	60	150	250	48	72	200	300
Aerobic glycolysis plus Krebs cycle plus ETS/OP (O_2)	7–19	32–37	30–80	135–155	360–1270	10,770–19,140	1500–5300	45,000-80,000

Source: Modified from Bouchard, Taylor, & Dulac;[13] Bouchard et al.[14]

activity of the enzymes responsible for the breakdown of ATP to ADP and the regeneration of ADP and ATP increase. Hence, the rate of turnover of ATP and PC increases. Taken together, the ATP-PC-LA changes indicate an increased anaerobic power and capacity with sprint type training.[56] Values for the ATP-PC, LA, and O_2 systems are presented in Table 12.1 contrasting the trained and untrained male. It can be seen that the LA system changes much more with training than does the ATP-PC system, but that the greatest change is in the O_2 system.[13, 14]

Work Output   Work output—measured as watts or kilocalories per kilogram of body weight on a bicycle test such as the 10-sec or 30-sec Wingate Anaerobic Test and/or a 90-sec test—shows improvements with training. This result is evidenced by higher scores of athletes when compared to nonathletes and by higher posttraining than pretraining scores in all populations. Furthermore, sprint or power type athletes typically show higher anaerobic values and greater adaptations than endurance athletes. Elite sprinters and power athletes score higher than do less successful competitors.[7, 8, 48, 58]

Aerobically, a trained individual can continue any given submaximal workload for a longer period of time than an untrained individual. The trained individual can also accomplish more total work to a higher absolute workload before achieving his or her maximum than an untrained individual can. Overall, the trained individual has a metabolic system capable of supporting enhanced performance, both at submaximal and at maximal levels. These changes, summarized in Table 12.2, are specific to the training employed.

The Influence of Age and Sex on Metabolic Training Adaptations

With the exception of $\dot{V}O_2$max (which is discussed in the cardiovascular unit), there is a scarcity of research data on most of the metabolic variables across the age spectrum. What scattered evidence is available indicates that training and detraining changes in children, adolescents, and the elderly are similar to changes for adults in the 20-to-50-yr range. This is especially true if the changes are considered relative to baseline values (that is, as a percentage of change) and not as absolutes.[2, 6, 18, 28, 34, 53, 60, 61]

Data concerning metabolic adaptations in females of all ages is also minimal, again with the exception of $\dot{V}O_2$max.[63, 67, 69] Studies have shown the following adaptations in females as a result of appropriate specific training:

1.   Fuel utilization shifts in favor of fat.

2. Lactic acid levels decrease during submaximal work and increase at maximal effort.

3. Enzyme levels change.

4. Submaximal $\dot{V}O_2$ consumption remains stable or decreases slightly.

5. Anaerobic power and capacity increase.[62, 69, 71]

TABLE 12.2 ■ Metabolic Training Adaptations

1. **FUEL SUPPLY**
   a. Carbohydrate.
      (1) ↑ Muscle and liver glycogen reserves.
      (2) ↓ Rate of muscle and liver glycogen depletion at absolute submaximal loads, that is, glycogen-sparing.
      (3) ↑ Velocity of glycogenolysis at maximal work.
   b. Fat
      (1) ↑ Mobilization, transportation, and beta oxidation of free fatty acids.
      (2) ↑ Fat storage adjacent to mitochondria.   *Intramuscular Fat*
      (3) ↑ Utilization of fat as fuel at same absolute and same relative workloads.
   c. Protein
      (1) ↑ Ability to utilize the BCAA leucine as fuel.   *Can perform longer & faster*
      (2) ↑ Capacity to form alanine and utilize it as a glyconeogenic precursor.
2. **ENZYME ACTIVITY**
   a. ↑ Hexokinase, phosphorylase, and probably phosphofructokinase activity.
   b. ↓ LDH activity with some conversion from the skeletal muscle to cardiac muscle form. *Pyruvate*
   c. ↑ Activity of the malate-aspartate shuttle enzymes but not the glycerol-phosphate shuttle enzymes.
   d. ↑ Number and size of mitochondria.
   e. ↑ Activity of most, but not all, of the enzymes of the Krebs cycle, electron transport, and oxidative phosphorylation due to greater mitochondrial protein amount.
3. **O_2 UTILIZATION**
   a. ↑ $\dot{V}O_2$max.
   b. = $\dot{V}O_2$ cost at absolute submaximal workload.
   c. ↑ Myoglobin concentration.
   d. ↓ Oxygen deficit.
   e. ↓ Oxygen drift.
4. **LACTIC ACID ACCUMULATION**
   a. ↓ La⁻ accumulation at same absolute workload and any given relative workload.
   b. ↑ Workload to achieve 2- and 4-mmol · L⁻¹ lactate thresholds.
   c. ↑ [La⁻] at maximum.
5. **ATP PRODUCTIONS, STORAGE, AND TURNOVER**
   a. = ATP from gram of precursor fuel substrate.
   b. ↑ ATP-PC storage.
   c. ↓ Depletion of PC and ATP degradation at same absolute workload.
   d. = Depletion of PC and ATP degradation at same relative workload.
   e. ↑ ATP-PC turnover.

↑ Power, ↑ Capacity

↑, increase; ↓, decrease; =, no change.

20 40 60 80

4 250

In short, both males and females respond to the same training with the same adaptation. This is not to say that sex differences are obliterated in equally trained males and females in the metabolic variables—just that both sexes are trainable and probably to the same extent.

Detraining also appears to operate in the same way and to the same extent for males and females.

The Impact of Genetics on Metabolic Trainability

Genetics impacts human physiological variables two ways. The first impact is directly on the expression of that variable. For example, at least 50% of an individual's endurance capacity, as measured by the maximal amount of work done on a cycle ergometer in 90 min, can be accounted for by heritability.[9] Other examples have been discussed for both anaerobic and aerobic metabolism in previous chapters.

The second way in which genetics impacts physiology is on the adaptation to training of any variable. Research in which multiple pairs of monozygous (MZ) twins have been trained under laboratory conditions has shown that for many of the variables examined the impact of genetics on trainability is stronger than the heritability of the trait itself in sedentary individuals. Furthermore, the influence of genetics is sometimes stronger the closer the individual is to achieving his or her maximal potential.

Although many of the energy system variables whose training adaptations have just been described have not been investigated to date, specific information is available on several.[9]

Submaximal Substrate or Fuel Utilization

Adaptations in substrate availability and utilization that occur as a result of aerobic endurance training are largely genetically based. In particular, data show that the change in epinephrine-stimulated lipolysis or breakdown of fat from isolated adipose cells that results from training is genetically dependent. The genetic influence on the training-induced ability to mobilize fat is also reflected in the ability to utilize fat during light submaximal exercise. Forty-four percent of the variance in the training adaptation of the respiratory exchange ratio can be attributed to genetics. Likewise, 42% of the variance of submaximal oxygen cost at the same absolute load depends on genetics.[12]

Maximal Work Output and Oxygen Consumption

Approximately 70% of the variance in the training adaptation increase in work output in 90 sec (primarily lactic anaerobic metabolism) can be accounted for by genetics. For training changes in $\dot{V}O_2$max and 90-min maximal work capacity, the amount of variance accounted for by genetics is approximately 75% and 80%, respectively. Both the training adaptations and the percentage of that work increase that can be accounted for by genetics are smaller for a 10-sec (alactic anaerobic) task: only about 30%. Maximal aerobic endurance capacity is about 60% more trainable than $\dot{V}O_2$max. Males show higher trainability in maximal aerobic endurance capacity than females.[9] Genetically dependent training changes in both glycolytic and oxidative muscle enzyme activity underlie these changes.[9, 42]

Genetic Variability

One of the most interesting aspects of the genetic impact on trainability is the wide range of adaptation. For example, following a 20-week endurance training program in which the mean improvement in endurance performance was about 50% of the pretraining work output, the range of improvement was from 16 to 97%.[12] Similarly wide ranges have been shown for other variables, suggesting that most of the individual differences in responding to the same training program are genetically determined.[10,11] Thus, it appears that there are both low and high responders. And there may be as much as a threefold to tenfold variation between high and low responders. Indeed, some people (probably less than 5% of the population) may be nonresponders. In addition, there are also early and late responders. Early responders show metabolic adaptations very quickly, within the first 5–7 weeks of a training program. Late responders may show little initial progress but after

8 weeks or so appear to make a major breakthrough. These variations, of course, are the basis for the individualization training principle.[11,42]

Unfortunately, there is no way at the present time to determine an individual's genetic training potential for either the aerobic or the anaerobic system. Thus, the physical educator, coach, or fitness leader must be alert for these variations and counsel those under their tutelage accordingly.[10]

SUMMARY

1. The most important consideration in applying each training principle to achieve metabolic adaptations is as follows:
   (a) For specificity, match the energy system of the activity.
   (b) For overload, manipulate time and distance or lactate level.
   (c) For adaptation, alternate hard and easy days.
   (d) For progression, reoverload if additional improvement is desired.
   (e) For individualization, evaluate the individual according to the demands of the activity and develop a training sequence, system, and load on the basis of your evaluation.
   (f) For maintenance, emphasize intensity.
   (g) For retrogression, plateau, and detraining, evaluate the training adaptations and modify as indicated.
   (h) For warm-up and cool-down, include activities that will actually elevate or reduce body temperature, respectively.

2. Properly prescribed training programs bring about adaptations in fuel supply, enzyme activity, oxygen utilization, lactate accumulation, and ATP production, storage, and turnover.

3. Most of the variation between individuals in metabolic training adaptation is genetically based. Long-term, lactic, anaerobic and aerobic metabolic training adaptations are influenced more by genetics than are short-term, alactic anaerobic adaptations.

Box 12.1 **Answers** *(cont.)*

Although there is undoubtedly some real difference between the contributions for the 4:37.32 and 4:25.57 times, this cannot be discerned from the graph in Figure 10.2. What can be seen is the greater LA contribution after puberty, when more glycogen and less fat is burned and the anaerobic (glycolytic) contribution to exercise approaches the adult level.

REVIEW QUESTIONS

1. Name and briefly describe the eight training principles. Select a sport or fitness activity and show how each of the training principles can be specifically applied to that activity.

2. Describe and explain the metabolic adaptations to exercise training for each of the following factors:
   (a) Substrate or fuel supply
   (b) Enzyme activity
   (c) Oxygen utilization
   (d) Lactate accumulation
   (e) ATP production, storage, and turnover

3. Discuss the impact of genetics on the metabolic adaptations to exercise training in terms of the following factors:
   (a) Submaximal substrate or fuel utilization
   (b) Maximal work output and oxygen consumption
   (c) Variability of response

Derive a practical application from this discussion, and provide a realistic example.

REFERENCES

1. Abernethy, P. J., R. Thayer, & A. W. Taylor: Acute and chronic responses of skeletal muscle to endurance and sprint exercise: A review. *Sports Medicine.* 10(6):365–389 (1990).
2. Adeniran, S. A., & A. L. Toriola: Effects of continuous and interval running programmes on aerobic and anaerobic capacities in schoolgirls aged 13 to 17 years. *Journal of Sports Medicine and Physical Fitness.* 28:260–266 (1988).
3. Allen, W. K., D. R. Seals, B. F. Hurley, A. A. Ehsani, & J. M. Hagberg: Lactate threshold and distance-running performance in young and older endurance athletes. *Journal of Applied Physiology.* 58(4):1281–1284 (1985).
4. Athletics Congress of the USA: *1989–1990 Competition Rules for Athletics: World and American Records.* Indianapolis: Author (1989).
5. Bailey, S. P., & R. R. Pate: Feasibility of improving running economy. *Sports Medicine.* 12(4):228–246 (1991).
6. Bar-Or, O.: *Pediatric Sports Medicine for the Practitioner: From Physiological Principles to Clinical Applications.* New York: Springer-Verlag, 1–65 (1983).

Box 12.1 **Answers**

	7:39	7:04	4:37.32	4:25.57
ATP-PC	2.5%	2.5%	≈3.5%	≈3.5%
LA	≈15%	≈15%	≈22%	≈22%
O_2	≈82.5%	≈82.5%	≈75%	≈75%

7. Bar-Or, O.: The Wingate Anaerobic Test: An update on the methodology, reliability and validity. *Sports Medicine.* 4:381–394 (1987).

8. Beld, K., J. Skinner, & Z. Tran: Load optimization for peak and mean power output on the Wingate Anaerobic Test. *Medicine and Science in Sports and Exercise* (Suppl. 164). 21(2):S28 (1989).

9. Bouchard, C.: Genetics of aerobic power and capacity. In R. M. Malina & C. Bouchard (eds.), *Sport and Human Genetics.* 1984 Olympic Scientific Congress Proceedings, Vol. 4. Champaign, IL: Human Kinetics Publishers, 59–88 (1986).

10. Bouchard, C.: Heredity and Health-Related Fitness. *Physical Activity and Fitness Research Digest.* Washington, DC: President's Council on Physical Fitness and Sports, 1(4) (1993).

11. Bouchard, C., M. R. Boulay, J.-A. Simoneau, G. Lortie, & L. Pérusse: Heredity and trainability of aerobic and anaerobic performances: An update. *Sports Medicine.* 5:69–73 (1988).

12. Bouchard, C., F. T. Dionne, J.-A. Simoneau, & M. R. Boulay: Genetics of aerobic and anaerobic performance. In J. O. Holloszy (ed.), *Exercise and Sport Sciences Reviews.* Baltimore: Williams & Wilkins, 20 (1992).

13. Bouchard, C., A. W. Taylor, & S. Dulac: Testing maximal anaerobic power and capacity. In J. D. MacDougall, H. W. Wenger, & H. J. Green (eds.), *Physiological Testing of the High-Performance Athlete* (2nd edition). Champaign, IL: Human Kinetics Publishers, 175–221 (1991).

14. Bouchard, C., A. W. Taylor, J. A., Simoneau, & S. Dulac: Testing anaerobic power and capacity. In J. D. MacDougall, H. A. Wenger, & H. J. Green (eds.), *Physiological Testing of the Elite Athlete* (1st edition). Hamilton, Ontario: Canadian Association of Sport Sciences Mutual Press Limited, 61–73 (1982).

15. Brooks, G. A.: Current concepts in lactate exchange. *Medicine and Science in Sports and Exercise.* 23(8):895–906 (1991).

16. Casaburi, R., T. W. Storer, I. Ben-Dov, & K. Wasserman: Effect of endurance training on possible determinants of VO_2 during heavy exercise. *Journal of Applied Physiology.* 62(1):199–207 (1987).

17. Chaloupka, E. C., & E. L. Fox: Physiological effects of two maintenance programs following eight weeks of interval training. *Federation Proceedings* (abstract). 34(3):443 (1975).

18. Clarke, H. H. (ed.): Exercise and aging. *Physical Fitness Research Digest.* Washington, DC: President's Council on Physical Fitness and Sports. 7(2) (1977).

19. Conconi, F., M. Ferrari, P. G. Ziglo, P. Droghetti, & L. Codeca: Determination of the anaerobic threshold by a noninvasive field test in runners. *Journal of Applied Physiology.* 52:869–873 (1982).

20. Conley, D., G. Krahenbuhl, & L. Burkett: Training for aerobic capacity and running economy. *Physician and Sportsmedicine.* 9(4):107–115 (1981).

21. Costill, D. L.: *Inside Running: Basics of Sport Physiology.* Indianapolis: Benchmark Press (1986).

22. Costill, D. L., D. S. King, R. Thomas, & M. Hargreaves: Effects of reduced training on muscular power in swimmers. *Physician and Sportsmedicine.* 13:94–101 (1985).

23. Coyle, E. F., W. H. Martin, D. R. Sinacore, M. J. Joyner, J. M. Hagberg, & J. O. Holloszy: Time course of loss of adaptations after stopping prolonged intense endurance training. *Journal of Applied Physiology: Respiratory, Environmental and Exercise Physiology.* 57(6):1857–1864 (1984).

24. Daniels, J., N. Oldridge, F. Nagle, B. White: Differences and changes in VO_2 among young runners 10 to 18 years of age. *Medicine and Science in Sports and Exercise.* 10(3):200–203 (1978).

25. Donovan, C. M., & G. A. Brooks: Endurance training affects lactate clearance, not lactate production. *American Journal of Physiology.* 244:E83–E92 (1983).

26. Dwyer, J., & R. Bybee: Heart rate indices of the anaerobic threshold. *Medicine and Science in Sports and Exercise.* 15(1):72–76 (1983).

27. Ekblom, B., P.- O. Åstrand, B. Saltin, J. Stenberg, & B. Wallström: Effect of training on circulatory response to exercise. *Journal of Applied Physiology.* 24(4):518–528 (1968).

28. Eriksson, B. O.: Physical training, oxygen supply and muscle metabolism in 11–13 year old boys. *Acta Physiologica Scandinavica.* Suppl. 384:1–48 (1972).

29. Fox, E. L., R. W. Bowers, & M. L. Foss: *The Physiological Basis of Physical Education and Athletics* (4th edition). Philadelphia: Saunders College (1988).

30. Fox, E. L., & D. K. Mathews: *Internal Training: Conditioning for Sports and General Fitness.* Philadelphia: W. B. Saunders (1974).

31. Fox, E. L., S. Robinson, & D. L. Wiegman: Metabolic energy sources during continuous and interval running. *Journal of Applied Physiology.* 27(2):174–178 (1969).

32. Franks, B. D.: Physical warm-up. In: M. H. Williams (ed.), *Ergogenic Aids in Sport.* Champaign, IL: Human Kinetics Publishers, 340–375 (1983).

33. Fry, R. W., A. R. Morton, & D. Keast: Overtraining in athletics: An update. *Sports Medicine.* 12(1):32–65 (1991).

34. Gaisl, G., & G. Wiesspeiner: Training prescriptions for 9– to 17–year-old figure skaters based on lactate assessment in the laboratory and on the ice. In: J. Rutenfranz, R. Mocellin, & F. Klimt (eds.) *Children and Exercise XII.* Champaign, IL: Human Kinetics Publishers, 17:59–65 (1986).

35. Galbo, H.: *Hormonal and Metabolic Adaptation to Exercise.* New York: Thieme-Stratton, Inc. (1983).

36. Gardner, A. W., E. T. Poehlman, & D. L. Corrigan: Effect of endurance training on gross energy expenditure during exercise. *Human Biology.* 61(4):559–569 (1989).

37. Gilman, M. B., & C. L. Wells: The use of heart rates to monitor exercise intensity in relation to metabolic variables. *International Journal of Sports Medicine.* 14(6):3334–3339 (1993).

38. Gollnick, P. D., W. M. Bayly, & D. R. Hodgson: Exercise intensity, training, diet, and lactate concentration in muscle and blood. *Medicine and Science in Sports and Exercise.* 18(3):334–340 (1986).

39. Gollnick, P. D., & L. Hermansen: Biochemical adaptations in exercise: Anaerobic metabolism. In J. H. Wilmore (ed.), *Exercise and Sport Sciences Reviews.* New York: Academic Press (1973).

40. Gutin, B., K. Stewart, S. Lewis, & J. Kruper: Oxygen consumption in the first stages of strenuous work as a function of prior exercise. *Journal of Sports Medicine and Physical Fitness.* 16(1):60–65 (1976).

41. Hagberg, J. M., J. P. Mullin, & F. J. Nagle: Oxygen consumption during constant-load exercise. *Journal of Applied Physiology: Respiratory, Environmental and Exercise Physiology.* 45(3):381–384 (1978).

42. Hamel, P., J.-A. Simoneau, G. Lortie, M. R. Boulay, & C. Bouchard: Heredity and muscle adaptation to endurance training. *Medicine and Science in Sports and Exercise.* 18(6):690–696 (1986).

43. Henritze, J., A. Weltman, R. L. Schurrer, & K. Barlow: Effects of training at and above the lactate threshold on the lactate threshold and maximal oxygen uptake. *European Journal of Applied Physiology.* 54:84–88 (1985).

44. Hickson, R. C., J. M. Hagberg, A. A. Ehsani, & J. O. Holloszy: Time course of the adaptive response of aerobic power and heart rate to training. *Medicine and Science in Sports and Exercise.* 13(1):17–20 (1981).

45. Holloszy, J. O.: Biochemical adaptations to exercise: Aerobic metabolism. In J. H. Wilmore (ed.), *Exercise and Sport Sciences Reviews.* New York: Academic Press, 1:45–71 (1973).

46. Holloszy, J. O., & E. F. Coyle: Adaptations of skeletal muscle to endurance exercise and their metabolic consequences. *Journal of Applied Physiology: Respiratory, Environmental and Exercise Physiology.* 56:831–838 (1984).

47. Hood, D. A., & R. L. Terjung: Amino acid metabolism during exercise and following endurance training. *Sports Medicine.* 9(1):23–35 (1990).

48. Horswill, C. A., J. R. Scott, & P. Galea: Comparison of maximum aerobic power, maximum anaerobic power, and skinfold thickness of elite and nonelite junior wrestlers. *International Journal of Sports Medicine.* 10:165–168 (1989).

49. Houmard, J. A., D. L. Costill, J. B. Mitchell, S. H. Park, R. C. Hickner, & J. M. Roemmich: Reduced training maintains performance in distance runners. *International Journal of Sports Medicine.* 11:46–52 (1990).

50. Janssen, P. G. J. M.: *Training Lactate Pulse-rate.* Oulu, Finland: Polar Electro Oy (1987).

51. Johns, R. A., J. A. Houmard, R. W. Kobe, T. Hortobagyi, N. J. Bruno, J. M. Wells, & M. H. Shinebarger: Effects of taper on swim power, stroke distance, and performance. *Medicine and Science in Sports and Exercise.* 24(10);1141–1146 (1992).

52. Karlsson, J., L. -O. Nordesjö, L. Jorfeldt, & B. Saltin: Muscle lactate, ATP, and CP levels during exercise after physical training in man. *Journal of Applied Physiology.* 33(2):199–203 (1972).

53. Massicotte, D. R., & R. B. J. MacNab: Cardiorespiratory adaptations to training at specified intensities in children. *Medicine and Science in Sports.* 6(4):242–246 (1974).

54. Mazzeo, R. S., G. A. Brooks, D. A. Schoeller, & T. F. Budinger: Disposal of blood $[1-^{13}C]$ lactate in humans during rest and exercise. *Journal of Applied Physiology.* 60(1):232–241 (1986).

55. McCafferty, W. B., & S. M. Horvath: Specificity of exercise and specificity of training: A subcellular review. *Research Quarterly.* 48(2):358–371 (1977).

56. Medbø, J. I., & S. Burgers: Effect of training on the anaerobic capacity. *Medicine and Science in Sports and Exercise.* 22(4):501–507 (1990).

57. Neufer, P. D.: The effect of detraining and reduced training on the physiological adaptations to aerobic exercise training. *Sports Medicine.* 8(5):302–321 (1989).

58. Patton, J. F., & A. Duggan: An evaluation of tests of anaerobic power. *Aviation and Space Environmental Medicine.* 58:237–242 (1987).

59. Ready, A. E., & H. A. Quinney: Alternations in anaerobic threshold as the result of endurance training and detraining. *Medicine in Sports and Exercise.* 14(4):292–296 (1982).

60. Rotstein, A., R. Dotan, O. Bar-Or, & G. Tenenbaum: Effect of training on anaerobic threshold, maximal aerobic power and anaerobic performance of preadolescent boys. *International Journal of Sports Medicine.* 7(5):281–286 (1986).

61. Rowland, T. W.: *Exercise and Children's Health.* Champaign, IL: Human Kinetics Publishers (1990).

62. Seals, D. R., B. F. Hurley, J. Schultz, & J. M. Hagberg: Endurance training in older men and women. II. Blood lactate response to submaximal exercise. *Journal of Applied Physiology: Respiratory, Environmental and Exercise Physiology.* 57(4):1030–1033 (1984).

63. Shepard, R. J.: *Physical Activity and Aging.* Chicago: Year Book Medical Publishers (1978).

64. Shepley, B., J. D. MacDougall, N. Cipriano, J. R. Sutton, G. Coates, & M. Tarnopolsky: Physiological effects of tapering in highly trained athletes. *Journal of Applied Physiology.* 72:706–711 (1992).

65. Sjödin, B., I. Jacobs, & J. Svedenhag: Changes in onset of blood lactate accumulation (OBLA) and muscle enzymes after training at OBLA. *European Journal of Applied Physiology.* 49:45–57 (1982).

66. Skinner, J. S., & D. W. Morgan: Aspects of anaerobic performance. In D. H. Clarke & H. M. Eckert (eds.), *Limits of Human Performance.* Champaign, IL: Human Kinetics Publishers, 131–144 (1985).

67. Tlusty, L.: Physical fitness in old age. II. Anaerobic capacity, anaerobic work in graded exercise, recovery after maximum work performance in elderly individuals. *Respiration.* 26:287–299 (1969).

68. Van de Graaff, K. M., & S. I. Fox: *Concepts of Human Anatomy and Physiology* (2nd edition). Dubuque, IA: Brown (1989).

69. Wells, C. L.: *Women, Sport and Performance: A Physiological Perspective* (2nd edition). Champaign, IL: Human Kinetics Publishers (1991).

70. Wells, C. L., & R. R. Pate: Training for performance of prolonged exercise. In D. R. Lamb & R. Murray (eds.), *Perspectives in Exercise Science and Sports Medicine. Vol. I: Prolonged Exercise.* Indianapolis: Benchmark Press, 357–388 (1988).

71. Weltman, A., R. J. Moffatt, & B. A. Stamford: Supramaximal training in females: Effects on anaerobic power output, anaerobic capacity, and aerobic power. *Journal of Sports Medicine and Physical Fitness.* 18(3):237–244 (1978).

72. Williams, C. G., C. H. Wyndham, R. Kok, & M. J. E. von Rahden: Effect of training on maximal oxygen intake and on anaerobic metabolism in man. *Internationale Zeitschrift fuer Angewandte Physiologie Einschliesslich Arbeitsphysiologie.* 24:18–23 (1967).

73. Wilmore, J. H., & D. L. Costill: *Training for Sport and Activity: The Physiological Basis of the Conditioning Process* (3rd edition). Dubuque, IA: Brown (1988).

74. Yoshida, T., S. Yoshihiro, & N. Takeuchi: Endurance training regimen based upon arterial blood lactate: Effects on anaerobic threshold. *European Journal of Applied Physiology.* 49:223–230 (1982).

13

Nutrition for Fitness and Athletics

After studying the chapter, you should be able to:

- List the goals for nutrition during training and for nutrition during competition and explain why they are different.

- Compare a balanced diet for sedentary individuals with a balanced diet for active individuals in terms of caloric intake; carbohydrate, fat, and protein intake; and vitamin, mineral, and fluid requirements.

- Discuss the positive and negative aspects of a high carbohydrate diet.

- Interpret the glycemic index; identify common high-, moderate-, and low-glycemic foods; and explain the best use of each classification.

- Discuss the situations where an increase in protein above the RDA is advisable and when it is not advisable.

- Describe a training situation when fat intake can be too low.

- Compare the theory behind the use of carbohydrate loading for endurance athletes to the theory behind its use for bodybuilders.

- Compare the classic versus the modified techniques of carbohydrate loading in terms of diet and exercise for endurance event competitors.

- Develop a preevent meal plan for athletic competition.

- Develop a plan for feeding during an endurance event and defend it.

- Describe optimal fluid ingestion during and after exercise.

- Judge the value of commercially available sport drinks.

- Differentiate among the eating disorders anorexia nervosa, bulimia nervosa, and anorexia athletica by definition and characteristics.

- Identify the risk factors for developing an eating disorder.

- Construct a list of guidelines to help prevent or deal with eating disorders in exercise settings.

Introduction

Proper nutrition and exercise are natural partners for health, fitness, and athletic performances. Consequently, many fitness enthusiasts pursue healthy diets, and athletes try to optimize athletic performance by identifying appropriate diets. Although these trends are very positive, they also have the potential to be taken to an extreme—an extreme that may simply involve spending money needlessly on "nutritional supplements" or an extreme that may actually be harmful—such as eating disorders. It is the responsibility of all fitness professionals to understand what constitutes optimal nutrition for fitness and athletics.

Nutrition education should be a part of physical fitness classes, community adult fitness and rehabilitation programs, and athletic training. Most individuals who are training regularly want to eat right, but they may confuse advertisements and media hype with factual information.

The issue of optimal nutrition for fitness and athletics must be considered for two different situations. The first is training, and the second competition, whether on the "fun run" or elite level. With the possible exception of youth sports, individuals typically spend more total time training than competing. Therefore, daily nutritional practices are the more critical. No amount of dietary manipulation the day of and/or the day before a competition can make up for poor nutritional habits otherwise.[12]

Nutrition and Training

Individuals involved in exercise training need to match their training regime with an appropriate diet. This attempt often involves consultation with a fitness professional, a complete diet analysis, and, many times, a trial-and-error technique to find what works best for a given individual.

The goals of an optimal training diet are:

1. To provide caloric and nutrient requirements.
2. To incorporate nutritional practices that promote good health.
3. To achieve and maintain optimal body composition and playing weight.
4. To promote recovery from training sessions and physiological adaptations.
5. To try variations of precompetition and competition fuel and fluid intake to determine bodily responses.[12]

There is almost universal agreement that poor nutritional status impairs work performance. There is also considerable, although not universal, agreement that good general nutrition (the balanced diet recommended for just about everyone; see Table 13.1) is adequate and probably even optimal for most active individuals as well as sedentary individuals.

Unfortunately, the typical American does not eat the recommended healthy balanced diet. Many still consume too much fat (37–42%) and too little carbohydrate (43–48%). If the recommended percentages (not more than 30% fat and 55–58% carbohydrate) are consumed, the vast majority of youth sport, middle and secondary school, and college athletes as well as fitness participants of all ages will not need any modification in their diet. For those athletes or fitness participants training very long, hard, and often and/or competing at an elite level, a few modifications may be beneficial.[2,3,6,9,12,36,45] Table 13.1 summarizes these recommendations, which are discussed in the following sections.

Kilocalories

The most obvious distinction between active and inactive individuals is the number of calories required per day. Everyone needs sufficient calories to support daily needs, and children need adequate calories for growth. In addition, an active individual can expend several hundred to several thousand kilocalories more per day than a sedentary individual. The actual amount depends on the size of the individual and the intensity, duration, and frequency of the workouts. Big football players doing two-a-days and smaller endurance athletes expend large amounts of energy, but golfers or softball and baseball players of any size expend much smaller amounts. Some athletes may actually increase their daily energy expenditure by 25–50% during the season.[3,9,12,31] Costill[19] cites figures of 900–2400 kcal·day^{-1} expended for elite distance runners, 6000 kcal·day^{-1} for cyclists, and 1250–3750

TABLE 13.1 ■ Balanced Diets

FOR SEDENTARY INDIVIDUALS	FOR ACTIVE INDIVIDUALS
Calorie balance to maintain acceptable body composition and weight	Adequate caloric intake to balance caloric expenditure of training and competition in excess of normal living while maintaining optimal body composition and playing weight
12–15% protein (1.2 g · kg^{-1} · day^{-1}, 7–10 yr; 1.0 g · kg^{-1} · day^{-1}, 11–14 yr; 0.9 g · kg^{-1} · day^{-1}, 15–18 yr; 0.8 g · kg^{-1} · day^{-1}, 19+ yr)	12–15% protein (1.2–2 g · kg^{-1} · day^{-1})
30% fat ($\frac{1}{3}$ saturated, $\frac{1}{3}$ unsaturated, $\frac{1}{3}$ polyunsaturated)	20–30% fat ($\frac{1}{3}$ saturated, $\frac{1}{3}$ unsaturated, $\frac{1}{3}$ polyunsaturated)
55–58% carbohydrate (4.5 g · kg^{-1} · day^{-1})	58–68% carbohydrate (8–10 g · kg^{-1} · day^{-1})
RDA for vitamins and minerals	RDA for vitamins and minerals
Fluid intake monitored by thirst	Fluids adequate to prevent dehydration

Source: Based on information from Brotherhood,[9] Haymes.[26]

kcal · day^{-1} for swimmers during training. These calories must be replaced.

Published reports indicate that male basketball and football players may consume as many as 9000–11,000 kcal · day^{-1}, triathletes 3500–6400 kcal · day^{-1} (female and male), cross-country skiers 4000–5500 kcal · day^{-1} (females and male), and track and field athletes (male) 3500–4700 kcal · day^{-1}, depending on the event. It is highly likely that these athletes are adequately resupplying their energy needs.[12]

On the other hand, in some sports (long-distance running, gymnastics, wrestling, and dance) an attempt is often made to maintain extremely low and, in some cases, "unnatural" body fat and body weight. Intake values as low as 600 kcal · day^{-1} for male gymnasts and 900 kcal · day^{-1} for female ballet dancers have been reported. It is equally likely that these athletes are *not* adequately resupplying their energy needs.[12]

If the relative proportion of nutrients remained the same as the calories increased to support training, the active individual would have an acceptable diet. However, some subtle shifting of percentages and/or amounts can be of benefit in certain situations. Chief among them is an increased percentage of carbohydrate ingestion for endurance athletes.

Carbohydrate

The earlier discussion of carbohydrate metabolism (Chapter 9) pointed out several important facts about carbohydrates as a fuel for exercise.[3,12,19,45]

1. The higher the intensity of exercise (whether continuous or intermittent; aerobic, anaerobic, or aerobic-anaerobic), the more important glycogen is as a fuel.

2. The body can only store limited amounts of carbohydrates. Training increases the ability to store carbohydrate and to spare carbohydrate. However, 60–90 min of heavy endurance work seriously depletes glycogen stores, and depletion can be complete in 120 min. Muscle glycogen can also be depleted by 15–30 min of near-maximal or supramaximal-intensity interval work.

3. Fat metabolism is linked to carbohydrate metabolism. Fatigue, "hitting the wall," and exhaustion are tied to glycogen depletion during high-intensity, long-duration activity. Thus, having an adequate supply of muscle glycogen is necessary if one is to avoid fatigue. Whatever glycogen is utilized, in training or competition, must be replenished before more heavy work can be done.

The storage of carbohydrate in liver and muscles depends on the level of activity (that is, the severity of glycogen depletion), the extent of muscle trauma, and the amount of dietary carbohydrate. Muscle glycogen resynthesis is highest when the muscle has been depleted, but not necessarily exhausted, and the diet is high in carbohydrate. Muscle fiber damage associated with exhaustive eccentric exercise (in which a contracting muscle is forcibly lengthened), such as running a marathon, may delay resynthesis for as long as 7–10 days despite elevated dietary carbohydrate.[12, 19]

How much carbohydrate should be included in the diet? The normal recommended intake of carbohydrate is 4.5 $g \cdot kg^{-1} \cdot day^{-1}$. For an individual utilizing high amounts of carbohydrate in training, 8–10 $g \cdot kg^{-1} \cdot day^{-1}$ are recommended. In some cases this may increase the percentage of carbohydrate to 70–80% of the dietary intake.

Particularly important is the intake of carbohydrate during recovery from exercise when the glycogen that has been used needs to be replenished. Carbohydrate ingestion (50–100 g) should begin as soon after the workout or competition as is practical (15–30 min) and continue at the rate of 50 g every 2 hr until a larger meal of solid food (150–250 g of carbohydrate) is desired and possible.[21] Does it matter which carbohydrates are ingested or if carbohydrates only are ingested? The answer to both questions is yes and no.

Liquid carbohydrate sources are as effective as solid carbohydrate sources. In fact, liquids may be even more useful, since many individuals are not hungry after an intense bout of exercise and fluid replacement is also important.[19, 20] Table 13.2 provides a comparison of some currently available liquid commercial products containing readily available carbohydrates. Figure 13.1 shows a cyclist ingesting one of these products. In addition, nutrition bars such as ATP Tour, Cross Trainer Bar, Gator Bar, Hard Body Sports Bar, Power Bar, Super Heavyweight Bar, and Tiger Sport Bar provide a readily available source of carbohydrates, usually consisting of at least two types.

Some forms of simple sugars appear to have different effects on glycogen resynthesis. Glucose and

TABLE 13.2 ■ Composition of Selected Sports Drinks (per 8 oz or 240 mL)

NAME	TYPE OF CHO*	kcal	CHO (g)	CHO† CONCENTRATION (%)	Na (mg)	K (mg)	OTHER
All Sport	F, G	88	22	9	55	55	Ca, Cl, P, vitamin C
Body Fuel 450	GP, F	40	10	4		20	—
Carbo Plus	GP	170	42.5	18	5	100	Mg
Exceed	GP, F	68	17	7	50	45	Ca, Mg, P, Cl
Gatorade	G, S	56	14	6	110	25	Cl, P
Gatorlode	G, GP	280	47	20	95	0	Vitamins
Gator Pro		360	58	24	180	630	Fat, protein, vitamins, minerals
Gookinade E.R.G.	G	45	11	5	70	100	—
Nutrament	F	240	34	14			Fat, protein
Power Burst	F	50	12	5	35	55	Ca, Cl, Mg, vitamins
R.P.M.		70	17.5	7	0	70	
Water		0	0	0	Low	Low	Depends on source

*F = fructose, G = glucose, GP = glucose polymer, and S = sucrose.
†% concentration = [CHO (g)] ÷ [volume (mL)] × 100, rounded to nearest whole percentage.

Source: Compiled from Applegate,[4] Murray,[41] Nieman,[45] Quaker Oats Company[50] and from brand labels.

FIGURE 13.1

Replenishment of carbohydrate during and after exercise training sessions can easily be accomplished by drinking specially formulated sports drinks. Such drinks provide both fuel and fluid.

sucrose promote muscle glycogen resynthesis, whereas fructose promotes liver glycogen resynthesis. Fructose alone is not recommended, because it must first be converted to glucose in the liver before muscles can store it as glycogen.[8, 19, 20] This conversion delays the process of replenishing muscle glycogen stores.

Ingesting protein along with the carbohydrates in the 4-hour time span after exercise has been shown to significantly increase the rate of glycogen storage.[63] Some of the liquid supplements listed in Table 13.2 and many of the solid nutrition bars include both carbohydrate and proteins.

Perhaps the most important criterion for selecting postexercise carbohydrates is the glycemic index.[20, 21, 53] The **glycemic index** compares the elevation in blood glucose caused by the ingestion of 50 g of any carbohydrate food with the elevation caused by 50 g of white bread.[62] The glycemic index cannot be predicted by knowing the chemical composition of the food, including whether it is a simple or a complex carbohydrate. Instead, the glycemic index depends upon the speed at which foods are digested and absorbed.[62] White bread has been assigned a glycemic index of 100. High-glycemic foods have a rating of 85 or greater; moderate-glycemic foods rate from 60 to 85; low-glycemic foods have a rating less than 60. Values greater than 100 are possible.

Foods with a high glycemic index cause a fast, high elevation in glucose and insulin; foods with lower indices cause a slower rise in both glucose and insulin. Table 13.3 gives examples of high-, moderate-, and low-glycemic foods. In general, sugars and sports drinks; syrups and jellies; and grain, pasta, and cereal products have high or moderate glycemic indices. Most fruits, legumes, and dairy products have low glycemic indices. Significantly greater glycogen resynthesis and storage results from the ingestion of high-glycemic foods over a 24-hr period than from the intake of low-glycemic foods.[13] Moderate-glycemic foods appear to promote glycogen resynthesis just about as effectively as high-glycemic goods.[21] Glycogen resynthesis occurs at about 5–6% per hour under optimal dietary conditions, thus even then requiring approximately 17–20 hr for complete recovery.[20, 21]

If replenishment of carbohydrates does not occur between training bouts, local muscle fatigue will result, and work output during succeeding training sessions will decline.[19, 20] Severe depletion followed by a nonoptimal diet will require more than one day of rest, which is one reason to alternate body parts and hard-easy exercise days. If the aim of carbohydrate ingestion is not quick glycogen replenishment but a slower sustained presentation of glucose into the system, as would be the case during a marathon or long hike, then low-glycemic foods are preferable.[21]

Although most individuals would benefit from increasing the percentage of carbohydrate ingested, levels as high as 70–80% are recommended only

Glycemic Index A measure that compares the elevation in blood glucose caused by the ingestion of 50 g of any carbohydrate food with the elevation caused by the ingestion of 50 g of white bread.

TABLE 13.3 ■ Glycemic Index of Selected Foods

HIGH-GLYCEMIC FOOD (85 OR GREATER)	MODERATE-GLYCEMIC FOOD (60–85)	LOW-GLYCEMIC FOOD (UNDER 60)
SUGARS, SYRUPS, AND JELLIES		**SUGARS, SYRUPS, AND JELLIES**
White table sugar		Fructose
Maple syrup		
Honey		
Sports drinks (6–20% CHO concentration)		
CEREAL PRODUCTS		
Bagel	Rice	Barley
Bread (white, wheat)	Pasta (spaghetti, macaroni)	
Corn flakes	Bread (whole grain, rye)	
Shredded wheat		
Oatmeal		
Puffed wheat and rice		
FRUITS		
Raisins	Grapes	Apples
Watermelon	Orange juice	Cherries
	Banana	Peach
		Pear
		Plum
		Grapefruit
VEGETABLES		
Potatoes (baked, microwaved, mashed)	Yams	
Carrots	Sweet corn	
Parsnips		
LEGUMES		
	Baked beans	Beans (butter, green, kidney, navy; dried)
	Beans (kidney, pinto; canned)	Lentils (green, red; dried)
	Peas (chick, green; canned or frozen)	
	Lentils (red, green; canned)	
DAIRY PRODUCTS		
	Ice cream	Milk (skim, whole)
		Yogurt
		Custard

Source: Compiled from Coyle & Coyle;[21] Jenkins et al.;[28] Singh, Pelletier, & Deuster;[53] Wolever.[62]

for athletes or fitness participants who are actually using high amounts of carbohydrate in their training regimens. Such individuals include long-distance runners, swimmers, cyclists, and soccer, hockey, or lacrosse players.[19, 20]

There is little advantage, and possibly some risk, for a nonendurance athlete such as a golfer, a softball or baseball player, or a fitness walker to ingest 70–80% carbohydrates, especially if much of this food has a high glycemic index. As mentioned earlier, absorption of a large dose of high glycemic carbohydrates results in temporary hyperglycemia and an increased insulin response. Glycogen storage is limited in sedentary and nonendurance-trained individuals, and the glycolytic pathway is overloaded. The result is a greater-than-normal reliance on a side pathway that converts the glucose to free fatty acids (and then triglycerides) and cholesterol.[19, 44] Absorption of the same amount of low-glycemic carbohydrates results in a smaller blood glucose and insulin rise and hence less lipid formation. High blood levels of triglycerides and, more definitively, cholesterol are frequently associated with an increased risk of cardiovascular disease.

Endurance-trained individuals demonstrate less hyperglycemia and a lower insulin response in relation to a given glucose load than do untrained individuals. Thus, endurance-trained individuals appear to be able to convert high dietary levels of carbohydrate, especially high-glycemic foods, into glycogen storage without an elevation of blood lipids. Carbohydrate should be the highest energy substrate in terms of percentage for all individuals, but an additional 10–20% above the normal 55–58% is not recommended for sedentary individuals nor for low-intensity nonendurance athletes.[19]

Protein

The optimal amount of dietary protein for individuals engaged in exercise training and competition has been debated practically forever, and it remains an area of controversy. The *recommended daily allowance* (RDA) of protein varies among countries for adults (United States: 0.8 g·kg⁻¹ for male and female; Australia: 1.0 g·kg⁻¹ for male and female; and Netherlands: 1.0 g·kg⁻¹ for female and 1.2 g·kg⁻¹ for male) and within countries for various ages. For example, the U.S. RDA decreases from 1.2 g·kg⁻¹ for 7–10-yr-olds to 1.0 g·kg⁻¹ for 11–14-yr-olds to 0.9 g·kg⁻¹ for 15–18-yr-olds. Pregnant or lactating females are encouraged to ingest higher levels of protein, but only the Netherlands officially recommends an increased intake (1.5 g·kg⁻¹·day⁻¹) for physically active individuals.[33, 34]

The reluctance of nutritional experts to advocate increased protein intake relative to body weight is based upon several factors.[36] First, because of the complexities of metabolism and the inaccuracies of measurement, the RDA for most nutrients, includ-

ing protein, has not been precisely determined. Second, the estimated recommendations for protein just given are thought to include a considerable safety margin (about 78%). Finally, this safety margin is generally assumed to be sufficient to cover any additional exercise-induced increase in protein requirement. However, in several situations this assumption is questionable.

The first such situation is activity involving large increases in muscle mass as a primary goal of the training.[29, 34, 35, 36] Individuals involved in resistance training—such as weight lifters, power lifters, bodybuilders, football players, sprinters, and wrestlers—strive for increased muscular strength and/or hypertrophy. Training of this type typically leads to increased protein in the muscle fibers (see Chapter 19). This increased muscle protein probably results from a decrease in the endogenous protein breakdown (which would decrease the need for dietary protein) and an increased protein synthesis from amino acids (which would increase the need for dietary protein). This balance between demand and supply, unfortunately, is generally not precise. In fact, there is evidence that for the body to maintain a positive nitrogen balance—and, hence, maintain the availability of indispensable amino acids—an increase above the RDA is needed. On the other hand, there is minimal scientific evidence that amino acid supplementation in excess of the additional amount needed to maintain a positive nitrogen balance will enhance muscle hypertrophy or strength attainment. The consensus of current evidence suggests that strength and speed athletes may need to consume 1.2–2.0 g·kg⁻¹·day⁻¹ of protein, which should be possible within the recommended 15% of total caloric intake.[3,9,26,33,34,35,59]

The second situation is endurance training. Surprising though it may be, both the need and the evidence for an increased protein intake are stronger here than for resistance and power athletes.[29] When an individual begins a training program, a situation called **sports anemia,** a transient decrease in red blood cells and hemoglobin level (grams per deciliter), may develop. During the initial two to

Sports Anemia A transient decrease in red blood cells and hemoglobin levels (grams per deciliter of blood).

three weeks of a training program, blood proteins, including erythrocytes (red blood cells, RBC), may be utilized to increase the myoglobin concentration, mitochondrial mass, and enzymes that are part of the training adaptation. An increased intake of dietary protein may minimize the destruction of red blood cells, promote their regeneration, and provide the protein needed for the other training adaptations to occur. However, there is an alternative explanation for sports anemia that involves plasma volume rather than protein (RBC) degradation. If plasma volume increases but hemoglobin and red blood cells do not (or they do not increase proportionally), a dilution effect may occur, resulting in decreased hemoglobin and red blood cell concentrations. Research supports blood volume changes. However, the two phenomena, increased dilution and protein degradation, are not mutually exclusive. Furthermore, research evidence is accumulating showing that experienced and not just novice endurance athletes may also suffer sports anemia.[3,26,35,59]

In addition, high-intensity long-duration training and competition result in increased amino acid oxidation as fuel, ranging from 5 to 15% of the total calories used, especially if the individual is depleted of carbohydrates.[9] Cool-temperature training (5–20°C, or 40–68°F) also utilizes more protein than warm-weather (30°C, or 86°F) training. Females utilize more protein during exercise in the midluteal phase of the menstrual cycle (approximately days 14–21) than during the follicular phase (approximately days 1–7).

Finally, additional protein may be needed to avoid overtraining or staleness for endurance athletes. The use of relatively large amounts of branched-chain amino acids (BCAA) as fuel during long endurance activity leads to increased levels of the neurotransmitter serotonin in the brain. High levels of serotonin, in turn, have been linked to many of the reported signs and symptoms of overtraining, including appetite suppression and weight loss, fatigue and performance decrement, increased resting heart rates, anemia, amenorrhea, and suppression of the immune system. Some preliminary research in which BCAA supplements were added to normal carbohydrate replacement drinks during ultraendurance triathlon performance and high-volume swim training has shown positive results.[29] Other studies have not shown a beneficial effect

from BCAA supplementation. There is also some concern regarding the size of the BCAA dosage needed, especially since gastrointestinal disturbances can result from high BCAA ingestion.[22] On the other hand, additional protein may also be beneficial to ensure repair of any damaged muscle fiber.[33, 34] For all of these reasons, a small increase in the intake of dietary protein to 1.2–1.4 $g \cdot kg^{-1} \cdot day^{-1}$ is recommended for high-intensity, long-duration aerobic endurance training. Individuals training at less than 50% $\dot{V}O_2$max for 20–60 $min \cdot day^{-1}$ do not need to increase their protein intake above the RDA.

At least two high-energy sport bars (the *Beta* Bar and the PR Bar) are formulated to include 40% carbohydrate, 30% protein, and 30% fat. This high protein percentage, eaten 30 min prior to a workout, is said to stimulate the release of glucagon and inhibit the release of insulin so that more fat is mobilized from adipose sites and used as fuel during exercise. Since glucagon does stimulate utilization of fat and insulin does inhibit fat burning in favor of fat storage, this is theoretically possible. However, research results from controlled studies are not available to support this claim.

Although these situations and recommendations call for an increased amount of protein per kilogram of body weight, the percentage should not be increased above the recommended 12–15% of the total calories ingested.[34, 47] Consider, for example, a 56-kg (123-lb) female triathlete. If her caloric intake goes from 1500 $kcal \cdot day^{-1}$ (12% protein) when sedentary to 2240 $kcal \cdot day^{-1}$ during heavy training while maintaining 12% protein ingestion, this increase now provides her with 1.2 $g \cdot kg^{-1}$ instead of 0.8 $g \cdot kg^{-1}$ of protein. At 15% of these calories 1.5 $g \cdot kg^{-1}$ of protein would be provided daily. The key point is that the *total* caloric intake must be increased. If the total energy intake is insufficient, then the percentages allotted to protein may be inadequate. For example, if the athlete increased her caloric intake to only 1900 $kcal \cdot day^{-1}$ at 12% protein intake, this increase would amount to only 1 $g \cdot kg^{-1} \cdot day^{-1}$. Also, if the athlete increased her carbohydrate to 70%, she would need to carefully select the remaining 30% of her foodstuffs to get an adequate protein intake.

The problem of ingesting too few calories and thus ingesting inadequate protein is especially evident where the athlete is concerned with percentage of body fat or making weight. The problem is compounded if the individual is a child or adolescent. As previously mentioned, individuals in this age range need more protein than adults. Inadequate protein intake at this age might adversely affect not only exercise performance but also growth.[33, 54] Of course, if the extra protein ingested is also excess calories, weight and fat will be gained, and that also is not desirable. For the elderly the interaction of protein need and exercise is unknown at the current time.

Before deciding to increase dietary protein, a complete nutritional analysis should be done. It should not be assumed that because an individual falls in one of the categories of strength or endurance athlete, that additional dietary protein or a protein supplement is needed.[33]

Can too much protein in the diet be harmful to the fitness participant or competitive athlete? In individuals with preexisting liver or kidney abnormalities a high-protein diet can lead to further deterioration of function.[3, 35] There is no evidence, though, that individuals with normal kidneys and livers are harmed from high-protein intake.

Two factors, however, require attention. The first is that the metabolism of protein requires more water than the metabolism of carbohydrate or fat does. Therefore, a concomitant increase in water intake is important for the individual to avoid dehydration if protein intake is increased. The second factor relates to calcium balance. There is evidence in sedentary individuals that increasing dietary protein levels leads to increased calcium excretion, suggesting a loss in bone calcium.[2, 36] If dietary protein intake is excessive, the result could be an accelerated loss of bone density (see Chapter 16). Many female endurance athletes already exhibit a profile of low bone mineral density (and the possible causative factors of low estrogen and low dietary calcium intake).[23] Whether exercise combined with a high-protein diet would exaggerate or protect against additional calcium loss has not been demonstrated experimentally. Until it is, the female endurance athlete should not conclude that if a high protein diet (12–15% as recommended) is good, then an even higher protein diet (greater than 15%) would be better.

Fat

As discussed earlier (Chapters 9 and 11), fat is a major fuel for exercises of low or moderate intensity,

and it is readily available in more-than-adequate storage amounts in most individuals. In addition, studies have documented (Chapter 12) that with endurance training more fat can be used as a fuel, hence sparing carbohydrate stores; and fat can be used at higher absolute levels of work intensity. The carbohydrate-loading studies described later in the section "Nutrition for Competition" have also shown that following glycogen depletion a high-fat, low-carbohydrate diet results in a decrement in exercise performance.[7]

In direct contrast to this last statement, however, are results from two types of studies. The first type has shown that both untrained obese individuals and well-trained athletes can adapt to a high-fat, low-carbohydrate diet and perform moderately intense (approximately 65% $\dot{V}O_2$max) exercise to exhaustion on a high-fat diet as well as they can when they ingest a normal amount of carbohydrates.[48, 49] This adaptation occurs within approximately four to five weeks and could be beneficial for continuous multiday ultraendurance events such as the cycling Race Across America competition. However, even endurance athletes following this regimen show elevated cholesterol levels. Such a diet is neither prudent nor healthy. High-cholesterol levels are a risk factor for coronary artery disease.

The second type of study has shown that too little fat can cause a decrement in physiological and performance variables. Muoio et al.[40] studied six collegiate distance runners under three dietary conditions: their self-selected normal diet, which consisted of 61% CHO, 24% FAT, and 14% PRO; a high-fat diet of 50% CHO, 38% FAT, and 12% PRO; and a high-carbohydrate diet of 73% CHO, 15% FAT, and 12% PRO. Both $\dot{V}O_2$max and running time to exhaustion were significantly higher following seven days on the high-fat diet than on either the high-carbohydrate or normal diets.

The explanation for these results is theoretically linked to intramuscular stores of triglycerides. Muscle triglycerides are significantly depleted during relatively high intensity submaximal exercise. If low concentrations of intramuscular triglycerides are present at the onset of such activity, there is a reduced availability of free fatty acid substrate for oxidative metabolism. To compensate for this an increased uptake of plasma free fatty acids would be necessary. The rate of exogenous free fatty acid delivery to the working muscle may not be sufficient to supply the needed substrate. Thus, just as glycogen can be depleted from muscle cells and bloodborne glucose not be sufficient to offset this depletion, so possibly can intramuscular free fatty acid depletion not be compensated for by bloodborne free fatty acid.

A low-fat, high-carbohydrate diet results in a reduced supply of intramuscular free fatty acid. However, because a diet that includes 38% fat, as in the study just cited, could represent a health hazard, this level is not recommended. Fat loading at the expense of carbohydrates should not be advised, but neither should any attempt be made to totally remove fat from the diet. The recommendation of between 20 and 30% fat for sedentary and moderately active individuals remains the best advice, but it may be that well-trained athletes doing endurance training should not drop below the 30% fat level in their diets. No more than 10% of the ingested fat should be saturated, regardless of activity level.[12, 31] There is no gram per kilogram per day recommended daily allowance for fat for either sedentary or active individuals of any age or either sex.

I w runner hits wall this

Vitamins

C, has exhausted m/glycogen

Thirteen compounds are now considered to be vitamins. **Vitamins** are organic substances of plant or animal origin which are essential for normal growth, development, metabolic processes, and energy transformations. For example, vitamin B_6 is important in amino acid metabolism and the breakdown of glycogen to glucose; thiamin (B_1) is important in carbohydrate metabolism. Riboflavin (B_2) and niacin are important as the hydrogen carriers FAD and NAD, respectively. Ascorbic acid (vitamin C) is necessary for the formation of connective tissues and the catecholamines (important in the stress response) and maintenance of capillary walls. Vita-

min E influences the flow of electrons within the mitochondrial respiratory chain.[6, 60, 61]

There is some evidence to suggest that exercise training may cause an increased need for vitamin C (especially in hot climates), B complex vitamins (particularly B_6 and B_2, also especially in hot climates), and vitamin E at high altitudes.[6, 8, 60, 61] These increased needs, as with the other nutrients, should be adequately covered if the exerciser concomitantly increases his or her total caloric intake with a balanced diet. The increased needs also mean that athletes who are concerned with restricting body weight or body fat or making weight (gymnasts, dancers, figure skaters, divers, wrestlers, boxers, jockeys) and hence restrict caloric intake could be at risk for an inadequate intake of vitamins. For these individuals a generic, one-a-day vitamin and mineral tablet might be appropriate to ensure adequate intake.[6]

After almost 50 years of research there is no evidence that vitamin supplementation, in an adequately nourished individual, improves exercise or athletic performance, speeds up recovery, or decreases injuries.[6, 26] Where deficiencies are present, supplementation to normal physiological levels can improve performance. This is another reason for a complete nutritional analysis for anyone training or competing. However, megadoses of vitamins are neither substitutes for vigorous training nor necessary for training adaptations.[60, 61] Furthermore, extremely large doses of vitamins (both water- and fat-soluble ones) can be toxic, can impair performance, and, more importantly, can cause health problems. Once again, if some is good, more is not necessarily better. For example, high doses of vitamin C have been linked with the formation of kidney stones and the breakdown of red blood cells, which causes a loss of hemoglobin. Megadoses of niacin inhibit fatty acid mobilization and utilization during exercise, thereby increasing the rate of glycogen usage.[45]

Minerals

Minerals are elements not of animal or plant origin that are essential constituents of all cells and of many functions in the body. Minerals are classified as microminerals (trace elements) or macrominerals on the basis of the amount contained in the body. Minerals are important in bone density, energy

---

Vitamins Organic substances of plant or animal origin which are essential for normal growth, development, metabolic processes, and energy transformations.

Minerals Elements not of animal or plant origin which are essential constituents of all cells and of many functions in the body.

metabolism enzyme function, muscle contraction, oxygen transport, insulin regulation, and ATP composition, to name just a few functions.

Microminerals Of the 14 essential microminerals only five (zinc, chromium, copper, selenium and iron) have been implicated as being affected by or potentially beneficial in enhancing exercise training and/or performance.

Exercise can cause a sizable loss of zinc in sweat and urine, and as a result, training may produce a zinc deficiency. However, excess zinc intake above the RDA (15 mg·day^{-1} for adult males, 12 mg·day^{-1} for adult females) can result in an impaired immune response and decreased iron and copper absorption. There is insufficient evidence to conclude that zinc status or zinc supplementation has any impact on exercise performance.[14, 17, 33, 35, 39]

There is speculation, but little evidence, that exercise and training may increase the requirements for chromium (50–200 μg·day^{-1}) and that active individuals should evaluate their chromium intake. Speculation that chromium can increase muscle mass and decrease the percentage of body fat in conjunction with resistance training remains just that—speculation.[32] Chromium supplementation (as chromium picolinate) has been shown in two studies to enhance lean body mass and in one study to decrease the percentage of body fat with weight training.[14, 15] A fourth study[25] using male and female college lifters, equally divided into two groups (those supplemented with chromium picolinate and those not), found the only treatment effect to be a greater gain in body weight in the female supplemented group without any concurrent gain in strength. Clearly, more research is needed in this area, including the safety of long-term chromium supplementation.[32]

There is no evidence that either selenium or copper has an impact on acute or chronic exercise responses, although copper may be lost in sweat. Neither of these trace minerals should be supplemented above the RDA (50–70 μg·day^{-1} for male adolescents and adults, 50–55 μg·day^{-1} for female adolescents and adults, for selenium; 1.5–3.0 mg for copper for everyone).[14, 17]

Iron deficiency can be a problem for the exercising or training individual, especially menstruating females. Iron deficiency exists in three stages: (1) iron depletion, or low-storage levels of iron;

(2) iron deficiency erythropoiesis, which is an impairment of the ability to produce red blood cells; and (3) iron deficiency anemia, or low-hemoglobin levels (less than 12 g·dL^{-1} for females and less than 13 g·dL^{-1} for males). Iron depletion is not associated with a decrement in performance, and the impact of iron deficiency erythropoiesis is marginal. However, iron deficiency anemia definitely impairs performance. Lower-hemoglobin levels mean lower oxygen transport, lower–blood iron levels due to a low iron absorption, and increased iron excretion (some in sweat). An inadequate dietary intake of iron can compound the problem. Moderate levels of exercise do not appear to affect iron status.

Iron supplementation given to individuals with iron deficiency anemia consistently improves iron status and exercise performance. Iron supplementation given to individuals with iron depletion or iron deficiency erythropoiesis shows variable but primarily nonsignificant changes in performance. Excessive iron intake can inhibit zinc and copper absorption. The iron status of an individual should be ascertained before supplementation exceeding the RDA (18 mg for everyone over the age of 4 yr) is undertaken.[3, 16, 26, 39]

Macrominerals Macrominerals include calcium, chlorine, magnesium, phosphorus, potassium, sodium, and sulfur. As macromineral electrolytes, chlorine, magnesium, potassium, and sodium are discussed in the section "Fluid Ingestion During Exercise." Sulfur has no direct importance for exercise.

The function of calcium in bone health is directly related to exercise training and is fully described in Chapter 16. Beyond its role in bone health, the relationship between exercise, training, and calcium level and supplementation is largely unknown.[15]

Magnesium is lost in sweat and has been linked with aerobic capacity and with aldosterone and cortisol function during exercise. However, there is no evidence that supplemental magnesium increases performance. At the same time, levels above the RDA (400–350mg·day^{-1} for adolescent and adult males, 300–280 mg·day^{-1} for adolescent and adult females) do not appear to be harmful.[39]

Several studies have shown that *phosphate loading*—increased phosphate ingestion for several days prior to an event—may improve performance by delaying the onset of anaerobic metabolism; other studies have shown no beneficial effects. Since phosphorus supplementation over an extended period of time can result in lowered blood calcium levels, it is not recommended. The RDA for phosphorus is 1200 mg·day⁻¹ for adolescent males and 800 mg·day⁻¹ for adult males and females.[15]

In summary, the pattern here is the same as the one for vitamins. The primary concern is that the exerciser ingest the RDA and, unless some deficiency has been diagnosed, only the RDA. For those who are strictly limiting their caloric intake, the combined generic, vitamin-and-mineral, one-a-day pill can be recommended.

Nutrition for Competition

The goals of an optimal competitive diet are:

1. To ensure adequate fuel supplies in the preevent time span.
2. To ensure adequate fuel supplies during the event, no matter what the duration.
3. To facilitate temperature regulation by preventing dehydration.
4. To achieve desired weight classifications while maintaining fuel and water supplies.
5. To avoid gastrointestinal discomfort during competition.

Depending on the event, precompetition dietary adjustment may be a matter of hours or days. Most manipulation centers around carbohydrate consumption.[12]

Carbohydrate Loading (Glycogen Supercompensation)

For individuals competing in continuous endurance events lasting at least 60–90 min at 65 to 85% V̇O₂max, **carbohydrate loading,** sometimes called **glycogen supercompensation,** may be utilized.[3, 9] Carbohy-

> **Carbohydrate Loading (Glycogen Supercompensation)** A process of nutritional modification that results in an additional storage of glycogen in muscle fiber that can be approximately three to four times the normal levels.

drate loading is a process of nutritional modification that results in an additional storage of glycogen in muscle fibers that can be approximately three to four times the normal level. As mentioned previously, the time to exhaustion in long-duration relatively high intensity activities is linked to initial levels of muscle glycogen. Although a high starting level of muscle glycogen will not enable an athlete to perform at a higher intensity (run faster per mile), it will allow him or her to maintain a given pace for a longer period of time.

Table 13.4 presents two carbohydrate loading techniques. The first, labeled as the classic technique, is based on studies by Swedish investigators in the 1960s.[7] This technique involves hard exercise to deplete muscle glycogen stores one week prior to the competitive event, followed by three days of hard training and three days of rest. During the first three days after the depletion run the individual is supposed to eat almost no carbohydrates; then for the next three days he or she eats almost exclusively carbohydrates.

This technique is effective but is not without its problems. The high-fat, high-protein ingestion after the exercise depletion phase is one problem. A diet with so little carbohydrate (less than 5%) means that an individual is ingesting high levels of fat, which is not healthy. Thus, this technique can cause high-blood lipid levels. In addition, the ingested fat is incompletely metabolized, and high levels of ketones appear in the blood (ketosis).[19,44] Hypoglycemia (abnormally low blood glucose levels) can also occur, leading to fatigue, restlessness, mental disturbances, irritability, and weakness. At the very least, it is difficult, if not impossible, to maintain the hard training recommended during this phase. At the same time, the 80–90% carbohydrate diet for the three days prior to competition can leave the athlete feeling stiff and heavy owing to water retention. Since approximately 2.7 g of water are stored with each gram of glycogen, water retention can add approximately 1–2 kg to the body weight. It has been theorized that this water could be important in delaying or preventing dehydration, but it has not been shown to have any beneficial effect on body temperature regulation or dehydration. Thus an athlete who had trained for months for an event such as a marathon could find him/herself down both psychologically and physiologically in the week prior to competition.

TABLE 13.4 ▪ **Carbohydrate Loading**

	Days Prior to Competition							DAY OF COMPETITION
	−7	−6	−5	−4	−3	−2	−1	
CLASSIC TECHNIQUE								
DIET	Mixed diet 50% CHO	<5% CHO or <2 g CHO · kg^{-1} · day^{-1}	Continue from previous day		80–90% CHO >10–12 g CHO · kg^{-1} · day^{-1}	Continue from previous day		High CHO pre-event meal Possible during event CHO feeding
EXERCISE	Exercise to exhaustion	90–120 min 65–85% $\dot{V}O_2$max	Continue from previous day	Continue from previous day or exercise to exhaustion	Rest	Rest	Rest	Continuous endurance event lasting 60–90 min, 65–85% $\dot{V}O_2$max
MODIFIED TECHNIQUE								
DIET	50% CHO or 4.5 g CHO · kg^{-1} · day^{-1}	Continue from previous day			70% CHO or 8–10 g CHO · kg^{-1} · day^{-1}	Continue from previous day		High CHO pre-event meal Possible during event CHO feeding
EXERCISE	90 min 75% $\dot{V}O_2$max	Continue from previous day	40 min 75% $\dot{V}O_2$max	Continue from previous day	20 min 75% $\dot{V}O_2$max or 30–60 min 50–70% $\dot{V}O_2$max	Continue from previous day	Rest	Continuous endurance event lasting 60–90 min 65–85% $\dot{V}O_2$max

Subsequent research has shown that neither the exhaustive glycogen depletion exercise nor the three days of high-protein, high-fat diet are necessary to maximize muscle glycogen storage.[51, 52] So the modified carbohydrate-loading technique presented in Table 13.4 emphasizes a slow downward taper in duration and/or intensity of the training regimen. This taper is accompanied by an always average, but increasing, percentage of carbohydrates in the diet. An athlete already modifying his or her training diet to include high levels of carbohydrate will have very few changes to make.

The practice of carbohydrate loading does not appear in any way to adversely affect the normal healthy individual.[3, 24, 51, 52] Obviously, diabetics should consult with a physician before attempting carbohydrate loading. There is no evidence to support the suggestion that carbohydrate loading is only effective if not done more than once or twice a year. Supercompensation may actually be occurring daily in an athlete undergoing strenuous training and eating 70% carbohydrate.

While carbohydrate loading was and is intended for the endurance athlete, bodybuilders often follow a version of the modified carbohydrate-loading technique.[29] The primary difference is a restriction of water intake during the high carbohydrate ingestion phase. This water restriction has nothing to do with energy requirements during competition; it is based on the belief that water will then be sucked from beneath the skin for storage with glycogen and lead to an increase in muscle size and definition for competition. Evidence in support of this consequence is primarily anecdotal.

Results from the only available scientific study are presented in Figure 13.2. Nine male bodybuilders had girth measurements taken after a normal dietary routine (55% CHO, 15% PRO, and 30% FAT) and after a traditional carbohydrate loading regimen (3 days of 10% CHO, 33% PRO, and 57% FAT, followed by 3 days of 80% CHO, 15% PRO, and 5% FAT). Identical weight-lifting workouts were followed during both dietary manipulations and prior to girth measurement. The trials were randomized. No measurement of muscle definition was made, but as the figure shows, diet prior to testing had no effect on muscle girth measurements.[5]

Pre-Event Meal

Most road races and other endurance events, unless scheduled for the convenience of the television audience such as during the Olympics, take place in the morning. Competing after an overnight fast is probably not a good idea for an athlete in any sport,

but it is most detrimental for the endurance athlete. Liver glycogen is the primary endogenous source of blood glucose, and an overnight fast reduces the liver's supply of glycogen. For this reason, approximately 50–100 g of carbohydrate should be included in the pre-event meal, with only enough fat and protein to ward off hunger pangs. A major question is the timing of this meal.

The ingestion of carbohydrate within one hour prior to exercise remains controversial. Theoretically, such a regimen should be detrimental to performance, for the following reasons. The ingestion of carbohydrate causes an increase in blood glucose. The increase of blood glucose causes a concomitant increase in insulin. Insulin favors the removal of blood glucose from the bloodstream, inhibits the release of glucose from the liver, and inhibits the mobilization of free fatty acids, which are used, along with carbohydrate, as fuel for exercise. These actions can cause hypoglycemia and may cause a greater dependency on muscle glycogen stores, depleting them at a faster rate.

Despite the popular acceptance of this reasoning the research literature is far from conclusive.[12,20] Eight studies conducted between 1979 and 1989 examined endurance performance following carbohydrate ingestion 1 hr or less (usually 30–45 min) before the exercise. One study reported a negative effect; four studies reported no significant effect, either positive or negative; and the other three reported improved performance. These results can be interpreted either as one against and three for or five against (one negative and four no difference) and three for carbohydrate feeding during this time frame. Other studies have shown that if the carbohydrate-feeding time is reduced to 5 min or less before the exercise, performance is improved.

The glucose or glycogen status of the individual prior to the feeding may also be important in determining whether or not the response is beneficial.[17] Fasted individuals may be more sensitive to glucose ingestion within this time span than those who have been recently fed and had followed a carbohydrate-loading regimen. And there may be other individual differences. Thus, eating within 1 hr of competition is something an athlete should experiment with in training before attempting it for competition.[12] When in doubt, don't ingest carbohydrates 30–45 min prior to competition.

FIGURE 13.2

Girth Measurements in Bodybuilders with and without Carbohydrate Loading

Source: Based on data from Balon, Horowitz & Fitzsimmons.[5]

A much more substantial case can be made in favor of a preevent meal 3–4 hr prior to competition.[12, 19, 20] For example, when Neufer et al.[43] fed subjects 200 g of cereal, bread, and fruit 4 hours prior to riding a bicycle ergometer, an 11% increase in power performance occurred. When the same protocol was followed with the addition of a candy bar 5 min before the exercise, the improvement was 22%. On the basis of this study and others, a light meal of 200–500 kcal, including 50–100 g of carbohydrate and plenty of fluid, is recommended 3–4 hr prior to an endurance event, with the option of a last-minute snack. Table 13.5 summarizes this information. It is important that this meal consist of foods that the individual likes and tolerates well. The absence or presence of gastrointestinal distress can be the difference between a PR (personal record) or a DNF (did not finish). High levels of fructose ingestion as the sole carbohydrate source prior to exercise have been associated with gastrointestinal distress and thus should be avoided.

Feeding During Exercise

When exercise begins, insulin release is suppressed and catecholamine secretion is increased. Thus, the potentially detrimental changes associated with carbohydrate ingestion are no longer of concern. Indeed, both theoretically and experimentally, there is support for the ingestion of carbohydrates once the activity begins. Even small amounts of carbohydrates (about 25 g · hr⁻¹) taken at 15–30 min intervals have been found to prevent a decline in blood glucose and delay fatigue during the latter portion of an endurance event longer than 1 hr. Note that fatigue can be caused by many factors, and carbohydrate feeding merely delays but does not prevent fatigue.

Carbohydrate feedings during intermittent exercise such as soccer or basketball have also been shown to be beneficial.[12,19,20] Oranges at half time may thus be more than a simple tradition, although modern-day carbohydrate beverages are probably more convenient. In addition, carbohydrates move through the stomach rapidly and are less likely than other nutrients to cause gastrointestinal and abdominal disturbances.[12, 20] The recommendation is to take in approximately 30–60 g of carbohydrates each hour, beginning early in the exercise. As noted, this can be accomplished at the same time as fluid replenishment.

No differences have been found when glucose, fructose, sucrose, or glucose polymer solutions (maltodextrins) have been compared in terms of rate of gastric emptying or impact on performance. Glucose, sucrose, and glucose polymers stimulate

TABLE 13.5 ■ Recommended Eating on Game Day

Sport	−3 to −4 hr	−30 min	−5–0 min	Event Begins	+15–+30 min Repeated for Duration of Event	Recovery (15–30 min past)
Nonendurance	Light balanced meal of high % CHO Fluid ingestion	Fluid ingestion	—	—	Water as desired	Fluid ingestion
Endurance	200–500-kcal meal with 50–100 g CHO Fluid ingestion	Fluid ingestion	CHO approximately 50 g (optional)		Fluid ingestion of CHO (optional): 30–60 g · hr⁻¹ and 6–10% CHO concentration Some Na	Fluid ingestion 50–100 g CHO Some Na

fluid absorption in the stomach, but fructose does not.[18] As for preexercise conditions, fructose ingestion (as the only carbohydrate source) during exercise has been associated with gastrointestinal distress and is not associated with performance improvement.

Research supports the position that beverages containing 2.5–10% carbohydrate are absorbed by the body as rapidly as water. A concentration of 6–8% is thought to be optimal. Drinks containing less than 5% carbohydrate do not provide enough energy to enhance performance, and drinks that exceed 10% carbohydrate (such as soda pop) are often detrimental since they tend to cause abdominal cramps, nausea, and diarrhea.[18]

Sometimes athletes eat energy bars during competition, but the fiber, protein, and fat they contain can slow down digestion and hence the quick availability of energy. An alternative to energy bars and sport drinks is energy gels. Generally, energy gels come in 1-ounce plastic or foil packets and consist of 70–100 kcal of carbohydrate with small amounts of electrolytes. As with energy bars, water should be ingested along with the energy gel. GU, Pocket Rocket, ReLode, and Squeezy are commercially available energy gels.

Fluid Ingestion During and After Exercise

As previously discussed (Chapter 11) the human body is only about 20–45% efficient, depending on how efficiency is calculated. The energy output that is not utilized as work appears as heat. Normal resting body temperature is in the range of 36.1–37.8°C. Thermal balance in this range is maintained by summing the factors of metabolic heat production, radiant heat exchange, conductive heat exchange, convective heat exchange, and evaporation (Chapter 7).[27]

In cool, dry weather heat generated by moderate exercise can be dissipated by radiation and convection. In moderately warm, dry weather, radiation and convection decrease, and sweating must be utilized. In hot weather, when the skin and environmental temperatures are nearly the same, radiation and convection cannot contribute to heat loss (and, indeed, may contribute to heat gain if the ambient temperature is higher), so evaporation alone can dissipate heat. The evaporative heat loss depends on environmental conditions (percentage of relative humidity and air movement), the rate of sweat secretion, and the electrolyte concentration of the sweat. The evaporation of 1 g of water from the skin surface removes slightly less than 0.6 kcal of heat.[42]

During heavy exercise metabolic heat production can increase as much as 100 times that of inactive muscle. If this heat is not dissipated, the internal temperature will rise 1°C every 5–8 min, resulting in overheating (hyperthermia) and collapse of the individual within 15–20 min. Thus, sweating under these conditions is absolutely essential.[42] However, sweating does not occur without a price, and that price is the removal of fluid from the body.[38] A 70-kg, 2:30 marathoner can lose 5 L of body water, or $1–2 \text{ L} \cdot \text{hr}^{-1}$. Sweat, of course, is not pure water; it includes the electrolytes sodium (Na^+), chloride (Cl^-), and potassium (K^+) and traces of amino acids, bicarbonate (HCO_3^-), carbon dioxide (CO_2), copper, glucose, hormones, iron, lactic acid, magnesium (Mg^+), nitrogen (N), phosphates (PO_4^{-2}), urea, vitamins, and zinc.[41] The exact proportion of these elements in sweat varies among individuals and within the same individual under different conditions.[27]

Although shifting occurs in the internal water compartments to provide the liquid portion of sweat, ultimately much of the water lost through sweating comes from blood plasma. If this water is not replaced, the individual may perform poorly and suffer from heat injuries (Chapter 7).

To avoid dehydration, adequate, and often forced, fluid intake is necessary.[3, 45] Thirst is an inadequate guide to the amount of water needed. Whether to supplement with plain water or a carbohydrate and/or electrolyte beverage (sports drink) is a matter of much debate. For the vast majority of sports or fitness workouts plain water is the beverage of choice. Again, however, endurance events may be the exception.[3]

The rate at which an ingested fluid actually enters the body's water supply depends upon the rate at which it leaves the stomach (called *gastric emptying*) and the rate at which it is absorbed across the intestinal membrane *(intestinal absorption)*. Both gastric emptying and intestinal absorption are influenced by the composition of the ingested fluid.

Three factors need to be considered for gastric emptying. First, the gastric-emptying rate decreases as the caloric content of the ingested fluid increases. However, the differences in the gastric-emptying rate of solutions between 2.5 and 10% carbohydrate are negligible between each other and compared to plain water.[18, 38] Second, the rate of gastric emptying is exponentially related to the volume of fluid in the stomach.[38, 41] That is, the amount of beverage emptied from the stomach is relatively large in the first minutes and then the rate slows down. Therefore, frequent ingestion of small amounts of fluid is preferable to the reverse. Thus, 200–400 mL of fluid should be ingested every 15–30 min, since approximately 400 mL can be cleared in 15 min.[3, 45] Third, the temperature of the fluid may be important. It has typically been suggested that any sports drink that is ingested should be cold to enhance gastric emptying. Recent evidence suggests, though, that the gastric-emptying rates of hot and cold beverages are the same.[38] The real advantage of a cold drink may simply be that it tastes better to a hot, sweaty athlete, thereby encouraging more drinking. Of course, a cold fluid also does not add heat to the body, which a hot fluid would.

Intestinal absorption is not influenced by as many factors as gastric emptying is. However, research has shown that the presence of glucose and sodium greatly increases intestinal fluid absorption over plain water. Thus, small percentages of glucose do not inhibit gastric emptying and will enhance intestinal absorption if accompanied by sodium.

In those situations where fluid replacement is more important than energy substrate supplementation (such as in a relatively short endurance event of 1–2 hr or an activity in high heat and humidity), the carbohydrate concentration should be low (2.5–8%) and the sodium content moderately high (30–110 mg). An 8-oz glass of 2% milk or tomato juice contains over 100 mg of sodium. The sodium is generally in the form of sodium chloride (common table salt). Conversely, in those situations where substrate provision is more important than fluid replacement (a long endurance event of over 2 hr in temperate environmental conditions), a more concentrated carbohydrate solution (6–10%) with sodium should be ingested.[38, 41]

If large quantities of plain water are ingested in events lasting longer than 4 hr, hyponatremia (low sodium, sometimes called "water intoxication") may occur. Hyponatremia is a serious condition that not only affects performance but also can lead to

brain damage and death. Thus, in ultraendurance events athletes are urged to drink electrolyte beverages. Conversely, there is no advantage to drinking beverages of any composition but water in activities lasting less than 30 min.[10, 38, 41]

Although it has been claimed that electrolytes make sports drinks more palatable and hence encourage drinking, the available evidence indicates that sodium, as mentioned earlier, is the only electrolyte that is physiologically beneficial when consumed during exercise.[38,41] Evidence does not indicate that matching the content of sweat—even if this were possible, considering its extreme variability—is necessary.[27] Despite the great amount of attention given to it, potassium loss in sweat is low and of little consequence during exercise. The general consensus is that electrolyte losses will be replaced through normal food intake after exercise. An exception again, may be sodium. Sodium appears to be important in postexercise beverages for reasons other than intestinal absorption. In the postexercise period, if drinks with little or no sodium are ingested, the plasma becomes diluted, stimulating urine production and fluid excretion. This also shuts off the thirst drive and rehydration is delayed.[38, 46] Once again, however, if some is good, more is not better. Salt tablets should never be ingested.[54] Such highly concentrated amounts of salt can lead to gastrointestinal discomfort, dehydration, and electrolyte loss.[54]

Since most sports drinks commercially available (Table 13.2) do contain varying amounts of electrolytes other than sodium, it must be asked whether these inclusions are harmful. A qualified "no" is the answer. There have been no cases of problems arising from the ingestion of commercial sports drinks reported in the literature.[46] One can only assume, given the ongoing debate about such products, that such occurrences would have been publicized had they occurred.

Do the problem outlined in Box 13.1 to together a package of fluids for ingestion by the indicated athlete. The answer is at the end of the chapter.

Eating Disorders

Whereas most individuals participating in fitness programs or athletics see nutrition as a partner with exercise to help them achieve their goals of

---

Box 13.1 A Question of Understanding

On the basis of the composition of the selected sports drinks given in Table 13.2 and from the text discussion, group the sports drinks into the indicated categories for a serious, but not world-class, marathoner (2:45–3:45). Support your groupings scientifically. Check your classifications against the answer at the end of the chapter.

1. Training replenishment and carbohydrate loading
   Drink   *Support*

2. Pre-event meal
   Drink   *Support*

3. During training runs and competition
   Drink   *Support*

---

health or successful competition, a few have a distorted view of food and develop eating disorders. Of course, eating disorders are not limited to physically active individuals, but symptoms of eating disorders are more prevalent among athletes than nonathletes. The problem occurs much more frequently in females than males, and typically has its onset after menarche but prior to age 25.[55]

Three types of eating disorders are of greatest concern for individuals working with active females: anorexia nervosa (AN), bulimia nervosa (BN), and anorexia athletica (AA). **Anorexia nervosa** is characterized by marked self-induced

---

Anorexia Nervosa An eating disorder characterized by marked self-induced weight loss accompanied by an intense fear of fatness and reproductive hormonal changes.

Bulimia Nervosa An eating disorder marked by an unrealistic appraisal of body weight and/or shape that is manifested by alternating bingeing and purging behavior.

Anorexia Athletica An eating disorder occurring primarily in young, female athletes that is characterized by a food intake less than that required to support the training regimen and by body weight no more than 95% of normal.

---

weight loss accompanied by an intense fear of fatness and reproductive hormonal changes. **Bulimia nervosa** is marked by an unrealistic appraisal of body weight and/or shape and is manifested by alternating bingeing and purging behavior. **Anorexia athletica,** occurring primarily in young female athletes, is characterized by a food intake that is less than that required to support the training regimen and body weight at least 5% below normal. The precise criteria for each are included in Table 13.6. Both anorexia nervosa and bulimia nervosa are among the eating disorders recognized by the American Psychiatric Association.[1] Anorexia athletica is characterized by elements of both of the other two disorders and individuals suffering from anorexia athletica may exhibit a variety of symptoms.[55, 58]

The specific causes of eating disorders are unknown.[55, 58] Psychological, genetic-biological, and sociocultural factors have been implicated but not proven. Individuals who are conscientious and achievement-oriented, who seek perfection, but who, at the same time, have a low self-esteem seem to have a psychological predisposition for an eating disorder. Eating disorders also appear to run in families and are more strongly associated in identical than fraternal twins. By the same token, our cultural obsession with thinness may be considered a social predisposition, although why some young girls succumb to the pressure but most don't is unknown.[37,55] Once an individual with a substantial predisposition begins a very restrictive diet, a cycling, self-perpetuating, self-reinforcing process begins; and the individual develops an eating disorder.

Sundgot-Borgen[58] identified a series of risk factors or trigger conditions for eating disorders. These results were obtained from a study that tested 522 elite female Norwegian athletes (out of a possible 603 in the entire country). Ninety-two athletes (17%) were found to have AN (N = 7), BN (N = 43), or AA (N = 42). The six risk factors included:

1. *Dieting at an early age.* Dieting is a risk factor especially if recommended by a coach who indicates that losing weight or fat would enable the athlete to improve her performance. Thus, the fact that athletes in weight-dependent sports (judo, karate) and aesthetic sports (gymnastics, diving, figure skating, dancing) have the highest incidence of eating disorders is not unexpected.[56]

TABLE 13.6 ■ Diagnostic Criteria for Selected Eating Disorders

ANOREXIA NERVOSA	BULIMIA NERVOSA	ANOREXIA ATHLETICA
Refusal to maintain body weight above that considered normal for height and age; marked self-induced weight loss	Recurrent episodes of binge eating (rapid consumption of large quantities of calorie-dense food, often secretly)	Weight loss (>5% below normal for age and height)[*]
		Absence of medical disorder to explain weight loss[*]
Intense fear of weight gain or becoming fat despite being underweight	Purging or compensating for bingeing by self-induced vomiting, use of diuretics or laxatives, vigorous exercise, and strict food restriction or fasting	Excess fear of becoming fat[*]
		Food intake < 1200 kcal $\cdot$ day^{-1}
Endocrine changes manifested by amenorrhea (for at least three consecutive cycles) in females and loss of sexual interest and potency in males		Delayed puberty
	Exhibiting bingeing or inappropriate compensatory behavior at least twice a week for three months	Primary or secondary amenorrhea or oligomenorrhea
		Binge eating that is not high in calories
	Unrealistic appraisal of body weight and shape	Purging
		Gastrointestinal complaints
		Distorted body image
		Compulsive exercise in addition to normal needed training

[*]Absolute criteria; others may or may not be present.

Source: Based on American Psychiatric Association,[1] Sundgot-Borgen.[55,58]

2. *Unsupervised dieting.* Athletes are rarely given guidance by someone trained in nutrition and knowledgeable about their sports' requirements. Those who are given such assistance often don't follow the good advice.

3. *Lack of acceptance of pubertal changes.* Young female athletes are often distressed at the bodily changes that occur as they mature—particularly menarche and the increasing levels of body fat. Many young athletes are also aware that a delayed menarche is often associated with athletic success (see Chapter 16).

4. *Early sport-specific training.* An individual's somatotype (body type) has a great influence on which sports she can successfully compete in. If this influence is disregarded, a young child may select a sport she enjoys (such as gymnastics) only to find that her body outgrows it. Being a generalist as a child allows more options later— although realistically, that becomes harder to do if one wishes to compete on the international level.

5. *A large increase in training volume accompanied by a significant weight loss.* Athletes do not always spontaneously increase energy intake when the energy expenditure increases. The weight loss is viewed as being good, and there is no incentive to eat more. Thus, the vicious cycle is in place.

6. *Traumatic events.* A traumatic event can be anything, but it is often associated with an illness or injury that prevents training (and increases the fear of gaining weight) and/or the loss of a coach who the athlete often sees as being vital to her career.

The consequences of an eating disorder can be dire. At the very least, the individual's nutritional status is compromised. Figure 13.3 shows a

FIGURE 13.3

Nutrient Intake in Elite Norwegian Female Athletes

AN = anorexia nervosa (N = 7); AA = anorexia athletica (N = 43); BN = bulimia nervosa (N = 92); C = control (N = 30).

Source: Based on data from Sundgot-Borgen.[56]

representative sample of nutrient intake in the Norwegian study of elite women athletes previously mentioned.[56] The control group (labeled C) was comprised of 30 athletes not classified as being at risk for developing an eating disorder. However, 27% of those athletes were on a diet. Except for the bulimics, all other groups had a lower total energy intake than recommended. The bulimics also had a diet that differed in composition from that of the other groups. They ate more fat (30% versus 20%) and less protein (10% versus 20%) than the other groups but an equal amount of carbohydrates as the other groups. Despite the equality of percentage of carbohydrates, only the bulimics were taking in sufficient amounts of carbohydrates in grams per kilogram per day. Those with anorexia nervosa showed the greatest nutritional disturbance. They were simply not ingesting enough of anything.

Although the bulimic group appears to be getting sufficient nutrients in terms of carbohydrates, protein, calcium, and iron, note that these values are prepurging intakes. The majority of the bulimia nervosa group and one-third of the anorexia athletica group vomited within 15 min of eating on a regular basis. Thus, the nutrients were ingested, but they were not absorbed. Individuals who purge by the use of diuretics or laxatives, in contrast, have minimal caloric loss; but they do lose electrolytes and can become dehydrated.

The loss of electrolytes, especially potassium, can have serious cardiac implications, whereas lack of fluid impacts blood pressure levels. Extensive hormonal changes, gastrointestinal complications, skin and hair problems, anemia, disordered thermoregulation, and dental abnormalities are just a few of the other medical problems associated with eating disorders. At times, these medical complications are severe enough to cause death.[11]

As a coach, physical educator, or exercise leader, your role is to be part of the solution, not part of the problem. To this end it is important to:

1. Encourage youngsters to try a variety of sports. As much as possible, try to guide them into more than one sport experience where they can potentially be successful.

2. Identify realistic, healthy weight goals appropriate for each youngster's stage of maturation.

3. Monitor weight and body composition to detect continued and unwarranted weight losses, or weight and fat fluctuations, without always equating weight loss as a positive outcome.

4. Provide proper nutritional guidance—if need be, in conjunction with a nutritionist—and emphasize nutrition for performance, not weight and fat control.

5. Provide a realistic, progressive training program to which the student, athlete, or fitness participant can gradually adjust both in terms of energy input and energy output.

6. Provide a realistic, progressive training program to avoid overtraining, illnesses, and injuries.

7. Provide an atmosphere that is supportive of pubertal changes and accept them so that young participants will see them in a positive light.

8. Be aware of symptoms of eating disorders.

9. Seek professional help in dealing with any individual you suspect of having an eating disorder. The first response to being questioned is often denial. Do not delay. The sooner treatment is started, the better the chances are for a full recovery.[54]

SUMMARY

1. There are five goals in an optimal training diet.
(a) To provide caloric and nutrient requirements.
(b) To incorporate nutritional practices that promote good health.
(c) To achieve and maintain optimal body composition and playing weight.
(d) To promote recovery from training sessions and for physiological adaptations.
(e) To try variations of precompetition and competition fuel and fluid intake to determine bodily responses.

2. A balanced nutritional diet composed of sufficient calories to maintain acceptable body weight and composition, with 12–15% protein, 30% fat, 55–58% carbohydrate, the RDA for vitamins and minerals, and sufficient fluid for hydration, is adequate and probably optimal for all but hard-training elite, competitive athletes.

3. Active individuals who are satisfied with their body weight and composition must ingest sufficient calories to balance those expended. This should proportionally increase nutrient intake.

4. For an individual utilizing high levels of carbohydrates in training, $8–10 \, g \cdot kg^{-1} \cdot day^{-1}$ are recommended. This value may increase the intake to 70–80% carbohydrate.

5. Carbohydrate ingestion should begin as soon after activity as possible to restore glycogen storage in the muscle. It should consist primarily of high– and moderate–glycemic index foods.

6. Excessive carbohydrate intake in individuals not training heavily in endurance activity can lead to elevated levels of blood lipids.

7. Strength, speed, and ultraendurance athletes may need to consume $1.2–2 \, g \cdot kg^{-1} \cdot day^{-1}$ of protein, up from the RDA of $0.8 \, g \cdot kg^{-1} \cdot day^{-1}$ for sedentary adults. This increased intake should not exceed 15% of the total caloric intake.

8. Excessive protein intake leads to calcium excretion, which may in turn lead to accelerated problems of osteoporosis in young amenorrheic female athletes.

9. Although endurance athletes can adapt to burning high amounts of fat as fuel, high levels of cholesterol also result from a high-fat diet. Therefore, fats should be maintained at no more than 30% of the calories ingested.

10. Vitamins are important in the production of energy. However, there is no evidence that vitamin supplementation in an adequately nourished individual improves performance, speeds up recovery, or reduces injuries. Where deficiencies are present, supplementation to normal physiological levels can improve performance.

11. Excessive levels of vitamins can be toxic.

12. There is insufficient evidence to conclude that supplementation of zinc, chromium, selenium, copper, iron, or any other micronutrient above normal levels has any impact on exercise performance. Iron supplementation given to individuals with iron deficiency anemia consistently improves performance, but supplementation should not be done unless needed clinically.

13. Excessive, unnecessary iron intake can inhibit zinc and copper absorption.

14. There is no evidence that supplementation of the macrominerals calcium and magnesium increases exercise performance. Phosphate loading may delay the onset of anaerobic metabolism effects.

15. Phosphate supplementation over an extended period of time can result in lowered blood calcium levels.

16. Nutritional analysis should always precede any supplementation to determine need and safety.

17. There are five goals of an optimal competitive diet.
(a) To ensure adequate fuel supplies in the preevent time span.
(b) To ensure adequate supplies during the event.
(c) To facilitate temperature regulation by prevention of dehydration.
(d) To achieve desired weight classifications while maintaining fuel and water supplies.
(e) To avoid gastrointestinal discomfort during competition.

18. Carbohydrate loading is beneficial only for individuals competing in endurance events of at least 60–90 min at 65 to 85% $\dot{V}O_2max$.

19. The modified carbohydrate-loading technique in which an individual increases the percentage of carbohydrate ingested from 50 to 70% while gradually tapering training the week before competition is the recommended procedure.

20. A light meal composed primarily of carbohydrate and accompanied by fluids is recommended 3–4 hr prior to competition. Fluid should continue to be ingested right up to the time of the event.

21. Carbohydrates ingested in small amounts (200–400 mL) at 15–30-min intervals during endurance activity can prevent a decline in glucose and delay fatigue. Beverages containing 6–8% carbohydrate are recommended for optimal benefit.

22. Thirst is not an adequate guide to the amount of water needed during activity. Plain water is recommended except in long endurance events (over 4 hr), where a sport beverage may be beneficial.

23. Electrolyte losses are usually replaced through normal food intake after exercise. However, sodium in a postexercise beverage may help with fluid retention.

24. Three types of eating disorders are of great concern for personnel working with active individuals: anorexia nervosa, bulimia nervosa, and anorexia athletica. Although there are technical differences among the three disorders, all involve a restriction of food intake or a purging of food ingested in a binge, a desire for more and more weight loss, and a denial of having a problem.

25. The exact cause of eating disorders is unknown. More athletes than nonathletes suffer from eating disorders, and most cases occur in weight-dependent or aesthetic sports. Far more females than males have eating disorders.

26. Personnel working with active individuals between the ages of 10 and 25 should be aware of and try to avoid situations that might trigger an eating disorder.

Box 13.1 Answers

The answer to the problem posed in Box 13.1 is:

1. Training replenishment and carbohydrate loading

Drink	Support
Gatorlode	High CHO; some Na
Nutrament	
Gator Pro	
Carbo Plus	

2. Pre-event meal

Drink	Support
Gatorlode	Light meal
Nutrament	50–100 g CHO
Gator Pro	200–500 kcal
Carbo Plus	

Box 13.1 Answers *(cont.)*

3. The drinks to be used during training runs and competition

Drink	Support
All Sport	Water (≈ 240 mL)
Body Fuel 450	2.5–10% concentration
Exceed	of CHO as G, GP, S, or
Gatorade	F combination (not F
Gookinade E.R.G.	alone); 6–8% is optimal
Power Burst	mal
R.P.M.	30–110 mg Na

REVIEW QUESTIONS

1. List the goals for nutrition during training and the goals for nutrition during competition. Explain why they are different.

2. Prepare a table comparing a balanced diet for a sedentary individual and one for an active individual. Include caloric intake, percentages, and grams per kilogram per day recommendations for the major nutrients, as well as similarities or differences in vitamin, mineral, and fluid ingestion.

3. Discuss the positive and negative aspects of a high-carbohydrate diet.

4. Define the glycemic index, and describe how foods are divided into high, moderate, and low categories. Using the glycemic index, develop a post-Century bike ride (100 mi) snack to be eaten approximately 30 min after the ride, and develop a snack to be eaten during a day of hiking on the Appalachian Trail. Explain your choices.

5. Discuss the situations in which an increase in protein above the RDA is advisable and situations in which such an increase is not advisable.

6. Describe a training situation and the theory behind when fat intake can be too low.

7. Compare the theory behind the use of carbohydrate loading for endurance athletes with the theory behind the use of carbohydrate loading for bodybuilders.

8. Compare the classic and the modified techniques of carbohydrate loading in terms of diet and exercise for endurance athletes. Explain the reasons for the modifications.

9. Prepare a table of a comprehensive fluid and nutrient intake for pre-event, during-the-event, and postevent diets for a football player and a triathlete.

10. Define and list the characteristics of anorexia nervosa, bulimia nervosa, and anorexia athletica.

11. Identify the risk factors for developing an eating disorder. Prepare a set of guidelines that might be useful in counteracting these risk factors or dealing with the disorder early in its progression.

REFERENCES

1. American Psychiatric Association: *Diagnostic and Statistical Manual of Mental Disorders* (4th edition). Washington, DC: American Psychiatric Association (1994).

2. Allen, L. H., E. A. Oddoye, & S. Margen: Protein-induced hypercalciuria: A longer term study. *American Journal of Clinical Nutrition.* (32):741–749 (1979).

3. American Dietetic Association: Nutrition for physical fitness and athletic performance for adults: Technical support paper. *Journal of the American Dietetic Association.* 87(7):934–939 (1987).

4. Applegate, L.: Drinks to your health. *Runner's World.* 26(7):24–26 (1991).

5. Balon, T. W., J. F. Horowitz, & K. M. Fitzsimmons: Effects of carbohydrate loading and weight-lifting on muscle girth. *International Journal of Sports Nutrition.* 2(4):328–334 (1992).

6. Belko, A. Z.: Vitamins and exercise—an update. *Medicine and Science in Sports and Exercise.* (Suppl.). 19(5): S191–S196 (1987).

7. Bergstrom. J., L. Hermansen, E. Hultman, & B. Saltin: Diet, muscle glycogen and physical performance. *Acta Physiologica Scandinavica.* 7:140–150 (1967).

8. Blom, P. C. S., A. T. Hostmark, O. Vaage, K. R. Kardel, & S. Maehlum: Effects of different post-exercise sugar diets on the rate of muscle glycogen synthesis. *Medicine and Science in Sports and Exercise.* 19(5):491–496 (1987).

9. Brotherhood, J. R.: Nutrition and sports performance. *Sports Medicine.* 1:350–389 (1984).

10. Brouns, F.: Heat-sweat-dehydration-rehydration: A praxis oriented approach. *Journal of Sports Sciences.* 9:143–152 (1991).

11. Brownell, K. D., J. Rodin, & J. H. Wilmore: *Eating, Body Weight and Performance in Athletics: Disorders of Modern Society.* Philadelphia: Lea & Febiger (1992).

12. Burke, L. M., & R. S. D. Read: Sport nutrition: Approaching the nineties. *Sports Medicine.* 8(2):80–100 (1989).

13. Burke, L. M., G. R., Collier, & M. Hargreaves: Muscle glycogen storage after prolonged exercise: Effect of the glycemic index of carbohydrate feedings. *Journal of Applied Physiology.* 75(2):1019–1023 (1993).

14. Campbell, W. W., & R. A. Anderson: Effects of aerobic exercise and training on the trace minerals chromium, zinc and copper. *Sports Medicine.* 4:9–18 (1987).

15. Clarkson, P. M.: Minerals: Exercise performance and supplementation in athletes. *Journal of Sports Sciences.* 9:91–116 (1991).

16. Clarkson, P. M.: *Tired Blood: Iron Deficiency in Athletes and Effects of Iron Supplementation.* Sports Science Exchange, vol. 3, no. 28. Chicago: Gatorade Sports Science Institute (1990).

17. Clarkson, P. M.: *Trace Mineral Requirements for Athletes: To Supplement or Not to Supplement.* Sports Science Exchange, vol. 4, no. 33. Chicago: Gatorade Sports Science Institute (1991).

18. Coleman, E.: *Sports Drink Update.* Sports Science Exchange, vol. 1, no. 5. Chicago: Gatorade Sports Science Institute (1988).

19. Costill, D. L.: Carbohydrates for exercise: Dietary demands for optimal performance. *International Journal of Sports Medicine.* 9(1):1–18 (1988).

20. Coyle, E. F.: Timing and method of increased carbohydrate intake to cope with heavy training, competition and recovery. *Journal of Sport Sciences.* (9):29–52 (1991).

21. Coyle, E. F., & E. Coyle: Carbohydrates that speed recovery from training. *The Physician and Sportsmedicine.* 21(2):111–123 (1993).

22. Davis, J. M.: Carbohydrates, branched-chain amino acids, and endurance: The central fatigue hypothesis. *International Journal of Sport Nutrition.* 5:S29–S38 (1995).

23. Drinkwater, B. L.: Relationship between altered reproductive function and osteoporosis. In J. L. Pohl & C. H. Brown (eds.), *The Menstrual Cycle and Physical Activity.* Champaign, IL: Human Kinetics Publishers, 117–127 (1986).

24. Goss, F. L., & C. Karam: The effects of glycogen supercompensation on the electrocardiographic response during exercise. *Research Quarterly for Exercise and Sport.* 58(1):68–71 (1987).

25. Hasten, D. L., E. P. Rome, B. D. Franks, & M. Hegsted: Effects of chromium picolinate on beginning weight training students. *International Journal of Sport Nutrition.* 2(4):343–350 (1992).

26. Haymes, E. M.: Protein, vitamins, and iron. In M. H. Williams (ed.), *Ergogenic Aids in Sports.* Champaign, IL: Human Kinetics Publishers, 27–55 (1983).

27. Haymes, E. M., & C. L. Wells: *Environment and Human Performance.* Champaign, IL: Human Kinetics Publishers (1986).

28. Jenkins, D. J. A., D. M. Thomas, M. S. Wolever, R. H. Taylor, H. Barker, H. Fielden, J. M. Baldwin, A. C. Bowling, H. C. Newman, A. L. Jenkins, & D. V. Goff: Glycemic index of foods: A physiological basis for carbohydrate exchange. *American Journal of Clinical Nutrition.* 34:362–366 (1981).

29. Kreider, R. B., V. Miriel, & E. Bertun: Amino acid supplementation and exercise performance: An analysis of the proposed ergogenic value. *Sports Medicine.* 16(3):190–209 (1993).

30. Kroculick, S. T.: Carb loading: How to look full and ripped on contest day. *Ironman.* December: 152–153 (1988).

31. Leaf, A., & K. B. Frisa: Eating for health or for athletic performance? *American Journal of Clinical Nutrition.* 49:1066–1069 (1989).

32. Lefavi, R. G., R. A. Anderson, R. E. Keith, G. D. Wilson, J. L. McMillan, & M. H. Stone: Efficacy of chromium supplementation in athletes: Emphasis on anabolism. *International Journal of Sports Nutrition.* 2(2):111–122 (1992).

33. Lemon, P. W. R.: Effects of exercise on protein requirements. *Journal of Sports Sciences.* 9:53–70 (1991).

34. Lemon, P. W. R.: *Influence of Dietary Protein and Total Energy Intake on Strength Improvement.* Sports Science Exchange, vol. 2, no. 14. Chicago: Gatorade Sports Science Institute (1989).

35. Lemon, P. W. R.: Nutrition for muscular development of young athletes. In C. V. Gisolfi & D. R. Lamb (eds.), *Perspectives in Exercise Science and Sports Medicine.* Indianapolis: Benchmark Press, 369–400 (1989).

36. Lemon, P. W. R., & F. J. Nagle: Effects of exercise on protein and amino acid metabolism. *Medicine and Science in Sports and Exercise.* 13(3):141–149 (1981).

37. Leon, G. R.: Eating disorders in female athletes. *Sports Medicine.* 12(4):219–227 (1991).

38. Maughan, R. J.: Fluid and electrolyte loss and replacement in exercise. *Journal of Sports Sciences.* 9:117–142 (1991).

39. McDonald, R., & C. L. Keen: Iron, zinc and magnesium nutrition and athletic performance. *Sports Medicine.* 5:171–184 (1988).

40. Muoio, D. M., J. J. Leddy, P. J. Horvath, A. B. Awad, & D. R. Pendergast: Effect of dietary fat on metabolic adjustments to maximal $\dot{V}O_2$ and endurance in runners. *Medicine and Science in Sports and Exercise.* 26(1):81–88 (1994).

41. Murray, R.: The effects of consuming carbohydrate-electrolyte beverages on gastric emptying and fluid absorption during and following exercise. *Sports Medicine.* 4:322–351 (1987).

42. Nadel, E. R.: *New Ideas for Rehydration During and After Exercise in Hot Weather.* Sports Science Exchange, vol. 1, no. 3. Chicago: Gatorade Sports Science Institute (1988).

43. Neufer, P. D.: The effect of detraining and reduced training on the physiological adaptations to aerobic exercise training. *Sports Medicine.* 8(5):302–321 (1989).

44. Newsholme, E. A., & A. R. Leech: *Biochemistry for the Medical Sciences.* New York: John Wiley & Sons (1983).

45. Nieman, D. C.: *Fitness and Sports Medicine: An Introduction.* Palo Alto, CA: Bull Publishing (1990).

46. Nose, H. M., G. W. Mack, X. Shi, & E. R. Nadel: Involvement of sodium retention hormones during rehydration in humans. *Journal of Applied Physiology.* 65(1):332–336 (1988).

47. Paul, G. L.: Dietary protein requirements of physically active individuals. *Sports Medicine.* 8(3):154–176 (1989).

48. Phinney, S. D., B. R. Bistrian, W. J. Evans, E. Gervion, & G. L. Blackburn: The human metabolic response to chronic ketosis without caloric restriction: Preservation of submaximal exercise capability with reduced carbohydrate oxidation. *Metabolism.* 32:769–776 (1983).

49. Phinney, S. D., E. S. Horton, E. A. H. Sims, J. S. Hanson, E. Danforth, & B. M. LaGrange: Capacity for moderate exercise in obese subjects after adaptation to a hypocaloric diet. *Journal of Clinical Investigations.* 66:1152–1161 (1980).

50. Quaker Oats Company: *The Science of Gatorade.* Barrington, IL: Author (1990).

51. Sherman, W. M.: Carbohydrates, muscle glycogen, and muscle glycogen supercompensation. In M. H. Williams (ed.), *Ergogenic Aids in Sport.* Champaign, IL: Human Kinetics Publishers, 3–26 (1983).

52. Sherman, W. M.: *Muscle Glycogen Supercompensation During the Week Before Athletic Competition.* Sports Science Exchange, vol. 2, no. 16. Chicago: Gatorade Sports Science Institute (1989).

53. Singh, A., P. A. Pelletier, & P. A. Deuster: Dietary requirements for ultraendurance exercise. *Sports Medicine.* 18(5):301–308 (1994).

54. Steen, S. N.: Nutrition for young athletes: Special considerations. *Sports Medicine.* 17(3):152–162 (1994).

55. Sundgot-Borgen, J.: Eating disorders in female athletes. *Sports Medicine.* 17(3):176–188 (1994).

56. Sundgot-Borgen, J.: Nutrient intake of female elite athletes suffering from eating disorders. *International Journal of Sport Nutrition.* 3(4):431–442 (1993).

57. Sundgot-Borgen, J.: Prevalence of eating disorders in elite female athletes. *International Journal of Sport Nutrition.* 3(1):29–40 (1993).

58. Sundgot-Borgen, J.: Risk and trigger factors for the development of eating disorders in female elite athletes. *Medicine and Science in Sports and Exercise.* 26(4):414–419 (1994).

59. Tarnopolsky, M. A., J. D. MacDougall, & S. A. Atkinson: Influence of protein intake and training status on nitrogen balance and lean body mass. *Journal of Applied Physiology.* 64(1):187–193 (1988).

60. vander Beek, E. J.: Vitamins and endurance training: Food for running or faddish claims? *Sports Medicine* 2:175–197 (1985).

61. vander Beek, E. J.: Vitamin supplementation and physical exercise performance. *Journal of Sports Sciences.* 9:77–89 (1991).

62. Wolever, T. M. S.: The glycemic index. In G. H. Bourne (ed.), Aspects of some vitamins, minerals and enzymes in health and disease. *World Review of Nutrition and Dietetics.* 62:120–185 (1990).

63. Zawadzki, K. M., B. B. Yaspelkis III, & J. L. Ivy: Carbohydrate-protein complex increases the rate of muscle glycogen storage after exercise. *Journal of Applied Physiology.* 72(5):1854–1859 (1992).

14

Body Composition: Determination and Importance

After studying the chapter, you should be able to:

- Describe the technique of hydrostatic weighing (densitometry) and explain its theoretical basis.

- Calculate body density and percent body fat.

- Discuss variations in the basic assumptions of densitometry apparent in children, adolescents, and the elderly; and show how these variations have practical meaning.

- List and identify the strengths and weaknesses of the field estimates of body composition.

- Compare the percent body fat estimated by skinfolds and bioelectrical impedance

with the percent body fat determined by hydrostatic weighing.

- Contrast the percent body fat and the patterns of fat distribution in an average adult male and in an average adult female.

- Differentiate between overweight and obesity.

- Describe what happens to adipose cells in obesity.

- List and discuss the health risks of being overweight or obese.

- Debate the importance of heredity in body composition.

*I*ntroduction

Answer the following questions to yourself. Is your body weight just right, a little high, very high, a little low or very low? Is your percent body fat just right, a little high, very high, a little low or very low? Do you like the way you look in a bathing suit? What mental images did you use as you answered the questions?

If you are a female, chances are that no matter what the reality of your body weight, composition, or shape, you feel that your values are too high and you are dissatisfied with your shape. You are probably incorrect in your assessment, but you are certainly not alone. For example, one study[40] presented active women with five figures that represented individuals who were 20% underweight, 10% underweight, average weight and size, 10% overweight, and 20% overweight. The subjects were asked to select the figure they would like to look like. Only 14% wanted the average shape; 44% wanted to be 10% underweight, and 38% wanted to be 20% underweight!

These feelings are, of course, a result of cultural expectations. There have been times in Western civilization (for example, in the seventeenth century) when plumpness was the norm for feminine attractiveness. Within our own century great changes have occurred in the idealization of the female body. An analysis of *Playboy* centerfolds and Miss America Pageant contestants from 1960 to 1980 showed that the percentage of average weight (average weight being based on mean population values) for these individuals declined steadily from approximately 90% to almost 80%. At the same time, average hip and bust values for these icons of beauty declined, while waist and height values increased. Thus, the ideal shape changed from the hourglass curve to a more tubular profile.[27]

If you are a male, chances are that no matter what the reality of your body weight, composition, or shape, you are not concerned with your body weight per se but would like larger muscles and greater muscle definition, which would imply a lower percent body fat and a more triangular shape. Data on Mr. America or Mr. Universe contestants are not available to substantiate this impression, but just look at the muscle magazines at any newsstand. You, also, are probably incorrect in your assessment,

but again, you are also not alone. What did you compare yourself with mentally? Hopefully standards that are consistent with good health, but most likely, with some image presented by the media.

If you, whether female or male, have a positive self-image and are content with your body, are eating right, and are exercising regularly, congratulations and keep up the good work. Unfortunately, as a physical education specialist, you will be dealing with a public that has more questions and concerns about body composition and weight control than just about anything else we deal with. These next two chapters are designed to present you with an understanding of these crucial areas.

*B*ody Composition Assessment

Laboratory Techniques

Although it is unpleasant to think about, the only way to directly assess body composition is by dissection of human cadavers. Not only are few bodies available for such studies, but the technique is also difficult and not without problems. From 1945 to 1984 (the time from the earliest to the latest reported studies) body composition analysis has been performed on only 40 cadavers. While the study of these bodies provided a great deal of information, particularly regarding the densities of body tissues, they were not used to determine the accuracy (validity) of the more commonly used laboratory techniques. Theoretically, direct cadaver analysis should be the most accurate technique; however, the newer cadaver studies have often been inconsistent with results from the earlier studies. Thus, when dealing with body composition analysis, keep in mind that some techniques are better than others, and none is likely to be 100% accurate.[5, 14]

Many methods are currently available for the laboratory assessment of body composition and could possibly serve as criterion measures. Techniques such as computed tomography, dual-energy absoptiometry, excretion of muscle metabolites, infrared reactance, isotope dilution, magnetic resonance imaging, neutron activation, ultrasound, and whole-body counting of potassium 40 are very accurate.[14, 15] Unfortunately, at this time they are also often expensive, cumbersome, and time-consuming, requiring sensitive instrumentation run by highly trained technicians. This discussion will therefore concentrate on techniques that are most practical and hence more commonly used in exercise physiology.

Hydrostatic (Underwater) Weighing: Densitometry

Hydrostatic, or underwater, **weighing** is generally considered to be the laboratory criterion measure for the determination of body composition through the calculation of body density.[5, 29] We have Archimedes, a Greek mathematician who lived in the second century B.C., to thank for this technique. When King Hieron of Syracuse commissioned a new crown, he suspected that the jeweler substituted silver for pure gold inside the crown. The king asked Archimedes to determine the composition of the crown without harming it in any way. Legend has it that as Archimedes was pondering this issue at the public baths, he solved the problem and went running through the streets naked, shouting, "Eureka!" ("I have found it!")

What Archimedes observed was that an amount of water was displaced from the bath equal to the volume of the body entering the bath. Archimedes also reasoned that the body (or any other object floating or submerged) is buoyed up by a counterforce equal to the weight of the water displaced. Thus **Archimedes' principle** states that a partially or fully submerged object experiences an upward buoyant force equal to the weight or the volume of fluid displaced by the object. Based on this principle, the volume of any object, including the human body, can be measured by determining the weight lost by complete submersion underwater. When Archimedes compared the amount of water displaced by a mass of pure gold and a mass of pure silver equal to the mass of the king's crown, he found that the crown displaced more water than the gold, but less than the silver. He confirmed this result by weighing, underwater, weights of gold and silver equal to the weight of the crown in air, and found the crown to have an intermediate value. Thus, the crown was not pure gold (only about 75%), and we can only speculate as to the fate of the jeweler.[5]

Even if you have never been weighed underwater, you probably have a basic understanding of the principle just described. Think back to a swimming class. Could you float easily, or were you a sinker who could walk on the bottom of the pool? How would you describe those who were either floaters or sinkers in terms of being lean or fat?

Whether you floated or sank depended on your body density, and *body density* (mass per unit volume) is determined to a large extent by the amount of body fat that is carried. The density of bone and muscle tissue is greater than the density of fat tissue; hence, the leaner, more muscular individual will weigh more underwater (and tend to sink) than an individual with a large amount of fat (who tends to float).

Whole-body **densitometry,** which is the measurement of mass per unit volume, is the foundation of hydrostatic weighing. It is based on dividing the body into two compartments: fat and fat-free weight. In Figure 14.1, rows A & B indicate this division. Row C lists the component parts of the **fat-free weight** (all of the tissues of the body minus the extractable fat) as muscle, bone, skin, blood, and organs and represents a second model. The fat compartment includes both storage and essential fats. *Storage fat* is the fat in the subcutaneous adipose tissues and the fat surrounding the various internal organs. *Essential fat* includes the fat in bone marrow, central nervous system, cell membranes, heart, lungs, liver, spleen, kidneys, intestines, and muscles.

Note that although the terms *lean body mass* (LBM) and *fat-free weight* (FFW; sometimes called the fat-free body, FFB, or fat-free mass, FFM) are used interchangeably, they are slightly different. Technically, LBM includes the essential fat, but FFW does not. Chemically, FFW is composed of water, proteins, and bone mineral (Figure 14.1, row D), and this represents a third model of compartmentalization or composition.[34] Although each of these models (B, C, and D) describes the composi-

---

Hydrostatic Weighing Criterion measure for determining body composition through the calculation of body density.

Archimedes' Principle The principle that a partially or fully submerged object will experience an upward buoyant force equal to the weight or the volume of fluid displaced by the object.

#6 **Densitometry** The measurement of mass per unit volume.

Fat-Free Weight The weight of body tissue excluding extractable fat.

A	Total body weight (mass) (TBW)					
B	Fat-free weight 55–96% of TBW					Fat 4–45% of TBW
C	Muscle 48%	Bone 16%	Skin 14%	Blood 9%	Organs 13%	Storage + essential fat
D	Water 72–74%		Protein 19–21%		Bone mineral 7%	Fat 100%

FIGURE 14.1

Models of Body Composition

Source: Lohman.[34]

tion of the body, when the term *body composition* is used in exercise physiology, it generally refers to model B. That is, **body composition** is defined as the partitioning of body mass into fat-free mass (weight or percentage) and fat mass (weight or percentage).

Compartmentalizing the body into only fat and fat-free weight (not water, mineral, protein, and fat) and using this two-compartment model to determine percent body fat (%BF) depends upon the following assumptions.

1. The densities of the fat and fat-free weight are known and additive.

2. The densities of water, bone mineral, and protein that make up the fat-free weight are known and relatively constant from individual to individual.

3. The percentage of each fat-free component is relatively stable from individual to individual.

4. The individual being evaluated differs from the assumptions of the equation being used only in the amount of storage fat.

Hydrostatic weighing determines body density (D_B), defined as mass (M) or weight (WT) divided by volume (V) according to the following formula:[4]

(14.1)	body density (g · cc^{-1}) = mass in air (g) ÷ {{[mass in air (g) − mass in water (g)] ÷ [density of water (g · cc^{-1})]} − [residual volume (L) + volume of gastrointestinal air (0.1 L)]}
or	$$D_B = \dfrac{M_A}{\dfrac{(M_A - M_W)}{D_W} - (RV + V_G)}$$

The mass of an individual in air (M_A) can be obtained either by weighing that individual nude on a sensitive, calibrated scale or by weighing the subject's bathing suit and then subtracting the weight of the suit from the weight of the subject wearing the suit. Obtaining the volume of the human body is based upon Archimedes' principle. In practice, the individual being weighed is submerged in water, attached in some way to a scale or strain gauge instrumentation (Figure 14.2). The subject then exhales as much air as possible and sits quietly for 3–7 sec while the weight is recorded. Multiple trials are usually necessary. The highest consistent weight is selected from the trials and the weight of the apparatus, called the tare weight, is then subtracted from the scale weight. The resultant weight is the underwater weight (M_W). Body weight may be measured in lb or kg, but calculations are typically done in metric units, so conversion may be necessary. All air cannot be expelled from the body, and air makes the body buoyant (hence lighter in weight). Therefore, the underwater weight must be corrected for residual volume (the volume of air remaining in the lungs following maximal expiration) and for gastrointestinal gases, the assumed constant equal to 100 mL, or .1 L in Equation 14.1. The weight lost underwater must also be corrected for the density of the water D_W, which in turn is temperature-dependent.

■ EXAMPLE

For example, the following measurements were obtained from a football player:

M_A = 225 lb (102.3 kg)   Water Temperature = 34°C

M_W = 6.07 kg   Water Density at 34°C = 0.9944

RV = 1.583 L

FIGURE 14.2

Hydrostatic Weighing
The technique for determining body density by hydrostatic (underwater) weighing is based upon Archimedes' principle.

Substituting into Eq. 14.1 we get

$$D_B \frac{102.3 \text{ kg}}{\left(\dfrac{102.3 \text{ kg} - 6.07 \text{ kg}}{0.9944}\right) - \left(1.583 \text{ L} + 0.1 \text{ L}\right)}$$

Remember that the numerator in this equation represents mass and the denominator represents volume. In the metric system 1 L of water (a volume measure) weighs 1 kg (a mass measure), and conversely 1 kg of mass occupies 1 L of volume (Appendix A). Therefore, the equation can be solved as written.

$$D_B = \frac{102.3 \text{ kg}}{96.77 - 1.683 \text{ L}}$$
$$= \frac{102.3 \text{ kg}}{95.089 \text{ L}} = 1.0758 \text{ kg} \cdot \text{L}^{-1}$$

Although $\text{kg} \cdot \text{L}^{-1}$ is an accurate unit, the D_B is usually reported in $\text{g} \cdot \text{cc}^{-1}$ units. Dividing the $\text{kg} \cdot \text{L}^{-1}$ unit by 1000 yields $\text{g} \cdot \text{mL}^{-1}$. Then, since 1 mL equals 1 cc (cubic centimeter) the cc designation can easily be substituted for the mL and typically is. ∎

Once body density has been obtained, percent body fat (%BF) can be calculated. The two most widely used formulas for converting body density to %BF were developed by Siri and by Brozek. They have been derived differently but, within the density units of 1.09 and 1.03 $\text{g} \cdot \text{cc}^{-1}$, agree within 1% on the %BF values calculated. At lower densities the Siri formula gives increasingly higher %BF values than the Brozek formula.[37]

(14.2)

$$\text{Brozek:} \quad \%\text{BF} = \left[\left(\frac{4.570}{D_B}\right) - 4.142\right] \times 100$$

(14.3)

$$\text{Siri:} \quad \%\text{BF} = \left[\left(\frac{4.950}{D_B}\right) - 4.5\right] \times 100$$

Brozek's formula assumes that the individual has neither lost nor gained substantial amounts of body weight recently.

■ **EXAMPLE**

If we use the body density results from the football player in the preceding example in Equation 14.2 and Equation 14.3 we get

$$\text{Brozek: } \% \text{ BF} = \left[\left(\frac{4.570}{1.0758}\right) - 4.142\right] \times 100 = 10.6\%$$

$$\text{Siri:} \quad \%\text{BF} = \left[\left(\frac{4.950}{1.0758}\right) - 4.50\right] \times 100 = 10.1\%$$

As expected, the %BF values are within 1% of each other with an actual difference of only 0.5% (10.6% − 10.1% = 0.5%). ∎

Once %BF has been determined, calculation of body weight at any selected fat percentage can be done using the following sequence of formulas. The first formula simply determines the amount of fat-free weight (FFW) an individual currently has (WT_1).

Body Composition The partitioning of body mass into fat-free mass (weight or percentage) and fat mass (weight or percentage).

(14.4)   fat-free weight = current body weight (lb or kg)

$$\times \left(\frac{100\% - \text{percent body fat}}{100} \right)$$

or $FFW = WT_1 \times \left(\dfrac{100\% - \%BF}{100} \right)$

The second formula calculates the desired weight (WT_2).

(14.5)   body weight at the selected percent of body fat (lb or kg) = [100 × fat-free weight (lb or kg)] ÷ (100% − selected percent body fat)

or $WT_2 = \dfrac{100 \times FFW}{100\% - \%BF}$

The third formula calculates the amount of weight to be gained or lost.

(14.6)   weight to gain or lose (1 lb or kg) = body weight at selected percent body fat − current body weight

or $\Delta WT = WT_2 - WT_1$

■ EXAMPLE

For example, an individual who currently weights 150 lb at a body fat of 25% wishes to reduce her body fat to 17%. Equation 14.4 is used to calculate her current fat-free weight.

$$FFW = 150\ lb \times \left(\frac{100\% - 25\%}{100} \right) = 112.50\ lb$$

Her current fat-free weight and selected %BF are then substituted into Equation 14.5 to obtain her weight goal.

$$WT_2 = \frac{100 \times 112.50\ lb}{100\% - 17\%} = 135.54\ lb$$

Comparing her current weight to her goal weight in Equation 14.6 we get

$$\Delta WT = 135.5\ lb - 150\ lb = -14.5\ lb$$

This means that if this individual wishes to be 17% BF she must reduce her current weight by 14.5 lb. Of course, these calculations assume that in the process of losing weight muscle mass is maintained. This is an assumption that is not always true.   ■

Now read Box 14.1 and complete the problems given. The data are presented as they would be recorded during an actual experiment. You will need to do some conversions and analysis to select the correct M_A and M_W. As you do each calculation, mentally review why each step needs to be done to assure yourself that you understand the underlying principles.

Box 14.1 A Question for Understanding

1. From the following information calculate M_A.
    Subject name _____ Phyllis Elizabeth Major _____
    Sex ____ F ____   Age ____ 18 ____
    Weight with bathing suit _112.5_ lb _____ kg
    Weight of bathing suit ____ 0.5 ____ lb _____ kg
    Nude weight (M_A) ____ 112 ____ lb _____ kg (M_A)
    Residual volume = 1.2774 L

2. Underwater weighing trials in kg
    Select the representative weight

    a. Highest obtained weight if obtained more than twice.

    b. Second-highest obtained weight if observed more than once.

    c. Third-highest obtained weight.

    Trial   1. 7.8   2. 8.25   3. 8.3   4. 8.35
              5. 8.275   6. 8.325   7. 8.3   8. 8.325
              9. 8.3   10. 8.275

    Tare weight* _____ 7.06 _____ kg
    Water temperature _____ 35 _____ °C
    Water density (D_W) _____ 0.9941 _____
    Underwater weight (M_W)
    = selected weight − tare weight
    M_W = _____ − _____ = _____ kg
    *Tare weight equals the weight of the apparatus without the subject in it.

3. From the information presented and calculated in 1 and 2, use Equation 14.1 to calculate D_B and Equation 14.2 to calculate %BF.

4. Phyllis would like to be 19% BF. Use Equation 14.4, Equation 14.5, and Equation 14.6 to determine if she needs to gain or lose weight to achieve this goal, and if so, how much.

Answers are presented at the end of the chapter.

When the measuring technique is properly conducted, the error of %BF determined by densitometry is approximately 2.7% for adults. This error is primarily due to variations in the composition of the fat-free mass.[37]

Densitometry: Children and Adolescents, and the Elderly

The previous section outlined the basic assumptions underlying hydrostatic weighing (densitometry). Recent research has cast doubt upon all of these assumptions with regard to children and adolescents.[39]

The values for the FFW or FFB components for adults (males and females) are assumed to be approximately 73% for water and 7% for mineral content, with an overall density of FFW of 1.100 g · cc⁻¹ (Figure 14.3 dashed lines).[8, 34] Protein, not shown on the graph, makes up about 20% of the FFW of adults.

Boileau et al.[8] have shown that the percentage of water in FFW decreases (Figure 14.3b) from 77–78% at ages 7–9 yr to 73% at approximately age 20 in a steady but slightly curvilinear fashion. Across the age span females have a slightly higher percentage of water in FFW than males. Conversely, the percentage of mineral content in FFW (Figure 14.3c) increases from approximately 5% at ages 7–9 to the 7% at age 20. This change is also slightly curvilinear, and the female values are consistently lower than the male values. The protein change is minimal (and therefore not presented in Figure 14.3), varying only about 1% (from 19 to 20%) over the age span. The result of these changes is that body density also increases in a curvilinear fashion from approximately 1.08 to 1.10 g · cc⁻¹ for adult males and to 1.095 g · cc⁻¹ for adult females. This means adult females never meet the 1.10-g · cc⁻¹ assumed value (Figure 14.3a).[34]

Because the components are constantly changing as children mature, no single formula can be used for children of different ages. Neither can one

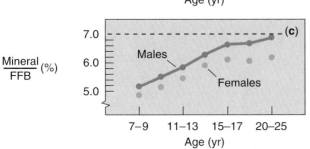

$\text{Density of FFB (g·cc}^{-1}\text{)}$

$\frac{\text{Water}}{\text{FFB}}$ (%)

$\frac{\text{Mineral}}{\text{FFB}}$ (%)

FIGURE 14.3

Estimated Changes in Fat-Free Body Composition as a Function of Age

The density of the fat-free body, also known as the fat-free weight, is much lower in both male and female children than in adults. FFB density increases as the child matures, but the female density is lower at each age than the male density and never reaches the assumed adult values of 1.1.

The percentage of the FFB that is composed of water is higher in both male and female children than in adults. As the child matures, the percentage of water in the FFB declines, but the female percentage is always higher than the male even after adulthood is reached.

The percentage of FFB that is composed of minerals is lower in both male and female children than in adults. As the child matures, the percentage of minerals in the FFB increases, but the female percentage is always lower than the male percentage even after adulthood is reached.

Source: T. G. Lohman. Applicability of body composition techniques and constants for children and youth. In K. B. Pandolf (ed.), *Exercise and Sport Science Reviews,* New York: Macmillan, 14:325–327 (1986). Reprinted by permission of Williams & Wilkins.

formula be used for boys and for girls. Table 14.1 shows the array of age and sex formulas needed.

The use of equations developed with the assumption of the composition of adult components will overestimate the %BF of the child or adolescent. This can be illustrated as follows. If the D_B of a 9-yr-old girl is determined to be 1.065 g · cc^{-1} by hydrostatic weighing, the %BF calculated by the Brozek formula (Equation 14.2) is

$$\left(\frac{4.570}{1.065}\right) - 4.142 \times 100 = 14.9\%$$

The Lohman[34] age- and sex-specific formula yields

$$\left(\frac{5.35}{1.065}\right) - 4.95 \times 100 = 7.3\% \quad \text{(see Table 14.1)}$$

The majority of research published to date for children and adolescents has been on normally active nonathletes. Further work is in progress to determine the effects of physical activity and/or athletic participation on bone mineral, hydration, and body density values throughout the growth years. Percent body fat values of young athletes, even if the appropriate age and sex formulas are used, must be interpreted cautiously. Although the pediatric formulas are better than adult formulas, even the pediatric formulas may need to be revised for young athletes. In addition, research in the area of body composition, on both sedentary and active youths, should directly measure water (W) and bone mineral content (M) of the FFW as well as body density in order to more accurately account

TABLE 14.1 ■ Formulas for Converting Body Density to Percent Body Fat in Children and Adolescents, by Sex

AGE (YR)	MALE	FEMALE
7–9	$\left(\dfrac{5.38}{D_B} - 4.97\right) \times 100$	$\left(\dfrac{5.43}{D_B} - 5.03\right) \times 100$
9–11	$\left(\dfrac{5.30}{D_B} - 4.89\right) \times 100$	$\left(\dfrac{5.35}{D_B} - 4.95\right) \times 100$
11–13	$\left(\dfrac{5.23}{D_B} - 4.81\right) \times 100$	$\left(\dfrac{5.25}{D_B} - 4.84\right) \times 100$
13–15	$\left(\dfrac{5.07}{D_B} - 4.64\right) \times 100$	$\left(\dfrac{5.12}{D_B} - 4.69\right) \times 100$
15–17	$\left(\dfrac{5.03}{D_B} - 4.59\right) \times 100$	$\left(\dfrac{5.07}{D_B} - 4.64\right) \times 100$
17–20	$\left(\dfrac{4.98}{D_B} - 4.53\right) \times 100$	$\left(\dfrac{5.05}{D_B} - 4.62\right) \times 100$

Calculated from the density FFW constant (D_1) reported by Lohman,[34] and a density of fat constant (D_2) of 0.9 g · cc^{-1} according to the formula

$$\%BF = \frac{1}{D_B}\left[\left(\frac{D_1 D_2}{D_1 - D_2}\right) - \frac{D_2}{D_1 - D_2}\right] \times 100$$

for all body compartments. These variables should be used in a more complex formula such as

(14.7)

$$\%BF = \left(\frac{2.747}{D_B} \right) - 0.714(W) + 1.146(M) - 2.0503$$

At the other end of the age continuum, the elderly, consideration needs to be given to the effect of the loss of bone mineral density owing to osteoporosis on the determination %BF. Theoretically, such a decrease would cause a decrement in body density and, thus, an overestimation of %BF if it were not accounted for.[2, 14, 34]

Field Tests of Body Composition

Skinfolds   The most widely used anthropometric estimation of body size or composition involves the measurement of skinfolds at selected sites. **Skinfolds** (or fatfolds) are the double thickness of skin plus the adipose tissue between the parallel layers of skin (see Figure 14.4). Since there are only slight variations in skin thickness among individuals, the resulting measure is taken as an indication of the thickness of the subcutaneous fat.[5] Technically, however, adipose tissue (and hence the subcutaneous fatfold) has both a fat and a fat-free component. The fat-free component is composed of water, blood vessels, and nerves. As the fat content of the adipose tissue increases (as in obesity), the water content decreases.[50]

The use of skinfold thicknesses to estimate body composition is based on two assumptions. The first is that the total subcutaneous adipose tissue mass is represented by the selected skinfold sites. In general, evidence supports this assumption.[37, 44, 50] The second assumption is that the subcutaneous tissue mass has a known relationship with total body fat. Table 14.2 shows the distribution of total body fat and the relative percentages of each storage site for a reference male and a reference female 20–24 yr old.

Most of the values in Table 14.2 are estimates. They indicate that approximately one-third of the total fat for both males (3.1 kg subcutaneous fat ÷ 10.3–10.5 kg total fat) and females (5.1 kg subcuta-

FIGURE 14.4

Measurement of Triceps Skinfold Using a Calibrated Skinfold Caliper

neous fat ÷ 13.4–17.2 kg total fat) is estimated to be subcutaneous. Other estimates put this value as high as 70% and as low as 20%. With advancing age a proportionally smaller amount of fat is stored subcutaneously. Thus, any given skinfold would then represent a smaller percentage of total body fat. It may also be that lean individuals and fat individuals store their fat in proportionally different ways. Additionally, females may store more or less fat subcutaneously than males.[37,44] There is little disagreement regarding the differences between essential fat amounts for males and females. The higher essential fat values in females are generally attributed to the energy requirements of pregnancy and lactation.

These variations in the estimation of subcutaneous fat percentage mean that the second assumption is not as firmly based as the first.[14] One way of

Skinfolds The double thickness of skin plus the adipose tissue between the parallel layers of skin.

TABLE 14.2 ▪ **Percentage of Fat Distribution in a Reference Male and a Reference Female**

DISTRIBUTION SITE	70 kg Male		56.8 kg Female	
	FAT kg	%	FAT kg	%
Total body	10.5	15	15.3	27
Essential	2.1	3	4.9–6.8	9–12
Storage	8.2–8.4	12	8.5–10.4	15–18
Subcutaneous	3.1	4	5.1	9
Intermuscular	3.3	5	3.5	6
Intramuscular	0.8	1	0.6	1
Abdominothoracic cavity	1.0	1	1.2	2

Source: Modified from Behnke & Wilmore,[5] Lohman.[37]

dealing with this problem is to make sure that the equations that are used are age-adjusted or generalized for sedentary individuals and population-specific for various athletic groups.

When skinfolds are taken by trained professionals and the appropriate equations are used, the accuracy of skinfold prediction of percent body fat is approximately 3–5% compared with underwater weighing. Improper techniques can result in large prediction errors. The greatest source of error arises from an improper location of the skinfold site to be tested. Therefore, anyone wishing to use this method to predict percent body fat should locate the site precisely and practice the technique repeatedly before using it. Table 14.3 presents equations that can be used to predict percent body fat from two to three skinfold sites. These equations are specific for sex and for age.

Skinfold or fatfold thickness values may be used in ways other than to predict percent body fat. First, the millimeter values of several sites (usually 5–7 from anatomically diverse locations) can be

TABLE 14.3 ▪ **Calculation of %BF from Skinfolds**

GROUP	EQUATION
Adult males	$\%BF = 0.39287(X_1) - 0.00105(X_1)^2 + 0.15772(X_2) - 5.18845$, where X_1 = sum of abdominal, suprailiac, and triceps skinfolds and X_2 = age
Adult females	$\%BF = 0.41563(X_1) - 0.00112(X_1)^2 + 0.03661(X_2) - 4.03653$, where X_1 = sum of abdominal, suprailiac, and triceps skinfolds and X_2 = age
Male children and adolescents (8–18 yr)	$\%BF = 0.735(X_1) + 1.0$, where X_1 = sum of triceps and calf skinfolds
Female children and adolescents (8–18 yr)	$\%BF = 0.610(X_1) + 5.1$, where X_1 = sum of triceps and calf skinfolds

Source: Based on information in Golding, Myers, & Sinning;[28] Jackson & Pollock;[33] Slaughter et al.[54]
Note: The last two equations were developed taking into account body density, percentage of water in FFW, and bone mineral content variations by age.

added to form a sum of skinfolds. Such a sum is an indication of the relative degree of fatness between individuals. Or it can be used to detect changes within a given individual, if measurements are taken repeatedly over time. Second, fatfolds may be used to determine the pattern of distribution of subcutaneous fat. Such a pattern has emerged as an important predictor of the health hazards of obesity.[30, 44, 50, 57]

Bioelectrical Impedance (Impedance Plethysmography)

The determination of body composition by *bioelectrical impedance analysis* (BIA) has gained a great deal of acceptance in fitness facilities due primarily to the ease with which the procedure can be conducted. In BIA four electrodes are attached to a quietly resting supine subject's hands and feet (two per limb either ipsilaterally or contralaterally) (see Figure 14.5). A harmless, sensationless, low-amperage (80 μA), radio frequency (50 kHz) electrical current is passed between the electrodes; and the resistance to the current is recorded. A reading of resistance (in ohms) is obtained. It is assumed that the body volume is defined as a cylinder of constant cross-sectional area and uniform density distribution. Body volume is more often defined as height squared divided by resistance (HT$^2 \div$ R).[3, 15, 58]

The ability to conduct the electrical current is directly related to the amount of water and electrolytes in the various body tissues. The flow of the

electrical current is easier in fat-free tissue (hence it offers less resistance) than fat tissue because the fat-free tissue contains a higher percentage of water and electrolytes. Therefore, individuals with large amounts of fat-free weight will show low resistance values, and those with large amounts of fat weight will show high resistance values.

Since the BIA technique is actually measuring total body water (TBW), estimates can be made of body density and fat-free weight on the basis of the obtained TBW and the known percentages of water in the body and in the FFW. Another technique is to derive regression equations from height, resistance, and/or other anthropometric variables (such as weight, age, sex, skinfolds, or circumferences) to directly predict FFW or %BF. In most cases hydrostatic weighing is used as the criterion measure. As with skinfolds, a number of equations have been generated in this manner.

As you might suspect from this discussion, the accuracy of BIA measurement depends highly upon the maintenance of a normal level of hydration. Either too much (hyperhydration) or too little (hypohydration or dehydration) fluid will affect the readings. The exact effect is controversial. Theoretically, an increase in body water should decrease resistance and %BF. There is some experimental evidence supporting this theory; however, other studies have shown the opposite result. That is, dehydration caused by exercise has decreased resistance, and hyperhydration from ingestion of replacement supplements has increased resistance. This variance may be related to whether the electrolyte content changes proportionally to water and to the shift in water between compartments. What is clear is that individuals should be measured 3–4 hr after the ingestion of a meal or after an exercise session and should not be under the influence of anything, such as caffeine, that might act as a diuretic.[3, 22, 56, 58]

The accuracy of BIA also depends upon both ambient and skin temperatures. Resistance is higher under cool temperatures than under warm ones. Thus, if an individual is tested repeatedly over a period of 15–20 min and is in an environment that permits body cooling to occur, the %BF estimate will go up as the skin temperature goes down. Care must therefore be taken that testing is done at a neutral temperature (27–29°C; 80–84°F) when the subject is neither overheated nor chilled.[20, 56]

FIGURE 14.5

Determination of Body Composition by Bioelectrical Impedance

A third factor that influences the accuracy of BIA estimates of body composition are the equations used. These equations include those for body geometry, cross-sectional area, and current distribution, as well as those used to convert resistance to TBW, body density, and %BF. Each of the electrical assumptions is violated by the human body but apparently not sufficiently to negate the use of BIA. However, these violations do limit the accuracy for estimating TBW, FFW, and %BF to individuals not at the extremes of leanness or fatness. Furthermore, if the criterion measure upon which the equation was based did not take into account the age-related differences in TBW, the inaccuracies would be confounded.[3, 15, 32]

BIA values under standard conditions will be consistent, but the accuracy is probably no better than that achieved by skinfolds.[3]

Height and Weight   In some situations, such as when large numbers of individuals are being evaluated, the only measures of body size that can easily be obtained are height and weight. These values are often used in conjunction with height and weight charts that include standards such as acceptable body weight (less than 10% over the chart weight), overweight (10–20% over the chart weight) and obese (more than 20% over the chart weight). Such use of height and weight charts is minimally acceptable for large group data, but is not recommended as a source of what one "should" weigh for individuals, for the following reasons.[18, 31, 45, 48]

1. The most commonly available height and weight charts were compiled from lowest mortality data on individuals who purchased life insurance in nongroup situations. The age range was 25–59 yr. Some people were included more than once when they purchased more than one policy. Thus, the sample was neither randomly drawn, as is necessary statistically, nor truly representative of the total American population, especially the elderly, lower-socioeconomic groups, and specific ethnic groups.

2. Individuals with known heart disease, cancer, and/or diabetes were excluded, but smokers were included. Thus, risk factors, other than body weight, were ignored in determining mortality ratios.

3. Only body weights at the time of purchasing the insurance, not at the time of death, were considered. This omission could greatly affect the values. In addition, in many cases height and weight were self-reported and not measured. The accuracy of self-reported data must be questioned.

4. The determination of frame size is not always defined. Even when it is, frame size is very difficult to defend and interpret in relation to body weight.

5. The 1983 Metropolitan Life Insurance height-weight chart shows higher weight values at a given height and frame size than the comparable 1959 chart, reflecting the trend of a national weight gain. The 1959 table values were listed as desirable weights (that is, weights associated with the lowest mortality), but not so the 1983 table values. If the Metropolitan tables are the only thing available for use, the 1959 (not the 1983) version should be selected, except for the elderly. Some evidence suggests that desirable weights are slightly higher in the elderly. Therefore, the 1983 tables can be used for this population.

6. Weight per se does not provide any information on body composition. What matters is the %BF, not the body weight, because %BF is related to health.

If height and weight are the only variables available, and if height and weight charts should not be used, a reasonable alternative is still available: the body mass index.

Body Mass Index   *Body mass index* (BMI) is a ratio of total body weight to height. Several ratios have been proposed, but the one used most frequently is weight (in kilograms) divided by height (in meters) squared [WT/HT^2 $(kg \cdot m^{-2})$]. This ratio is also known as the Quetelet index.[14,49,51] Calculated BMI can then be compared against standard values to determine whether the individual has acceptable body weight, is overweight, or is obese (see Table 14.4).

■ EXAMPLE

For example, if a female subject (age = 30 yr) weighs 165 lb and is 5 ft 8 in. tall, calculation of her BMI first requires conversion to metric units. Dividing 165 lb by 2.2 kg/lb gives a weight of 75 kg. Multiplying 68 in. by 2.54 cm/in. gives 172.7 cm (1.73

m). The meter value squared is 2.98 m². Thus, BMI = 75 ÷ 2.98 = 25.2. Check Table 14.4 to see whether this is an acceptable, overweight, or obesity value for this individual. ∎

Note that the table gives both upper and lower ranges of acceptable values. Being too lean is no more desirable than being too fat in a normal, nonathletic population. Athletes often have body composition values below these standards, but as we discussed in the previous chapter in terms of eat-ing disorders, too lean can be a problem or the sign of one. Body composition for athletes will be discussed later in this chapter.

The selection of BMI values of 27.8 for males and 27.3 for females as the upper limit of acceptable is based on the data graphed in Figure 14.6. The figure shows that for adults there is a curvilinear increase in excess mortality (a greater number of deaths than expected in a given population) with an increasing BMI. Significant increases in risk begin at a BMI of 27.3 for females and 27.8 for males.[12]

TABLE 14.4 ∎ Commonly Used Standards for Acceptable Body Weight, Overweight, and Obesity in Nonathletes

	Acceptable Body Weight		Overweight		Obesity	
	MALE	**FEMALE**	**MALE**	**FEMALE**	**MALE**	**FEMALE**
BMI (kg · m⁻²)						
5 yr	14.7–20	16.2–21	> 20	> 21		
6 yr	14.7–20	16.2–21	> 20	> 21		
7 yr	14.9–20	16.2–22	> 20	> 22		
8 yr	15.1–20	16.2–22	> 20	> 22		
9 yr	15.2–20	16.2–23	> 20	> 23		
10 yr	15.3–21	16.6–23.5	> 21	> 23.5		
11 yr	15.8–21	16.9–24	> 21	> 24		
12 yr	16.0–22	16.9–24.5	> 22	> 24.5		
13 yr	16.6–23	17.5–24.5	> 23	> 24.5		
14 yr	17.5–24.5	17.5–25	> 24.5	> 25		
15 yr	18.1–25	17.5–25	> 25	> 25		
16 yr	18.5–26.5	17.5–25	> 26.5	> 25		
17 yr	18.8–27	17.5–26	> 27	> 26		
18+ yr	19–27.8	18–27.3	> 27.8	> 27.3	30–40 > 40	30–40 Grade 2* Massive obesity > 40 Grade 3 Morbid obesity
%BF						
5–18 yr	10–20%	14–25%	20–25%	26–31%	≥ 25%	≥ 32%
> 18 yr	12–18%	16–25%	19–24%	26–31%	≥ 25%	≥ 32%
SKINFOLDS†						
5–18 yr	10–25	16–30	25–31	31–36	> 32	> 36
> 18 yr					> 45	> 69

Source: Based on Bray,[13] Bubb,[17] Lohman,[36, 38] Nieman,[45] Simoupoulos.[52]

†Sum of triceps and calf for children and adolescents; sum of triceps and subscapular for adults.

*BMI 25–30 kg · m⁻² is sometimes called Grade I obesity.

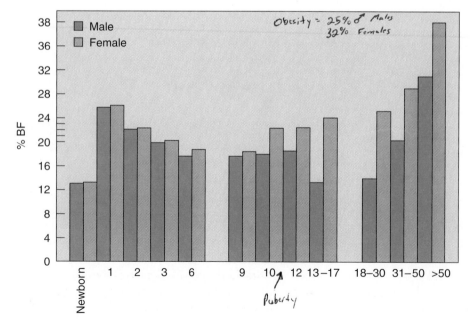

FIGURE 14.6

The Relationship Between Body Mass Index and Mortality

The risk of excess mortality (depicted as a mortality ratio where 100 represents normal mortality) from increasing values for body mass index (BMI) is described by a J-shaped curve. BMI values from 15–25 represent no excess mortality risk. BMI values from 25–30 represent a low risk, from 30–40 a moderate risk, and over 40 a high risk of excess mortality.

Source: G. A. Bray. Complications of obesity. *Annals of Internal Medicine.* 103:1052–1062 (1985). Reprinted by permission of American College of Physicians.

BMI has been shown to correlate highly with %BF derived from skinfold measures (r = 0.74) and hydrostatic weighing (r = 0.58–0.85). These correlations indicate a moderate relationship, but they also suggest that there is considerable measurement error in using BMI as an estimate of body adiposity. In situations where the same group of individuals were evaluated, skinfolds generally predicted %BF better than BMI did. Nevertheless, BMI is often used as an indication of overweight or obesity, particularly when mass screening is done.

Overweight and Obesity

Although being overweight is what concerns most people, it is really %BF that should be of concern. Excess weight can be caused by high levels of lean muscle mass and additional muscle mass is beneficial. Except in rare instances, such as providing protection from the cold water for an English Channel swimmer, excess fat is not beneficial.

Figure 14.7 shows average %BF values for males and females across the age spectrum from infancy to 50 yr. Prior to puberty (which begins at approximately 10 yr for females and 12 yr for males) there is very little sex difference in %BF. The 10–20% range, representing acceptable body weight and

FIGURE 14.7

Percent Body Fat Changes with Age

Source: Boileau et al.;[8] Dietz;[23] Forman et al.;[25] Friiz-Hansen;[26] Malina et al.;[42] McArdle et al.;[44] Plowman et al.[47]

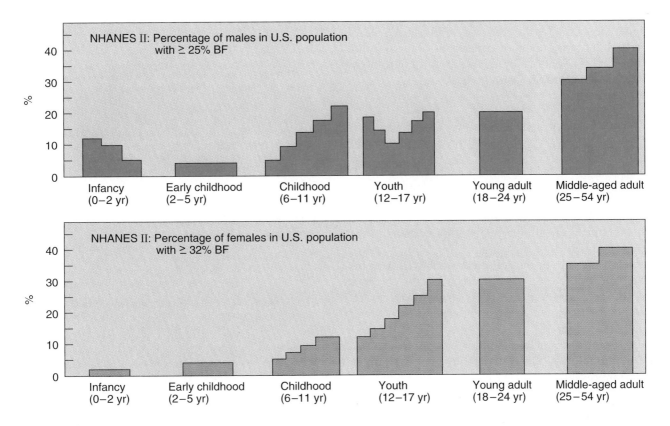

FIGURE 14.8

Prevalence of Obesity in U.S. Population

Obesity was defined in the National Health and Nutrition Examination Survey-II as 25% BF for males and 32% BF for females. The values were calculated from triceps plus subscapular skinfold measures taken on a representative sample of Americans. The percentage of individuals who are classified as obese shows an inconsistent but definite increasing trend from infancy to adulthood for both males and females. By late middle age (last bar) almost 40% of the American population is estimated to be obese.

Source: "Assessment of body composition in children" by T. G. Lohman, *Pediatric Exercise Science,* (Vol. 1, No. 1), p. 26. Copyright 1989 by Human Kinetics Publishers. Reprinted by permission.

composition, is very close to actual measured values during this time span. After puberty male values drop until approximately 30 yr of age and then rise; female values rise slowly and then tend to jump. By age 30 both male and female averages fall in the overweight category, and by age 50 they fall into the obesity category.

The data used to construct Figure 14.7 were not based on a random sampling of the United States population but on available published sources. In contrast, Figure 14.8 presents the results from the 1976–1980 National Health and Nutrition Exami-

nation Survey–II (NHANES II), which can be considered representative of the population. In this survey obesity was also defined as 25% BF for males and 32% BF for females. It depicts not average %BF levels but the percentage of obesity across the age spectrum.[35] As shown, the incidence of obesity increases rather steadily as both males and females age, being a problem for females earlier than it is for males. By middle age fully one-third of the U.S. population can be considered obese. Although these data are not shown on the graph, another 25–30% of adults are estimated to be overweight. Thus, despite what appears to be a national obsession with thinness, diets and weight control, large numbers of Americans of all ages are either overweight or obese; and the problem intensifies as the calendar years go by.[60]

What Happens to Adipose Cells in Obesity? The Cellular Basis of Obesity

Adipose tissue is composed of a matrix of connective tissue in which white adipose cells (adipocytes) appear singularly or in small clusters. A typical cell (Figure 14.9) looks something like a signet ring: a metal band with some type of stone or jewel at the top. The nucleus of the cell appears as the stone or jewel of the ring in the cell membrane which forms the band of the ring. The space within the confines of the cell is where the triglyceride droplets are stored.[43] The brown adipose cell in Figure 14.9 will be discussed later.

There are about 30–50 billion fat cells in an adult of acceptable weight. Females have approximately 50% more fat cells than males. Adipocytes can change in size about tenfold if needed to store triglycerides. Apparently, this increase in size (or hypertrophy) is the way in which increasing levels of fat are first stored. Sometimes when the fat cell size is enlarged, the increased size causes a bulging between the fibrous tissue strands, causing a dimply, waffled appearance. These lumpy areas are often labeled as *cellulite*. As can be seen from this discussion, though, cellulite is simply fat.[6, 7]

Once the upper limit of fat storage by hypertrophy is approached (somewhere around 30 kg of fat), fat cell hyperplasia occurs. **Hyperplasia** in general is growth in a tissue or organ through an increase in the number of cells. In fat tissue hyperplasia is the development of new adipocytes from immature precursor cells. Adipocytes themselves do not divide and multiply, but hypertrophy in adipocytes stimulates cell division and maturation in precursor cells.[41] Thus, a newly overweight adult is likely to have the same number of fat cells as when he or she was of normal weight, but these adipocytes will be larger than before. An obese individual may have

White Adipose Cell

Nucleus
Mitochondria
Lipid vacuole

Brown Adipose Cell

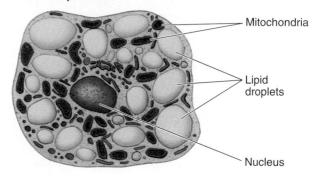

Mitochondria
Lipid droplets
Nucleus

FIGURE 14.9

Adipose Cells

White and brown adipose cells both store lipid as triglyceride, but do so in slightly different ways. White adipose cells contain one large fat droplet; brown adipose cells contain many small fat droplets. Most of the fat stored in the human body is stored in white adipose cells.

Source: Growth, Maturation and Physical Activity (p. 134) by Robert M. Malina and Claude Bouchard. Champaign, IL: Human Kinetics Publishers. Copyright 1991 by Robert Malina and Claude Bouchard. Reprinted by permission.

enlarged adipocytes, an increased number of adipocytes, or both. Obese individuals may have as many as 75–80 billion fat cells. Once created, fat cell numbers are not naturally reduced, even if body weight and body fat are lost.[53] Liposuction—the surgical removal of adipose tissue—is the only way to get rid of adipocytes. The maintenance of large numbers of adipocytes may be one reason why it is so difficult for obese individuals to maintain a weight/fat loss once it occurs.

These facts emphasize the importance of avoiding the maturation of extra fat cells. Overweight or obese infants, children, or adolescents tend to be-

---

Hyperplasia Growth in a tissue or organ through an increase in the number of cells.

come overweight or obese adults, although adolescent obesity is more predictive of adult obesity than are obesity at birth or in infancy.[21, 23, 35]

Figure 14.10 indicates the typical pattern in cell size (Figure 14.10a) and number (Figure 14.10b) that occurs in normal (nonobese) children and adolescents.[41] From birth to young adulthood the average cell size doubles or even triples. Most of this increase in size happens during the first year after birth. From 1 yr to the onset of puberty there is no significant increase in size and no sex difference. At puberty cell size increases in females but remains fairly constant in males. Not all adipose cells are the same size; internal (visceral) fat cells are generally smaller than subcutaneous fat cells. Furthermore, not all subcutaneous cells are equal in size. For example, gluteal adipocytes tend to be larger than abdominal adipocytes, which in turn are larger than subscapular cells.

At birth the number of adipocytes is approximately 5 billion. For the number to increase to the average adult value of 30 billion, considerable change must occur. However, little increase in number occurs during the first year after birth when the cell size is changing so drastically (see Figure 14.10b). From 1 yr to the onset of puberty there is a gradual but steady increase in number, with no difference appearing between the sexes. This gradual increase can double or even triple the number of fat cells. At puberty the cellularity of adipose tissues increases greatly in both males and females, but the female increase far exceeds the male increase. This increase in fat cell number plateaus in late adolescence and early adulthood and ideally remains at that level. In reality, however, hyperplasia can and often does occur in adulthood.[41] Thus, although there are two critical periods—infancy and adolescence—in the development of adipocytes, this should not be interpreted as meaning that fat cells cannot be added during adulthood.

Some individuals produce more adipocytes than others during growth, and this can amount to billions of cells. During the growth changes males tend to accumulate more subcutaneous fat on the trunk and females on the extremities.

Fat Distribution Patterns

The location of fat storage varies among individuals. In general, humans distribute fat in three basic patterns: android, gynoid, and intermediate pat-

Hypertrophy Table (handwritten)

* Adolescents is best predictor of obesity. (handwritten)

FIGURE 14.10

Adipose Cell Size and Number Changes with Growth

(a) The greatest change in adipose cell size occurs before age 5. Until approximately age 10, cell size is similar in males and females. After age 10 the difference between males and females gradually widens, and individual variations (indicated by the vertical lines) become more apparent. (b) The number of adipose cells gradually increases over the childhood years in males and females at a similar rate. At approximately age 10 in both sexes, the rate of increase in fat cell number accelerates, but females far exceed males. Individual differences indicated by vertical bars (labeled SD for standard deviation) increase considerably with age.

Source: Growth, Maturation and Physical Activity (pp. 138, 139) by Robert M. Malina and Claude Bouchard. Champaign, IL: Human Kinetics Publishers. Copyright 1991 by Robert Malina and Claude Bouchard. Reprinted by permission.

terns (Figure 14.11). The *android pattern*, also known as the abdominal or apple pattern, is predominately found in males. It is characterized by the storage of

(a)   (b)   (c)

Figure 14.11

Patterns of Fat Distribution
Android (a); Gynoid (b);
Intermediate (c).

fat in the nape of the neck, shoulders, and abdomen (upper part of the body). In this pattern the largest quantity of fat is stored internally, not subcutaneously. The result is the classic potbelly shape. Individuals with potbellies often make the claim that they are not fat and occasionally challenge others to hit them in the stomach as hard as possible to prove their superior musculature. In fact, the hardness of the abdominal region is caused by the excess fat in the abdominal cavity pushing against the abdominal muscles and stretching them taut, not by muscle tone or hypertrophy. Once the amount of fat to be stored exceeds the capacity of the abdominal cavity, subcutaneous sites are loaded.[19, 55]

The *gynoid pattern*, also called the gluteofemoral or pear pattern, is found predominantly among females. It is characterized by the storage of fat in the lower part of the body, specifically, in the thighs and buttocks, with the largest quantity being stored subcutaneously. No pseudohardness is apparent. These sites tend to be soft and to jiggle.[19, 55]

There is a growing body of evidence that the deposition of fat in the gluteal-femoral region by females is linked to reproductive function. In particular, gluteal-femoral fat may furnish energy for the development of the fetus primarily during the latter states of pregnancy and for the newborn child during lactation. As would be expected, these fat deposits are controlled by the steroid hormones.

The third type of fat pattern is known simply as the *intermediate pattern*. In this pattern, fat is stored in both the upper and the lower parts of the body, giving a somewhat rectangular cubic appearance. Note that all three patterns are found in both males and females, despite the sex-specific predominance associated with android and gynoid shapes.[19, 55]

Abdominal fat deposits are easily mobilized; therefore it is possible to reduce fat accumulation in this area relatively easily. Conversely, glutealfemoral fat deposits are not easily mobilized, and so it is not possible to reduce fat accumulation in these areas easily. The potential for reshaping the gluteofemoral fat pattern is extremely limited.[19, 55]

The reason behind the variation in fat deposit mobilization is hormonally based. Two different receptors, alpha and beta, have been identified in fat cells; they vary in their ability to facilitate or inhibit fat incorporation into the cell or fat mobilization out of the cell. Alpha-receptors inhibit fat transfer to and from the adipocytes, and beta-receptors enhance these transfers. Enzyme activity is concomitantly increased or decreased. Alpha-receptors predominate in the lower body and are thus more abundant in the gynoid pattern. Beta-receptors are concentrated in the upper body and are more abundant in the android pattern. Thus, the adipose cells in the abdominal region are more unstable.

Under the influence of epinephrine (released from the adrenal medulla), fat from the abdominal cells is easily mobilized and dumped into the circulatory system. If the free fatty acids and glycerol can be used (directly or indirectly) as fuel to support exercise, there is no problem. However, when epinephrine is released in times of emotional stress, there is no need for the excess fuel; the fatty acids and glycerol are then routed to the liver, where they are primarily converted to low-density lipoproteins (LDLs). LDLs are largely composed of cholesterol and are associated with atherosclerosis and an increased risk of coronary artery disease (CAD). (See Chapter 8 for an in-depth discussion of CAD risk factors.)

In addition, abdominal fat cells tend to be larger than fat cells found in other parts of the body. Larger fat cells are associated with glucose intolerance (the inability to dispose of a glucose load effectively), coupled with insulin resistance and hyperglycemia, and an excess of insulin in the blood (hyperinsulinemia). These conditions are associated with diabetes mellitus (a CAD risk factor) and hypertension (a CAD risk factor). The latter occurs because of the action of insulin in promoting reabsorption of sodium by the kidneys.[16, 19, 55]

Table 14.5 summarizes the differences between android and gynoid fat patterns.

Waist-to-Hip Ratio

Simply looking in the mirror while naked is probably the best way to determine whether you are android, gynoid, or intermediate in terms of fat distribution. Computation of a waist-to-hip ratio is suggested as a way to estimate the health risk of the pattern of fat distribution. Research has shown that the waist-to-hip ratio (W/H) is a stronger predictor for diabetes, coronary artery disease, and overall death risk than body weight, body mass index, or percent body fat.[16, 24]

Waist circumference is measured with a tape measure, to the nearest centimeter, at the level of the natural indentation or at the navel if no indentation is apparent. Hip circumference is measured at the largest site. Both measures should be taken while the individual is standing and is without clothes. The average value for females ages 17–39 is 0.80, and this value increases with age to above 0.90. Comparable averages for males range from 0.90 to 0.98. Values above these averages raise the health risks for individuals of both sexes.[55]

Health Risks of Overweight and Obesity

Individuals who are overweight from an excess of body fat, but are not obese, incur mild to moderate health risks. Individuals who are obese possess an excess of body fat that represents a significant health risk. The amount of fat and the distribution of that fat are linked to higher risks of major diseases. These diseases, discussed in the following sections, lead to increased mortality or decreased longevity.

TABLE 14.5 ▪ Patterns of Fat Distribution

FACTOR	ANDROID	GYNOID
Sex it predominates in	Males	Females
Regional fat storage	Upper body (neck, abdomen)	Lower body (thighs, buttocks)
Fat storage site	Internal ($\uparrow$ LDL levels)	Subcutaneous
Characteristic of fat deposit	Hard	Soft
Adipose tissue receptors	Beta	Alpha
Adipose cell size	Large	Small
Fat mobilization	Easy	Difficult
Major risk	Coronary artery disease, glucose intolerance, diabetes, hypertension	Psychological

Cardiovascular Disease Framingham, Massachusetts, has been the site of a longitudinal study investigating the risk factors for heart disease in more than 5000 residents. Data from 26–30 yr of follow-up have shown that overweight or obesity is a significant predictor of cardiovascular disease, independent of age, cholesterol, systolic blood pressure, cigarette smoking, and glucose tolerance. The Framingham investigators have concluded that if everyone were at or within 10% of his or her desirable weight, there would be 25% less coronary heart disease and 35% less congestive heart failure and stroke. The risk is greater for those who become obese early in life rather than in old age.[13, 18, 46, 52] And as mentioned in the previous section, the degree of risk is higher for those who store their fat in the android pattern than in the gynoid pattern.

Hypertension (High Blood Pressure) There is a strong association between elevated blood pressure and excess body weight and fat. The relationship varies directly, and a reduction in blood pressure usually follows weight loss.[13, 18, 46] Hypertension is also a very strong and independent risk factor for coronary heart disease.

Gallbladder Disease and Hypercholesterolemia (High Cholesterol) In the Framingham study mentioned previously individuals who were 20% or more above the average weight for their height were about twice as likely to develop gallbladder disease as those who were 10% less than the average weight. In another study the frequency of gallbladder disease was largely explained by weight, age, and, in females, the number of viable pregnancies (parity). Obese females between 20 and 30 yr of age had a 600% greater chance of having gallbladder disease than average-weight females. Within all age groups the frequency of gallbladder disease increased with the level of body weight. The body weight of males with gallstones has also been shown to be significantly more than the body weight of men without gallstones.[13, 46]

At least part of the explanation for the increased gallbladder disease in overweight or obese individuals can be linked to the effect of increased body weight and fat on cholesterol. There is a significant relationship between fatness and cholesterol level that is direct and positive. Cholesterol production is also related to body weight such that 1 excess kg of body weight increases cholesterol production 20–22

mg $\cdot$ dL^{-1}. Bile is produced in the liver and stored in the gallbladder and always contains some cholesterol. The bile of obese individuals is more saturated with cholesterol than that of nonobese individuals. This increased presence of cholesterol in bile is the likely cause of the increased risk of gallbladder disease.[13]

Diabetes Mellitus Diabetes is a disorder of carbohydrate (glucose) metabolism. Overweight or obesity appears to cause a deterioration in glucose tolerance (leading to high levels of blood glucose) and to aggravate the appearance of diabetes. Weight loss reduces this risk, and adult onset diabetes can thus often be controlled by diet and weight loss.[13,18,46]

Cancer The American Cancer Society has published data on 750,000 individuals studied between 1959 and 1972. In these studies, as BMI increased, so did the incidence of death from cancer, even independent of cigarette smoking. Overweight males were particularly susceptible to prostate and colorectal cancer; overweight females showed increased rates of breast, cervical, endometrial, uterine, and ovarian cancer. The suspected link, at least for the females, is the level of estrogen. Adipose tissue is a site for estrogen formation in all females and the major site in postmenopausal females. Estrogen formation is increased in overweight and obese individuals owing to the increased number of adipose cells.[13, 21, 46, 52]

Miscellaneous Disorders In addition to the specific diseases just discussed, overweight or obesity has been linked to respiratory dysfunction, joint problems and gout, endocrine disorder, problems in the administration of anesthetics for surgery, and an impaired physical work capacity.[1, 46] The increase in prevalence of these diseases applies to adults, but overweight or obese children also show increased risk factors, though not the actual diseases, compared with normal-weight children.[59]

*H*eredity and Body Composition

There is evidence in humans that both obesity and localized fat deposition are determined solely by genetic transmission in some individuals. Thirteen genetic syndromes have been identified in the medical literature, but all are considered to be pathological disorders and are extremely rare. Even the most common has an incidence rate of only about 1 in 25,000. For the vast majority of us the contribution of genetics to our body composition is not nearly so absolute, despite what our experience tells us about familial resemblance.[8]

Studies conducted to determine the contribution of genetics to body composition show the expected pattern of very low relationships between biological siblings, whether born separately or together (dizygotic twins), and moderate relationships between monozygotic twins. Despite these moderate relationships, Bouchard et al.[10] have concluded the following:

1. Only about 5% of the total variation in BMI and skinfold thickness is genetically transferable.

2. About 25–30% of the variance in %BF, FFW, and fat distribution patterning is genetically transferable.

3. About 30% of the transmission of body composition variables is linked to cultural factors, defined as the environment established by the family (such as the role and amount of food consumed, the types of food eaten, and activity patterns).

4. About 45–65% of the variance in body composition is genetically nontransferable.

The first two conclusions may mean that the storage of internal fat is influenced by genetics more than the storage of subcutaneous fat is.

These low to moderate contributions of biological transferability do not mean that heredity does not play a critical role in an individual's body composition. For example, when six pairs of male monozygotic twins were overfed by 1000 kcal · day^{-1} for 22 days, all responded with significant gains in body weight, skinfold thickness, and fat mass. There were large interpair (between-pair) differences in these gains, but not intrapair (between-twin) differences. These data indicate that some individuals are genetically programmed for fat gain in response to excess calories, but others are not. A follow-up study lasting for 100 days showed the same response, with some of the pairs exhibiting more of a tendency to gain fat-free mass than fat mass. This tendency to gain fat or fat-free tissue is called *nutrient partitioning*. At the present time there is no way to identify who falls into which category.[9,11] The best advice, therefore, seems to be to avoid consistently ingesting more calories than are utilized—which, of course, is easier said than done for most people.

SUMMARY

1. Hydrostatic, or underwater, weighing is generally considered to be the laboratory criterion measure for the determination of body composition. It is based on densitometry.

2. Densitometry usually divides the body into two components, fat and fat-free weight. Fat-free weight is composed of water, protein, and bone mineral. The components are known and relatively stable in adults but not in children and adolescents. Thus, no single equation, and especially not the adult equations of Brozek or Siri, can be used for children.

3. Skinfolds, bioelectrical impedance, and height and weight indices are frequently used field tests for assessing body composition.

4. Reasonable values for assessing overweight as a risk to health are 26–31% BF or a BMI of > 27.3 kg · m^{-2} for adult females and 19–24% BF or a BMI of > 27.8 kg · m^{-2} for adult males. Comparable standards for obesity are over 32% BF (BMI > 30) for females and over 25% BF (BMI > 30) for males.

5. The size and number of adipocytes increase as a child grows to adulthood. Adult fat gain first involves hypertrophy of the adipocytes and then hyperplasia of precursor cells.

6. The health risks of overweight and obesity include cardiovascular disease, hypertension, gallbladder disease and hypercholesterolemia, diabetes mellitus, and cancer.

7. Heredity influences total percent body fat, fat-free mass, the tendency to gain or lose one or the other, and fat distribution.

Box 14.1 Answers

1. $M_A = 112$ lb $\div 2.2$ lb · kg^{-1} = 50.91 kg

2. Selected weight from underwater trials. 8.35 kg (trial 4) is the highest weight, but it was only obtained once, not more than twice as listed in the selection criteria, so it cannot be used. 8.325 kg is the second-highest obtained weight and it is observed more than once (trials 6 and 8), so it is the selected representative weight. 8.325 kg – 7.06 kg = 1.265 kg M_W.

Box 14.1 Answers *(cont.)*

3. $D_B =$

$$D_B = \cfrac{50.91\ \text{kg}}{\left(\cfrac{50.91\ \text{kg} - 1.265\ \text{kg}}{0.9941}\right) - (1.2274\ \text{L} + 0.1\ \text{L})}$$

$D_B \quad = 1.0473$

$\%BF = \dfrac{4.570}{1.0473} - 4.142 \times 100 = 22.2\%$

4. $FFW = 112\ \text{lb} \times \left(\dfrac{100 - 22.2}{100}\right) = 87.14\ \text{lb}$

$WT_2 = \dfrac{100 \times 87.14}{100\% - 19\%} = 107.58\ \text{lb}$

$\Delta WT = 107.58\ \text{lb} - 112\ \text{lb} = -4.42\ \text{lb}$

Phyllis needs to lose approximately 4.5 lbs to have 19% BF, assuming she maintains her muscle mass (FFW).

REVIEW QUESTIONS

1. Define densitometry. Relate densitometry to hydrostatic weighing.

2. Explain the assumptions that must be met in order for hydrostatic weighing to be accurate. What variations in these basic assumptions occur in children, adolescents, and the elderly? State two practical applications of this information.

3. List and identify the strengths and weaknesses of the field estimates of overweight and obesity. Which technique would you select to use in a field setting? Explain why.

4. Compare the accuracy of %BF determined by skinfolds and bioelectrical impedance with %BF determined by hydrostatic weighing.

5. Compare and contrast the %BF, %BF distribution, and patterns of fat distribution between males and females.

6. Differentiate between overweight and obesity.

7. What happens to adipose cells as an individual becomes overweight and then obese?

8. List and briefly discuss the health risks of being overweight or obese.

9. Debate the importance of heredity in body composition.

REFERENCES

1. American College of Sports Medicine: Proper and improper weight loss programs. *Medicine and Science in Sports and Exercise.* 15:xi–xiii (1983).
2. Ballor, D. L., V. L. Katch, M. D. Becque, & C. R. Marks: Resistance weight training during caloric restriction enhances lean body weight maintenance. *American Journal of Clinical Nutrition.* 47:19–25 (1988).
3. Baumgartner, R. N., W. C. Chumlea, & A. F. Roche: Bioelectrical impedance for body composition. In K. B. Pandolf (ed.), *Exercise and Sport Sciences Reviews.* Baltimore: Williams & Wilkins, 18, 193–224 (1990).
4. Beeson, V., C. Ray, R. A. Coxon, & S. Kreitzman: The myth of the yo-yo: Consistent rate of weight loss with successive dieting by VLCD. *International Journal of Obesity.* 13:135–139 (1989).
5. Behnke, A. R., & J. H. Wilmore: *Evaluation and Regulation of Body Build and Composition.* Englewood Cliffs, NJ: Prentice-Hall (1974).
6. Bjorntorp, P. A.: Fat cell distribution and metabolism. In R. J. Wurtman & J. J. Wurtman (eds.), *Annals of the New York Academy of Science.* New York: New York Academy of Science, 499:66–72 (1987).
7. Bjorntorp, P. A.: Sex differences in the regulation of energy balance with exercise. *American Journal of Clinical Nutrition.* 49:958–961 (1989).
8. Boileau, R. A., T. G. Lohman, M. H. Slaughter, T. E. Ball, S. B. Going, & M. K. Hendrix: Hydration of the fat-free body in children during maturation. *Human Biology.* 56(4): 651–666 (1984).
9. Bouchard, C.: Heredity and the path to overweight and obesity. *Medicine and Science in Sports and Exercise.* 23(3): 285–291 (1991).
10. Bouchard, C., & L. Perusse: Heredity and body fat. *Annual Review of Nutrition.* 8:259–277 (1988).
11. Bouchard, C. T., A. Tremblay, A. Nadeau, J. Dussault, J. P. Depres, G. Theriault, P. J. Lupien, O. Serresse, M. R. Boulay, & G. Fournier: Long-term exercise training with constant energy intake. 1. Effect on body composition. *International Journal of Obesity.* 14:57–73 (1990).
12. Bray, G. A.: Complications of obesity. *Annals of Internal Medicine.* 103(6 pt 2):1052–1062 (1985).
13. Bray, G. A.: Overweight is risking fate: Definition, classification, prevalence, and risks. *Annals of the New York Academy of Science.* New York: New York Academy of Science, 499:14–28 (1987).
14. Brodie, D. A.: Techniques of measurement of body composition: Part I. *Sports Medicine.* 5:11–40 (1988).
15. Brodie, D. A.: Techniques of measurement of body composition: Part II. *Sports Medicine.* 5:74–98 (1988).
16. Brownell, K. D., S. N. Steen, & J. H. Wilmore: Weight regulation practices in athletes: Analysis of metabolic and health effects. *Medicine and Science in Sports and Exercise.* 19(6):546–556 (1987).
17. Bubb, W. J.: Relative leanness. In E. T. Howley & B. D. Franks (eds.), *Health Fitness Instructor's Handbook* (2nd edition). Champaign, IL: Human Kinetics Publishers (1992).
18. Burton, B. T., W. R. Foster, J. Hirsch, & T. B. van Itallie: Health implications of obesity: An NIH consensus development conference. *International Journal of Obesity.* 9:155–169 (1985).

19. Campaigne, B. N.: Body fat distribution in females: Metabolic consequences and implications for weight loss. *Medicine and Science in Sports and Exercise.* 22(3):291–297 (1990).

20. Caton, J. R., P. A. Mole, W. C. Adams, & D. S. Heustis: Body composition analysis by bioelectrical impedance: Effect of skin temperature. *Medicine and Science in Sports and Exercise.* 20(5):489–491 (1988).

21. Charney, E., H. C. Goodman, M. McBride, B. Lyon, & R. Pratt: Childhood antecedents of adult obesity. *New England Journal of Medicine.* 295(1):6–9 (1975).

22. Deurenberg, P. W., I. Paymans, & K. vander Kooy: Factors affecting bioelectrical impedance measurements in humans. *European Journal of Clinical Nutrition.* 42:1017–1022 (1988).

23. Dietz, W. H.: Childhood obesity. In R. J. Wurtman & J. J. Wurtman (eds.), *Annals of the New York Academy of Science.* New York: New York Academy of Science, 499:47–54 (1987).

24. Folsom, A. R., S. A. Kaye, T. A. Sellers, C.-P. Hong, J. R. Cerhan, J. D. Potter, & R. J. Prineas: Body fat distribution and 5-year risk of death in older women. *Journal of the American Medical Association.* 269(4):483–487.

25. Fomon, S., J. Haschke, E. E. Ziegler, & S. E. Nelson: Body composition of reference children from birth to age 10 years. *American Journal of Clinical Nutrition.* 35:1169–1175 (1982).

26. Friiz-Hansen, B.: Hygrometry of growth and aging. In J. E. Brozek (ed.), *Human Body Composition.* Oxford, England: Pergaman Press, 191–209 (1965).

27. Garner, D. M., P. E. Garfinkel, D. Schwartz, & M. Thompson: Cultural expectations of thinness in women. *Psychological Reports.* 47:483–491 (1980).

28. Golding, L. A., C. R. Myers, & W. E. Sinning: *The Y's Way to Physical Fitness* (3rd edition). Champaign, IL: Human Kinetics Publishers (1989).

29. Goldman, R. F., & E. R. Buskirk: Body volume measurement by under water weighing: Description of a method. In J. Brozek & A. Henschel (eds.), *Techniques for Measuring Body Composition.* Washington, DC: National Academy of Sciences—National Research Council, 78–89 (1961).

30. Harrison, G. G., E. R. Buskirk, J. E. L. Carter, F. E. Johnston, T. G. Lohman, M. L. Pollock, A. F. Roche, & J. Wilmore: Skinfold thickness and measurement technique. In T. G. Lohman, A. F. Roche, & R. Martorell (eds.), *Anthropometric Standardization Reference Manual.* Champaign, IL: Human Kinetics Publishers, 55–70 (1988).

31. Himes, J. H., & R. A. Frisancho: Estimating frame size. In T. G. Lohman, A. F. Roche, & R. Martorell (eds.), *Anthropometric Standardization Reference Manual.* Champaign, IL: Human Kinetics Publishers, 122–124 (1988).

32. Hodgdon, J. A., & P. I. Fitzgerald: Validity of impedance predictions at various levels of fatness. *Human Biology.* 59(2):281–298 (1987).

33. Jackson, A. S., & M. L. Pollock: Practical assessment of body composition. *Physician and Sportsmedicine.* 13:76–90 (1985).

34. Lohman, T. G.: Applicability of body composition techniques and constants for children and youth. In K. B. Pandolf (ed.), *Exercise and Sport Sciences Reviews.* New York: Macmillan, 14:325–357 (1986).

35. Lohman, T. G.: Assessment of body composition in children. *Pediatric Exercise Science.* 1:19–30 (1989).

36. Lohman, T. G.: Body composition. In J. R. Morrow, H. B. Falls, & H. W. Kohl (eds.), *FITNESSGRAM Technical Reference Manual.* Dallas: Cooper Institute for Aerobics Research (1994).

37. Lohman, T. G.: Skinfolds and body density and their relation to body fatness: A review. *Human Biology.* 53(2): 181–225 (1981).

38. Lohman, T. G.: The use of skinfold to estimate body fatness on children and youth. *Journal of Physical Education, Recreation and Dance.* 58(9):98–102 (1987).

39. Lohman T. G., R. A. Boileau, & M. H. Slaughter: Body composition in children and youth. In R. A. Boileau (ed.), *Advances in Pediatric Sport Sciences.* Champaign, IL: Human Kinetics Publishers, 29–57 (1984).

40. Lutter, J. M.: Is your attitude weighing you down? *Melpomene Journal.* 13(1):13–16 (1994).

41. Malina, R. M., & C. Bouchard: *Growth, Maturation and Physical Activity.* Champaign, IL: Human Kinetics Publishers (1991).

42. Malina, R. M., B. W. Meleski, & R. F. Shoup: Anthropometric, body composition, and maturity characteristics of selected school-age athletes. *Pediatric Clinics of North America.* 29(6):1305–1323 (1982).

43. Marieb, E. N.: *Human Anatomy and Physiology.* Redwood City, CA: Benjamin-Cummings (1989).

44. McArdle, W. D., F. I. Katch, & V. L. Katch: *Exercise Physiology: Energy, Nutrition, and Human Performance* (3rd edition). Philadelphia: Lea & Febiger (1991).

45. Nieman, D. C.: *Fitness and Sports Medicine: An Introduction.* Palo Alto, CA: Bull Publishing (1990).

46. Pi-Sunyer, F. X.: Medical hazards of obesity. *Annals of Internal Medicine.* 119(7 pt 2):655–660 (1993).

47. Plowman, S. A., N. Y. Liu, & C. L. Wells: Body composition and sexual maturation in premenarcheal athletes and nonathletes. *Medicine and Science in Sports and Exercise.* 23(1):23–29 (1991).

48. Powers, S. K., & E. T. Howley: *Exercise Physiology: Theory and Application to Fitness and Performance.* Dubuque, IA: Brown (1990).

49. Revicki, D. A., & R. G. Israel: Relationship between body mass indices and measures of body adiposity. *American Journal of Public Health.* 76:992–994 (1986).

50. Roche, A. F.: Some aspects of the criterion methods for the measurement of body composition. *Human Biology.* 59(2):209–220 (1987).

51. Satwanti, B. S., I. P. Singh, & H. Bharadwaj: Body fat from skinfold thicknesses and weight-height indices: A comparison. *Zeitschrift für Morpholgie und Anthropologie.* 71(1): 93–100 (1980).

52. Simopoulos, A. P.: Characteristics of obesity: An overview. In R. J. Wurtman & J. J. Wurtman (eds.), *Annals of the New York Academy of Science.* New York: New York Academy of Science, 499 4–13 (1987).

53. Sjöström, L., & P. Björntorp: Body composition and adipose tissue cellularity in human obesity. *Acta Medica Scandinavica.* 195:201–211 (1974).

54. Slaughter, M. H., T. G. Lohman, R. A. Boileau, C. A. Horswill, R. J. Stillman, M. D. Van Loan, & D. A. Bemben: Skinfold equation for estimation of body fatness in children and youth. *Human Biology.* 60(5):709–723 (1988).

55. Stamford, B.: Apples and pears: Where you "wear" your fat can affect your health. *The Physician and Sportsmedicine.* 19(1):123–124 (1991).

56. Stump, C. S., L. B. Houtkooper, M. H. Heweitt, S. B. Going, & T. G. Lohman: Bioelectrical impedance variability with dehydration and exercise. *Medicine and Science in Sports and Exercise.* 20(2):S82 (1988).

57. Van Itallie, T. B.: Topography of body fat: Relationship to risk of cardiovascular and other diseases. In T. G. Lohman, A. F. Roche, & R. Martorell (eds.), *Anthropometric Standardization Reference Manual.* Champaign, IL: Human Kinetics Publishers, 143–149 (1988).

58. Van Loan, M. D.: Bioelectrical impedance analysis to determine fat-free mass, total body water and body fat. *Sports Medicine.* 10(4):205–217 (1990).

59. Williams, D. P., S. B. Going, T. G. Lohman, D. P. Harsha, S. R. Srinivasau, L. S. Webber, & G. S. Beneuson: Body fatness and risk for elevated blood pressure, total cholesterol, and serum lipoprotein ratios in children and adolescents. *American Journal of Public Health.* 82:358–363 (1992).

60. Williamson, D. F.: Descriptive epidemiology of body weight and weight change in U.S. adults. *Annals of Internal Medicine.* 119(7 pt 2):646–649 (1993).

15

Body Composition and Weight Control

After studying the chapter, you should be able to:

- State the caloric balance equation, and define and explain its components.

- Discuss the impact of diet, as caloric restriction, on the components of the caloric balance equation.

- Discuss the impact of an exercise session on the components of the caloric balance equation.

- Discuss the impact of exercise training on the components of the caloric balance equation.

- Compare and contrast the effects of diet alone, exercise alone, and diet plus exercise combined on body weight and composition control.

- Apply the training principles to body weight and composition control.

- Compose guidelines for making weight in a sport.

The Caloric Balance Equation

At its most basic level weight control follows the first law of thermodynamics. The **first law of thermodynamics,** sometimes called the **law of conservation of energy**, states that energy can neither be created nor destroyed, but only changed in form. This law was described fully in Chapter 9.

When the body converts the potential chemical energy of food into other chemical, mechanical, or heat energy, it follows the law of conservation of energy. Theoretically, if the amount of energy taken in equals the amount of energy expended, the body is in balance and the weight remains stable. If an excess of energy is ingested, that energy is neither destroyed nor lost; rather, weight (mass) is gained. If insufficient energy is ingested in relation to expenditure, the needed energy cannot be created but must be provided from storage sites, and weight (mass) is reduced.

Energy, in the forms involved in the human body, is most frequently described in terms of kilocalories (kcal) or kilojoules (kJ). One **kilocalorie** is the amount of heat needed to raise the temperature of 1 kg of water 1°C. One kilocalorie is equal to 4.186 kJ. A calorie is equal to 0.001 kcal. The term *calorie* is often used generically, however, as in the statement "Caloric intake should be equal to caloric output," even though the units would be kilocalories. The caloric equivalent of 1 lb of fat is 3500 kcal.

The **caloric balance equation,** the mathematical summation of the caloric intake (+) and energy expenditure (–) from all sources, quantifies the law of conservation of energy. It describes the source of potential energy as food ingested and the various uses of that energy. The input and output can be partitioned into the following elements:

caloric balance = + food ingested (kcal)

– basal or resting metabolic rate (kcal)

– thermogenesis (kcal)

– work or exercise metabolism (kcal)

– energy excreted in waste products (kcal)

Food intake represents the only positive factor in the caloric balance equation. It is the only way that energy can be added to the system. Energy is expended in three ways. The first is basal or resting metabolic rate, the second is thermogenesis, and the third is work or exercise. These are the negative factors in the caloric balance equation.

Figure 15.1 indicates that the basal or resting metabolic rate accounts for the majority of the total energy expenditure, varying from approximately 60 to approximately 75% in active and sedentary individuals, respectively. Thermogenesis accounts for a relatively stable 10% in both sedentary and active individuals. The thermic effect of exercise is obviously higher in active individuals, and it depends on the intensity, duration, and frequency of exercise.[63]

If the amount of energy in the food ingested exceeds the energy expended, the body is in a positive balance. If the amount of energy in the food ingested is less than the energy expended, the body is in a negative balance. The amount of energy excreted in waste products is insignificant and rarely measured. It need not be considered here further. The other elements have considerable impact on body weight (mass) and body weight control. In the pages that follow each of these elements will be defined and discussed. The impact of diet, exercise, and exercise training on each of the elements will be emphasized.

Food Ingested

Little needs to be said about food intake per se. We all eat, and lists of the potential energy (calorie) content of foods are readily available. Labels on packaged foods at the grocery store have printed kilocalorie values as well as a nutrient breakdown. Getting into the habit of reading food labels is a good idea and should enable you to make wise food choices in terms of both nutritional and energy content.

First Law of Thermodynamics or the Law of Conservation of Energy Energy can neither be created nor destroyed but only changed in form.

Kilocalorie The amount of heat needed to raise the temperature of 1 kg of water 1°C.

Caloric Balance Equation The mathematical summation of the caloric intake (+) and energy expenditure (–) from all sources.

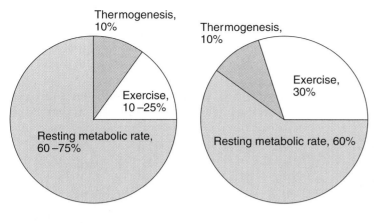

Sedentary Individual   Active Individual

FIGURE 15.1

Energy Expenditure
Resting metabolic rate accounts for the largest percentage of energy expended in both inactive and active individuals although the exact percentage varies between the two groups. The percentage of energy expended during exercise is higher in active than in inactive individuals. Thermogenesis accounts for about 10% of the energy expended in both active and inactive individuals.
Source: Modified from Poehlman.[63]

Impact of Diet on Food Intake   The term **diet** may mean many things, including the food regularly consumed during the course of normal living. It is also used to mean a restriction of caloric intake. This second meaning is how the term is being used in this chapter. Therefore, "going on a diet" should, by definition, mean a reduction in food intake.

Impact of Exercise and Exercise Training on Food Intake   The relationship between exercise, exercise training, appetite, and energy intake is complex and difficult to discern. Appetite and the amount of food ingested are influenced by physiological, nutritional, behavioral, and psychological factors in humans. It is not just a matter of a physiological drive to balance energy demand and supply.[79,87] People eat or don't eat for a variety of reasons. For example, when you are upset, do you cease eating, or do you consume everything in sight?

It is also very difficult to accurately measure food intake. Feeding individuals in a controlled setting where food can be measured may cause changes in eating behavior. Asking individuals to write down everything they eat necessitates a faith that they are neither over- nor (more likely) under-reporting. For these reasons conducting studies on the effects of exercise and/or exercise training on appetite in humans is difficult. Despite the difficulties, the following generalizations can be drawn from the studies that are available.

1.   Neither a transient reduction nor an increase in energy intake immediately following a single bout of exercise has been clearly established in humans. In one study the subjective rating of appetite was lowered in female subjects following 30 min of exercise at 50% $\dot{V}O_2$max. Despite this decreased subjective rating, food intake at the postexercise meal and for two days after was not affected. A chemical known to have anorectic (loss of appetite) properties in rats is also known to increase in response to exercise in humans; however, it has not been shown to actually decrease the human appetite.

2.   Physically active males, females, adults, and children (such as heavy manual laborers and athletes) consume more calories than sedentary individuals. Yet the active individuals generally maintain their body weight and composition at or below normal levels.

3.   Energy intake in both males and females generally increases or remains unchanged in response to exercise training. Which response occurs appears to depend on the fitness and body composition status of the individual. Highly trained athletes and lean individuals usually increase their energy intake in response to increased training loads. Untrained and/or obese individuals most often do not change energy intake in response to exercise training.

Diet (a) The food regularly consumed during the course of normal living; (b) a restriction of caloric intake.

4. When chronic exercise training ceases, energy intake in humans is spontaneously reduced. Unfortunately, this reduction does not appear to be matched to the reduced energy expenditure. The result is often a positive energy balance, a regain of lost body weight, and a concomitant elevation of body fat.

Resting or Basal Metabolism

Basal energy expenditure, more commonly called **basal metabolic rate (BMR),** is defined as the level of energy required to sustain the body's vital functions in the waking state. Technically, this definition means that the individual is resting quietly in a supine position, has not eaten for 8–18 hr, is at normal body temperature (37°C) and neutral ambient temperature (27–29°C; 80–84°F), and is without feelings of psychological stress. Because of the difficulty of obtaining truly basal conditions in most laboratory settings, the term resting metabolic rate is probably a more accurate descriptor. **Resting metabolic rate (RMR)** is defined as the energy expended while an individual is resting quietly in a supine position. The two terms are often used interchangeably, since the measured differences are small. That practice will be followed here, with the term RMR used primarily but not exclusively.[22]

A variety of organs and processes are responsible for energy consumption at rest. The liver is the largest consumer of energy at rest (29–32%), followed by the brain (19–21%), muscles (18%), heart (10%), lungs (9%), and kidneys (7%). The muscle energy is primarily for the maintenance of tonus or tension, necessary even in sleep. On the cellular level the energy is used to fuel ion pumps (particularly the sodium-potassium pump), synthesize and degrade cellular constituents, conduct electrical im-

pulses, and secrete various substances, including hormones.[12, 22]

Basal or resting metabolism is usually related to body surface area and expressed in $kcal \cdot m^{-2}$. It may also be expressed in $kcal \cdot day^{-1}$ or $\dot{V}O_2$ $mL \cdot min^{-1}$. The choice of measurement unit depends on the intended use of the information. If the interest lies in comparing submaximal or maximal oxygen values, then the choice is $\dot{V}O_2$ $mL \cdot min^{-1}$. In many cases, however, the interest lies in determining caloric needs, and then one of the kilocalorie units is utilized. Tables or graphs are available that allow one to estimate body surface area (BSA, in square meters) from height and weight (Table 15.1) and standard BMR values per BSA (Figure 15.2). From these values BMR ($kcal \cdot day^{-1}$) can be computed.

(15.1) basal metabolic rate ($kcal \cdot day^{-1}$) = standard basal metabolic rate ($kcal \cdot m^{-2} \cdot hr^{-1}$) × body surface area ($m^2$) × 24 hr · day^{-1}

or   BMR = standard BMR × BSA × 24

FIGURE 15.2

Standard Basal Metabolic Rate Across the Age Span

Standard basal metabolic rates decline steeply during childhood and adolescence and then more gradually during the adult years. At every age male values are higher than female values despite being prorated to body surface area.

Source: Calculated from Bursztein, Elwyn, & Askanazi;[21] Kinney.[22]

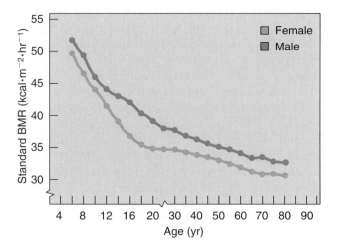

Basal Metabolic Rate (BMR) The level of energy required to sustain the body's vital functions in the waking state, when the individual is in a fasted condition, at normal body and room temperature, and without psychological stress.
the energy exp. while and indvdual's resting qu
Resting Metabolic Rate (RMR) The energy expended while an individual is resting quietly in a supine position.

TABLE 15.1 ■ Surface Area in Square Meters for Different Heights and Weights

Height (cm)	25	30	35	40	45	50	55	60	65	70	75	80	85	90	95	100	105
200							1.84	1.91	1.97	2.03	2.09	2.15	2.21	2.26	2.31	2.36	2.41
195						1.73	1.80	1.87	1.93	1.99	2.05	2.11	2.17	2.22	2.27	2.32	2.37
190				1.56	1.63	1.70	1.77	1.84	1.90	1.96	2.02	2.08	2.13	2.18	2.23	2.28	2.33
185				1.53	1.60	1.67	1.74	1.80	1.86	1.92	1.98	2.04	2.09	2.14	2.19	2.24	2.29
180				1.49	1.57	1.64	1.71	1.77	1.83	1.89	1.95	2.00	2.05	2.10	2.15	2.20	2.25
175	1.19	1.28	1.36	1.46	1.53	1.60	1.67	1.73	1.79	1.85	1.91	1.96	2.01	2.06	2.11	2.16	2.21
170	1.17	1.26	1.34	1.43	1.50	1.57	1.63	1.69	1.75	1.81	1.86	1.91	1.96	2.01	2.06	2.11	
165	1.14	1.23	1.31	1.40	1.47	1.54	1.60	1.66	1.72	1.78	1.83	1.88	1.93	1.98	2.03	2.07	
160	1.12	1.21	1.29	1.37	1.44	1.50	1.56	1.62	1.68	1.73	1.78	1.83	1.88	1.93	1.98		
155	1.09	1.18	1.26	1.33	1.40	1.46	1.52	1.58	1.64	1.69	1.74	1.79	1.84	1.89			
150	1.06	1.15	1.23	1.30	1.36	1.42	1.48	1.54	1.60	1.65	1.70	1.75	1.80				
145	1.03	1.12	1.20	1.27	1.33	1.39	1.45	1.51	1.56	1.61	1.66	1.71					
140	1.00	1.09	1.17	1.24	1.30	1.36	1.42	1.47	1.52	1.57							
135	0.97	1.06	1.14	1.20	1.26	1.32	1.38	1.43	1.48								
130	0.95	1.04	1.11	1.17	1.23	1.29	1.35	1.40									
125	0.93	1.01	1.08	1.14	1.20	1.26	1.31	1.36									
120	0.91	0.98	1.04	1.10	1.16	1.22	1.27										

Source: D. DuBois & E. F. DuBois. Clinical calorimetry: A formula to estimate the approximate surface area if height and weight be known. *Archives of Internal Medicine* 17:863–871 (1916). Reprinted by permission of *Archives of Internal Medicine.*

■ EXAMPLE

A 22-yr-old female is 5 feet 5 inches (165 cm) tall and weighs 143 lb (65 kg). According to Table 15.1 her BSA is 1.72 m². The number closest to her age on Figure 15.2 is 20 yr. Since this individual is female the lower line is used to estimate a standard BMR of 35.1 kcal · m⁻² · hr⁻¹. Substituting these values into Equation 15.1 we get

$$\text{BMR kcal} \cdot \text{day}^{-1} = 35.1 \text{ kcal} \cdot \text{m}^{-2} \cdot \text{hr}^{-1} \times 1.72 \text{ m}^2$$
$$\times 24 \text{ hr} \cdot \text{day}^{-1}$$
$$\text{BMR} = 1448 \text{ kcal} \cdot \text{day}^{-1} \qquad ■$$

Somewhat less cumbersome is the use of prediction equations such as those presented in Table 15.2. For the individual in the previous example the calculation becomes RMR = 447.593 + (3.098 × 165) + (9.247 × 65) – (4.330 × 22) = 1464.6 kcal·day⁻¹. Although the two techniques do not agree exactly, they are very comparable for practical use.

Eighty-five percent of all normal subjects have estimated RMR values within 10% of measured values. The other 15% of the population have either higher or lower values. The range of variation may exceed 20%. Thus an individual who has a 20% higher RMR than average is able to ingest more calories without gaining weight, but the individual with a 20% lower RMR must ingest less or gain weight.[22,33]

Two criterion measures are available for RMR. The first is open-circuit indirect calorimetry, which was described in Chapter 11. The second is a blood test for the determination of protein-bound iodine (PBI). The iodine comes from thyroxine (T4), the hormone secreted by the thyroid gland, which has the greatest impact on BMR. This test gives a relative indication of BMR, not a direct kcal·day⁻¹ value.[12]

The prediction equations in Table 15.2 give an indication of the primary nonhormonal factors that

TABLE 15.2 ■ **Estimation of Basal (Resting) Metabolic Rate**

MALES

$$RMR = 88.362 + (4.799 \times HT)$$
$$+ (13.397 \times WT) - (5.677 \times AGE)$$

FEMALES

$$RMR = 447.593 + (3.098 \times HT)$$
$$+ (9.247 \times WT) - (4.330 \times AGE)$$

where HT = height (in centimeters), WT = weight (in kilograms), AGE = age (in years).

Source: Based on Roza & Shizgal.[66]

influence RMR. What are they? If you said body size, age, and sex, you are absolutely correct. RMR relates best to body surface area externally and to cell mass internally. Obese individuals have a larger surface area and a larger cell mass (both fat and fat-free) than average-weight individuals. Hence, not surprisingly, the RMR of obese individuals is higher than that of the normal-weight individuals.[40]

The influence of age and sex can be seen in Figure 15.2. RMR is highest in infants and young children. The drop from age 6 to 18 is approximately 25%, or 2% per year. The decline then slows to about 2–3% per decade after that age. Part of this decline in RMR may be attributed to and be responsible for the increment in %BF that usually occurs as people age.

Figure 15.2 also clearly shows that at all ages average-weight females have lower RMR than do average-weight males. The difference, which is least in young children, is accentuated at puberty and then tends to remain at about 5–6% through middle age and old age. In terms of calories the RMR of adult males averages between 1500 and 1800 kcal·day^{-1} and the RMR of adult females averages between 1200 and 1450 kcal·day^{-1}. The lower female values are partially because females have smaller internal organs than males and tend to be smaller in terms of total body mass, on average, than males. However, the most obvious explanation is the difference in body cell mass, particularly muscle tissue. Females on average have a higher %BF than do males. At any body weight, for each 1% increase in body fat the RMR decreases 0.6 kcal·hr^{-1}

or 14.4 kcal·day^{-1}. If we assume a 10% difference in %BF between the average male and average female, the result can amount to 144 kcal·day^{-1}. When RMR is expressed relative to FFW, the sex differences disappear.[12,22]

Another factor that influences resting metabolic rate is body core temperature. For each degree increase in Celsius or Fahrenheit temperature, metabolic rate increases 13 or 7.2%, respectively. Similarly, a decrease in body temperature, at least until the point where shivering is induced, reduces energy expenditure.

A genetic effect has been documented for RMR. Correlations for RMR measured in kilojoules per kilogram of body weight were found to be 0.38 for dizygotic (DZ) twins and 0.78 for monozygotic (MZ) twins of both sexes. The genetic effect (heritability) was deemed to account for approximately 40% of the variance between individuals after adjustments for age, sex, and body composition. By itself, this genetic effect has considerable potential for predisposing an individual to gaining or losing fat over time.[14, 15]

The Impact of Diet on Resting Metabolic Rate   The amount and the type of food ingested affect RMR. The effect of caloric restriction on RMR is well documented and clear-cut. Severe caloric restriction decreases RMR.[4,18,21,31,49] Since resting metabolism represents the greatest percentage of daily caloric expenditure in sedentary individuals, the result is a discouraging effect of slowing the weight loss that would be expected from the amount of dietary restriction and negative balance.

■ EXAMPLE

One lb (0.45 kg) of body fat contains the energy equivalent of approximately 3500 kcal. In order for a person to lose 1 lb of weight according to the caloric balance equation, the amount of calories expended must exceed the amount ingested by 3500 kcal. If an individual expends 2000 kcal·day^{-1} and ingests 2000 kcal·day^{-1}, weight should be maintained. If that same individual maintains this activity level but reduces his/her caloric intake to just 1000 kcal·day^{-1}, a weight loss of 2 lb per week would be anticipated (2000 kcal·day^{-1} − 1000 kcal·day^{-1} = −1000 kcal·day^{-1}; −1000 kcal·day^{-1} x

7 days $\cdot$ week^{-1} = -7000 kcal; -7000 kcal $\div$ 3500 kcal = -2 lbs), assuming that approximately 75% of the 2000 kcal $\cdot$ day^{-1} expenditure or 1500 kcal $\cdot$ day^{-1} is expended by RMR.

However, within 2–3 weeks of such a restricted diet, the RMR will have been reduced by approximately 15% (the range is typically 10–20%) to 1275 kcal $\cdot$ day^{-1}. The difference is now -1775 kcal $\cdot$ day^{-1} expended + 1000 kcal $\cdot$ day^{-1} ingested = -775 kcal $\cdot$ day^{-1}; -775 kcal $\cdot$ day^{-1} $\times$ 7 days $\cdot$ week^{-1} = -5425 kcal; -5425 kcal $\div$ 2500 kcal $\cdot$ lb^{-1} = -1.5 lb instead of -2 lb per week. As the drop in RMR continues with severe caloric restriction, the weight loss becomes progressively slower.[49]   ■

Researchers speculate that this decline in RMR is the body's protective response to energy restriction. Conversely, a short-term excessive ingestion of food and calories results in an elevation of RMR.[4] This elevation has been seen as protection against an increase in the body's "natural" weight.[21, 63]

The Impact of Exercise on Resting Metabolic Rate
The energy cost of exercise, in oxygen or calorie units, includes a resting component. METs (Chapter 11) express the energy cost of activity in multiples of the resting metabolic rate. Therefore, although metabolism is definitely elevated by exercise, it is not the resting metabolism itself that is elevated. The resting metabolism is assumed to remain constant; the increase in energy consumption is attributed solely to the activity demands and responses.

Immediately after exercise the metabolic rate remains elevated. This rate is called the excess post-exercise oxygen consumption (EPOC) and was discussed in Chapter 11. This recovery oxygen utilization represents additional calories that are expended as a direct result of the response to exercise. These calories are typically not included in the measured caloric cost of the activity. Thus, if an individual expends 250–300 kcal walking or jogging 3 mi an additional 20–30 kcal may be expended during the hour or two after exercise until complete recovery is achieved. This expenditure, however, also does not mean that the resting metabolic rate itself has been affected.

In order for it to be concluded that the resting metabolism is changed by exercise, the change would have to be evident 24 or 48 hr after exercise.

Research evidence for such a change is mixed and difficult to interpret. The inconsistency of the evidence can partially be attributed to the intensity and duration of the exercise involved. Mild to heavy exercise of moderate duration (35–86% $\dot{V}O_2$max for 20–80 min) has generally been shown to cause no long-term metabolic elevation in RMR, whereas longer, moderate exercise (50–70% $\dot{V}O_2$max; 80–180 min) has.

There is a problem, however, in interpreting metabolic changes 24 or 48 hr after exercise as being caused by the exercise. Studies showing an increase in resting metabolic rate over the long term, even after heavy exercise, have not controlled for the ingestion of food. The elevated metabolism observed was probably due, at least in part, to the thermic effect of the meals taken. (The thermic effect of a meal will be fully explained later in this chapter.) Consequently, it is unlikely that exercise causes any permanent change in resting metabolic rate per se— at least not light or moderate aerobic endurance exercise nor dynamic resistance activity.[9,38,47,63]

Exercise Training and Resting Metabolic Rate
The effect of exercise training on RMR is controversial. Some studies have shown that trained individuals exhibit higher RMRs than sedentary individuals or that training programs bring about an increase in RMR, but others have not. An occasional study has even shown a decrease in RMR when exercise training was added to severe caloric restriction.[63]

Recent cross-sectional studies have reported higher RMRs (adjusted for body size) in trained individuals or athletes than in untrained individuals. In some cases the difference amounted to 200 kcal $\cdot$ day^{-1}. The difference persisted when the subjects were matched not only on body weight but also on fat-free weight or body fat content. These results suggest that the role of exercise training in the elevation of RMR is separate from its influence in maintaining muscle mass or decreasing body fat. This conclusion is supported by the fact that muscles account for only 18% of the RMR.

In addition, a significant, direct rectilinear relationship ($r = 0.77$) has been shown to exist between the level of training or fitness as measured by $\dot{V}O_2$max and RMR. In one study moderately trained men ($\dot{V}O_2$max $\leq$ 55 mL $\cdot$ kg^{-1} $\cdot$ min^{-1}) and untrained men had similar RMRs, but highly trained men

($\dot{V}O_2$max 55–80 mL $\cdot$ kg^{-1} $\cdot$ min^{-1}) had significantly higher RMRs than both the moderately trained and the untrained individuals.[63] Thus, one reason why some studies have not revealed differences between trained and untrained individuals may be that the trained individuals were simply not trained enough. In these studies neither the trained nor the untrained individuals were restricted calorically. It may also be that what is being seen is simply an elongated exercise response to RMR (a last-bout effect) by those training at high levels rather than a true training adaptation of an increased RMR.[47]

Longitudinal studies investigating the impact of exercise training on RMR usually add the exercise component after several weeks of severe caloric restriction in an attempt to reverse the decline in RMR. Again, the results are inconclusive. Here, also, the intensity of the exercise and possibly even the frequency of exercise make a difference. High-intensity programs performed daily have not only brought about a return to baseline in RMR but also, in some instances, caused an elevation of 7–10%. Unfortunately, insufficient work has been done to state exactly what threshold of intensity is needed. In those studies showing a reversal of the decline in RMR, the change began within just a few days, which is well before any change would be expected in body composition. Thus the conclusion again is that the effect of training on RMR is over and above any change in muscle mass or body fat.[21,49,55,63]

In those studies that have shown an additional decline in RMR when exercise was added to caloric restriction, the decline is often explained as being part of the body's protective mechanism. If RMR declines when calories are restricted, burning additional calories in activity simply makes matters worse. Therefore, it is logical that the RMR would decrease even further. It has been suggested that this decline occurs in individuals (such as some athletes) who are attempting to maintain body weights below their natural level.[21]

It is important to realize that if diet and/or exercise results in a loss of body weight (mass), then a proportional long-term reduction in RMR should be expected. Despite the claims of many overweight individuals to the contrary, overweight or obese people have higher RMRs than normal-weight individuals of similar age, sex, and height to begin with. With weight loss this higher RMR should not be expected to be maintained.[26, 82]

Because RMR is highly correlated with or related to fat-free weight (FFW), but not entirely dependent upon it, it might be expected that resistance weight training would bring about an increase in RMR. Again, the data are not definitive. Perhaps the most impressive evidence for this idea comes from a study with males 50–65 yr old. After 16 weeks of heavy resistance strength training these subjects exhibited no change in total body weight but showed a decrease in %BF, an increase in FFW, and an increase in RMR. This increase in RMR remained significant even when expressed per kilogram of FFW. Resting norepinephrine levels also increased. The researchers concluded that the increase in RMR with strength training was only partially due to the increase in FFW and may also have been linked to an increase in basal sympathetic nervous system activity.[64] This conclusion reinforces the idea that RMR is not totally dependent on muscle mass.

Most of the studies that have been done relative to exercise training and RMR have been conducted using men as subjects. What limited data are available on women show the same trends.

Weight Cycling   A special concern regarding the influence of diet on RMR is weight cycling. **Weight cycling** is defined as repeated bouts of weight loss and regain.[67] Sometimes this cycling is called the rhythm method of girth control or the yo-yo effect. Most dieters repeatedly lose weight and then gain weight again, despite their best intentions not to. Some athletes (wrestler, jockeys, and the like) lose and gain weight purposely as they make weight for competition and then make up for missed meals by eating large quantities. Dieters may take months or years to complete each cycle; weight class athletes will do the same thing in two or three days. Furthermore, dieters may lose and gain 20–100 lb or more in each cycle, but athletes generally lose or gain less than 20 lb.

It has been theorized that weight cycling slows down the RMR, increases the difficulty of subsequent weight loss, and enhances abdominal fat.[10, 51]

Weight Cycling Repeated bouts of weight loss and regain.

Despite the theory, experimental evidence from studies testing the influence of weight cycling on RMR has presented inconclusive results. High school wrestlers who weight-cycled exhibited a 15% lower RMR than those who did not.[76] However, college wrestlers who weight-cycled had RMRs similar to those of non-weight-cycling wrestlers, and both wrestling groups had higher RMR values than non-wrestling controls.[68] Perhaps an initially lower RMR necessitated weight cycling in the high school wrestlers and not the reverse. These results cannot be considered conclusive evidence one way or the other.

Studies using dieters, whether initially obese or overweight, are also conflicting, with two of three studies[7, 80, 81] finding no evidence that a history of weight cycling affected RMR. One study that has received a great deal of attention did find that prior weight cycling made subsequent weight loss harder.[10] This study followed two groups (hospital inpatients and outpatients) of obese individuals who exhibited weight cycling over a 9-yr period. During the first attempt at supervised weight loss the outpatients lost an average of 0.19 kg·day^{-1} or 11 kg in 72 days. After regaining 120% of the weight loss these individuals underwent the same regimen again and lost an average of 0.15 kg·day^{-1} or 8 kg in 72 days. Results for the inpatients were even more definitive. During the first weight loss cycle these individuals lost an average of 0.47 kg·day^{-1} in 31 days for a total of 12 kg. They regained 115% of their weight loss. The second time around the weight loss average was only 0.37 kg·day^{-1} for a total loss of 6 kg in 20 days.[10]

These data suggest a slowing of the rate of weight loss with successive dieting. However, the subjects in this study were also older during the second weight loss cycle, and age does decrease RMR. Furthermore, there was less adherence to the diet during the second weight loss cycle than during the first, which would affect both the rate and the amount of weight loss.[89] Finally, three other studies found no relationship between weight loss in one cycle and the subsequent rate or amount of weight loss in later cycles.[7, 80, 81]

One other study[65] found that weight cycling was associated with upper-body (abdominal) fat deposition. However, three similar studies found no difference in fat distribution or waist-to-hip ratio as a function of weight-cycling history.[39, 80, 81] There is no evidence that weight cycling leads to increased abdominal visceral fat deposition.

Neither body fat distribution nor body composition appear to be adversely affected by a history of weight cycling in humans.[52] Remaining overweight or obese is not preferable, from a physiological standpoint, to undergoing repeated attempts at weight loss.[52] Taken together, the research does not support any of the theoretical concerns mentioned at the beginning of this discussion.[89]

Thermogenesis

Think about this. The temperature is 100°F (38°C) with a relative humidity of 80%. Your apartment air conditioner is not working. You are hungry, but you can't afford to go out to eat. In your food stock are ground beef, red beans and rice, tuna, and the ingredients for both a fruit and a tossed salad. Which do you select?

In all probability you will pick one or both of the salad options, intuitively going for the meal that will not add to your heat load. Actually, though, following ingestion of any meal, energy metabolism is enhanced. This energy increase is due, in part, to the energy-requiring processes of digestion, absorption, assimilation, and synthesis of protein, fat, and carbohydrate.

However, more energy is expended than can be accounted for by these processes. The extra energy expenditure usually peaks in 30–90 min but, depending on the size and content of the meal, may last as long as 4–6 hr. This energy all appears in the form of heat. The production of heat is called **thermogenesis.** For any given meal the increased heat production as a result of food ingestion is called the **thermic effect of a meal (TEM).** Cumulatively, the energy expenditure associated with the ingestion of all food during a day is called the *thermic effect of feeding* (TEF). TEF is what is depicted as thermogenesis in Figure 15.1 as constituting approximately 10% of daily energy expenditure.[11, 63]

Thermogenesis   The production of heat.

Thermic Effect of a Meal (TEM)   The increased heat production as a result of food ingestion.

There is some evidence for a link between thermogenesis and the control of body weight. TEF is thought to be a survival technique. When stimulated, TEF allows the individual to adapt to a diet low in nutrients by the ingestion of more food without gaining weight. When suppressed, TEF allows the body to maintain its weight during fasting or starvation situations. The stimulus or suppression appears to be mediated through the sympathetic nervous system.[11]

Precisely how thermogenesis occurs has not been determined, but probably some mechanism for the uncoupling of oxidative phosphorylation is involved. That is, energy substrates are oxidized, but ATP is not produced. Instead, heat is produced. This process may occur at specific steps in the metabolic pathways (known as substrate or futile cycling) or in brown adipose tissue (BAT)[37] (see Figure 14.9). Humans, however, have only about 1% of body weight as BAT after early postnatal life. Changes in the sodium-potassium pump activity have also been proposed.[11] These mechanisms may, in part, be responsible for why some individuals can seemingly eat everything in sight and not gain weight, while others eat much less proportionately and gain weight. Most studies comparing the thermic response of lean and obese individuals to a test meal do indeed show a blunted TEM in the obese.[11, 40, 53, 69, 70, 71, 72, 73, 75]

The Impact of Diet on the Thermic Effect of a Meal   Both the total caloric content and the percent composition of a meal have an impact on the thermic effect of the meal. The greatest thermic effect occurs with protein (15–25%). Carbohydrate and fat show only about half the thermic increase shown by protein, with carbohydrate's increase being slightly higher than fat's. These differences would seem to indicate that a high-protein diet would be valuable for individuals wishing to expend extra calories. However, as mentioned in Chapter 13, high-protein diets can exacerbate kidney and liver problems in individuals with preexisting conditions and may result in excessive losses of calcium. For these reasons diets exceeding 15% protein are not recommended no matter what the thermic effect.[8, 30, 50, 61, 77]

If the percentages of protein, fat, and carbohydrate are kept constant and close to those values recommended for a healthy diet (55% CHO, 30% FAT,

15% PRO), a direct relationship is found between the caloric content of a meal and TEM. That is, higher-caloric meals cause a higher thermic effect. As a result, an individual on a restricted caloric diet will burn fewer calories through dietary-induced thermogenesis than he or she would when eating larger meals.[8, 22]

The Impact of Exercise on the Thermic Effect of a Meal   Both meal ingestion and exercise stimulate the sympathetic nervous system and thermogenesis. Since many people are interested in maximizing energy expenditure, it was deemed of interest to determine whether a combination of exercise plus a meal in close temporal proximity would potentiate (or increase) the singular effect of either exercise or food. A number of studies have been completed following two basic sequences. After a period of rest the subjects eat a meal, and then exercise. Or conversely, after a period of rest the subjects exercise and then eat a meal. In both sequences some studies have shown that TEM was enhanced due to exercise[8,71,72,73,90] while others have shown that TEM was not enhanced due to exercise.[23,57,85,86] The studies have been so diverse in terms of subjects, meal composition and energy value, exercise mode, intensity, and duration that it is not possible to determine a pattern for when the effect appeared to be additive and when it did not.

Exercise Training and the Thermic Effect of a Meal   Studies investigating the effects of training, either cross-sectionally or longitudinally have shown that aerobic-trained individuals have a larger, smaller, or similar TEM response. As in the studies dealing with the acute effects of exercise, there is a wide diversity of subjects (especially in training level), meal composition, and meal energy value. However, a pattern is evident here. The level of fitness or training is the key, and the pattern follows that of an inverted U. Moderate levels of fitness (around 50–55 mL $\cdot$ kg^{-1} $\cdot$ min^{-1} $\dot{V}O_2$max for males; unknown for females) in young nonobese adults appear to enhance TEM above that of unfit subjects. High levels of fitness (greater than 65 mL $\cdot$ kg^{-1} $\cdot$ min^{-1} $\dot{V}O_2$max) appear to decrease TEM.

In both cases the results are probably good news. They mean that the individual beginning a physical fitness program to get in shape and lose a few pounds will benefit from an enhanced thermic effect. By expending more calories in that way, he or she may lose weight slightly faster. The highly trained and active individual, on the other hand, is able to preserve energy needed to sustain his or her exercise training. The reduced stimulation of the sympathetic nervous system and catecholamines that accompanies exercise training has been suggested as the reason for a lower TEM in highly trained individuals.[63] If the intent in highly trained individuals is to preserve energy for activity, it is unclear why they also exhibit an elevated RMR (see "Exercise Training and Resting Metabolic Rate"). For whatever reason, it seems that moderate levels of exercise training, which are probably attainable by large numbers of individuals, may enhance TEM but not RMR. Conversely, high levels of exercise training decrease TEM, but elevate RMR.[63]

Only one study has compared the thermic effect of a meal-exercise combination in resistance-trained individuals. In this study the $\dot{V}O_2$max was similar between the resistance-trained (52 mL $\cdot$ kg^{-1} $\cdot$ min^{-1}) and untrained (51.1 mL $\cdot$ kg^{-1} $\cdot$ min^{-1}) subjects and within the range of the moderately fit just cited; but the untrained subjects had a significantly higher TEM.[29]

Genetics may also play a part in explaining the interaction of TEM and training. For example, when six pairs of male monozygotic twins underwent a 22-day exercise training program, four sets showed a decreased TEM after training, and the remaining two showed an increase. Despite this wide between-pair difference, the intrapair resemblance was high (r = 0.72). Both the degree and the direction of response to TEM following training may in large part be hereditary. Thus, heredity may be one of the factors contributing to individual variations in body composition and weight change.[16]

The Impact of Diet, Exercise, and Exercise Training on Energy Expenditure

The last element in the caloric balance equation is the amount of energy expended in manual work or exercise. Restricting calories does not change the energy expended in any activity except as it influences body weight. However, individuals on calorically restrictive diets may have insufficient energy and may not be able to do as much physical work or exercise.

By definition, exercise will increase energy expenditure and the effects of training will be cumulative. Unless efficiency and/or body weight change, the caloric expenditure of any activity will not change with exercise training.

Table 15.3 summarizes all that has been discussed about the impact of diet, exercise, and exercise training on all of the elements of the caloric balance equation.

The Effect of Diet, Exercise Training, and Diet Plus Exercise Training on Body Composition and Weight

Many people wish to lose weight strictly for aesthetics (to look better) without caring what is lost. The concern from a physiological standpoint, however, is fourfold:

1. To lose body fat.
2. To preserve fat-free weight.
3. To maintain or improve health.
4. To maintain or improve performance, in the case of athletes.

Many factors influence whether these goals can be and are met. These factors include the following:

1. The initial status of the individual (Is he or she a few pounds overweight, or is he or she obese? What are his or her genetic predispositions?).
2. The type of diet selected (Is the caloric restriction minimal, moderate, severe, or maximal? What are the percentages of the basic nutrients included in the diet?).
3. The length of time of the weight-reducing program (24–48 hr, 5–20 weeks, or longer).
4. Whether or not exercise training is included as part of the program, and if so, the amount and type of exercise (dynamic aerobic endurance, weight-bearing or non-weight-bearing, or dynamic resistance training).

Exact responses to all possible combinations of these factors are not available. But some generalizations can be made.

The Effects of Diet on Body Composition and Weight   The vast majority of individuals on a weight-reducing regimen elect to diet. Caloric

TABLE 15.3 ■ Impact of Diet, Exercise, and Exercise Training on the Caloric Balance Equation

CALORIC BALANCE FACTOR	DIET	EXERCISE	EXERCISE TRAINING
Food ingested (+)	By definition, a reduction occurs	No clearly established effect; appetite does not decrease	Energy intake increases (highly trained and lean individuals) or remains constant (untrained and obese individuals); when training ceases, food intake spontaneously decreases but does not match the decrease in expenditure
BMR and/or RMR (−)	Severe caloric restriction causes a 10–20% decrease; weight cycling does not decrease	Unchanged per se but metabolic rate postexercise remains elevated	No consistent effect is evident
Thermogenesis (TEM) (−)	Decreases because fewer calories are being ingested; dependent on composition of meals	No consistent additive effect in either a sequence of food-exercise or exercise-food	Inverted U response, dependent on fitness level; moderate levels of fitness and training increase TEM; high levels of fitness and training decrease TEM
Work or exercise expenditure (−)	If calories are insufficient, may voluntarily do less exercise; but no direct effect on caloric cost	By definition, an increase occurs	A cumulative increase occurs

restriction may be minimal (a deficit of about 250–500 kcal·day^{-1}), moderate (a total intake of 1200–1500 kcal·day^{-1}), severe (a total intake of 400–800 kcal·day^{-1}, or maximal (fasting, or zero caloric intake). Strictly adhered to, all will bring about a weight loss.

Figure 15.3 shows that in dietary restriction approximately 28% of the lost total body weight is fat-free weight and 72% is fat weight. These values, however, are composites primarily from studies with severe caloric restriction. The percentages will vary on the basis of the caloric content of the diet. Thus, body weight loss from total fasting is split equally between body fat (50%) and fat-free weight (50%); from very low (400–800 kcal·day^{-1}) or low- (800–1200 kcal·day^{-1}) calorie diets the split is approximately 75% body fat and 25% fat-free weight;

and from 1200–1500 kcal·day^{-1} diets 90% body-fat and only 10% fat-free weight.[54] Fasting, which is obviously incompatible with life over the long haul, is not recommended as a dietary technique. The use of low-calorie and very low calorie diets should only be undertaken in extreme situations and only under the direct supervision of a physician. This technique is typically reserved for extremely obese individuals and is often conducted on a live-in basis in a metabolic ward of a hospital. The 1200–1500 kcal·day^{-1} regimen is often recommended, but even that does not totally preserve lean body mass.[2]

The importance of the FFW loss may depend on how much excess weight the individual started with. Obese individuals have an excess of both body fat and FFW. That is, their excess body weight is composed of 62–78% fat and 22–38% FFW. The ex-

FIGURE 15.3

Effects of Diet, Exercise, Training, and Diet Plus Exercise on the Composition of Weight Loss

Almost 30% of the weight lost by dietary restriction is fat-free weight. When exercise is added to dietary caloric restriction, the loss of fat-free weight is reduced. The smallest loss of fat-free weight occurs if the caloric deficit is achieved by exercise alone.

Source: Based on data from Donnelly, Jakicic, & Gunderson;[25] Walberg;[83] Hagan;[34] Heymsfield et al.;[36] Zuti & Golding;[91] Hagan et al.;[35] Depres et al.;[24] Bouchard et al.;[16] Ballor et al.[5]

*Diets were generally very low calorie or low-calorie (400–1000 kcal · day^{-1}).

cess of FFW is necessary to support and move the large bulk that accompanies obesity. Therefore, as one loses total body weight, less FFW would be needed; and its loss would therefore not be unexpected. Thus, loss of some FFW in such an individual may not be critical, but its preservation would also not be detrimental from a health standpoint. Therefore, individuals with less weight to lose need to protect their FFW.[20, 25, 40, 58, 59]

Recall that fat-free weight is composed of water, protein, and bone mineral (Figure 14.1). There is no indication that bone mineral content changes with a loss of body weight. The relative proportions of the loss of water and protein when dieting varies with the time course of the diet. During the first several days of a diet the majority of any weight loss (55–70%) is water loss. But by the end of the first month this percentage is considerably reduced

(to ≈ 40%) and after seven to eight months it may be as low as 5%. The protein (primarily the component of muscle tissue) loss is a consistent 5% in a nonexercising dieter.[31,36] What does this say about the proportion of fat loss? Simply that the percentage of fat loss is a mirror image of the percentage of water loss: little fat is lost at first and then progressively more fat is lost as caloric restriction continues.

Given these facts alone, would you recommend a series of short, VLCD regimens for quick weight loss or a slow steady approach? Why? Check your thinking in the section on the application of training principles section under the subsection "Adaptation."

Strangely enough, restricting water intake while dieting causes a higher proportion of water to be lost, not less, which could lead to dehydration. More total weight is lost if water is restricted, but not more fat. Water intake should not be restricted when dieting.[32, 36]

The Effects of Exercise Training on Body Composition and Weight   On the one hand, few people wishing to lose body weight would set out to do it entirely by exercising. You will come across some of these people in Y's and health clubs across the country, but they are a minority. On the other hand, there are many individuals who consciously or unconsciously do control their body weight through exercise training. These are, of course, athletes. If we ignore the fact that some athletes also closely watch their caloric intake, indirect evidence of the role of exercise on body composition can be inferred from the %BF values measured on various groups of athletes. Figure 15.4 presents a compilation of available data.

Keeping in mind that the average %BF for a young adult male is 13–15% and that for a young adult female it is 25% (Figure 14.7), several conclusions are discernible from the graph. First, even in the athletic population, the male-female difference in %BF is maintained. Second, athletes in different sports, both male and female, vary considerably in their %BF, from much leaner than average to slightly above average. Third, the %BF values appear to have a direct relationship to the demands of the sport. Athletes in sports where body aesthetics play a part in success (dance, figure skating, body building, gymnastics) tend to have low %BF values.

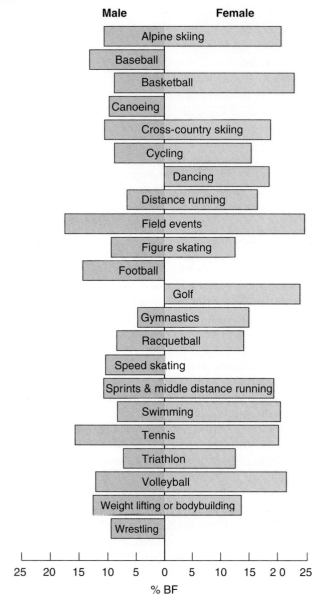

Male   **Female**

Alpine skiing
Baseball
Basketball
Canoeing
Cross-country skiing
Cycling
Dancing
Distance running
Field events
Figure skating
Football
Golf
Gymnastics
Racquetball
Speed skating
Sprints & middle distance running
Swimming
Tennis
Triathlon
Volleyball
Weight lifting or bodybuilding
Wrestling

25 20 15 10 5 0 5 10 15 20 25

% BF

FIGURE 15.4

Average Percent Body Fat of Male and Female Athletes (17–35 yr) in Selected Sports

Source: Based on a literature review presented in Wilmore & Costill.[88]

Endurance athletes (cyclists, cross-country skiers, distance runners, triathletes) also tend to have low %BF values. Athletes in predominantly motor skill sports (baseball, golf, volleyball) tend to be just about average. The only athletes consistently at or above average %BF values are the field event participants.

These data tend to support the value of exercise training in maintaining a low %BF, since athletes in activities known to have high caloric costs and engaged in for long periods of time have the lowest %BF values. However, the problem of self-selection arises when dealing with studies of this type. That is, we do not know whether individuals who are genetically programmed for leanness and success in these sports naturally gravitate to them, or whether the training demands of the sport determine the body composition of the performer. Both factors are probably operating.

Although the mean values cited show a definite pattern, a wide range of variability exists among successful athletes in any given event. For example, successful female distance runners have an average measured %BF value of 16.5%. Included in that group, however, is an athlete who won six consecutive international cross-country championships and another who held the 1972 world best time for the marathon; both of these runners had only 6%BF. At the other end of the range, the mid-1970s world record holder for the 50-mi run tested at 35.8%BF.[21] These extremes point out the importance of not establishing a specific %BF value for all athletes in any sport. The average values should not be interpreted as values that all athletes competing in a particular sport should achieve. If %BF values are suggested to athletes, they should be in the form of a range of values. The health and the performance of the athlete need to be monitored within that range, and individual adjustments should be made on the basis of this monitoring.

Figure 15.3 includes the results of four studies that were designed to determine whether weight could be lost but FFW maintained by exercise training without caloric restriction. The column is labeled "exercise training only." In the studies that make up this pool, less than 5% of the weight lost could be attributed to FFW. Indeed, only one study showed any FFW loss. In the other three FFW was gained. Only in those studies where a caloric deficit was achieved did a body weight loss occur.

Wilmore[87] compiled a list of body weight and body composition changes from 55 training studies whose general purpose was to improve physical fitness. The average body fat change was a decrease of only 1.6%, but at the same time a 1% increase occurred in FFW. No information was provided about the caloric balance in these studies. It must be emphasized that the key to weight and fat loss is not exercise per se but the achievement of a caloric deficit through exercise.[25, 83] Diet alone can also achieve a caloric deficit; but when weight is lost through dieting alone, it includes a greater percentage of FFW. The evidence discussed earlier is strong for the conclusion that exercise can maintain or even increase FFW, no matter what the caloric balance, but a substantial weight and fat loss will be achieved only when a negative caloric balance is achieved. Dynamic aerobic endurance activity is most helpful in increasing caloric expenditure; dynamic resistance activity (which is low in caloric cost) acts more directly to increase muscle mass.

Recent evidence has shown that overweight individuals (both male and female) benefit from exercise even if they remain overweight. Active overweight persons have better risk profiles for the diseases identified earlier and lower rates of morbidity and mortality than their sedentary counterparts. These health gains are related to the beneficial changes in glucose-insulin responses and lipoprotein values. Thus, the value of exercise training for overweight individuals goes far beyond the sometimes minor contribution to weight loss.[17]

Children and adolescents appear to be similar to adults in relation to the influence of exercise training on body composition. Comparisons of young athletes with their sedentary counterparts typically show that the athletes, both boys and girls, have a lower percent body fat and higher fat-free weight values. The variation among sports is similar to that for adults. There is also evidence from training studies that a decrement in percent body fat results from systematically applied exercise programs.[13, 62]

The Effects of Diet Plus Exercise Training on Body Composition and Weight
Studies that have combined diet and exercise seem to suggest that this approach is best for positive, long-term changes. Body weight is not lost faster in combined exercise-plus-diet programs than in diet-alone programs. However, the desirable maintenance of FFW is achieved. Figure 15.3 shows (from a composite of studies) that when exercise is added to caloric restriction, 20% of the total weight loss is FFW and 80% is fat. This is more FFW loss than

when exercise is used alone to achieve the caloric deficit, but less than when diet is used alone. In some cases muscle mass can actually be gained, as shown in Figure 15.5. Note that despite the increase of lean tissue when an exercise component is included, the total weight loss is very similar in all three groups of women in this study.[91]

The key to weight loss while maintaining FFW is probably the total caloric deficit and the nutrient content (PRO and CHO) of the calories ingested.[83] One advantage of adding exercise to a weight loss regimen may simply be that it allows an individual to ingest more kilocalories and still be in a negative caloric balance. Eating a moderately restricted diet allows for adequate nutrition and lifestyle changes that can be tolerated for a lifetime; in contrast, a

FIGURE 15.5

Weight Loss Is Similar but Body Composition Changes Vary Depending on the Means of Achieving a Caloric Deficit

Total weight loss was very similar in three groups of women who achieved their caloric deficit by diet, diet plus exercise, or exercise alone. Both exercise groups not only maintained lean muscle mass tissue but added some.

Source: W. B. Zuti & L. A. Golding. Comparing diet and exercise as weight reducing tools. *The Physician and Sports Medicine.* 4:49–53 (1976). Reprinted by permission of McGraw-Hill Inc.

VLCD can seldom be sustained for a prolonged time.

A study by Pavlou et al.[59, 60] illustrates that another benefit of adding exercise to a restricted caloric diet is the ability to maintain a weight loss. In this study (the results are depicted in Figure 15.6), 56 policemen lost an average of 10.1 kg by four preselected, calorically restricted, liquid and solid food diets over an 8-week period. Another 56 policemen lost an average of 12.2 kg when 90 min of supervised walk-jog-run plus calisthenics and relaxation exercises three times per week (for a total of 1500 kcal of work) were added to the same four diet routines. Subjects were reassessed at 8 and 18 months after the 8-week program.

Follow the lines in Figure 15.6 by the number of subjects at each time point to understand the follow-up results. At the 8-month follow-up 52 of the 56 dieters had regained all but 3.75 kg (≈63%) of their lost weight. Ten of the diet-plus-exercise group had ceased the exercise program and also regained all but about 3.5 kg (≈71%) of their lost weight. Conversely, the 44 who continued to exercise maintained their entire weight loss, and 4 of the diet group who added exercise lost an additional 3 kg.

At 18 months 47 of the original dieters and 8 of the 10 original diet-plus-exercise group continued to be sedentary and had regained all of their weight loss. The 2 diet-plus-exercise individuals who went back to exercising lost approximately 2 kg again. Their net loss was then approximately 5 kg, the same as 8 individuals who had stopped exercising between the 8th and 18th month.

Five men who had originally been just dieters became exercisers between the 8th and 18th month and reduced their weight to the level of the original loss. One of the 4 individuals from the diet group who began to exercise at the 8th month stopped and regained 5.5 kg. The 36 men in the original diet-plus-exercise group and 3 of the 4 from the diet-only group who began to exercise immediately at the end of the 8-week session maintained their entire weight loss.

Thus, all subjects—no matter how they had originally lost weight—regained the weight lost 1½ yr later if they did not exercise consistently during the intervening time. Conversely, all subjects—no matter how they had originally lost weight—maintained their weight loss after 1½ yr if they did exercise.

Regardless of how successful an initial weight loss diet is, most individuals regain at least a third of the lost weight within a year. Therefore, the contribution of exercise just described is extremely ben-

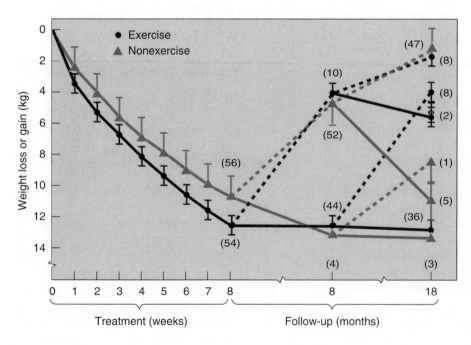

FIGURE 15.6

The Importance of Exercise in Maintaining Weight Loss

Subjects who exercised and dieted lost only slightly more weight than those who only dieted over an 8-week period. However, only those individuals who continued to exercise were able to maintain or regain their weight loss over a follow-up period of 18 months.

Source: K. N. Pavlou, S. Krey, & W. P. Steffee. Exercise as an adjunct to weight loss and maintenance in moderately obese subjects. *American Journal of Nutrition.* 49:1115–1123 (1989). © *American Journal of Nutrition.* American Society of Clinical Nutrition. Reprinted by permission.

eficial.[67] This study used an exercise program that totaled approximately 1500 kcal·week⁻¹ in just three sessions. This exercise could just as effectively be divided into five sessions of 300 kcal or six of 250 kcal. The calories expended in exercise are cumulative and the effect is the same no matter how long it takes as long as a deficit is ultimately achieved.

Why is it so hard to keep weight off once it has been lost? There is no definite answer to that question. Interest is currently centered on the enzyme lipoprotein lipase as a possible culprit. Lipoprotein lipase is the enzyme responsible for fat synthesis and storage in adipose tissue. It has been theorized that lipoprotein lipase notifies the brain when fat cells have shrunk, as they would when the body is losing weight. In response, appetite increases and fat cells refill. In other words, starving leads to stuffing. Not only does the appetite increase, but also it appears to be selectively predisposed to disproportionately increase the amount of fat ingested. Fat, of course, is calorically dense. Furthermore, after restrictive dieting the individual can more easily convert other excess food nutrients to fatty acids.

Previously or currently obese individuals seem to be more susceptible to the stimulus and response of lipoprotein lipase. In these individuals lipoprotein lipase activity may be twice as high as in nondieting individuals. That is the bad news. The good news is that when people who are not obese but mildly or moderately overweight diet, the changes in lipoprotein lipase activity are minimal. It may be that a certain amount of weight (approximately 15% of total body weight) must be lost before lipoprotein lipase activity becomes a counterproductive factor.[27, 28, 51, 67]

A change in food efficiency may be another factor that complicates the problem of maintaining weight loss. **Food efficiency** is an index of the amount of calories an individual needs to ingest in order to maintain a given weight or percent body fat. Food efficiency increases when the calories needed to sustain a certain weight (or percent fat) decrease. This response could be protective if food were scarce. Food efficiency decreases when the number of calories needed to sustain a certain weight (or percent fat) increases. This is what every dieter would like to have happen, but which does not happen.[19]

Several studies exemplify what appears to happen. In one study a group of obese individuals lost an average of 52 kg (114.4 lb) but remained 60%

overweight (39 kg or 85.8 lb, excess) when compared with a normal weight control group. The daily caloric needs (2171 kcal·day⁻¹) of the reduced-weight obese individuals to maintain their weight were found to be 25% lower than the value estimated from their body size and almost 5% lower than the value needed by much lighter normal-weight controls (2280 kcal·day⁻¹). These and other data suggest an increased food efficiency, an RMR that has remained depressed, or other compensatory changes in energy expenditure that oppose the maintenance of a body weight lower than usual.[43, 44]

Finally, several studies in which dietary and activity analysis were done indicate that some female distance runners ingest only between 1400 and 1990 kcal·day⁻¹ while training as much as 65 mi·week⁻¹. These caloric intake values are much lower than those for comparably sized, inactive females of the same age. Again, these results suggest that food efficiency is operating. It may be that food efficiency operates at the two extremes of obesity and excessive thinness when the body reacts to protect against what is perceived as starvation and a wasting away. Food efficiency may not be much of a factor for those losing a moderate amount of weight. More information is needed on this phenomenon.[21]

Application of the Training Principles for Weight and Body Composition Loss and/or Control

On the basis of the previous discussion of the impact of diet, exercise training, and diet plus exercise training on body weight and composition, the following guidelines are presented for the application of the training principles to achieve weight and body composition loss, change, and/or control. These guidelines are intended for the mildly or moderately overweight and overfat individuals that the physical educator or fitness leader is likely to

---

Food Efficiency An index of the amount of calories an individual needs to ingest in order to maintain a given weight or percent body fat.

encounter; they are not meant for the more severely obese individuals, who require more drastic reductions and medical supervision.

Specificity

The general goals of weight and body composition control should be as stated previously: to maximize the decrease in body weight or body fat while minimizing fat-free weight loss and supplying adequate nutrition. Such a program should become a lifestyle and not be just a temporary test of willpower and discipline.

In order to achieve these goals, a program that combines dietary caloric restriction and both dynamic aerobic endurance exercise and dynamic resistance training exercise is recommended. The combined caloric deficit should bring about a weight loss of no more than 0.5–1 lb (0.23–0.45 kg) per week.[67] This amount is less than the previously recommended 1–2 lb (0.45–0.9 kg) per week since new evidence suggests that slow weight losses are healthier and easier to maintain than fast weight losses. For the caloric equivalent of 3500 kcal $\cdot$ lb^{-1} of fat a deficit of 1750–3500 kcal per week or 250–500 kcal $\cdot$ day^{-1} is needed to achieve the 0.5–1 lb desired weight loss.

The endurance exercise modality selected (walking, jogging, cycling, swimming, aerobic dancing, stair stepping or stair climbing) should not matter if it is used in conjunction with a weight resistance program. However, for reasons that are neither known nor understood, swim training used by itself does not usually bring about changes in body composition. This is unfortunate, since non-weight-bearing activities such as swimming or cycling may be the least stressful orthopedically for overweight individuals beginning an exercise program. Exercise in water also overcomes other problems often seen when overweight individuals exercise, such as joint immobility, body instability, and heat intolerance. Because of these positive aspects, activity in water (aqua aerobics, walking-jogging, or swimming) may still be the exercise of choice. The addition of dynamic resistance training to water-based training is of even greater importance than it is to land-based exercise modalities.[42, 74]

Another way to interpret specificity in relation to weight control might be a desire to reduce body fat from a specific location, called *spot reduction*. The idea behind spot reduction is that fat will be selec-

tively mobilized and hence reduced from the area that is exercised. Thus, an individual wishing to reduce his or her abdominal region would concentrate on pelvic tilts, curls, and sit-ups.

Consistent training of specific muscles can increase muscle tone, which may give a slimming appearance (or if hypertrophy occurs, give a more defined appearance). However, there is no experimental evidence that fat (in the form of fatty acids) is mobilized preferentially from adipose cells located near active muscles.[46] That is, spot reducing may be an attractive idea, but in reality, it does not work, either for males or for females. In one study 27 women who performed calisthenics for the abdomen, hips, and thighs were compared with 29 women who performed aerobic activities.[55] Both groups worked out three times per week for 30 min for 10 weeks. Although %BF did not decrease significantly in either group, several girth and skinfold measures did decrease in both groups. There was no indication of any preferential site reduction in the specifically selected areas, however. Likewise, when 13 men underwent a 27-day training program during which 5004 sit-ups were performed, no significant changes occurred in %BF, skinfold, or girth measurements either as a result of training in the same subjects or in comparison with six nonexercising controls. Adipose biopsy measures did show significant decreases in all diameters; however, there was no significant difference in these changes between the heavily exercised abdominal site and the nonexercised gluteal and subscapular locations.[41]

Fat is mobilized to be used as a fuel by hormonal action. Hormones circulate to all parts of the body via the bloodstream. The distribution of body fat in the android (abdominal), gynoid (gluteofemoral), or intermediate pattern does not appear to affect the amount of weight lost by caloric deficit, nor is the relative distribution of fat altered by the weight loss. That is, the general shape of the individual is preserved despite a reduction in the total amount of fat and despite any attempt at spot reduction. Because spot reduction does not work, any activity that burns enough calories to cause a negative caloric balance can be utilized.

Overload

In the situation where weight loss is the goal, overload really means the attainment of a net deficit.

However, the general guidelines for the application of the training principles for dynamic aerobic endurance training outlined in Chapters 6 and 12 also apply here. The one exception is a shift in the importance of intensity and duration. The bottom line is that burning large numbers of calories is what is most important.

Previously sedentary, unfit, and overweight or overfat individuals cannot work at high-intensity levels for even short periods of time, and they should not try to. Instead, low-intensity activities continued for a long duration are recommended. A study by Milesis et al.[48] exemplifies the importance of duration. Fifty-nine young adult male subjects were divided into four roughly equal groups: a control group whose lifestyle remained unchanged and three exercise groups who engaged in a progressive walk-jog program for 15, 30, or 45 minutes three times per week for 20 weeks. The intensity level was the same for all groups, and no dietary restrictions were involved. Skinfold thickness and percent body fat were significantly reduced in all experimental groups, compared with the controls, but were proportional to the duration of training. Body weight decreased significantly only in the 30- and 45-min exercise groups.

The American College of Sports Medicine[3] recommends that the threshold level for total body weight and fat weight reduction is an aerobic program 20–60 min in duration with a combination of intensity and duration that will expend at least 300 kcal per session three times per week. If the frequency is raised to four times per week, then a 200-kcal expenditure each session is deemed to be sufficient. Thus, the recommendation for weight loss is any combination of frequency, duration, and intensity of exercise that will burn sufficient calories to obtain a deficit.

This recommendation is contrary to an often mentioned misconception that the way to lose fat is to burn fat doing long-duration, low-intensity exercise. Although it is true that fat is the dominant fuel in long-duration, low-intensity exercise, the important factor in weight loss is to establish a caloric deficit, regardless of the fuel being used. This principle is exemplified in a study by Ballor et al.[6] on two groups of obese women on equally restricted caloric intakes (1200 $kcal \cdot day^{-1}$). One group exercised on the cycle ergometer at 51% of their peak $\dot{V}O_2max$ for 50 min and the other at 85% of their peak $\dot{V}O_2max$ for 25 min. The low-intensity group

expended an average of 283 kcal per session at an RER of 0.80, and the high-intensity group expended an average of 260 kcal per session at an RER of 0.92. The estimated fat utilization was 26% for the high-intensity group and 66.6% for the low-intensity group. Although the high-intensity group did improve their cardiovascular fitness more, both groups lost equal amounts of body weight, fat-free mass, fat mass, and percent body fat, and decreased the sum of five skinfold thicknesses.

The advantage of the low-intensity exercise was not an increased loss of fat but a better initial tolerance to the exercise sessions. Individuals who are overweight or obese are also frequently out of shape, and low-intensity work at the initiation of an exercise program is probably more appropriate and less likely to bring about muscle and joint problems than is a high-intensity program. On the other hand, more active or higher fit individuals need not be concerned that in order to reap the weight control benefits of exercise, they need to slow down. The intensity and duration can be manipulated to best suit each individual interested in body weight or composition control.

Increasing caloric expenditure above 300 kcal of exercise and increasing the frequency of the exercise will enhance the fat and weight loss. An individual combining dynamic aerobic endurance and resistance weight training can alternate days (three each) and still have a rest day or can combine sessions on each of three or four days. The caloric cost of dynamic resistance exercise is less than that of dynamic endurance exercise and this difference needs to be taken into account when designing the exercise program.

In calculations of the energy cost of an activity session the net, not the gross, value should be used. That is, the calories that would have been burned anyway, had the individual been sedentary, should be subtracted from the cost of the exercise.[58] For example, if the energy cost of playing tennis is 7.1 $kcal \cdot min^{-1}$ but the individual would have expended 1.3 $kcal \cdot min^{-1}$ at rest the net cost is 5.8 $kcal \cdot min^{-1}$. Thus, it would take almost 52 min of tennis to burn 300 excess calories, not 42 min.

Adaptation

The importance of adaptation in caloric deficit lies in the fact that the composition of the weight loss varies the longer the deficit is maintained. Thus, the answer to the question previously posed regarding whether a series of short, very calorically restricted diets or one consistent, moderate-deficit diet is better is definitely the latter. The individual must get past the early water loss stages and into the stage where fat loss is proportionally the greatest. This adaptation will occur in addition to the specific adaptations to the exercise training.

Progression

The greatest progression will be made in the amount of calories that can be expended in exercise as the individual adapts to the training. When the calories expended in exercise increase, the amount of food ingested can be kept at the same level, hence increasing the deficit and/or possibly offsetting the decrease in RMR that may occur. Another possibility is to increase the amount of food ingested proportionally to maintain the same relative deficit. Progression should not be interpreted as an attempt to exercise more and more while eating less and less.

Individualization

In order to tailor a weight or fat loss program for an individual, several evaluations and calculations are helpful. The first is the direct measurement or estimation of the RMR. Formulas such as those presented earlier in the chapter (Table 15.2) enable RMR to be estimated fairly easily. The second is a dietary analysis of the nutrient and caloric intake of the individual. Computer programs are available for this analysis. The third is an analysis of the amount of calories normally expended in daily activity. Lists of the caloric cost per kilogram of activities, such as the list presented in Chapter 11, Table 11.6, are available for this calculation.

Once these numbers are available, the relative proportion of the caloric deficit to come from food intake and from energy expenditure can be determined. How much comes from which category should depend on the intake and fitness levels of the individual.

■ EXAMPLE

If an individual is sedentary, unfit, ingests 2000 kcal·day^{-1} and expends 1800 kcal·day^{-1}, 1350 kcal

of which is RMR, then an initial 450-kcal decrement makes sense (2000 − 1800 = 200 kcal to get to a caloric balance, and a 250-kcal deficit for a 0.5-lb weight loss per week). If the individual is really unfit, 100 kcal·day^{-1} of exercise may be all he or she is able to do; the other 350 kcal will need to come from the calories ingested. This diet would still allow for a caloric ingestion of 1650 kcal. If, on the other hand, the individual is relatively fit, a higher number of calories can be expended in exercise and either a greater intake of food allowed or a greater deficit achieved. ■

The caloric ingestion should not fall below the RMR. Although the flat values of 1200 and 1500 kcal·day^{-1} (female and male, respectively) are often suggested as a lower limit of caloric intake,[2] a more individualized system is to calculate a value halfway between RMR and 30% above RMR.[67]

Retrogression/Plateau/Reversibility

Weight loss tends to be uneven, even if caloric intake and output remain the same. Weight loss is fastest in the early stages of caloric deficit and then tends to level off. This pattern occurs, at least in part, because of the early loss of large amounts of glycogen and water. Later, RMR may decrease, and food efficiency may become a factor.[18] Although few who are attempting to lose weight will want to hear about these patterns, they need to be informed in order to get mentally prepared to deal with them. Reverting to old habits of food intake and a sedentary lifestyle (in a sense, detraining) will result in a rapid retrogression or complete reversal, exemplified by regaining lost weight, as was seen in the study described by Pavlou et al.[59, 60]

Maintenance

As discussed previously, many more people manage to lose weight than to maintain that weight loss. The key to the maintenance of a weight or fat loss is exercise training. Although the amount of food ingested cannot be disregarded, those who continue to exercise are able to eat enough to satisfy their physiological and psychological need for food without creating a positive balance. Those who do not exercise often cannot handle the food deprivation needed; as a result, they overeat for their activity level. The level of food intake and exercise output at the weight the individual wishes to maintain must be continued for life.

Making Weight for Sport

Although athletes in many sports are concerned with maintaining a low body weight and/or a low percent body fat,[21] only a few sports organize the competition around weight classes. The original intention was to make the competitions as fair as possible by matching individuals of approximately the same size. However, in practice, many participants manipulate their body weights and drop down to lower-weight classes under the assumption that they will then have an advantage over their opponents. One wonders what possible advantage there can be when both competitors are following the same strategy (although each athlete will always think he or she can drop down more than his or her opponent) and, more importantly, what the health and performance implications are. Despite the concerns, dropping into a lower-weight class is routinely done, often by individuals in their growth years. Boxers, wrestlers, and jockeys all engage in making weight, but by far the most research attention has been directed toward wrestlers (Figure 15.7).

In 1976 the American College of Sports Medicine[1] published the "Position Stand on Weight Loss in Wrestlers." The techniques typically utilized by wrestlers and the physiological consequences were detailed in that paper, as well as a number of suggestions for "making weight" in a healthier manner. Unfortunately, these recommendations appear to have had little impact on the patterns of weight loss and regain in wrestlers.

Over a decade later a study of 63 college and 368 high school wrestlers reported that 44% of the college wrestlers had weight fluctuations between 2.7 and 4.5 kg (6–10 lb) and 41% had fluctuations between 5.0 and 9.1 kg (11–20 lb) per week.[76] The majority of the high school wrestlers fluctuated slightly less, with 49% reporting variations of 1.4–2.3 kg (3–5 lb), 23% reporting variations of 2.7–4.5 kg (6–10 lb), and 21% reporting variations of 0–1 kg (0–2 lb). Techniques utilized still included fluid and food restriction (including fasting), vomiting, laxatives, diuretics, time in a sauna, and exercise in a rubber suit. Thirty-five percent of the college sample had

FIGURE 15.7

Making weight by following sound scientific guidelines should be an important goal for wrestlers at all levels of competition.

lost between 5.0 and 9.1 kg over 100 times in their lives!

Another 1990 study confirmed the detrimental effects of weight loss on physiological parameters (strength, peak aerobic power, anaerobic power, anaerobic capacity, and lactate threshold).[84] The wrestlers in this study elected to lose weight by 1–2 hr of exercise in a rubber suit after a 1.5-hr practice session combined with food restriction. The negative work responses were probably the result of dehydration and glycogen depletion. Thus, the conflict between tradition and science continues.

The key to changing the situation appears to be convincing coaches, athletes, trainers, parents, and officials in charge of the sports that a proper weight can and should be determined based on percent body fat, not just body weight at the time of weigh-in. Body fat should be determined in the preseason, and a minimal weight should be determined on the basis of the guideline of not less than 7%BF for competitors younger than 16 yr and not less than 5%BF for those 16 yr or older. Total body weight loss should not exceed 7%. Body fat should be lost gradually over a period of weeks to achieve the desired wrestling weight. Consideration should be given to allowing the wrestler to compete in a higher-weight class as the season goes on if a substantial increase in height (0.5 in. or more) and/or lean body mass occurs.[78]

It is important that the %BF determinations be accurate. Coaches and/or trainers can learn to take accurate skinfold and other anthropometric measurements and utilize these in sport-specific equations such as the one that follows. This equation is recommended on the basis of studies with wrestlers.[45]

(15.2) body density (g · cc^{-1} = 1.0982 – {[0.000815 × sum of triceps + subscapular + abdominal skinfolds (mm)] + [0.0000084 × sum of triceps + subscapular + abdominal skinfolds squared (mm)]}

$$D_B = 1.0982 - (0.000815 \text{ sum of skinfolds}$$
$$+ 0.0000084 \text{ sum of skinfolds}^2)$$

■ EXAMPLE

If a 17-yr-old wrestler weighed 165 lb and his sum of skinfolds for the selected sites was 46 mm, the calculation would be:

$$D_B = 1.0982 - [0.000815 (46) + 0.0000084(2116)]$$

$$= 1.0429 \text{ g} \cdot \text{cc}^{-1}$$

The D_B value is then substituted into the age-appropriate formula presented in Table 14.1 for a male adolescent to determine %BF. For a 17-yr-old this is

$$\%BF = \left(\frac{5.03}{D_B} - 4.59\right) \times 100 = 23.31$$

Equations 14.4, 14.5, and 14.6 are then used to determine the wrestler's most appropriate competitive weight. Using Equation 14.4

$$FFW = 165 \text{ lb} \times \left(\frac{100\% - 23.3\%}{100}\right) = 126.6 \text{ lb}$$

Using Equation 14.5

$$WT_2 = \frac{100 \times 126.6}{100\% - 16.3\%} = 151.3 \text{ lb}$$

Note: 16% is used here as the desirable %BF not 5%, which is the lowest recommended %BF for a wrestler of this age. The 16.3% complies with the recommendation that weight loss not exceed 7% of body weight. To get down to 5%BF this wrestler would need to lose 18.3% of his body weight and that is too much. Using Equation 14.6

$$151.3 \text{ lb} - 165 \text{ lb} = -13.7 \text{ lb}$$

Box 15.1 A Question of Understanding

Calculate the weight at which the following 14-yr-old wrestler should compete.

Name: Zachary   Triceps skinfold: 8 mm
Weight: 138 lb   Subscapular skinfold: 9 mm
                   Abdominal skinfold: 12 mm

How much weight does Zachary need to gain or lose to achieve this weight?

To achieve his recommended body weight, this wrestler needs to lose 13.7 lb.   ■

Complete the problem in Box 15.1 and check your answer at the end of the chapter.

Specific guidelines for making weight have not been established for other sports, but the principles discussed here can and should be applied.

SUMMARY

1. Weight gain, loss, and stabilization follow the first law of thermodynamics as expressed in the caloric balance equation. The components of this equation are food ingestion (+), resting or basal metabolic rate (–), thermogenesis (–) and exercise (–).

2. Diet, acute exercise, and exercise training can have an impact on the components of the caloric balance equation.

3. The goal of weight or fat control should be to lose body fat, to preserve fat-free weight, to maintain or improve health, and in the case of athletes to maintain or improve performance.

4. Twenty-eight percent of the total weight lost by diet alone is FFW, 72% is fat; 20% of the total weight loss by diet plus exercise is FFW, 80% is fat; only 4.5% of the weight lost by exercise alone is FFW, 95.5% is fat. Thus exercise helps to preserve FFW during times of caloric deficit.

5. A combination of diet plus exercise is the preferred technique for body composition and body weight control both in accomplishing an initial loss and in the maintenance of a weight loss.

6. The exercise training component of weight and fat control should include both an aerobic endurance portion (to burn at least 200–300 kcal per session) and a resistance weight training portion (to maintain and/or build fat-free weight).

7. Proper weight for wrestling should be determined based on %BF. The %BF should not be less than 7% for competitors under the age of 16 yr nor less than 5% for older competitors. Body weight loss should not exceed 7%, and this weight should be maintained throughout the season, except for allowing for more weight if height increases more than 0.5 in.

Box 15.1 Answer

Zachary's weight should be 132 lb. He needs to lose 6 lb. These results are computed as follows using Equation 15.2.

$$D_B = 1.0982 - [0.000815\ (8+9+12) \\ + 0.0000084\ (8+9+12)^2]$$
$$= 1.0982 - [0.023635 + 0.0070644]$$
$$= 1.0982 - 0.0306994 = 1.0675\ g \cdot cc^{-1}$$

For a 14-yr-old male the %BF formula from Table 14.1 is

$$\%BF = \left(\frac{5.07}{1.0675} - 4.64\right) \times 100 = 10.9$$

Using Equation 14.4

$$FFW = 138\ lb \times \left(\frac{100\% - 10.9\%}{100}\right) = 123\ lb$$

Zachary should wrestle at no less than 7%BF with a weight loss not exceeding 7% of body weight. Using Equation 14.5

$$WT_2 = \frac{100 \times 123\ lb}{100\% - 7\%} = 132.26\ lb$$

Using Equation 14.6

$$132\ lb - 138\ lb = -6\ lb$$

REVIEW QUESTIONS

1. State the caloric balance equation, and relate it to the first law of thermodynamics. Define and explain the components of the caloric balance equation.

2. Discuss the impact of dietary restriction on the components of the caloric balance equation.

3. Discuss the impact of exercise on the components of the caloric balance equation.

4. Discuss the impact of exercise training on the components of the caloric balance equation.

5. Compare and contrast the effects of diet alone, exercise alone, and diet and exercise combined on body weight and composition control.

6. List the training principles. Explain how each should be specifically applied for body weight or body composition control or maintenance.

7. Defend or refute the following statements, using evidence provided in this chapter.

   (a) Weight cycling makes subsequent weight loss physiologically more difficult.

   (b) The most important reason to add exercise or exercise training to a weight loss or maintenance program is that exercise decreases appetite.

   (c) If food is eaten near the time of exercise (either directly prior to or after), the thermic response is potentiated (made more effective), so that more calories are burned and weight is lost faster.

   (d) The maintenance of, increase in, or decrease in resting metabolic rate depends on the maintenance or change in lean body mass.

   (e) To lose fat, burn fat by doing long-duration, low-intensity exercise.

8. Prepare a set of weight control guidelines for a jockey.

REFERENCES

1. American College of Sports Medicine: Position stand on weight loss in wrestlers. *Medicine and Science in Sports.* 8(2):xi–xiii (1987).

2. American College of Sports Medicine: Proper and improper weight loss programs. *Medicine and Science in Sports and Exercise.* 15:xi–xiii (1983).

3. American College of Sports Medicine: The recommended quantity and quality of exercise for developing and maintaining cardiorespiratory and muscular fitness in healthy adults. *Medicine and Science in Sports and Exercise.* 22(2):265–274 (1990).

4. Apfelbaum, M., J. Bostarron, & D. Lacatis: Effect of caloric restriction and excessive caloric intake on energy expenditure. *American Journal of Clinical Nutrition.* 24:1405–1409 (1971).

5. Ballor, D. L., V. L. Katch, M. D. Becque, & C. R. Marks: Resistance weight training during caloric restriction enhances lean body weight maintenance. *American Journal of Clinical Nutrition.* 47:19–25 (1988).

6. Ballor, D. L., J. P. McCarthy, & E. J. Wilterdink: Exercise intensity does not affect the composition of diet- and exercise-induced body mass loss. *American Journal of Clinical Nutrition.* 51:142–146 (1990).

7. Beeson, V., C. Ray, R. A. Coxon, & S. Kreitzman: The myth of the yo-yo: Consistent rate of weight loss with successive dieting by VLCD. *International Journal of Obesity.* 13:135–139 (1989).

8. Belko, A. Z., T. F. Barbier, & E. C. Wong: Effect of energy and protein intake and exercise intensity on the thermic effect of food. *American Journal of Clinical Nutrition* 43:863–869 (1986).

9. Bingham, S. A., G. R. Goldberg, W. A. Coward, A. M. Prentice, & J. H. Cummings: The effect of exercise and im-

proved physical fitness on basal metabolic rate. *British Journal of Nutrition*. 61:155–173 (1989).

10. Blackburn, G. L., G. T. Wilson, B. S. Kanders, L. J. Stein, P. T. Lavin, J. Adler, & K. D. Brownell: Weight cycling: The experience of human dieters. *American Journal of Clinical Nutrition*. 49:1105–1109 (1989).

11. Blanchard, M. S.: Thermogenesis and its relationship to obesity and exercise. *Quest*. 34(2):143–153 (1982).

12. Bogert, L. J., G. M. Briggs, & D. H. Calloway: *Nutrition and Physical Fitness* (9th edition). Philadelphia: Saunders (1973)

13. Boileau, R. A., T. G. Lohman, & M. H. Slaughter: Exercise and body composition in children and youth. *Scandinavian Journal of Sport Sciences*. 7:17–27 (1985).

14. Bouchard, C.: Heredity and the path to overweight and obesity. *Medicine and Science in Sports and Exercise*. 23(3):285–291 (1991).

15. Bouchard, C. T., A. Tremblay, A. Nadeau, J. P. Despres., G. Theriault, M. R. Goulay, C. Lortie, C. Leblanc, & G. Fournier: Genetic effect in resting and exercise metabolic rates. *Metabolism*. 38(4):364–370 (1989).

16. Bouchard, C. T., A. Tremblay, A. Nadeau, J. Dussault, J. P. Depres, G. Theriault, P. J. Lupien, O. Serresse, M. R. Boulay, & G. Fournier: Long-term exercise training with constant energy intake. 1. Effect on body composition. *International Journal of Obesity*. 14:57–73 (1990).

17. Bray, G. A.: Complications of obesity. *Annals of Internal Medicine*. 103(6 pt 2):1052–1062 (1985).

18. Bray, G. A.: Effect of caloric restriction on energy expenditure in obese patients. *Lancet*. 2:397–398 (1969).

19. Brodie, D. A.: Techniques of measurement of body composition: Part I. *Sports Medicine*. 5:11–40 (1988).

20. Brown, M. R., W. J. Klish, J. Hollander, M. A. Campbell, & G. B. Forbes: A high protein, low calorie liquid diet in the treatment of very obese adolescents: Long-term effect on lean body mass. *The American Journal of Clinical Nutrition*. 38:20–31 (1983).

21. Brownell, K. D., S. N. Steen, & J. H. Wilmore: Weight regulation practices in athletes: Analysis of metabolic and health effects. *Medicine and Science in Sports and Exercise*. 19(6):546–556 (1987).

22. Bursztein, S. E., D. H. Elwyn, J. Askanazi, & J. M. Kinney: *Energy Metabolism, Indirect Calorimetry and Nutrition*. Baltimore: Williams & Wilkins (1989).

23. Dallasso, H. M., & W. P. James: Whole-body calorimetry studies in adult men. 2. The interaction of exercise and over-feeding on the thermic effect of a meal. *British Journal of Nutrition*. 52:65–72 (1984).

24. Despres, J. P., C. Bouchard, A. Tremblay, R. Savard, & M. Marcotte: Effects of aerobic training on fat distribution in male subjects. *Medicine and Science in Sports and Exercise*. 17(1):113–118 (1985).

25. Donnelly, J. E., J. Jakicic, & S. Gunderson: Diet and body composition: Effect of very low calorie diets and exercise. *Sports Medicine*. 12(4):237–249 (1991).

26. Garrow, J. S.: Energy balance in man: An overview. *American Journal of Clinical Nutrition*. 45:1114–1119 (1987).

27. Gershoff, S. N. (ed.): Ask the experts. *Tufts University Diet & Nutrition Letter*. 9(7):8 (1991).

28. Gershoff, S. N. (ed.): Ask the experts. *Tufts University Diet & Nutrition Letter*. 9(11):7 (1992).

29. Gilbert, J. A., J. E. Misner, R. A. Boileau, L. Ji, & M. H. Slaughter: Lower thermic effect of a meal post-exercise in aerobically trained and resistance-trained subjects. *Medicine and Science in Sports and Exercise*. 23(7):825–830 (1991).

30. Glickman, N. M., H. H. Mitchell, E. H. Lambert, & W. Keeton: The total specific dynamic action of high-protein and high-carbohydrate diets of human subjects. *Journal of Nutrition*. 36:41–57 (1948).

31. Grande, F. A., J. T. Anderson, & A. Keys: Changes of basal metabolic rate in man in semistarvation and refeeding. *Journal of Applied Physiology*. 12(2):230–238 (1958).

32. Grande, F. T., H. L. Taylor, J. T. Anderson, E. Buskirk, & A. Keys: Water exchange in men on a restricted water intake and a low calorie carbohydrate diet accompanied by physical work. *Journal of Applied Physiology*. 12(2):202–210 (1958).

33. Guyton, A. C.: *Textbook of Medical Physiology* (7th edition). Philadelphia: Saunders (1986).

34. Hagan, R. D.: Benefits of aerobic conditioning and diet for overweight adults. *Sports Medicine*. 5:144–155 (1988).

35. Hagan, R. D., S. J. Upton, L. Wong, & J. Whittam: The effects of aerobic conditioning and/or calorie restriction in overweight men and women. *Medicine and Science in Sports and Exercise*. 18(1):87–94 (1986).

36. Heymsfield, S. B., K. Casper, J. Hearn, & D. Guy: Rate of weight loss during underfeeding: Relation to level of physical activity. *Metabolism*. 38(3):215–233 (1989).

37. Himms-Hagen, J.: Thermogenesis in brown adipose tissue as an energy buffer. *The New England Journal of Medicine*. 311(24):1549–1558 (1984).

38. Horton, E. S.: Metabolic aspects of exercise and weight reduction. *Medicine and Science in Sports and Exercise*. 18(1):10–18 (1985).

39. Jeffery, R. W., R. R. Wing, & S. A. French: Weight cycling and cardiovascular risk factors in obese men and women. *American Journal of Clinical Nutrition*. 55:641–644 (1992).

40. Jequier, E.: Energy, obesity, and body weight standards. *American Journal of Clinical Nutrition*. 45:1035–1047 (1987).

41. Katch, F. I., P. M. Clarkson, W. Kroll, T. McBride, & A. Wilcox: Effects of sit-up exercise training on adipose cell size and adiposity. *Research Quarterly for Exercise and Sport*. 55(3):242–247 (1984).

42. Kieres, J., & S. Plowman: Effects of swimming and land exercises versus swimming and water exercises on body composition of college students. *Journal of Sports Medicine and Physical Fitness*. 31(2):189–195 (1991).

43. Leibel, R. L., & J. Hirsch: Diminished energy requirements in reduced-obese patients. *Metabolism*. 33(2):164–170 (1984).

44. Leibel, R. L., M. Rosenbaum, & J. Hirsch: Changes in energy expenditure resulting from altering body weight. *The New England Journal of Medicine*. 332:621–628 (1995).

45. Lohman, T. G.: Skinfolds and body density and their relation to body fatness: A review. *Human Biology*. 53(2):181–225 (1981).

46. McArdle, W. D., F. I. Katch, & V. L. Katch: *Exercise Physiology: Energy, Nutrition, and Human Performance* (3rd edition). Philadelphia: Lea & Febiger (1991).

47. Melby, C., C. Scholl, G. Edwards, & R. Bullough: Effect of acute resistance exercise on postexercise energy expenditure and resting metabolic rate. *Journal of Applied Physiology*. 75(4):1847–1853 (1993).

48. Milesis, C. A., M. L. Pollock, M. D. Bah, J. J. Ayres, A. Ward, & A. C. Linnerod: Effects of different durations of physical training on cardiorespiratory function, body composition, and serum lipids. *Research Quarterly*. 47(4):716–725 (1976).

49. Mole, P. A., J. S. Stern, C. L. Schultz, E. M. Bernauer, & B. J. Holcomb: Exercise reverses depressed metabolic rate produced by severe caloric restriction. *Medicine and Science in Sports and Exercise*. 21(1):29–33 (1989).

50. Nair, K. S., D. Halliday, & J. S. Garrow: Thermic response to isoenergetic protein, carbohydrate or fat meals in lean and obese subjects. *Clinical Science*. 66:307–312 (1983).

51. Nash, J. D.: Eating behavior and body weight: Physiological influences. *American Journal of Health Promotion.* 1(3):5–15 (1987).

52. National Task Force on the Prevention and Treatment of Obesity: Weight cycling. *Journal of the American Medical Association.* 272(15):1196–1202 (1994).

53. Newsholme, E. A.: A possible metabolic basis for the control of body weight. *New England Journal of Medicine.* 302(7):400–405 (1980).

54. Nieman, D. C.: *Fitness and Sports Medicine: An Introduction.* Palo Alto, CA: Bull Publishing (1990).

55. Nieman, D. C., J. L. Haig, E. D. DeGuis, G. P. Dizon, U. D. Register: Reducing diet and exercise training effects on resting metabolic rates in mildly obese women. *Journal of Sports Medicine and Physical Fitness.* 28(1):79–88 (1988).

56. Noland, M., & J. T. Kearney: Anthropometric and densitometric responses of women to specific and general exercise. *Research Quarterly.* 49(3):322–328 (1978).

57. Pacy, P. J., N. Barton, J. D. Webster, & J. Garrow: The energy cost of aerobic exercise in fed and fasted normal subjects. *American Journal of Clinical Nutrition.* 42:764–768 (1985).

58. Pacy, P. J., J. Webster, & J. S. Garrow: Exercise and obesity. *Sports Medicine.* 3:89–113 (1986).

59. Pavlou, K. N., S. Krey, & W. P. Steffee: Exercise as an adjunct to weight loss and maintenance in moderately obese subjects. *American Journal of Clinical Nutrition.* 49:1115–1123 (1989).

60. Pavlou, K. N., W. P. Steffee, R. H. Lerman, & B. A. Burrows: Effects of dieting and exercise on lean body mass, oxygen uptake, and strength. *Medicine and Science in Sports and Exercise.* 17(4):466–471 (1985).

61. Pillet, P. H., P. H. Gygaz, & E. Jequier: Thermic effect of glucose and amino acids in man studied by direct and indirect calorimetry. *British Journal of Nutrition,* 31:343–349 (1974).

62. Plowman, S. A.: Maturation and exercise training in children. *Pediatric Exercise Science* 1:303–312 (1989).

63. Poehlman, E. T.: A review: Exercise and its influence on resting energy metabolism in man. *Medicine and Science in Sports and Exercise.* 21(5):515–525 (1989).

64. Pratley, R., B. Nicklas, M. Robin, J. Miller, A. Smith, M. Smith, B. Hurley, & A. Goldberg: Strength training increases resting metabolic rate and norepinephrine levels in healthy 50- to 65-yr-old men. *Journal of Applied Physiology.* 76(1):133–137 (1994).

65. Rodin, J., N. Radke-Sharpe, M. Rebuffe-Scrive, & M. R. C. Greenwood: Weight cycling and fat distribution. *International Journal of Obesity.* 14:303–310 (1990).

66. Roza, A. M., & H. M. Shizgal: The Harris Benedict equation reevaluated: Resting energy requirements and the body cell mass. *American Journal of Clinical Nutrition.* 40:168–182 (1984).

67. Schelkun, P. H.: The risks of riding the weight-loss roller coaster. *The Physician and Sportsmedicine.* 19(6):149–156 (1991).

68. Schmidt, W. D., D. Corrigan, & C. L. Melby: Two seasons of weight cycling does not lower resting metabolic rate in college wrestlers. *Medicine and Science in Sports and Exercise.* 25(5):613–619 (1993).

69. Schutz, Y. B., T. Bessard, & E. Jequir, E.: Diet-induced thermogenesis measured over a whole day in obese and nonobese women. *American Journal of Clinical Nutrition.* 40:542–552 (1984).

70. Schwartz, R. S., J. B. Halter, & E. L. Bierman: Reduced thermic effect of feeding in obesity: Role of norepinephrine. *Metabolism.* 32:114–117 (1983).

71. Segal, K. R., B. Gutin, J. Albu, & F. Pi-Sunyer: Thermic effects of food and exercise in lean and obese men of similar lean body mass. *American Journal of Physiology.* 252:E110–E117 (1987).

72. Segal, K. R., B. Gutin, A. M. Nyman, & F. X. Pi-Sunyer: Thermic effect of food at rest, during exercise, and after exercise in lean and obese men of similar body weight. *Journal of Clinical Investigation.* 76:1107–1112 (1985).

73. Segal, K. R., E. Presta, & B. Gutin: Thermic effect of food during graded exercise in normal weight and obese men. *American Journal of Clinical Nutrition.* 40:995–1000 (1984).

74. Sheldahl, L. M.: Special ergometric techniques and weight reduction. *Medicine and Science in Sports and Exercise.* 18(1):25–30 (1985).

75. Shetty, P. S., R. T. Jung, W. P. James, M. A. Barrand, & B. A. Callingham: Postprandial thermogenesis in obesity. *Clinical Science.* 60:519–525 (1981).

76. Steen, S. N., R. A. Oppliger, & K. D. Brownell: Metabolic effects of repeated weight loss and regain in adolescent wrestlers. *Journal of the American Medical Association.* 260(1):47–50 (1988).

77. Swaminathan, R. K., R. F. King, J. Holmfield, R. A. Siwek, M. Baker, & J. K. Wales: Thermic effect of feeding carbohydrate, fat, protein, and mixed meal in lean and obese subjects. *American Journal of Clinical Nutrition.* 42:177–181 (1985).

78. Tipton, C. M.: Making and maintaining weight for interscholastic wrestling. *Sports Science Exchange.* 2(22) (1990).

79. Titchenal, C. A.: Exercise and foot intake: What is the relationship? *Sports Medicine.* 6:135–145 (1988).

80. van Dale, O., & W. H. M. Saris: Repetitive weight loss and weight regain: Effects on weight reduction, resting metabolic rate, and lipolytic activity before and after exercise and/or diet treatment. *American Journal of Clinical Nutrition.* 49:409–416 (1989).

81. Wadden, T. A., S. Bartlett, & K. A. Letizia: Relationship of dieting history to resting metabolic rate, body composition, eating behavior and subsequent weight loss. *American Journal of Clinical Nutrition.* 56:206S–211S (1992).

82. Wadden, T. A., G. D. Foster, K. A. Letizia, & J. L. Mullen: Long-term effects of dieting on resting metabolic rate in obese outpatients. *Journal of the American Medical Association.* 264(6):707–711 (1990).

83. Walberg, J. L.: Aerobic exercise and resistance weight-training during weight reduction: Implications for obese persons and athletes. *Sports Medicine.* 47:343–356 (1989).

84. Webster, S. R., & R. Weltman: Physiological effects of a weight loss regimen practiced by college wrestlers. *Medicine and Science in Sports and Exercise.* 22(2):229–234 (1990).

85. Welle, S.: Metabolic response to a meal during rest and low intensity exercise. *American Journal of Clinical Nutrition.* 40:990–994 (1984).

86. Willms, W. L., & S. A. Plowman: The separate and sequential effects of exercise and meal ingestion on energy expenditure. *Annals of Nutrition and Metabolism.* 35(6):347–356 (1991).

87. Wilmore, J. H.: Appetite and body composition consequent to physical activity. *Research Quarterly for Exercise and Sport.* 54(4):415–425 (1983).

88. Wilmore, J. H., & D. L. Costill: *Training for Sport and Activity: The Physiological Basis of the Conditioning Process* (3rd edition). Dubuque, IA: Brown (1988).

89. Wing, R. R.: Weight cycling in humans: A review of the literature. *Annals of Behavioral Medicine.* 14(2):113–119 (1992).

90. Zahorska-Markiewicz, B.: Thermic effect of food and exercise in obesity. *European Journal of Applied Physiology.* 44:231–235 (1980).

91. Zuti, W. B., & L. A. Golding: Comparing diet and exercise as weight reducing tools. *The Physician and Sportsmedicine.* 4:49–53 (1976).

Neuromuscular-Skeletal System

16

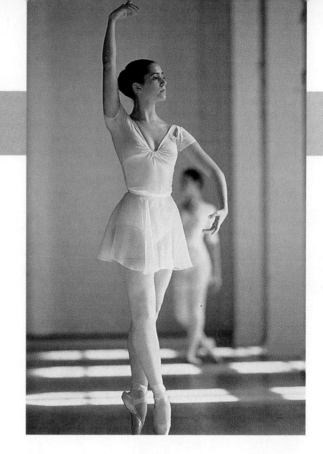

Skeletal System

After studying the chapter, you should be able to:

- Differentiate between cortical and trabecular bone.

- Define bone remodeling, and explain how bone mineral density is effected by the balance of bone resorption and deposition.

- Describe the hormonal control of bone remodeling and growth.

- Explain the criterion method of assessing bone mineral density.

- Identify age-related changes in bone mineral density.

- Identify sex-related differences in bone mineral density.

- Discuss the factors involved in the attainment of peak bone mineral density.

- Discuss the factors involved in the rate of bone loss in adults.

- Apply the training principles to the development of an exercise program to enhance bone health.

- Describe the skeletal adaptations that occur as a result of an exercise training program.

- Identify the risk to bone health associated with athletic amenorrhea.

- Describe micro- and macrotrauma skeletal injuries, and suggest ways of minimizing their prevalence.

Introduction

The skeletal system includes the bones and cartilage that provide the framework for the muscles and organs of the body. The skeletal system is not only taken for granted but also generally neglected in exercise physiology textbooks. This neglect is no longer acceptable: Research indicates that the skeletal system adapts to exercise training in much the same way as other body systems and that a healthy skeleton is important in the prevention of major health problems, including osteoporosis.

Exercise physiologists are concerned with such issues as the prevention and treatment of osteoporosis (in amenorrheic athletes and the elderly) and the impact of heavy training on the skeleton of growing prepubescent athletes. This chapter will address these important issues. But first, we must review the basic concepts of skeletal physiology in order to understand the influence of activity on bone.

Skeletal Tissue

Bone tissue, also called *osseous tissue*, is a dynamic, living tissue that is constantly undergoing change. In fact, 10–30% of an adult's skeleton and 100% of an infant's skeleton is typically replaced each year by the process of bone remodeling.[20] **Bone remodeling** refers to the continual process of bone breakdown (resorption) and formation (deposition of new bone). Bone remodeling plays an important role in regulating blood calcium levels and in replacing old bone with new bone to ensure the integrity of the skeletal system. The mass and shape of the bones depend largely upon the stress placed upon them. The more the bones are stressed (by mechanical loading in the form of activity), the more they increase in volume and mass, specifically at the site of mechanical loading.

Functions

The skeletal system provides a number of important functions that can be classified as either structural or physiological. Structurally, the skeletal system provides rigid support and protection for the vital organs and allows for locomotion. Physiologically, skeletal tissue provides a site for blood formation (hematopoiesis), plays a role in the immune function (by providing the site for white blood cell formation), and serves as a dynamic storehouse for calcium and phosphate, which are essential for nerve conduction, heart and muscle contraction, blood clotting, and energy formation.[3]

The ability of the bone to perform its structural functions is directly related to its role as a storehouse for calcium. Because calcium is essential for many processes within the body, bone will be broken down (resorbed) to maintain blood calcium levels. That is, the body will sacrifice bone mineral (calcium) if it is needed to maintain blood calcium levels.

Levels of Organization

An understanding of the functions of the skeletal system and the way that the skeletal system responds to training is best pursued by examining the three organizational levels of the skeletal system: organs, tissues, and cells.

Bones as Organs   The human body contains over 200 different bones joined together at articulations known as joints. *Joints* aid in movement by providing junctions for bones whereby they move when muscles exert force on them. The skeleton is typically divided into two categories: the central or axial skeleton includes the bones of the skull, vertebral column, ribs, and sternum; and the peripheral or appendicular skeleton includes the bones of the hips, shoulders, and extremities. There are several different shapes of bones—long, short, flat, and irregular—and each shape is specific to its function. Furthermore, each bone's shape reflects its response to the stress placed on it.

Bone Tissue   There are two types of bone tissue: cortical and trabecular bone. *Cortical bone,* also called compact, dense, or lamellar bone, is densely packed and makes up the majority of the

---

Bone Remodeling The continual process of bone breakdown (resorption) and formation (deposition of new bone).

skeleton (around 80%). *Trabecular bone,* also called spongy or cancellous, is more porous and surrounded by cortical bone. Individual bones are composed of both types of bone tissue; however, the relative proportion of trabecular and cortical bone varies. Table 16.1 presents relative percentages of trabecular and cortical bone tissue in various bones of the body. In general, bones of the axial skeleton have a much greater percentage of trabecular bone, whereas bones of the appendicular skeleton have a greater percentage of cortical bone.

Figure 16.1 is a diagram of a typical long bone. Note that it is composed of both cortical and trabecular bone. The shaft is composed primarily of cortical bone, and the epiphyses have a greater percentage of trabecular bone.

Cortical bone is composed of *osteons,* which are the functional units of bone (Haversian system). Osteons are organized into concentric layers of matrix called lamellae, which are surrounded by widely dispersed cells. The matrix is the intercellular space, and it is made up of organic and inorganic substances.

Trabecular bone is composed of branching projections or struts, called *trabeculae,* which form a latticelike network of interconnecting spaces. Its appearance is responsible for another one of its names, spongy bone. Trabecular bone has the same cells and matrix elements as cortical bone, but it has a greater degree of porosity. About 80–90% of the volume of cortical bone is calcified; only 15–25% of trabecular bone is calcified (the remaining volume is occupied by bone marrow, blood vessels, and connective tissue).[4] Therefore, cortical bone is best suited for structural support and protection, and trabecular bone is best suited for bone's physiological functions.

Owing to its large surface area, trabecular bone is able to remodel more rapidly than cortical bone. It is also in the trabecular bone that the greatest age-related loss in bone mineral density occurs. Therefore, the most common sites of osteoporotic fractures occur in areas composed predominantly of trabecular bone (wrist, hip, and spine).

Bone Modeling The process of altering the shape of bone by bone resorption and bone deposition.

TABLE 16.1 ■ Composition of Various Bones

MEASUREMENT SITE	CORTICAL PERCENTAGE	TRABECULAR PERCENTAGE
Culcaneus	5	95
Lumbar spine		
Anterior-posterior view	50	50
Lateral view	10	90
Proximal femur	60	40
Total body	80	20

Source: Highet.[23]

Bone Development

Bone development can be divided into three processes: bone growth, bone modeling, and bone remodeling. Each process occurs at different times throughout an individual's life.

Growth Bone growth refers to the increase in size of bone owing to an increasing number of bone cells.[18] There are two types of bone growth. The first is called *appositional growth,* which indicates that a bone increases in thickness or mass. The second type of bone growth, *longitudinal growth,* occurs at the epiphyseal plate prior to a person's reaching adult height. This is an area of interest owing to the concern of stunting a child's growth as a result of excessive exercise.

The longitudinal growth of bones is not directly due to bone growth but, rather, to the longitudinal growth of cartilage, which is later replaced by bone. During the process of growth, bone is also remodeling itself—that is, it is changing its shape and thickness. Think of growth and remodeling as two processes that are distinct but closely related. In general, *growth* refers to the longitudinal growth of bone, and *remodeling* describes the balance between bone resorption and bone formation. If bone formation exceeds resorption, this process would also represent *growth.*

Modeling **Bone modeling** is the process of altering the shape of bone by bone resorption and bone formation.[18] *Micromodeling* is the microscopic level of cell organization that occurs during for-

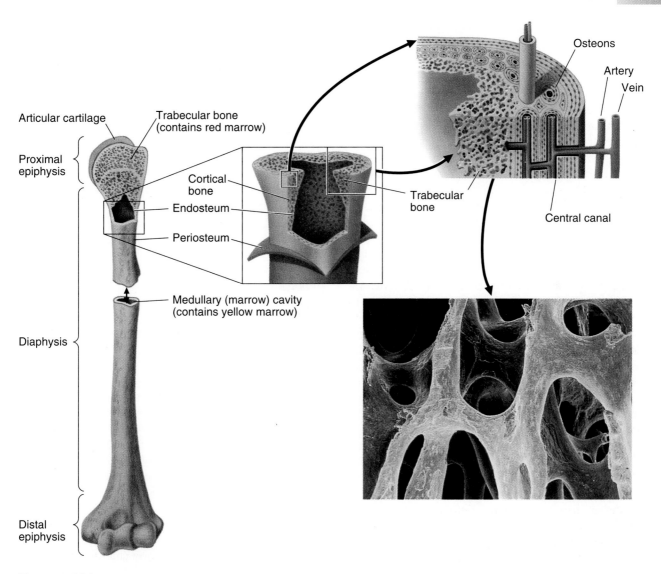

FIGURES 16.1

Typical Long Bone
Structure and cross-sectional view of bone.

mation; it determines what kind of tissue will be formed.[18] *Macromodeling* controls if, when, and where new tissue will form or old tissue will be removed.[18] This process ensures that the shape of the bone is matched to the role that bone will serve.[17, 18, 19, 33, 41]

Remodeling   As noted earlier, bone remodeling refers to the continual process of bone turnover, maintenance, replacement, and repair.[18] It reflects the balance between the coupled processes of bone resorption and bone formation. This ongoing process occurs because of the coupled action of bone cells.

Bone Cells.   There are three types of bone cells: osteoclasts, osteoblasts, and osteocytes. The cells are the living part of bone. Although the cells represent a small fraction (less than 2%)[60] of the total composition of bone, they are responsible for its remodeling.

Osteoclasts are large, multinucleated bone cells that cause the resorption of bone tissue (bone-destroying cells). These cells secrete digestive enzymes that destroy and disintegrate (phagocytize) bone matrix. As the bone is degraded, the mineral salts (primarily calcium and phosphate) are dissolved and move into the bloodstream. **Osteoblasts** are bone cells that cause the deposition of bone tissue (bone-forming cells). Osteoblasts are cells that produce an organic bone matrix that will become calcified and harden when minerals are deposited in it. The hardening of the bone matrix is known as ossification. **Osteocytes** are mature osteoblasts surrounded by calcified bone that help regulate the process of bone remodeling. Osteocytes appear to initiate the process of calcification.

The actions of the osteoclasts and the osteoblasts are coupled; they work together to remodel bone. In fact, osteoclasts must first cause bone resorption before the osteoblasts can form new bone. Figure 16.2 outlines the major events of a bone-remodeling cycle.[41, 49, 60] First, the osteoclasts are stimulated and cause the resorption of bone, resulting in a cavity (Figures 16.2b and 16.2c). Osteoblasts then appear and deposit bone matrix where the cavity exists (Figure 16.2d). The matrix is called *osteoid* until it is calcified (Figure 16.2e). Calcification of the new bone occurs as calcium and phosphate minerals are deposited in the osteoid (Figure 16.2f). The bone then returns to the resting or quiescent phase (Figure 16.2a).

Bone remodeling may result in greater bone mass, the same bone mass, or a reduction in bone mass. Through young adulthood, typically, more bone is formed than is resorbed; thus, there is an increase in bone mass. This increased mass strengthens the bone and accounts for the increase in bone mineral density that occurs during this period of life. When bone remodeling is in equilibrium, the amount of bone resorbed is equal to the amount of bone formed; thus, bone mineral density remains relatively constant. In the elderly and as a result of some disease conditions the amount of bone resorbed is greater than the amount of bone formed, and a decrease in bone mineral density occurs.

The remodeling of bone just discussed provides the means for skeletal growth, particularly during developmental years, and for the constant turnover of bone that occurs throughout life. Bone remodeling is a complex process that is regulated by hormonal and local factors, which in turn affect bone cells and the process of bone resorption and formation.[7]

Hormonal Control. Bone remodeling reflects the interrelationship between the structure and physiological function of bone. Not only is calcium necessary to provide structural integrity of bone, but it is also essential to the proper functioning of the heart, skeletal muscles, and nervous tissue. Only about 1 g of calcium (less than 1%) is present in the extracellular fluid of the body, compared to approximately 1150 g of calcium present in bone tissue.[3]

The skeletal system, the digestive system, and the urinary system operate together, under hormonal control, to maintain blood calcium levels. Because of the importance of calcium in so many vital processes of the body, bone mass is broken down to maintain blood calcium within normal limits. Thus, blood calcium is the variable that is closely regulated. The primary hormones involved in regulating blood calcium levels and bone remodeling are parathyroid hormone (PTH), calcitonin, and vitamin D (calcitrol).

Excess calcium in the blood leads to the release of calcitonin (from the thyroid gland), which causes deposition of calcium in the bone.[43] This deposition has the effect of decreasing blood calcium levels and simultaneously increasing bone mineral density. Conversely, when blood calcium drops below normal values, parathyroid hormone stimulates osteoclast activity, causing calcium to be released from its

Osteoclasts Bone cells that cause the resorption of bone tissue (bone-destroying cells).

Osteoblasts Bone cells that cause the deposition of bone tissue (bone-forming cells).

Osteocytes Mature osteoblasts surrounded by calcified bone that help regulate the process of bone remodeling.

Hydroxyapatite Calcium and phosphate salts that are responsible for the hardness of the bone matrix.

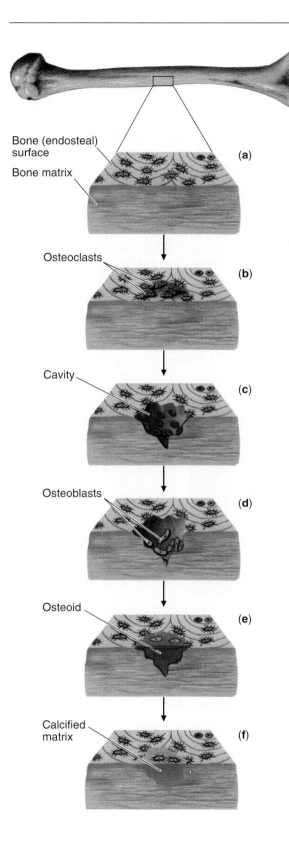

Bone (endosteal) surface
Bone matrix
(a)

Osteoclasts
(b)

Cavity
(c)

Osteoblasts
(d)

Osteoid
(e)

Calcified matrix
(f)

FIGURE 16.2

Stages of Bone Remodeling

(a) Resting cell surface. (b) Osteoclasts (multinucleated) are activated and begin dissolving bone (minerals released to the blood). (c) Osteoclasts produce a cavity in the blood matrix. (d) Osteoblasts appear. (e) Osteoblasts secrete the osteoid (uncalcified matrix). (f) The matrix is calcified.

storage site, the skeletal system. This release of calcium from the bone causes blood calcium levels to increase and bone mineral density to decrease. Vitamin D (calcitrol) is important for the absorption of calcium from the intestines. Thus, it leads to an increased blood level of calcium.

Other hormones that play an important role in skeletal health are the sex steroids (estrogen and testosterone) and growth hormone. These hormones stimulate the protein formation necessary for bone growth and are responsible for the closure of the epiphyseal plate, which will ultimately determine bone length and thus a person's height.[3] Estrogen is important in promoting calcium retention and acts as an inhibiting agent of parathyroid hormone. The loss of the protective role of estrogen on the skeletal system has important consequences for women after menopause or during secondary amenorrhea. A decrease in estrogen has the net result of increasing bone resorption. Hormones are themselves stimulated by other factors, including physical activity.

*A*ssessment of Bone Health

Measures of bone mass and bone mineral density are used to describe bone health. *Bone mineral content* refers to the absolute amount of **hydroxyapatite**—calcium and phosphate salts that are responsible for the hardness of the bone matrix—measured in grams. *Bone mineral density* is defined as the relative value of bone mineral per measured bone area, expressed as grams per centimeter squared ($g \cdot cm^{-2}$) or milligrams per centimeter cubed ($mg \cdot cm^{-3}$), depending upon the technology used to assess area. Bone mineral density is used clinically to provide an operational definition of osteopenia and osteo-porosis.[27] **Osteopenia** is a condition of decreased bone mineral density (BMD) and is diagnosed when BMD is greater than one standard deviation below (but not more than 2.5 standard deviations below) values for young, normal adults. **Osteoporosis** is a condition of porosity and decreased BMD that is defined as BMD greater than 2.5 standard deviations below values for young, normal adults. Established osteoporosis refers to the condition of osteoporosis as defined above, and one or more fractures.[28]

Laboratory Measures

Bone mineral content and bone mineral density are measured only in laboratory or clinical settings, primarily because of the cost of equipment and safety considerations. The results, however, are worth the effort, since they have dramatically increased the amount of information that is available to re-searchers, clinicians, and those involved in fitness professions. Two laboratory measures are absorp-tiometry and biochemical markers.

Absorptiometry During the past 30 yr there have been a large number of studies investigat-ing bone mineral density using the accurate, non-invasive techniques of single- and dual-photon absorptiometry (SPA and DPA, respectively). How-ever, dual-energy, X-ray absorptiometry (DXA) has become the standard or criterion measure to assess bone mineral density, and most investigations now rely on this technique.[21] Dual-energy X-ray absorp-tiometry (DXA) uses an X-ray beam to measure regional and whole-body mineral content. This technology decreases the time necessary for a scan and also decreases the subject's exposure to radia-tion. Figure 16.3 provides a computer-generated printout of whole-body bone mineral density (BMD) and various regions of the body for a 37-yr-old active

(a)

(b)

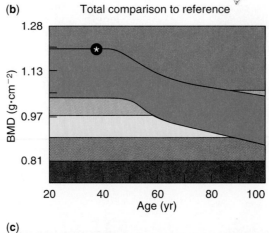

FIGURE 16.3

Computer-Generated Printout of Whole Body BMD for Young, Healthy Female

Source: Data from the University of Connecticut Health Center, Osteo-porosis Research Center. Photo courtesy of LUNAR.

(c)

Bone results

Standard analysis – DEXA calibration

Region	BMD g·cm^{-2}	% young adult	% age matched
Head	2.323	—	—
Arms	0.977	116	117
Legs	1.229	106	108
Trunk	0.971	106	108
Ribs	0.711	—	—
Pelvis	1.217	110	112
Spine	1.289	113	116
Thoracic	1.185	—	—
Lumbar	1.507	—	—
Total	1.197	106	108

female. Figure 16.3a represents regions of the body that are individually analyzed for BMD. The total body BMD is compared with standard references in Figure 16.3b. The dark area represents an average range across the age span of 20–100 yr. Notice that the individual in the example is above average for total body BMD as represented by the asterisk (located at the intersection of age 37 yr and BMD 1.197 g · cm^{-2}).

Regional BMDs are provided in Figure 16.3c along with comparisons with young adult normative data. Notice that each region of the body has a unique BMD value because of the composition of the bone and the stress (load) placed upon it. For example, the legs have a BMD of 1.229 g · cm^{-2}, whereas the pelvis has a BMD of 1.217 g · cm^{-2}. These values correspond to 106 and 110% of young adult values, respectively.

Figure 16.4 provides an example of an individual with low BMDs. Work through the problem in Box 16.1 to be sure than you understand the differences in total body and regional BMDs in these examples.

These techniques enable researchers to investigate differences in bone mineral density at various sites, among various individuals, and as a result of adaptation to long-term exercise training.

Biochemical Markers   Some researchers are using sophisticated blood analysis techniques in an attempt to quantify changes in blood levels of hormones, ions, and proteins (for example, osteocalcin) unique to bone following an acute bout of exercise.[47] For example, osteocalcin may be an indicator of bone formation, and as such, it could be used as a marker of bone turnover. The use of biochemical markers represents an exciting area of bone research, but it is in the very early stages of development.

Field Tests

There are currently no field tests to measure bone mineral density. However, because the actions and adaptations of muscles and bones are so interdependent, some scientists speculate that measures of muscular strength might also give an indication of bone mineral density.

Significant positive correlations have been found between lumbar spine BMD and back extensor strength, grip strength and forearm BMD, back

strength and hip BMD, and hip adductor strength and hip BMD.[57] These relationships make intuitive sense, since the action of the muscle on bone would be expected to be site-specific. However, significant positive relationships have also been found between biceps brachii strength and spine BMD, biceps strength and hip BMD, and dominant grip strength and spine BMD.[56] These relationships imply that site specificity is not absolute.

Arm activity may require sufficient simultaneous trunk stabilization so that enough force is exerted on the spine and hips to cause bone density to increase. Unfortunately, these relationships are not very strong, with correlations falling in the range of 0.35–0.50.

Since strength measures are relatively easy to do as part of a physical fitness assessment, it would be convenient to be able to get an estimate of BMD from strength tests. However, the relationships are simply not strong enough as currently assessed to be able to do so. The relationships between muscle strength and BMD do hold some promise for yielding estimates of BMD; but for now, we cannot assume that muscle strength indicates BMD.

*F*actors Influencing Bone Health

Bone health is determined largely by the attainment of peak bone mass and the rate of bone loss. Both of these processes are influenced by age and sex.

Age-Related Changes in Bone

Bone is a dynamic tissue that changes in density throughout its life. As shown in Figure 16.5, a char-

---

Osteopenia A condition of decreased bone mineral density (BMD), diagnosed when BMD is greater than one standard deviation (SD) below (but not more than 2.5 SD below) values for young, normal adults.

Osteoporosis A condition of porosity and decreased bone mineral density that is defined as a BMD greater than 2.5 standard deviations (SD) below values for young, normal adults.

(a)

(b)

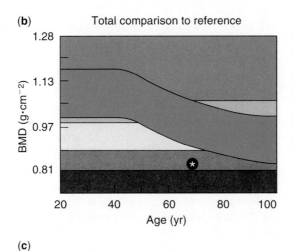

Total comparison to reference

(c)

Bone results			
Standard analysis – DEXA calibration			
Region	BMD g·cm^{-2}	% young adult	% age matched
Head	1.897	—	—
Arms	0.631	75	88
Legs	0.733	63	76
Trunk	0.677	74	88
Ribs	0.575	—	—
Pelvis	0.717	65	80
Spine	0.718	63	78
Thoracic	0.710	—	—
Lumbar	0.732	—	—
Total	0.847	75	88

FIGURE 16.4

Computer-Generated Printout of Whole Body BMD for an Old, Osteopenic Female

Source: Data from the University of Connecticut Health Center, Osteoporosis Research Center. Photo courtesy of LUNAR.

acteristic pattern exists between bone mass and age for males and females.[48] Approximately the first 20 yr of life are characterized by active growth in bone

---

Box 16.1 A Question of Understanding

Figure 16.3 gives bone mineral data for a 37-yr-old active female. Figure 16.4 gives bone mineral data for a 69-yr-old osteoporotic woman. Study these printouts carefully and answer the following questions.

1. What is the BMD and percentage of young healthy values for the (a) arms, (b) pelvis, (c) spine, and (d) total body for each of these individuals?

2. What implications do these results have for the likelihood of each individual having an osteoporotic fracture?

---

mass. The skeletal consolidation phase occurs during early adulthood, and this is the time when peak bone mass occurs. Shortly after the attainment of peak bone mass, a loss of bone mass begins. Following the rapid-loss phase, the rate of bone loss decreases.[60]

Sex Differences in Bone Mineral Density

There are systematic differences in bone mineral density between males and females. As shown in Figure 16.5, bone mineral density changes throughout the life span for both sexes. Bone mineral density increases throughout childhood and early adult life for males and females; however, the peak bone mineral density achieved by females is less than that achieved by males.[48] Additionally, at the time of menopause women lose the protective influence of estrogen, and the rate of bone loss is accelerated if

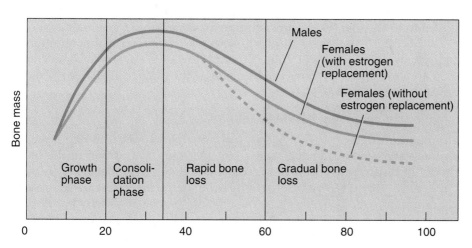

FIGURE 16.5

Comparison of BMD for Females and Males

estrogen is not pharmacologically replaced. The loss of the protective influence of estrogen explains the prevalence of osteoporotic fractures in women.

Development of Peak Bone Mass

Peak bone mass is developed during young adulthood and is influenced by mechanical factors, nutrition, hormonal levels, and genetics.[48] The mechanical factors affecting bone are physical activity and gravity. These forces are generally accepted as necessary stimuli for bone formation and growth.[39] Although there is still much research to be done before specific exercise prescriptions can be developed for the skeletal system, children and adolescents should be encouraged to engage in physical activity to promote bone health as well as to promote other positive changes and development within the body. Specifically, children and adolescents should be encouraged to participate in high-impact activities for bone development.[22]

Adequate nutrition is necessary in order to develop a strong skeletal system. A nutrient that is essential to bone health, and often deficient in young athletes, is calcium. Table 16.2 shows the recommended optimal dietary intake of calcium. Unfortunately, many individuals fall well below recommendations, particularly young women who are concerned about weight control. For instance, they may eliminate dairy products from their diet because they are high in fat. But dairy products also are an excellent source of calcium. Thus, while trying to maintain weight, these athletes may be negatively affecting the attainment of peak bone mass. Exercise professionals should be careful to consider the need for dietary calcium when counseling young athletes (particularly females) about weight management.[37] The availability of the many low-fat

TABLE 16.2 ▪ NIH Consensus Statement: Optimal Daily Calcium Intake

AGE GROUP	OPTIMAL CALCIUM INTAKE (mg)
INFANT	
Birth–6 months	400
6 months–1 yr	600
CHILDREN	
1–5 yr	800
6–10 yr	800–1200
ADOLESCENTS AND YOUNG ADULTS	
11–24 yr	1200–1500
MEN	
25–65 yr	1000
Over 65 yr	1500
WOMEN	
25–60 yr	1000
Postmenopausal (under 65 yr), on estrogen	1000
Postmenopausal, not on estrogen	1500
Over 65 years	1500
Pregnant or nursing	1200–1500

Source: NIH Consensus Conference.[46]

dairy products makes including calcium in the diet easier.

As mentioned previously, adequate levels of the hormone estrogen are also needed to attain peak bone mass. Thus, athletes who are amenorrheic are likely to develop a lower peak bone mass than athletes with normal menstrual function.

Finally, genetic makeup is an important determinant of BMD. In other words, there are genetically determined limits to the amount of BMD that an individual can attain. But the only way to achieve genetic potential is to pay careful attention to the factors that an individual can modify, namely, nutritional status, hormonal status, and activity level.

Exercise Response

There is skeletal adaptation to exercise training; therefore, logic implies that there must also be an exercise response occurring within the skeletal system to bring about training adaptations. Unfortunately, researchers have not yet found a way to quantify the acute effects of exercise on the skeletal system. Limited research has been conducted on the effects of exercise on biochemical markers of bone activity and the response of hormones known to be involved with bone remodeling.[35, 47] However, human research has yet to yield data describing the acute skeletal exercise response.

Application of the Training Principles

Since exercise physiologists generally agree that physical activity has a positive effect on bone health, the logical question is: What is an appropriate exer-

cise prescription for increasing or maintaining bone health? Unfortunately, the answer to that question is not fully known. However, several recommendations can be made on the basis of available research.

Specificity

The specificity principle applies to the specific bones being stressed, the composition of the bone being stressed (cortical versus trabecular), and the type of activity being performed. Research data suggests that the type of exercise or activity performed greatly influences skeletal adaptations. **Weight-bearing exercise** refers to movement in which the body weight is supported by muscles and bones thereby working against the pull of gravity. **Non-weight-bearing exercise,** on the other hand, refers to movement in which the body is supported or suspended and thereby working against the pull of gravity. Weight-bearing or impact-loading activities, such as running, gymnastics, stair climbing, or volleyball, are more likely to stimulate an increase in bone mass than non-weight-bearing activities, such as swimming or cycling.[10, 22, 25] The type of activity that should be chosen depends upon the health and preference of the individual. A major concern when one is considering exercise for individuals with low bone mineral content is the risk of falling and causing a fracture. Activities that carry a high risk of falls or collisions should not be recommended for certain segments of the population, such as the elderly. Table 16.3 provides some general guidelines for the type of activity that should be considered for various groups.[10]

Since resistance training has been associated with positive adaptations in skeletal tissue, as well as muscular fitness, exercise physiologists recommend that individuals engage in resistance training exercise as a way of maintaining both muscular and skeletal health. A general resistance training program that works all the major muscles of the body should benefit the total skeleton.

Box 16.2 is included to allow you the opportunity to apply the information presented in this section.

Overload

As mentioned earlier, weight-bearing exercises result in positive adaptations to the skeleton. How-

Weight-Bearing Exercise A movement performed in which the body weight is supported by muscles and bones.

Non-Weight-Bearing Exercise A movement performed in which the body weight is supported or suspended and thereby not working against the pull of gravity.

TABLE 16.3 ■ Recommended Activities for Skeletal Health

	CHILDREN AND YOUNG ADULTS	ADULTS, PREMENOPAUSAL	ADULTS, BELOW-NORMAL BMD	ADULTS, VERY LOW BMD
Goal	To attain peak bone mass	To slow the rate of bone loss and prevent musculoskeletal injury	To decrease risk of injury	To avoid injury
Type of activity	High-impact-loading movements	Moderate-impact-loading movements	Low- to moderate-impact-loading movements	Low-impact-loading movements
Example	Sprinting, jumping, track and field, volleyball, basketball, gymnastics, soccer, weight training, rope skipping	Walking, jogging, running, hiking, stair climbing, stepping (machines), dancing, weight training, rope skipping, skiing	Stair climbing (machine), hiking, cross-country skiing, weight training	Walking, water aerobics, swimming, stationary cycling

ever, the load that is necessary for positive bone adaptation is not known. Impact loads can be manipulated by increasing repetitions or by increasing the intensity as measured by ground reaction force or joint force. For example, a runner would load the bones by high repetition whereas a power lifter would overload primarily by intensity. For adaptations to skeletal tissue, intensity is apparently more important than repetition.

Until the amount and type of exercise needed to impose an overload is known, we cannot determine the rate of adaptation or the progression necessary to induce additional gains in bone density. However, any type of exercise overload (intensity, duration, or frequency) must begin at a level the individual can handle and progress gradually.

Box 16.2 **A Question of Understanding**

Use Table 16.3 to answer the following questions.

1. What type of activities would you recommend for your 45-yr-old aunt who has just found out that she has low BMD? How is this program consistent with the goals for this population?
2. Because of your aunt's diagnosis of low BMD, what physical activities and dietary recommendations would you give to your 15-yr-old cousin (your aunt's daughter)? Why?

Individualization

The individual response principle applies to bone as well as to other systems of the body. That is, different people will respond to the same exercise stress differently, depending upon their genetic makeup, hormonal and nutritional status, and so on. Therefore, the guidelines for applying this principle as described for dynamic aerobic and dynamic resistance activities should be employed.

Retrogression/Plateau/Reversibility

The reversibility principle suggests that if you cease exercising for a period of time, you will lose the benefits of exercising. Studies of immobilized patients[11,32,61] and discontinued training[9] indicate that this principle also applies to bone. However, neither the level of activity needed to maintain bone mineral density, the threshold at which bone loss occurs, nor the rate of bone loss is known. Additional research is necessary to determine the level of activity necessary to maintain improvements in bone mineral density that have resulted from exercise training.

Warm-Up and Cool-Down

The effect of warming up and cooling down on bone density is not known. However, warming up and stretching are important to the ligaments and tendons, which are part of the skeletal system.

In summary, the exact exercise prescription for skeletal health is not currently known. However, this should not be used as an excuse not to exercise. Some weight-bearing or impact-loading exercise is better than none. Furthermore, since dynamic aerobic and dynamic resistance activities are recommended, it is prudent to use the guidelines given for these modalities until guidelines more specific to skeletal health are developed.

Skeletal Adaptations to Exercise Training

The adaptation of the skeletal system to exercise training is depicted by the continuum in Table 16.4. As the table indicates, the adaptation of bone depends on the amount of activity. In addition, skeletal adaptation depends on the type of bone being measured (trabecular or cortical) and the type of activity employed.

Research clearly indicates that a lack of weight-bearing exercise is detrimental to the skeleton (that is, results in a loss of bone mineral density). This effect has been shown in astronauts and in patients confined to bed rest or immobilized in a cast. Studies have consistently indicated that weight-bearing bones are affected to a greater degree and that trabecular bone (measured in the spine) is lost at a greater rate than cortical bone.

Despite the fact that the exact amount and type of exercise needed to develop and maintain a healthy or enhanced skeletal system are unknown, there is evidence that suggests that physical activity, within a reasonable range, does have a positive effect on bone density. There is no consistent evidence that suggests that exercise training affects either skeletal maturation (measured by ossification) in growing children or bone length. Although isolated studies have shown both retarded and accelerated growth in stature in young athletes, the consensus is that youngsters involved in exercise training grow at the same rate and to the same extent as do their sedentary counterparts.[6, 40, 51, 58]

One approach to studying the effect of increased physical activity on bone density is to compare the dominant limb to the nondominant limb in sports such as tennis and baseball. These studies report that the dominant arm has greater bone mineral density or mass than the nondominant arm.[24, 26] This result appears to be true for both females and males and across a wide age span.

Another approach has been to compare different athletic groups with one another and with control groups. These studies collectively suggest that individuals who are involved in athletics or participate in vigorous fitness training have greater bone mineral density than sedentary controls. Furthermore, individuals who are involved in weight-bearing or impact-loading sports tend to have higher

TABLE 16.4 ▪ Effects of Physical Activity and Exercise Training on Bone Health

No or Too Little Activity	Acceptable Amounts of Activity	Too Much, High-Intensity, Long-Duration, Rapid Increment Activity
	Amount of Activity	
←		→
Low mineralization and density	Adequate mineralization or enhanced mineralization and density	Osteopenia or osteoporosis in amenorrheic athletes
Aging-associated osteoporosis	Normal rate of growth, stature, and proportion	Fragile bones; increased risk of fracture
Fragile bones; increased fracture potential	Delayed aging-associated osteoporosis	Overuse injuries include those to the elbow (bony spurs or bone disruption at joint surface), the vertebrae (microfractures leading to slippage), the knees (Osgood-Schlatter diseases: inflammation of the bones or cartilage), and the legs and feet (stress reactions and/or fractures)

bone mineral density than those involved in non-weight-bearing activities.[25, 53]

Training studies have also been conducted in which sedentary individuals initiated an exercise program. Measurements of bone mineral density were compared prior to and following the exercise training. In a study that investigated changes in bone mineral content with training and subsequent detraining, Dalsky and colleagues[9] reported that 22 months of weight-bearing exercise caused a significant increase (6.2%) in lumbar bone mineral content. When subjects discontinued exercise training (or trained less than three days per week), however, bone mineral content returned to baseline values. After 1 year of detraining, bone mineral content was only 1.1% above baseline values. These data suggest that the increase in bone mineral that results from exercise is lost if exercise is not continued; bone responds to activity and inactivity.

If some is good, more is not necessarily better when it comes to exercise training and bone health. As indicated in Table 16.4, excessive amounts of physical activity can potentially exceed the adaptive ability of bone, resulting in decreased bone density and/or overuse injuries.

Special Applications to Health and Fitness

This section will discuss several topics related to the practical implications of skeletal health of special interest to those involved in health and fitness. These topics include osteoporosis, amenorrhea, and skeletal injuries.

Osteoporosis

Osteoporosis is a serious health problem that affects over 20 million Americans.[2] Osteoporosis means "porous bones," and the condition is characterized by a loss of bone mineral density, resulting in bones that are weak and susceptible to fracture. This disease represents an imbalance between bone resorption and bone formation: Resorption occurs faster than formation, leading to a decrease in bone mineral density. Osteoporosis, as defined earlier, is a condition in which the bone mineral density is greater than 2.5 SD below the young normal adult average.[28] Figure 16.6 present photographs of nor-

(a)

(b)

FIGURE 16.6

Trabecular Bone
(a) Normal. (b) Osteoporotic.

mal and osteoporotic trabecular bone. Note the more porous trabeculae in the osteoporotic bone, which weakens the bone.

The most common sites of fracture related to osteoporosis are the hip, spine, and wrist. Approximately 275,000 hip fractures each year in the United States are related to osteoporosis. Most hip fractures require surgery, and there is a 15–20% mortality rate following such surgeries. The monetary cost of these operations exceeds $8 billion a year.[31] Spinal vertebral fractures occur when a osteoporotic bone is literally crushed by the weight of the body, resulting in a loss of height, curvature of the spine, and considerable pain.

The cause of osteoporosis is not known. However, several risk factors have been identified, and they are outlined in Table 16.5.[31,35,37] Genetic factors related to the development of osteoporosis include race, sex, family history, and body size. Nutritional factors associated with increased risk of osteoporosis include low calcium intake, excessive alcohol consumption, and consistently high protein intake.

Lifestyle factors associated with osteoporosis include lack of physical activity, smoking, and inadequate levels of estrogen (related to a delayed menarche, amenorrhea, or an early menopause). Several research studies have indicated that the rapid loss of bone mineral density following menopause is related to the decrease in estrogen levels at this time. These findings have led to an increase in the use of estrogen replacement therapy (ERT) for women who are at a higher risk of developing osteoporosis. The low activity levels of females in this country, particularly older women, also contribute to the risk of developing osteoporosis. Bone mineral content is positively related to long-term physical activity.

In addition to having a positive effect on bone mineral density, exercise may also be helpful in preventing fractures by increasing muscular strength and coordination and thereby decreasing the risk of falling. Individual factors that affect the risk of falling include coordination, sight, and muscular strength. Environmental factors that influence the risk of falling include lighting, floor surface, and footwear. Exercise leaders have a specific responsibility to provide an exercise area that reduces the risk of falling for the elderly.

Physical Activity, Altered Menstrual Function, and Bone Density

The elderly and postmenopausal females are not the only people at risk for developing osteoporosis and subsequent bone fractures; so too are young amen-

TABLE 16.5 ▪ Risk Factors Associated with Osteoporosis

Risk Factors	Relationship to Disease	Possible Explanations
Genetic		
Race	Whites are more likely to develop disease than African Americans	Unknown
Sex	Women are four times more likely to develop osteoporosis than men	Lighter bones of females; rapid bone loss following menopause; longer life span
Heredity	There appears to be a genetic predisposition to the disease	Unknown
Body build	Petite individuals are at greater risk	Less peak bone mass to lose
Lifestyle		
Lack of physical activity	Lack of weight-bearing activity increases risk of disease	No weight-bearing activities to stimulate bone formation
Smoking	Smoking increases risk of disease	May lower serum estrogen or cause early menopause
Sex hormones (late menarche, amenorrhea, or menopause)	Decrease in sex hormones is associated with increased risk	Loss of protective effect of estrogen on bone
Nutritional		
Calcium intake	Low calcium level interferes with bone formation	Insufficient calcium to adequately ossify bone
Alcohol use	Alcohol use may be damaging to bone	Resulting poor diet from excessive alcohol consumption

muscle is manipula
refers to the ability
ing length after bei
tics of muscles func
movement.

Macroscopic
Skeletal M

There are ov
human body, and
adult male body w
male body weigh
gether in a rema
integrated movem
ties, many of whic
Muscle action also
fitness activities,
seen in Figure 17.1
of bodybuilding.
tion in bodybuild
it is necessary to l

Organization

Skeletal muscles
ion, as depicted i
zation is appare
aspects of this org
muscle fibers are
electron microsco
Skeletal mus
dons, an arrange
a muscle to mov
gether by a thick
called the *fascia*. J
icate layer of con
directly covers t
The interior
bundles of musc
is *fasciculus* or *f*
by connective tis
that separates th
is called *perimys*
many individua
is surrounded b
called *endomysi*
The three la
sium, the perim

orrheic athletes. **Amenorrhea** is the absence of menses and may be classified as either primary or secondary. *Primary amenorrhea* refers to a late or delayed menarche. Mean menarcheal age in the United States is between 12.3 and 12.8 yr. Menarche is attained later in athletes than in the general population, although the degree of delay varies among sports. In general, swimmers show the least delay (a matter of a couple of months); dancers and gymnasts show delays of approximately 2 yr. Athletes who have been the most successful exhibit the greatest delays in menarche. Furthermore, the higher the level of competition, the higher the percentage of delayed menarche in the athletic population. The cause of the delay in menarche in young athletes has not yet been clearly established.[16, 50, 62]

Delayed menarche has not been associated with either increased or decreased bone mineral density, but it has been weakly (although inconclusively) linked with both secondary amenorrhea and high levels of stress fractures.[62] *Secondary amenorrhea* refers to the cessation of menstruation or menstrual periods that occur at intervals greater than 90 days after an established periodicity has been achieved. The exact incidence of secondary amenorrhea in athletes is unknown; however, it is generally acknowledged that young, competitive, lean female athletes engaged in high-intensity training are at a greater risk for developing amenorrhea than their sedentary counterparts. Like delayed menarche, this phenomenon is somewhat sport-specific, with those at the highest level of international competition showing the greatest vulnerability. In addition, as with delayed menarche, the cause of secondary amenorrhea has not yet been determined.[23, 29, 54, 55, 62]

Although the cause of secondary amenorrhea is not known, its effect on bone is quite clear. Amenorrheic athletes often have osteopenia, or decreased levels of bone mineral density.[8,12,34,42,52] The first study to show this effect did so quite accidently when one subgroup of amenorrheic women being studied for spinal mineral content just happened to be athletes.[8] Prior to this study, on the basis of the positive protective influence of exercise training on the bone density of postmenopausal women and the findings of enhanced bone mineralization in male athletes, exercise physiologists had simply assumed that female athletes, regardless of their menstrual status, would show the same benefits. When the re-

search study just cited showed that the amenorrheic athletes had 29% less spinal mineralization than normal controls, research in the area was stimulated.

The average results from subsequent studies of amenorrheic athletes are presented in Figure 16.7. The decrease in bone mineralization appears to be in vertebral bone, which is composed primarily of trabecular bone. Indeed, as shown in Figure 16.7, bone density measured at the cortical radius site is not distinguishable among amenorrheic athletes, normally cycling athletes, and sedentary controls, all of which exhibit values in the normal range. But no matter which unit is used to express body density ($g \cdot cm^{-2}$ or $mg \cdot cm^{-3}$), the bone density at the spinal site is different among the three groups. Other trabecular sites have not shown this deficit in bone mineral density. Therefore, vulnerability is not determined just by whether a bone is cortical or trabecular but is also specific to certain bones; the spine appears to be most vulnerable.[13] Although the differences may not appear to be great, a 25-year-old amenorrheic athlete's values in one study were equivalent to those of 51-yr-old women![12]

Note that the spinal trabecular values for the normally cycling athletes are not only higher than those for the amenorrheic athletes but are also at or above the normal expected values. Thus, if an athlete who trains hard maintains a normal menstrual cycle, the expected effect of enhanced bone density is maintained.

The factor that is most suspected as the causal link or mechanism in amenorrhea is a deficiency in estrogen (that is, a hypoestrogenic state).[8,23,42,52] Numerous studies have shown that a deficiency in estrogen is associated with both cessation of menstruation and low bone mineral density. Until the late 1980s when estrogen receptors were discovered on bone, researchers had speculated that estrogen exerted its influence on bone by its effect on calcium balance.[12] Increased amounts of calcium intake are needed in individuals who are hypoestrogenic. Highly trained hypoestrogenic female athletes often do not take in sufficient calcium. With the discovery of estrogen receptors on bone, however, a direct link

Amenorrhea The absence of menses.

Introduction

Muscle contra
human movemen
movement occurs
interactions amo
body. For instance
able to produce a
ergy for contract
process requires t
docrine, and card
tively to provide
and nutrients the
For the purposes
these other syste
properly.

Overview

Muscle tissu
teraction of its b
ments), which a
The function of
pends upon the
skeletal, smooth
contraction may
muscle), the mo
tubes such as t
(smooth muscle
(cardiac muscle)
ability to prod
characteristics
will focus on sk

Because sk
teristics, physi
names. That is
conscious contr
untary muscles

Irritability T
respond to sti

Contractility
a stimuli by s

Extensibility
stretched or

(a)

Tendons

Biceps brachii

Ulna

Radius

(b)

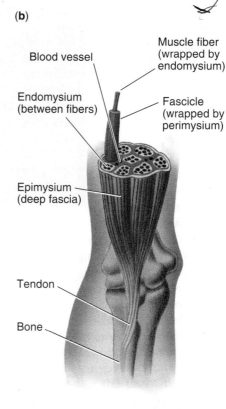

Blood vessel

Endomysium (between fibers)

Epimysium (deep fascia)

Tendon

Bone

Muscle fiber (wrapped by endomysium)

Fascicle (wrapped by perimysium)

FIGURE 17.2

Organization of Skeletal Tissue

(a) Intact skeletal muscle. Biceps brachii are attached to bones through tendons. (b) Connective tissue. The entire muscle is surrounded by connective tissue called epimysium. The muscle is organized into bundles called fasciculi, which are surrounded by connective tissue called perimysium. Each fasciculus contains many individual fibers surrounded by connective tissue called endomysium. Muscle fibers are long fibers with a striated appearance owing to the arrangement of their subunits.

Microscopic Structure of a Muscle Fiber

The individual muscle fibers that comprise the fasciculi are further subdivided into smaller units called myofibrils, which are in turn made up of myofilaments. This organization of skeletal muscle is shown in Figure 17.4, which should be referred to as you read the following sections.

Muscle Fibers

A muscle cell is also called a muscle fiber. *Muscle fibers* are long, cylinder-shaped cells ranging from 10 to 60 μm in diameter and from 1 to 400 mm in length.[16] As an overview of the muscle fibers, the major structures of a muscle fiber and their functions are summarized in Table 17.1 (p. 429).

A skeletal muscle fiber contains many nuclei, which are located just below the cell membrane. The *polarized plasma membrane* of a muscle cell is referred to as the *sarcolemma,* and it is the properties of this membrane that account for the irritability of muscle. The *sarcoplasm* of a muscle cell is similar to the cytoplasm of other cells, but it has specific adaptations to serve the functional needs of muscle cells, namely, increased amounts of glycogen and the oxygen-binding protein myoglobin.

The muscle fiber contains the organelles found in other cells (including a large number of mitochondria) along with some specialized organelles. The organelles that are of specific interest are the transverse tubules, the sarcoplasmic reticulum, and the myofibrils. The myofibrils are composed of the protein myofilaments and are responsible for the contractile properties of muscles.

Classification	Example	Diagram
Longitudinal	Sartorius	
Fusiform	Biceps brachii	
Radiate	Gluteus medius	
Unipennate	Tibialis posterior	
Bipennate	Gastrocuemius	
Circular	Orbicular oculi (and sphincters)	

FIGURE 17.3

Arrangement of Fasciculi

Sarcoplasmic Reticulum and Transverse Tubules   Figure 17.4 illustrates the relationship among the myofibrils, the sarcoplasmic reticulum and the transverse tubules. The **sarcoplasmic reticulum (SR)** is a specialized organelle that stores calcium. It is an interconnecting network of tubules running parallel with and wrapped around the myofibrils. (Notice in Figure 17.4 that the sarcolemma has been partially removed in order to illustrate the SR and myofibrils.) The major significance of the sarcoplasmic reticulum is its ability to store, release, and take up calcium and thereby control muscle contraction. Calcium is stored in the portion of the sarcoplasmic reticulum called the *lateral sacs* or *cisterns.*

The **transverse tubules (T tubules)** are organelles that carry the electrical signal from the sarcolemma to the interior of the cell. T tubules are continuous with the sarcolemma and protrude into the sarcoplasm of the cell. Although the T tubules run in close proximity to the sarcoplasmic reticulum and interact with it, they are anatomically separate organelles. As the name implies, the T tubules run perpendicular (transverse) to the myofibril. The spread of depolarization through the T tubules causes the release of calcium from the lateral sacs of the sarcoplasmic reticulum as an electrical signal is carried into the interior of the cell.

Myofibrils and Myofilaments   Each muscle fiber contains hundreds to thousands of smaller cylindrical units, or rod-like strands, called myofibrils (Figure 17.4). **Myofibrils** are contractile structures composed of myofilaments. These myofibrils, or simply fibrils, typically lie parallel to the long axis of the muscle cell and extend the entire length of the cell. Myofibrils account for approximately 80% of the volume of a muscle fiber.

As shown in Figure 17.4, each myofibril is composed of still smaller myofilaments (or filaments) that are arranged in a repeating pattern along the length of the myofibril. **Myofilaments** are contractile proteins (thick and thin) that are responsible for muscle contraction. It is the myofilaments that account for the majority of muscle protein. The repeating pattern of these myofilaments along the length of the myofibril gives skeletal muscle its striated appearance. Each repeating unit is referred to as a *sarcomere.*

Sarcoplasmic Reticulum (SR)   The specialized muscle cell organelle that stores calcium.

Transverse Tubules (T tubules)   Organelles that carry the electrical signal from the sarcolemma into the interior of the cell.

Myofibril   Contractile structures composed of myofilaments.

Myofilaments   Contractile (thick and thin) proteins that are responsible for muscle contraction.

FIGURE 17.4

Organization of a Muscle Fiber

The anatomical relationship among the organelles, specifically the myofibrils, T tubules, and sarcoplasmic reticulum (SR) is close. The repeating pattern of the myofibrils is due to the arrangement of the myofilaments.

Sarcomeres A **sarcomere** is the functional unit (contractile unit) of a muscle fiber. As illustrated in Figure 17.5 (p. 430), each sarcomere contains two types of myofilaments: *thick* filaments, composed primarily of the contractile protein myosin, and *thin* filaments, composed primarily of the contractile protein actin. Thin filaments also contain

Sarcomere The functional unit (contractile unit) of muscle fibers.

the regulatory proteins, troponin and tropomyosin. When myofilaments are viewed under an electron microscope, their arrangement gives the appearance of alternating bands of light and dark striations. The light bands are called *I bands* and contain only thin filaments. The dark bands are called *A bands* and contain thick and thin filaments, with the thick filaments running the entire length of the A band. Thus, it is the length of the thick filament that determines the length of the A band.

The names for the various regions of the sarcomere are not arbitrary; they are derived from the

TABLE 17.1 ■ Summary of Major Components of a Skeletal Muscle Cell

CELL PART	DESCRIPTION	FUNCTION
Nucleus	Multinucleated	Is the control center for the cell
Sarcolemma	Polarized cell membrane	Is capable of receiving stimuli from the nervous system
Sarcoplasm	Intracellular material	Holds organelles and nutrients; provides the medium for glycolytic enzymatic reactions
Organelles		
Myofibrils	Rodlike structures composed of smaller units called myofilaments; account for 80% of muscle volume	Contains contractile proteins (myofilaments), which are responsible for muscle contraction
T tubules	Series of tubules that run perpendicular to the cell and are open to the external part of cell	Spreads polarization from the cell membrane into the interior of cell, which triggers the sarcoplasmic reticulum to release calcium
Sarcoplasmic reticulum	Interconnecting network of tubules running parallel with and wrapped around the myofibrils	Stores and releases calcium
Mitochondria	Sausage or spherical-shaped organelles; numerous in a muscle cell	Is the major site of energy production

first letter of the German word that describes their appearance. The names for the bands describe the refraction of light through the respective bands. The I band is abbreviated from the word *isotropic,* which means that this area appears lighter because more light is able to pass through it. The A band is so named because of its *anisotropic* properties, meaning that it appears darker because it does not allow as much light to pass through. These properties are directly related to the type of filament present. The I bands allow more light to pass through them because they are composed of thin filaments. The A bands do not allow as much light to pass through because they are composed of both thick and thin filaments.

Each A band is interrupted in the midsection by an *H zone* (from the German *Hellerscheibe,* for "clear disc"), where there is no overlap of thick and thin filaments. Running through the center of the H zone is a dense line called the *M line* (from the German *Mittelscheibe,* for "middle disc"). The I bands are also interrupted at the midline by a darker area called the *Z disc* (from the German *Zwischenscheibe,* for "between disc"). A sarcomere extends from one Z disc to the successive Z disc. The Z disc serves to anchor the thin filaments to adjacent sarcomeres.

Note that the myofilaments occupy three-dimensional space. The arrangement of the myofilaments at different points in the sarcomere is shown in Figure 17.5d–17.5f. Notice that in regions where the thick and thin filaments overlap, each thick filament is surrounded by six thin filaments, and each thin filament is surrounded by three thick filaments.

A sarcomere consists of more than just contractile and regulatory proteins. Proteins of the cytoskeleton provide much of the internal structure of the muscle cell. Figure 17.6 (p. 431) diagrams the cytoskeleton of the sarcomere and its relationship to the contractile proteins.[3] The M line and the Z disc hold the thick and the thin filaments in place, respectively. The elastic filament helps keep the thick filament in the middle between the two Z discs during contraction.

Molecular Structure of the Myofilaments

The contractile proteins of the myofilaments slide over one another during muscular contraction.

(a)

(b)

Sarcomere

(c)

FIGURE 17.5

Arrangement of Myofilaments in a Sarcomere

(a) Photo of sarcomeres. (b) Model of sarcomeres. (c) Relationship between thick and thin filaments. (d) Cross-sectional view of thin filaments. (e) Cross-sectional view of thick filaments. (f) Cross-sectional view of thick and thin filaments.

Sliding Filament Theory of Muscle Contraction
The theory that explains muscle contraction as the result of the myofilaments sliding over one another.

Hence, **sliding-filament theory of muscle contraction** explains how muscles contract. Therefore, it is essential to pay careful attention to the structure of the myofilaments.

Thick Filaments

Thick filaments are composed primarily of myosin molecules (Figure 17.7). Each molecule of myosin has a rodlike tail and two globular heads (Figure 17.7a). A typical thick filament contains approximately 200 myosin molecules.[15] These molecules are oriented so that the tails form the central rodlike structure of the filament (Figure 17.7b). The globular myosin heads extend outward and will form *cross-bridges* when they interact with the thin filaments. The myosin heads have two reactive sites: One allows it to bind with the actin filament, and one binds to ATP.[10] It is only when the myosin heads bind to the active sites on actin, forming a cross-bridge, that contraction can occur.

The myosin subunits are oriented in opposite directions along the filament, forming a central section that lacks projecting heads (Figure 17.7c). The result is a bare zone in the middle of the filament, which accounts for the H zone seen in the middle of the A band (Figure 17.7d).

Thin Filaments

Thin filaments are composed primarily of the contractile protein actin. As illustrated in Figures 17.8a and 17.8b, actin is composed of small globular subunits (G actin) that form long strands called fibrous actin (F actin). A filament of actin is formed by two strands of F actin coiled about one another to form a double-helical structure; it resembles two strands of pearls wound around each other and may be referred to as a *coiled coil* (Figure 17.8c). The actin molecules contain an active site to which myosin heads will bind during contraction.

The thin filaments also contain the regulatory proteins called tropomyosin and troponin, which regulate the interaction of actin and myosin. *Tropomyosin* is a long, double-stranded, helical protein that is wrapped about the long axis of the actin backbone (Figure 17.8d). Tropomyosin serves to block the active site on actin, thereby inhibiting actin and myosin from binding under resting conditions.

Troponin is a small, globular protein complex composed of three subunits that control the position

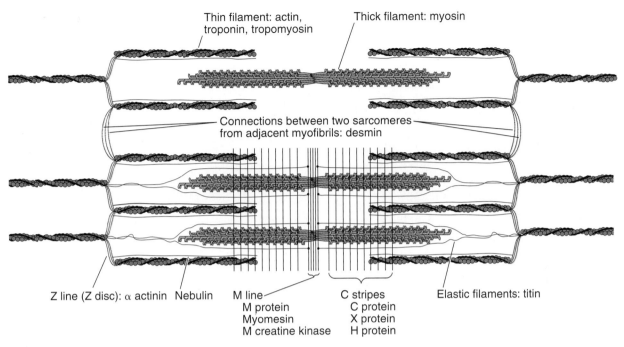

Thin filament: actin, troponin, tropomyosin

Thick filament: myosin

Connections between two sarcomeres from adjacent myofibrils: desmin

Z line (Z disc): α actinin   Nebulin

M line
M protein
Myomesin
M creatine kinase

C stripes
C protein
X protein
H protein

Elastic filaments: titin

FIGURE 17.6

Representation of Auxiliary Proteins in the Sarcomere

Source: From "Muscular Basis of Strength" by Rudolf Billeter and Hans Hoppeler. In *Strength and Power in Sport* (p. 45) by P. V. Komi (ed.). Champaign, IL: Human Kinetics Publishers. Copyright 1992 by International Olympic Committee. Reprinted by permission.

of the tropomyosin (Figure 17.9). The three units of troponin are troponin C (Tn-C), troponin I (Tn-I), and troponin T (Tn-T). Tn-C contains the calcium-binding sites, Tn-T binds troponin to tropomyosin, and Tn-I inhibits the binding of actin and myosin in the resting state (Figure 17.9b). When calcium binds to the Tn-C subunit, the troponin complex undergoes a configurational change, which causes tropomyosin to be removed from its blocking position, thus exposing the active sites on actin.[10,15] Once the active sites are exposed, the myosin heads are able to bind to the actin forming the cross-bridges (Figure 17.9c). Thus, calcium is the key to controlling the interaction of the filaments and, therefore, muscle contraction.

Contraction of a Muscle Fiber

In order for a muscle to contract, an *action potential* must be generated in the motor neuron. The message from the motor neuron must then be passed to the muscle fiber through the neuromuscular junction. Finally, the action potential must be conducted along the sarcolemma and into the interior of the muscle fiber to stimulate movement of the myofilaments. The process whereby electrical events in the sarcolemma are linked to the movement of the myofilaments is called *excitation-contraction coupling.*

As we describe the specific changes that occur during contraction, pay careful attention to three factors: the position of the myofilaments, the location of calcium ions, and the role of ATP.

The Sliding-Filament Theory of Muscle Contraction

A great deal of data has been amassed since the 1950s on the basis of X-ray, light microscopic, and electron microscopic studies to support the sliding-filament theory of muscle contraction. The basic principles of this theory are summarized in three statements:

(d)

FIGURE 17.7

Molecular Organization of Thick Filaments

(a) Individual myosin molecules have a rod-like tail and two globular heads. (b) Individual molecules are arranged so that the tails form a rod-like structure and the globular heads project outward to form cross-bridges. (c) Myosin subunits are oriented in opposite directions along the filament forming a central bare zone in the middle of the filament (H zone). (d) Thick filament (myosin) within a single sarcomere showing the myosin heads extending toward the thin filament.

1. The force of contraction is generated by the process that slides the actin filament over the myosin filament.

2. The lengths of the thick and the thin filaments do not change during muscle contraction.

3. The length of the sarcomere decreases as the actin filaments slide over the myosin filaments and pull the Z discs toward the center of the sarcomere.

Excitation-Contraction Coupling

Excitation-contraction coupling refers to the sequence of events by which an action potential in the

> **Excitation-Contraction Coupling** The sequence of events by which an action potential in the sarcolemma initiates the sliding of the myofilaments, resulting in contraction.
>
> **Cross-Bridging Cycle** The cyclic events that are necessary for the generation of force or tension within the myosin heads during muscle contraction.

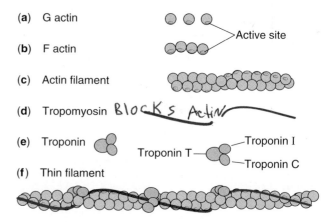

FIGURE 17.8

Molecular Organization of Thin Filaments

(a) Individual actin subunits (globular, G actin) shown with active site for binding to myosin heads. (b) Fibrous actin (F actin). (c) Actin filament with two strands of fibrous actin wound around itself to form a coiled coil. Active sites are exposed. (d) Tropomyosin is a regulatory protein that covers the binding site of actin. (e) Troponin is a regulatory protein that when bound to Ca++ removes tropomyosin from its blocking position on actin (f) The thin filament is composed of actin, tropomyosin, and troponin.

sarcolemma (an electrical event) initiates the sliding of the myofilaments, resulting in contraction (a mechanical event). Excitation-contraction coupling can be categorized into three phases:

1. The spread of depolarization

2. The binding of calcium to troponin

3. The generation of force

Figure 17.10 summarizes the events that occur during each phase of excitation-contraction coupling. Excitation-contraction coupling begins with depolarization and spread of an action potential (AP) along the sarcolemma (labeled 2 in Figure 17.10) and continues with the propagation of the action potential into the T tubules (labeled 2), causing the subsequent release of calcium from the lateral sacs of the sarcoplasmic reticulum (labeled 3). When calcium is released from the sarcoplasmic reticulum (the second phase), it binds to the troponin molecules, which undergo a configurational change, thereby removing tropomyosin from its blocking position on the actin filament (labeled 4 in the figure).

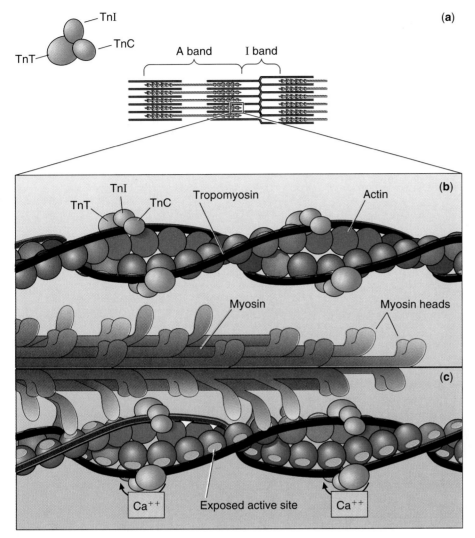

(a)

FIGURE 17.9

Regulatory Function of Troponin and Tropomyosin

(a) Tropomyosin is a small globular protein with three subunits. (b) Resting condition: Tropomyosin under resting conditions blocks the active sites of actin, preventing actin and myosin from binding. (c) Contraction: When troponin binds with Ca^{++}, it undergoes a configurational changes and *pulls* tropomyosin from the blocking position on the actin filament, allowing myosin heads to form cross-bridges with actin.

The third phase of excitation-contraction coupling is the cross-bridging cycle (labeled 5 in Figure 17.10). The **cross-bridging cycle** describes the cyclic events that are necessary for the generation of force or tension within the myosin heads during muscle contraction. The generation of tension within the contractile elements results from the binding of the myosin heads to actin and the subsequent release of stored energy in the myosin heads. As shown in Figure 17.11 (p. 435), four individual steps are necessary for the cross-bridging cycle.[2, 10, 15]

1. Binding of myosin heads to actin (cross-bridge formation)

2. Power stroke

3. Dissociation of myosin and actin

4. Activation of myosin heads

The first step in the cross-bridge cycle occurs when activated myosin heads (*M) bind with the active sites on actin, forming cross-bridges. In Figure 17.11 a centered dot (·) is used to indicate binding, and an asterisk (*) is used to indicate activated myosin heads. Thus, A · *M indicates that the activated myosin heads are bound to actin (A), whereas A + M indicates that actin and myosin are unbound.

The second step in the cross-bridging cycle is the power stroke. It is during this step that activated myosin heads swivel from their high-energy, activated position to a low-energy configuration (M

FIGURE 17.10

**Phases of Excitation-
Contraction Coupling**

❶ Resting

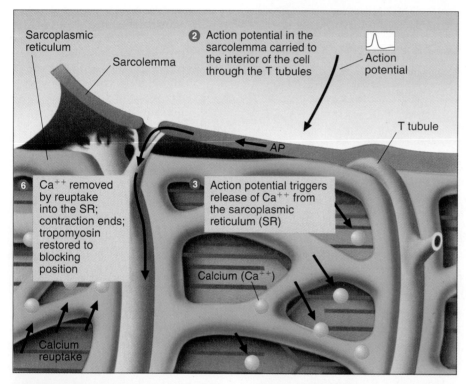

Sarcoplasmic reticulum

Sarcolemma

❷ Action potential in the sarcolemma carried to the interior of the cell through the T tubules

Action potential

T tubule

AP

❻ Ca^{++} removed by reuptake into the SR; contraction ends; tropomyosin restored to blocking position

❸ Action potential triggers release of Ca^{++} from the sarcoplasmic reticulum (SR)

Calcium (Ca^{++})

Calcium reuptake

Tropomyosin removed from blocking position on actin

Ca^{++}

❺ Activated myosin head binds to active site pulling the actin over the myosin and contracting the sarcomere

❹ Calcium binds to TnC subunit of troponin, causing exposure of the actin active site

with no *). This movement of the myosin cross-bridges results in a slight displacement of the thin filament over the thick filament toward the center of the sarcomere. As shown in Figure 17.11, during the second step ADP and P_i are released from the myosin heads, providing the energy for the power stroke. This results in myosin bound only to actin ($A \cdot M$).

FIGURE 17.11

Force Generation of the Contractile Elements: The Cross-Bridging Cycle

The third step involves the binding of ATP to the myosin heads and the subsequent dissociation of the myosin cross-bridges from actin, thus producing $A + M \cdot ATP$.

Note the role of ATP in steps 3 and 4. It is the *binding of ATP* molecules, in step 3, that allows the cross-bridges to detach. In the fourth step *it is the breakdown of ATP* that provides the energy to activate the myosin heads (*M). The activation of the myosin head is extremely important because it provides the cross-bridges with the stored energy to move the actin during the power stroke. The breakdown of ATP at this step depends upon the presence of myosin ATPase (also known as myofibrillar ATPase), as depicted in the following reaction:

$$\underset{\substack{\text{myosin} \\ \text{ATPase}}}{M \cdot ATP \longrightarrow {}^{*}M \cdot ADP + P_i}$$

Notice that the products of ATP hydrolysis, ADP + P_i, remain bound to the myosin cross-bridges and that the myosin is now in its high-energy or activated state.

The cross-bridging cycle will continue as long as calcium is bound to troponin (T_nC), causing the active sites on actin to be exposed, and ATP is available. On the other hand, activated myosin will remain in the resting state awaiting the next stimulus if calcium is not available in sufficient concentration to remove the inhibition of the regulatory protein [(4b) in Figure 17.11]. Since each cycle of the myosin cross-bridges barely displaces the actin, the myosin heads must bind to the actin and be displaced many times for a single contraction to occur. Thus, myosin will make and break its bond with actin hundreds or even thousands of times during a single muscle twitch. In order for this make-and-break cycle to occur, myosin heads must detach from actin and then be reactivated. This detaching and reactivating process requires the cycle to be repeated and requires the presence of ATP (step 3).

An analogy may be helpful for an understanding of the role of ATP in providing energy to activate the myosin head. Visualize a spring-loaded mousetrap. It takes energy to set the trap, just as it takes the splitting of ATP to set or activate the myosin. Once set, however, the trap will release energy when it is sprung. In a similar manner, the myosin head possesses stored energy, which will be released when the myosin heads bind to actin and swivel.

Admittedly, this process is complex (and perhaps intimidating at first). Take time to go through the cycle of events presented in Figure 17.11 several times. Try paying attention to different aspects of the figure (the symbols, the wording, the diagrams, the role of ATP) with each review of it.

Also, keep in mind that ATP plays several important roles in muscle contraction. The breakdown of ATP provides the energy to activate and reactivate the myosin cross-bridge prior to the binding with actin. ATP binding to the myosin head is also necessary to break the cross-bridge linkage between the myosin heads and the actin so that the cycle can be repeated. In addition, ATP is used for the return of calcium into the sarcoplasmic reticulum and restoration of the resting membrane potential once contraction has ended.

The final phase of muscular contraction is muscular relaxation. Relaxation occurs when the nerve impulse ceases and calcium is pumped back into the sarcoplasmic reticulum by active transport. In the absence of calcium tropomyosin returns to its blocking position and myosin heads are not able to bind to actin. Note that although we often place considerable emphasis on muscle contraction, the ability to relax a muscle following contraction is just as important.

Changes in the Sarcomere During Contraction

Much of the evidence supporting the sliding-filament theory comes from observation of changes in the length of a sarcomere during muscular contraction. Figure 17.12 provides diagrams of the sarcomere during rest (Figure 17.12a) and during contraction (Figure 17.12b) and also provides a photograph of the sarcomere during rest (Figure 17.12c). Notice that during contraction the A bands of adjacent sarcomeres move closer together, but the length of each A band does not change. Length is preserved because the A band is comprised of both thick and thin filaments of which the thick filaments are not compressible. The I band, however, shortens and may disappear as the actin is pulled over the myosin toward the center of the sarcomere. The greater amount of overlap of the thick and the thin filaments also causes the central H zones to disappear.

The shortening of the sarcomere is the result of the attachment of the myosin heads with the active site on actin and the subsequent release of stored energy that swivels the myosin cross-bridges. This step causes the actin to pull the Z disc toward the center of the sarcomere, which, in turn, causes the sarcomere length to decrease.

All-or-None Principle

According to the **all-or-none principle**, when a motor neuron is stimulated, all of the muscle fibers in that motor unit contract to their fullest extent or they do not contract at all. The minimal amount of stimuli necessary to initiate that contraction is referred to as the *threshold stimulus*. That is, if the threshold of contraction is reached, a muscle fiber will contract to its fullest extent. This phenomenon is related to the electrical properties of the cell membrane and refers to the contractile properties of a motor unit or a single muscle fiber only, not to the entire muscle.

To better understand this principle, consider the analogy of turning on a light switch. If sufficient

All-or-None Principle When a motor neuron is stimulated, all of the muscle fibers in that motor unit contract to their fullest extent or they do not contract at all.

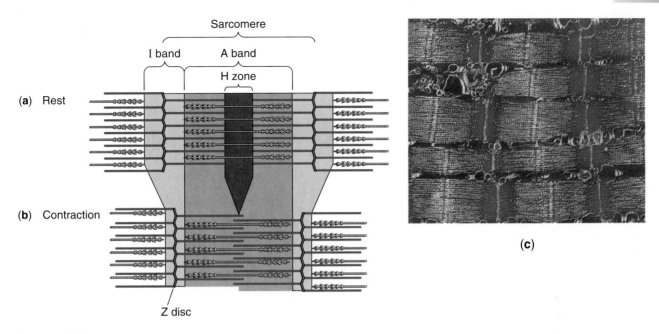

FIGURE 17.12

Changes in a Sarcomere During Contraction

(a) Sarcomere at rest. (b) During contraction of the sarcomere the lengths of actin and myosin filaments are unchanged. Sarcomere shortens because actin slides over myosin, pulling Z discs toward the center of the sarcomere. The H zone disappears, the I band shortens, and the A band remains unchanged. (c) Micrograph of sarcomere at rest.

pressure is applied to the switch (to reach a threshold for flipping it on), the lights will be turned on to their fullest extent. Expanding the analogy to a motor unit, when you turn on a light switch that controls a group of lights (such as the overhead lights in a classroom), all of the lights connected to it will turn on to their fullest extent. You cannot cause the lights to be brighter by pulling (or pushing) the light switch harder. It is an-all-or-none response. Either you produce enough force to turn the lights on, or you do not. The same is true for an individual muscle fiber or a motor unit: Either a threshold stimulus is reached and contraction occurs, or a threshold stimulus is not reached and contraction does not occur.

Muscle Fiber Types

Muscle fibers are typically described by two characteristics: their contractile properties and their metabolic properties (Figure 17.13). On the basis of

FIGURE 17.13

Properties of Motor Units

Muscle Fibers			
Twitch properties	Slow	Fast	
Metabolic properties	Oxidative	Oxidative/ glycolytic	Glycolytic
Name based on twitch and metabolic properties	SO	FOG	FG
Other nomenclature	ST, Type I	FTa, FTA, Type IIA	FTb, FTB, Type IIB
Motor Neurons			
Neuron type	α_2	α_1	α_1
Neuron size	Small	Large	Large
Conduction velocity	Slow	Fast	Fast
Recruitment threshold	Low	High	High

differences in *contractile properties*, human muscle fibers can be divided into two types, *slow-twitch* (ST) and *fast-twitch* (FT) *fibers.* Slow-twitch fibers are sometimes called Type I fibers; fast-twitch fibers are correspondingly called Type II fibers. The difference between ST and FT fibers appears to be almost ab-solute—like the difference between black and white. Some FT fibers contract and relax slightly faster than other fast-twitch fibers, but both of them are clearly much faster than ST fibers. To understand the dif-ference between twitch speeds, we must consider the integration of muscles and nerves.

Striated muscle fibers as described in this chap-ter are sometimes referred to as extrafusal muscle fibers. Extrafusal muscle fibers are innervated by alpha (α) motor neurons, which are subdivided into two categories, α_1 and α_2. The α_1 neurons innervate FT fibers, and the α_2 neurons innervate ST fibers. Figure 17.14 shows an experiment in which the in-nervation of muscle fibers was manipulated: The α_1 neuron was severed from the FT fibers and con-nected to the ST fibers, and the α_2 neuron was cut from the ST fibers and connected to the FT fibers. What conclusion can we draw from this diagram re-garding why a muscle fiber is either ST or FT? Since the ST fiber became an FT fiber when the α_1 neuron replaced the α_2 neuron and vice versa, it is logical to conclude that the contractile property of muscle de-pends on the type of motor neuron that innervates the muscle fiber.[11]

What cannot be seen from the experiment is that other elements in the muscle, especially the con-tractile enzyme myosin ATPase, also contribute to twitch speed and account for some of the variation

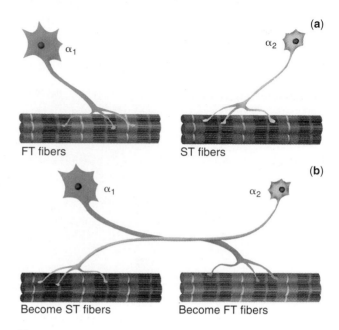

FIGURE 17.14

Results of Cross Innervation

(a) Under normal conditions α_1 neurons innervate FT fibers and α_2 neurons innervate ST fibers. (b) If the neurons supplying the muscles are switched (cross-innervated), the muscle fibers acquire the properties of the new motor neuron.

Slow Oxidative (SO) Fibers Slow-twitch muscle fibers that rely primarily on oxidative metabolism to produce energy.

Fast Oxidative Glycolytic (FOG) Fibers Fast-twitch muscle fibers that have the ability to work under oxidative and glycolytic conditions.

Fast Glycolytic (FG) Fibers Fast-twitch muscle fibers that perform primarily under glycolytic con-ditions.

Motor Unit A motor neuron and the muscle fibers it innervates.

---

in twitch speed.[14] Indeed, when muscle fibers are typed, it is often the amount of stain for myosin ATPase that is used to distinguish twitch speed, since the motor neurons are not typically biopsied. Note that α_2 motor neurons are the smaller of the two nerves and innervate the ST muscles fibers; the α_1 motor neurons are the larger nerves and inner-vate the FT muscle fibers. The size difference is im-portant because small motor neurons have low excitation thresholds and slow conduction veloci-ties. Because of the properties of the motor neuron that innervates them, ST fibers are recruited at low-work intensities. The reverse is true for the larger (α_1) motor neurons.

On the basis of differences in *metabolic properties,* human muscle fibers can be described as *glycolytic, oxidative,* or a combination of both. All muscle fibers can produce energy both anaerobically (that is, without oxygen, labeled as glycolytic) and aerobi-cally (that is, with oxygen, labeled as oxidative).

These processes and terms are fully explained in the unit on metabolism, but this general understanding is sufficient at this point if you have not yet covered that unit.

Despite the ability of all muscle fibers to produce energy by both glycolytic and oxidative processes, one or the other may predominate or the production may be balanced. Thus, the metabolic properties of muscle fibers do not represent discrete entities as much as a continuum (oxidative to glycolytic) of shades of gray, as opposed to the black-and-white type of dichotomy seen for twitch speed (slow or fast twitch). The metabolic properties are determined by staining for key enzymes in the muscle specimen [often phosphofructokinase (PFK) for glycolytic processes and succinate dehydrogenase (SDH) for oxidative processes].[12]

Slow-twitch fibers rely primarily on oxidative metabolism to produce energy and are therefore referred to as **slow oxidative (SO) fibers.** Fast-twitch fibers that have the ability to work under both oxidative and glycolytic conditions are called **fast oxidative glycolytic (FOG) fibers.** These fibers are also referred to as fast-twitch A (FTa, FTA, or Type IIA) fibers. Other fast-twitch fibers that perform predominantly under glycolytic conditions are called **fast glycolytic (FG) fibers.** These fibers are also called fast-twitch B (FTb, FTB, or Type IIB) fibers. A third type of fast-twitch fiber (between FTa and FTb, called unclassified, undifferentiated, Type IIC, or FTc) appears to represent a small percentage of total muscle fibers primarily in infants. By the end of the first year of life these Type IIC fibers have largely become differentiated, and by age 6 a normal adult pattern has been established.[1] Figure 17.13 and Table 17.2 summarize the properties of motor units on the basis of muscle fibers and various properties of their motor neurons.

A **motor unit** is defined as a motor neuron (α_1 or α_2) and the muscle fibers it innervates. As we have just seen, the twitch speed of a muscle fiber depends largely on the motor neuron that innervates

TABLE 17.2 ■ **Structural and Functional Characteristics of Muscle Fibers**

	Type I	Type II	
CONTRACTILE:	ST	FTa	FTb
METABOLIC:	SO	FOG	FG
STRUCTURAL ASPECTS			
Muscle fiber diameter	Small	Largest	Large
Mitochondrial density	High	High	Low
Capillary density	High	Medium	Low
Myoglobin content	High	Medium	Low
FUNCTIONAL ASPECTS			
Twitch (contraction) time	Slow	Fast	Fast
Relaxation time	Slow	Fast	Fast
Force production	Low	High	High
Fatigability	Fatigue-resistant	Fatigable	Most fatigable
METABOLIC ASPECTS			
Phosphocreatine stores	Low	High	High
Glycogen stores	Low	High	High
Triglyceride stores	High	Medium	Low
Myosin-ATPase activity	Low	High	High
Glycolytic enzyme activity	Low	High	High
Oxidative enzyme activity	High	High	Low

it. Thus, all muscle fibers within a motor unit will be either FT or ST. In addition, since all muscle fibers in a motor unit are recruited to contract together, they will require the same metabolic capabilities as well. Therefore, a motor unit is composed exclusively of SO, FOG, or FG muscle fibers. Thus, when reference is made to muscle fiber types, it also means motor unit types.

Table 17.2 further compares the different muscle fiber types in reference to important structural, neural, functional, and metabolic characteristics. As the table indicates, the diameters of the individual muscle fibers differ between ST and FT fibers. The size of the muscle fiber is related to the size of the nerve fiber innervating it but primarily reflects the amount of contractile proteins. ST fibers are smaller than FT fibers and have smaller motor neurons. The larger size of the FT fibers is the result of their having more contractile proteins, which, in turn, enables them to produce greater force. Figure 17.15 indicates differences in force production, twitch speed, and fatigue curve for the different fibers.[7]

Other structural differences exist between fiber types that can be related directly to their predominant metabolic pathway for energy production. The SO fibers, which rely mainly on oxidative pathways for energy production, have a high number of mitochondria, high capillary density, high myoglobin content, and high oxidative enzyme activity. The FG fibers, which rely primarily on glycolytic pathways for energy production, have few mitochondria, low capillary density, low myoglobin content, and high glycolytic enzyme activity. The FOG fibers require the most attention because they possess not only characteristics common to both SO and FG but also characteristics unique to themselves. Specifically, the FOG fibers have high mitochondrial density, moderate or medium capillary density and myoglobin content, and both high glycolytic and high oxidative enzyme activity.

FIGURE 17.15

Force Production and Fatigue Curves of Fiber Types
Source: Adapted from Edington & Edgerton.[7]

(a) Force Production

(b) Fatigue Curves

The metabolic differences both require and reflect differences in energy substrate availability. All muscles store and utilize glycogen; but since glycogen is the only substrate (along with its constituent parts—glucose) that can be used to fuel glycolysis, it makes sense that the FOG and FG fibers would have higher glycogen stores than SO fibers have. Conversely, since triglycerides can only be broken down and used oxidatively, it would be anticipated that SO fibers would have more triglyceride storage than either FG or FOG fibers. Furthermore, FOG fibers would have an intermediate amount—more than FG but less than SO fibers.

Because SO fibers are so well supplied by the cardiovascular system and either have or can get ample fuel supplies (that is, energy substrate), particularly from triglycerides, they are very resistant to fatigue. Because the FOG fibers have a substantial oxidative capability and the FG fibers do not, the FG fibers are the quickest to fatigue. The FOG fibers are somewhat less resistant to fatigue than the SO fibers and somewhat more resistant to fatigue than the FG fibers.

Table 17.2 is a convenient way to make logical sense of all of this information and to check your understanding of the characteristics of each fiber type. Take a few minutes now to study this table and interrelate all of the information. Remember that although the fiber types have been labeled at the top of the columns separately for their contractile and metabolic properties, in practice the designations ST and SO, FTa and FOG, FTb and FG are used interchangeably.

Assessment of Muscle Fiber Type

The determination of muscle fiber type is typically an invasive procedure that involves needle biopsy of skeletal muscle. A core sample is withdrawn and frozen in liquid nitrogen; then the sample is sliced into thin cross sections, and each is stained with a chemical preparation. Although muscle fibers can be typed noninvasively by nuclear magnetic resonance spectroscopy (NMR), this is still an expensive, little-used laboratory technique.[4] Attempts to use the vertical jump as a field measure of fiber type have proven unsuccessful.[6]

Despite the lack of ability to easily determine fiber types, knowledge about fiber types is important for at least three reasons.

1. Fiber type differences help explain individual differences in performance and response to training.

2. Fiber type differences help explain what training can and cannot do.

3. The relationship between fiber types, training, and performance in elite athletes helps in the design of training programs for others who wish to be successful in specific events even if they do not know their exact fiber type percentages or distribution.

Distribution of Fiber Types

All of the muscles of the human body are composed of a combination of slow-twitch and fast-twitch muscle fibers arranged in a mosaic pattern. This arrangement is thought to reflect the variety of tasks that human muscles must perform. The relative distribution of these fibers, however, may vary greatly from one muscle to another. For example, the soleus muscle may have as much as 85% ST fibers, and the triceps and ocular muscles may have as few as 30% ST fibers. The distribution may also vary from one individual to another for the same muscle group.[12] In general, the following statements describe the distribution of fiber types.

1. Although distribution of fiber type varies within and between individuals, most individuals posses between 45 and 55% ST fibers.

2. The distribution of fiber types is not different for males and females, although males tend to show greater extremes or variation than females.

3. After early childhood the fiber distribution does not change significantly as a function of age.

4. Fiber type distribution is primarily genetically determined.

5. Muscles that are involved in sustained postural activity have the highest number of slow-twitch muscle fibers.

Fiber Type in Athletes

Few topics have caused as much interest and debate as the topic of fiber type in athletes. Figure 17.16 shows the distribution of fiber types for male and female athletes. Athletes involved in endurance ac-

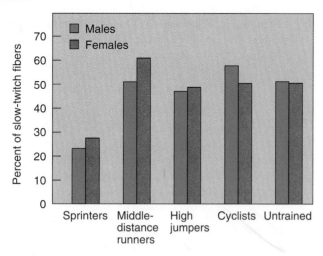

FIGURE 17.16

Fiber Type Distribution Among Athletes

Source: Data from Fox et al.[8]

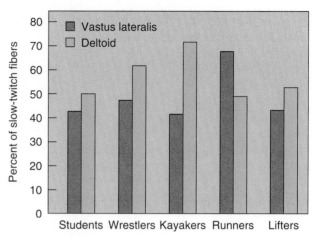

FIGURE 17.17

Fiber Type Distribution of Different Muscle Groups Among Athletes

Source: Tesch & Karlsson.[13]

tivities typically have a higher percentage of slow-twitch fibers; athletes involved in power activities have a higher percentage of fast-twitch muscle fibers. Note, however, that there is a large range of fiber type in each group, indicating that athletic success is not determined solely by fiber type.

Not only do endurance athletes differ in general fiber type from power or resistance athletes, but often these differences are site-specific within athletic groups. The results of one study of fiber type distribution are reported in Figure 17.17.[13] According to the study, the vastus lateralis muscles of the legs possess a greater percentage of ST fibers in endurance athletes who rely heavily upon the legs for their activity (such as runners). On the other hand, athletes whose sport requires endurance of the upper body possess a greater percentage of ST fibers in the deltoid muscle.

An interesting question arises when looking at the fiber type distribution of various athletes: Did training for and participating in a given sport influence the fiber type, or did fiber type influence the type of athletic participation? Available evidence indicates that the distribution of fiber types based on contractile properties (ST or FT) is genetically determined and is not altered in humans by exercise training.[12,16] There is evidence, however, that training can alter the metabolic properties of the cell (enzyme concentration, substrate storage, and so on). These changes may lead to a conversion of FT fiber

subdivisions. Indeed, with endurance training the oxidative potential of FOG and FG fibers can exceed that of SO fibers of sedentary individuals.[12]

In summary, the distribution of fiber types varies considerably within the muscle groups of an individual and between individuals. The basic distribution of fiber type appears to be genetically determined. Training may alter the metabolic capabilities of muscle fibers (but not the contractile properties), and there remains the possibility that this alteration could be significant enough to change the classification of the FT fibers.

SUMMARY

1. Skeletal muscles provide for locomotion and manipulation, maintain body posture, and play an important role in heat generation.

2. The characteristics that allow a muscle to produce movement include irritability, contractility, extensibility, and elasticity.

3. A motor neuron and the muscle fibers it innervates is called a motor unit. Because each muscle fiber in a motor unit is connected to the same neuron, the electrical activity in the motor neuron controls the contractile activity of all the muscle fibers in a given motor unit.

4. Skeletal muscle fibers are bundled together into groups of fibers called fasciculi. A muscle fiber is itself comprised of smaller units called myofibrils, which are, in turn, made up of myofilaments.

5. There are two types of myofilaments: thick and thin filaments. It is the repeating pattern of these myofilaments along the length of the myofibril that gives skeletal muscle its striated appearance.

6. Each repeating unit is referred to as a sarcomere and represents the functional unit of the muscle.

7. Tropomyosin is a regulatory protein that serves to block the active site on actin, thereby inhibiting actin and myosin from binding under resting conditions. The position of tropomyosin is controlled by troponin.

8. Excitation-contraction coupling refers to the sequence of events by which an action potential in the sarcolemma initiates the contractile process of the myofilaments.

9. Excitation-contraction coupling has three phases: the spread of depolarization, the binding of calcium to troponin, the generation of force. The cross-bridging cycle describes the generation of force. This cycle consists of the binding of myosin to actin, the powerstroke, the dissociation of myosin and actin, and the activation of myosin heads.

10. The spread of depolarization (action potential) is carried into the interior of the muscle fiber by the T tubules. As the electrical signal is carried into the cell, it causes the release of calcium, which is stored in the lateral sacs of the sarcoplasmic reticulum.

11. When calcium is released from the sarcoplasmic reticulum, it binds to the troponin molecules, which undergo a configuration change, thereby removing tropomyosin from its blocking position on the actin filament. This removal of tropomyosin allows the myosin cross-bridges (heads) to bind with the actin filaments.

12. The generation of tension within the contractile elements results from the binding of actin and myosin, which causes the release of stored energy in the myosin heads.

13. ATP plays several important roles in muscle contraction. The hydrolysis of ATP provides the energy to activate or reactivate the myosin head prior to binding with actin. ATP binding is also necessary to break the linkage between the myosin cross-bridge and actin so that the cycle can be repeated. ATP is also used to return calcium to the sarcoplasmic reticulum and to restore the resting membrane potential.

14. During relaxation calcium is pumped back into the sarcoplasmic reticulum (by active transport), and troponin no longer keeps tropomyosin from its blocking position.

15. When a muscle fiber or motor unit is stimulated to contract, it contracts to its fullest extent, or it does not contract at all. This response is referred to as the all-or-none principle.

16. Human muscle fibers can be divided into two different types, ST and FT, on the basis of contractile properties. The FT fibers can be further subdivided into FOG and FG fibers on the basis of metabolic properties.

17. Athletes involved in endurance activities typically have a higher percentage of slow-twitch fibers. Athletes involved in power activities typically have a higher percentage of fast-twitch muscle fibers.

18. Training may alter the metabolic capabilities of muscle fibers (but not the contractile properties), and there remains the possibility that this alteration could be significant enough to change the classification of the FT fibers.

REVIEW QUESTIONS

1. List, in order of largest to smallest, the major components of the whole muscle.

2. What causes the striated appearance of skeletal muscle fibers?

3. What are the T tubules and the sarcoplasmic reticulum? What is the function of each?

4. Relate each region of the sarcomere to the presence of thick and thin myofilaments.

5. Diagram a sarcomere at rest and at the end of a contraction, and identify each of the areas.

6. Describe the role of the regulatory proteins in controlling muscle contraction.

7. Describe the sequence of events in excitation-contraction coupling.

8. Identify the role of ATP in the production of force within the contractile unit of muscle.

9. What is the role of calcium in muscle contraction?

10. Describe the all-or-none principle as it relates to the contraction of a single muscle fiber.

11. Diagram the force production, twitch speed, and fatigue curve for the different fiber types.

12. Discuss the possibility of influencing fiber type distribution by exercise training.

REFERENCES

1. Baldwin, K. M.: Muscle development: neonatal to adult. In R. L. Terjung (ed.), *Exercise and Sport Sciences Reviews*. Baltimore: Williams & Wilkins. 12:1–19 (1984).

2. Berne, R. B., & M. N. Levy: *Physiology*. St. Louis: Mosby, 315–342 (1988).

3. Billeter, R., & H. Hoppler: Muscular basis of strength. In P. V. Komi (ed.), *Strength and Power in Sport*. Oxford: Blackwell Scientific, 39–63 (1992).

4. Boicelli, C. A., A. M. Baldassarri, C. Borsetto, & F. Conconi: An approach to noninvasive fiber type distribution

by nuclear magnetic resonance. *International Journal of Sports Medicine.* 10:53–54 (1989).

5. Costill, D. L.: *Inside Running: Basics of Sports Physiology.* Indianapolis: Benchmark Press, 1–29 (1986).

6. Costill, D. L.: Muscle biopsy research: Application of fiber composition to swimming. *Proceedings from Annual Clinic of American Swimming Coaches Association, Chicago.* Ft. Lauderdale: American Swimming Coaches Association (1978).

7. Edington, D. W., & V. R. Edgerton: *The Biology Of Physical Activity.* Boston: Houghton Mifflin (1986).

8. Fox, E. L., R. W. Bowers, & M. L. Foss: *The Physiological Basis for Exercise and Sport.* Dubuque, IA: Brown & Benchmark, 94–135 (1993).

9. Fox, S.: *Human Physiology.* Dubuque, IA: Brown (1987).

10. Marieb, E.: *Human Anatomy and Physiology* (2nd edition). Redwood City, CA: Benjamin/Cummings (1992).

11. Noth, J.: Motor units. In P. V. Komi (ed.), *Strength and Power in Sport.* Oxford: Blackwell Scientific, 21–28 (1992).

12. Saltin, B., J. Henriksson, E. Nygaard, P. Anderson, & E. Jansson: Fiber types and metabolic potentials of skeletal muscles in sedentary man and endurance runners. *Annals of the New York Academy of Sciences.* 301:3–29 (1977).

13. Tesch, P. A., & J. Karlsson: Muscle fiber types and size in trained and untrained muscles of elite athletes. *Journal of Applied Physiology.* 59:1716–1720 (1985).

14. Van deGraaff, K. M., & S. I. Fox: *Concepts of Human Anatomy and Physiology* (2nd edition). Dubuque, IA: Brown, 291–355 (1989).

15. Vander, A. J., J. H. Sherman, & D. S. Luciano: *Human Physiology: The Mechanisms of Body Function* (4th edition). New York: McGraw-Hill (1985).

16. Williams, J.: Normal musculoskeletal and neuromuscular anatomy, physiology, and responses to training. In S. M. Hasson, *Clinical Exercise Physiology.* St. Louis: Mosby-Year Book Publishers (1994).

18

Muscular Contraction and Human Movement

After studying the chapter, you should be able to:

- Differentiate between force and load.

- Identify the different types of muscle contraction, and indicate the proper use of the terms to describe muscle fiber contraction or whole-muscle contraction.

- Compare and contrast concentric and eccentric dynamic contractions.

- Describe neural and mechanical factors that affect force development.

- Differentiate between the length-tension relationship as it applies to a muscle fiber and as it applies to a whole muscle.

- Identify possible causes of muscle fatigue.

- Outline the two primary models that explain delayed-onset muscle soreness,

and discuss a possible integration of these two models.

- Refute the popular belief that delayed onset muscle soreness is caused by an accumulation of lactic acid in the muscle.

- Identify the different laboratory and field methods for assessing muscular function.

- Describe the basic pattern of strength development.

- Compare and contrast the expression of strength in males and in females.

- Describe the factors that affect age-related loss of muscular strength.

- Discuss the heritability of muscle function.

*E*xercise—The Result of Muscle Contraction

The definition of exercise in *Taber's Cyclopedia Medical Dictionary* is "performed activity of the muscles."[38] In other words, the contraction of muscles is exercise. Therefore, it is impossible to discuss the exercise response of the neuromuscular system in the same way that it is discussed for the cardiovascular-respiratory or metabolic systems.

Nonetheless, there are enough differences in the contraction of muscles that an endless number of exercises result. For example, imagine a basketball player taking off from the foul line for a slam dunk, a bodybuilder flexing in a pose, a swimmer slicing through the water doing a front crawl stroke, the movement of your eyes across the pages of this book. All of these activities require different muscle actions—explosive dynamic power; controlled static activity; constant force against a resistance through a large range of motion; highly coordinated, rapid, but minimal force movement. In fact, the list of individual actions involving muscle contractions is practically endless; yet some generalities are apparent, and hence, some classifications can be made. But first, some terms must be clarified.

Tension Versus Load

The force developed when a contracting muscle acts on an object is called *muscle tension.* The force exerted on the muscle by the object is called the *load.* The load and muscle tension are opposing forces.

The term *contraction* refers to the initiation of the tension-producing process of the contractile elements within muscle. However, not all contractions

---

Torque The capability of a force to produce rotation.

Isotonic Contraction A muscle fiber contraction in which the tension generated by the muscle is constant through the range of motion.

Dynamic Contraction A muscle contraction in which the force exerted varies as the muscle shortens to accommodate change in muscle length and/or joint angle throughout the range of motion while moving a constant external load.

---

produce movement; movement depends on the magnitude of the load exerted and the tension produced by the muscle. In order for a muscle to move a load, the force of muscle tension must exceed the force of the load. Furthermore, muscle tension developed experimentally in an isolated muscle fiber, a motor unit, or even a whole muscle is not necessarily the same as the force developed by an intact muscle in the human body.

All human motion involves rotation of body segments about their joint axes. The capability of a force to produce rotation is referred to as **torque.**[16] Thus, torque is force applied at some distance away from the center of the joint, causing the limb to rotate around the joint. Torque changes as a muscle moves bone through the range of motion.

Classification of Muscle Contractions

A classification of muscle contractions is presented in Table 18.1. This classification is based upon three component characteristics: time (as duration and/or velocity), displacement (length change), and force production. The type of muscle contraction affects how much force can be produced by a given muscle.

As shown in Table 18.1, at the muscle fiber or motor unit level three basic types of contraction are possible: isotonic, isokinetic, and isometric. The name *isotonic contraction* indicates that the force production (or tonus) is unchanged (*iso* means "same") when the muscle contracts, causing movement of an external load. An **isotonic contraction** is a muscle fiber contraction in which the tension generated by the muscle is constant throughout the range of motion. In the intact human system such a contraction is practically impossible. What actually happens is that the muscle force varies as the muscle contracts. This variation is necessary to accommodate changes in muscle length and/or joint angles as limbs move through their ranges of motion. Thus, the load is constant, but the force produced to move it through the range of motion is not. Therefore, the term *dynamic,* or *isotorque,* is more accurate to describe contraction within the intact human.

A **dynamic contraction** is a muscle contraction that produces movement of the skeleton. If the movement results from a dynamic muscle contraction that produces tension during shortening, it is a **concentric contraction.** Concentric contractions result in positive external work and are primarily re-

TABLE 18.1 ▪ Classification of Contractions

Type of Contraction		External Work in Intact Muscle in Humans	Function of Contraction
Muscle Fiber or Motor Unit	**for Intact Muscle in Humans**		
Isotonic: constant-force production: shortening, or lengthening	**Dynamic concentric (isotorque):** muscle force varies as muscle shortens to accommodate change in muscle length and/or joint angles as limb moves through ROM while moving a constant external load	Positive: (work = force × distance); external load can be overcome	Acceleration
	Dynamic eccentric: see above, except muscle lengthens	(work = force × negative distance); external load assists lengthening	Deceleration
Isokinetic: constant velocity of lengthening or shortening	**Isokinematic (dynamic):** rate of limb displacement or joint rotation is constant. Velocity varies with joint angle.	Positive or negative: see above	Acceleration or deceleration
Isometric: constant muscle length	**Static:** limb displacement or joint rotation does not occur; little muscle fiber shortening occurs	Zero: (work = force × distance, where distance = 0); external load cannot be overcome	Fixation

Source: Komi;[25] Williams.[41]

Note: ROM = range of motion.

sponsible for acceleration in movement. The lifting action of the biceps in curling a barbell is an example of a concentric dynamic contraction. The discussion in Chapter 17 of the sliding-filament theory describes this type of contraction.

If movement occurs as a result of a dynamic muscle contraction that produces tension while lengthening, the contraction is referred to as an **eccentric contraction.** Eccentric contractions result in negative work and are primarily responsible for deceleration in movement. The lowering action of the biceps in curling a barbell is an example of an eccentric dynamic contraction. During an eccentric contraction the cross-bridges are cycling as the filaments are being pulled apart. Because of this action of being pulled apart, strenuous eccentric activities can cause damage to myofibrils. However, strenuous eccentric contractions also allow for a greater force of contraction at a lower energy cost than do concentric contractions.[37]

Why can an eccentric contraction produce more force than a concentric one? During a concentric contraction only about half of the available cross-bridges cycle. During an eccentric contraction some of the cross-bridges do not cycle, but are continually pulled backward. Because the cross-bridges are pulled backward, the myosin heads do not rotate forward, and the actin and myosin remain bound.[37] As the contraction continues, additional cross-bridges are formed in an amount that may exceed the number of cross-bridges in a concentric contraction. Hence, more tension can be produced.

Why does eccentric (negative) work have a lower energy cost than concentric (positive) work? The answer to this question is not completely

Concentric Contraction A dynamic muscle contraction that produces tension during shortening.

Eccentric Contraction A dynamic muscle contraction that produces tension (force) while lengthening.

known, but two possibilities have been suggested.[37] First, fewer muscle fibers are recruited during eccentric than during concentric contractions; fewer fibers use less oxygen, which translates to a smaller energy cost. Second, because some of the cross-bridges do not cycle, less ATP is broken down and used as energy. Researchers estimate that positive work uses three to nine times more energy than negative work. All you have to do is think about climbing up the stairs in a high-rise building and then think about walking down them to believe this estimate.

Isokinetic contractions are also dynamic contractions in that movement occurs; the force generated is sufficient to overcome the external load. What differentiates isokinetic contractions from other forms of dynamic contractions is that the rate of shortening or lengthening (*kinesis* means "motion") is constant (*iso* means "same"). An **isokinetic contraction** is a muscle fiber contraction in which the velocity of contraction is kept constant. In the intact human the velocity of the movement actually varies with the joint angle; however, the rate of limb displacement or joint rotation can be held constant with the help of special exercise equipment. Thus, the term **isokinematic** is technically more accurate; the term *isokinetic* is more likely to be used, though.

A muscle fiber contraction that does not result in a length change in muscle fiber is termed an **isometric contraction.** In an isometric contraction the cross-bridges are cycling—hence producing tension—but sliding of the filaments does not occur.

Isokinetic Contraction A muscle fiber contraction in which the velocity of the contraction is kept constant.

Isokinematic Contraction A muscle contraction in which the rate of limb displacement or joint rotation is held constant with the use of specialized equipment.

Isometric Contraction A muscle fiber contraction that does not result in a length change in muscle fiber.

Static Contraction A muscle contraction that produces an increase in muscle tension but does not cause meaningful limb displacement or joint displacement and therefore does not result in movement of the skeleton.

This kind of action is possible in an isolated fiber because the fiber can be stabilized at both ends in an experimental apparatus before being stimulated. However, an intact fiber has an elastic element (in connective tissue and joints) to contend with, and so some fiber shortening actually does occur even though no limb displacement or joint rotation occurs. A **static contraction** is a muscle contraction that produces an increase in muscle tension but does not cause meaningful limb displacement or joint rotation and therefore does not result in movement of the skeleton. Thus, the term *static*, meaning "not in motion," is a better descriptor when describing a contraction that occurs in a human. No external work is done by static contractions, but they often perform the important task of fixation or stabilization. For example, gripping a tennis racket or suitcase handle is a static contraction.

Force Development and Gradation of Response

Dynamic, isokinetic, and static contractions all exert tension; however, the tension that can be generated is not the same for the three types of contractions. Eccentric dynamic contractions produce the greatest force, followed by static contractions, and finally, by dynamic concentric contractions. The amount of force produced by each type of contraction depends on both neural and mechanical factors.[25]

Neural Activation If a single muscle fiber or motor unit is stimulated to contract, it will contract maximally or not contract at all (according to the all-or-none principle of muscle contraction). If a muscle fiber is stimulated to contract, it will produce a twitch and then relax (Figure 18.1a). If a second stimulus is applied before the fiber has completely relaxed, temporal summation results, producing slightly greater tension. If the frequency of stimulation is increased to a sufficient level (so that relaxation is prohibited), the individual contractions blend together to form first an irregular (or unfused) tetanus and then a smooth (fused) tetanus (Figure 18.1b). Unfused tetanic contractions produce greater tension than both single twitches and summations, and fused tetanic contractions produce the highest tension. Movement in the intact human is based on tetanic contractions of motor units, not of single muscle fibers.[33] Once estab-

FIGURE 18.1

Muscle Fiber Response to Electrical Stimulation

(a) Myogram of a single muscle twitch. (b) Myogram of a series of twitches.

lished, these tetanic contractions continue until the stimuli are removed or fatigue occurs. This control of force output of a motor unit is called *rate coding*.[16]

The second neural way of controlling force output is by varying the number of motor units activated, which is called *number coding*. In the intact human some motor units, on an alternation basis, are always contracting. These contractions maintain what is called *muscle tone*, or tonus. When greater tension is needed, more motor units are recruited by the central nervous system. Such activation or recruitment, and the subsequent deactivation or derecruitment, occurs according to the size principle.

From your knowledge of the fiber types, what order of recruitment would you expect? Remember that smaller motor neurons are easier to stimulate than larger ones. Therefore, in accordance with the size principle, the small α_2 motor neurons innervat-

ing SO motor units are recruited first. As the stimulus increases, the larger α_1 motor neurons that innervate the FOG muscle fibers will be activated, followed by the recruitment of FG fibers as the stimulus continues to increase. Thus, the speed continuum of walk, jog, and run is paralleled by a muscle fiber recruitment continuum of SO, FOG, and FG recruitment.

All motor units in a given muscle are probably recruited at submaximal levels.[16] That is, if the **maximal voluntary contraction** (MVC) is taken as the maximal force (100%) that a muscle can exert, the recruitment of all available motor units would have occurred at a value less than 100%, possibly 30–85% depending on the specific muscle. Deactivation, once the neural stimulation has been removed, proceeds in reverse sequence. The larger, faster fibers (FG, then FOG) are inactivated first; finally, the slower, smaller fibers are deactivated until only muscle tonus remains.

Mechanical Factors Influencing Muscle Contractions   There are several mechanical factors that influence muscle contractions in the human body. This section will discuss four of them: length-tension-angle relationships, force-velocity relationships, the elasticity-force relationship, and architectural design.

Length-Tension-Angle Relationships.   One mechanical factor that influences the expression of muscle tension and resultant torque is the initial length of the muscle fibers.[15] On the cellular level the amount of tension that can be exerted by a muscle is related to the initial length of the sarcomere. As shown in Figure 18.2a, this relationship can basically be described as an inverted U.[15]

The amount of tension produced is directly related to the degree of overlap of the thick and thin filaments (Figure 18.2c). In elongated fibers there is little overlap of the actin and myosin filaments, making it hard for cross-bridges to form. In shortened fibers, where the thick and thin filaments

Maximal Voluntary Contraction The maximal force (100%) that a muscle can exert.

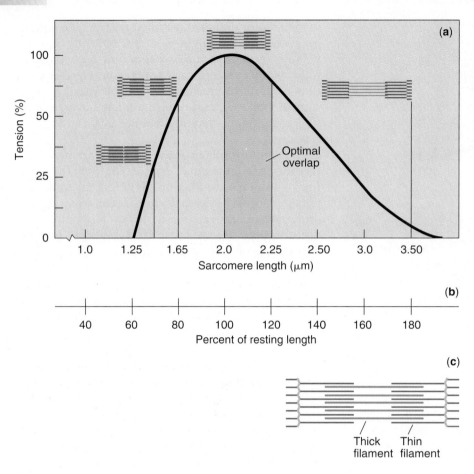

FIGURE 18.2

Length-Tension Relationship in Skeletal Muscle Fibers

Source: From "Contractile Performance of Skeletal Muscle Fibres" by K. A. Paul Edman. In *Strength and Power in Sport* (p. 103) by P. V. Komi (ed.). Champaign IL: Human Kinetics Publishers. Copyright 1992 by International Olympic Committee. Reprinted by permission.

already overlap almost completely, there is little room for further shortening. Thus, less force is produced in both the elongated and shortened position. On the other hand, the maximum number of cross-bridges coincides with the highest force production, which occurs at approximately 100–120% of the resting sarcomere length (Figure 18.2b).[35]

Although this length-tension relationship holds true in intact muscle, its expression in human movement is complicated by many factors. These factors include the cross-sectional area of the muscle, the arrangement of the sarcomere to the line of pull, the level of neural muscle activation, the degree of fatigue, the involvement of the elastic components of muscle, and the biomechanical aspects of how a muscle exerts force at a joint. The biomechanical aspects are most notable and will be considered here.

When muscle tension (measured as muscle force or torque) is plotted against the joint angle at which it occurs, *strength curves* are generated. Again, imagine the muscle action involved in performing a bicep curl. As the barbell is lifted through the range of motion, different amounts of force are generated in order to compensate for biomechanical differences in joint angle. Of course, the force produced is related to the length of the sarcomere, but force production is also greatly influenced by biomechanical aspects of the joint.

Figure 18.3 provides a schematic of a strength curve for this bicep curl (elbow flexion) example. The joint angle is plotted along the horizontal axis, and the force produced by the contracting muscle is plotted along the vertical axis. Notice along the top of the figure that the action of raising the barbell proceeds from right to left. That is, the joint angle is greatest in the lowered position (~170°) and least when the barbell is in the raised position (~30°). In this example peak force occurs at approximately 100–120°.

FIGURE 18.3

Example of a Strength Curve

curve is one where force initially increases and then decreases as a function of joint angle.

Figure 18.5 presents a generalized strength curve for knee flexion (most studies describe this as an ascending curve, although there is some disparity in the findings).[26] As shown in the figure, when the joint angle is greatest, the greatest force is exerted. This point also corresponds to the time when the muscles of the hamstrings are longest.

Figure 18.6 presents a generalized strength curve for hip abduction.[26] These curves are generally described as descending. In this case larger joint angles correspond to lower forces. In this example the tensor fasciae latae (the muscle responsible for hip abduction) is longest at the lowest joint angle.

Both of these situations—Figures 18.5 and 18.6—are really consistent: The longer the muscle length, the greater the force that is exerted. However, remember that it is not just, or even primarily, the length of the muscle itself that causes this variation.

There is general agreement that both elbow flexion (Figure 18.7) and knee extension (Figure 18.8) exhibit ascending and descending strength curves.[26] The strongest angles for elbow flexion seem to be between 90° and 130°; for knee extension the strongest angles are between 100° and 130°. As with the other configurations, the joint angle that coincides with the greatest force production is partially, but not entirely, a result of the muscle length and degree of overlap of the thick and thin filaments.

Although there are some differences, by and large the shapes of the strength curves are consistent for males and females, the young and the old. Injuries typically result in low strength curve values; thus, preinjury strength curves or strength curves from a comparable healthy individual are

As indicated in Figure 18.4, strength curves can take one of three forms: ascending, descending, or ascending and descending. An ascending strength curve is characterized by an increase in torque as the joint angle increases. A descending strength curve is characterized by a decrease in torque as the joint angle increases. An ascending and descending

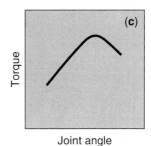

FIGURE 18.4

Classification of Strength Curves

(a) Ascending. (b) Descending. (c) Ascending and descending.

Source: K. Kulig, J. G. Andrews, & J. G. Hay. Human strength curves. In R. Terjung (ed.), *Exercise and Sport Sciences Reviews* (Vol. 12). Lexington, MA: Collamore Press, 417–466 (1984). Reprinted by permission of Williams & Wilkins.

FIGURE 18.5

Strength Curves for Knee Flexion

Source: K. Kulig, J. G. Andrews, & J. G. Hay. Human strength curves. In R. Terjung (ed.), *Exercise and Sport Sciences Reviews* (Vol. 12). Lexington, MA: Collamore Press, 417–466 (1984). Reprinted by permission of Williams & Wilkins.

sometimes used as goals in rehabilitation. Agreed-upon norms for strength curves are not generally available.

Knowledge of strength curves has another practical application. If an individual is going to lift an external load—for example, a barbell through the range of elbow flexion (biceps curl exercise)—he or she is limited by the weight that can be handled at the weakest point. Thus, the stronger angles are not overloaded to the same extent as the weaker angles,

and the muscle is taxed maximally only at its "sticking point."

Finally, strength curves have been used in the design of strength training equipment—specifically, variable-resistance equipment.[26] Nautilus developed the variable-radius cam to mimic the strength curve of selected single-joint exercises. The aim is to compensate for changes in mechanical leverage throughout the range of motion of a joint, thereby matching the load to the strength curve so that all angles, not just the sticking point, are taxed maximally. Although this reasoning appears to be logical, training

FIGURE 18.6

Strength Curve for Hip Abduction

Source: K. Kulig, J. G. Andrews, & J. G. Hay. Human strength curves. In R. Terjung (ed.), *Exercise and Sport Sciences Reviews* (Vol. 12). Lexington, MA: Collamore Press, 417–466 (1984). Reprinted by permission of Williams & Wilkins.

studies have not demonstrated that greater benefits are derived from variable-resistance training programs than from traditional free weight programs.

Force-Velocity and Power-Velocity Relationships. The second major mechanical factor that influences the expression of muscle force or torque is the velocity at which the shortening occurs. On the cellular level the maximal velocity of shortening varies among individual muscle fibers, but within the same fibers it is constant regardless of the sarcomere length (Figure 18.9).[15] Compare Figure 18.9 with Figure 18.2 (the length-force curve). From the comparison, it is apparent that the length of the sarcomere influences force production, but it does not affect the velocity of force production. The maximum velocity of shortening does not depend on the

FIGURE 18.7

Strength Curve for Elbow Flexion

Source: K. Kulig, J. G. Andrews, & J. G. Hay. Human strength curves. In R. Terjung (ed.), *Exercise and Sport Sciences Reviews* (Vol. 12). Lexington, MA: Collamore Press, 417–466 (1984). Reprinted by permission of Williams & Wilkins.

FIGURE 18.8

Strength Curve for Knee Extension

Source: K. Kulig, J. G. Andrews, & J. G. Hay. Human strength curves. In R. Terjung (ed.), *Exercise and Sport Sciences Reviews* (Vol. 12). Lexington, MA: Collamore Press, 417–466 (1984). Reprinted by permission of Williams & Wilkins.

FIGURE 18.9

Velocity-Length Curves

Source: Reprinted with permission from Edman.[15]

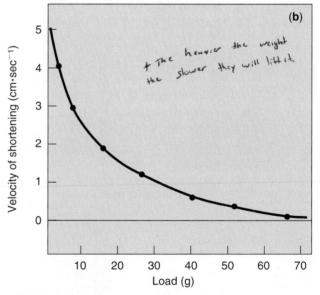

FIGURE 18.10

Force-Velocity Curves

(a) In a single muscle fiber. (b) In a whole muscle.

Source: From "Contractile Performance of Skeletal Muscle Fibres" by K. A. Paul Edman. In *Strength and Power in Sport* (p. 105) by P. V. Komi (ed.). Champaign, Il: Human Kinetics Publishers. Copyright 1992 by International Olympic Committee. Reprinted by permission.

number of cross-bridges between the thick and thin filaments but on the maximal cycling rate of the cross-bridges.[15]

The relationship between force and velocity is similar for a single muscle fiber (Figure 18.10a) and for an intact whole muscle (Figure 18.10b). The single muscle fiber does not exhibit the smooth hyperbolic curve that an intact muscle does, but both show the basic relationship: The shortening velocity of a muscle increases as the force developed by the muscle decreases. Maximal velocity occurs in an unloaded (zero force) situation, and a maximal load results in no movement (zero velocity). In between these two extremes the velocity gradually decreases in a curvilinear fashion as the load increases. To apply this information, consider a simple example of swinging a bat. As the weight of the bat is increased, the speed with which it can be swung decreases.

If the external force overcomes the ability of the muscle to resist it, the muscle lengthens (eccentric contraction), but only after producing additional tension.[37] The eccentric contraction is seen in Figure 18.10a where the force curve dips below the horizontal axis. Notice that the force produced continues to increase during this eccentric phase. This result is consistent with the information presented earlier in this chapter concerning eccentric dynamic contractions.

Figure 18.11 shows the relationship between torque and velocity (Figure 18.11a) and the relationship between power and velocity (Figure 18.11b). These relationships were derived from a study of two different groups of subjects: one group of subjects with more than 50% FT muscle fibers (average = 58.5%) and one group with less than 50% FT fibers (average = 38.3%).[10] Several conclusions can be drawn from these graphs. First, power is positively related to velocity, whereas torque is negatively related to velocity (as previously noted for load). The shape of the relationship is curvilinear for both torque and power, but the curves are practically upside down from each other. Consider what this power-velocity relationship means if a heavier (as opposed to lighter) bat can be swung quickly enough to contact a fast pitch.

The graphs in Figure 18.11 show that the percentage of torque and power that can be generated at any given velocity varies with the predominant fiber type. At any given velocity of movement the torque (force) that can be generated and the power that results is higher in individuals with more than 50% FT fibers than in individuals with less than 50% FT fibers. Thus, individuals with high percentages of FT fibers would seem to be genetically predisposed (given sufficient training and practice) to be successful in power events such as sprinting, power lifting, and jumping, and in field events such as shot, javelin, and discus.

The power curve of the predominantly ST fiber individuals (those with less than 50% FT) not only levels off but also makes a downturn at the higher velocities. Although such a downturn is not evident at the tested speeds for the FT group, it is likely that there is an optimal speed of movement for the generation of power that is fiber-type-specific.

Elasticity-Force Relationship. Elasticity is the third mechanical factor that must be considered in a description of the force development capabilities of muscles. Both the muscle fibers and their tendinous attachments contain elastic components. When a muscle fiber is stretched and then contracted, the resultant contraction is stronger than it would have been had there been no prestretching. In the intact human, the relationship between prestretch and force of contraction is expressed as a *stretch-shortening cycle* (SSC).[24] Stretch-shortening cycles do not occur in all human movements. They

FIGURE 18.11

Influence of Fiber Type on Velocity

(a) Expressed as a percentage of torque. (b) Expressed as power.

Source: Coyle, Castill, & Lesmes.[10]

are most evident in activities such as running, jumping, and (to a lesser extent) bicycling. Figure 18.12 shows that the calf muscles and Achilles tendon are stretched while contracting eccentrically as the foot of a runner impacts the ground.[24] The push-off or concentric-shortening phase is aided by the release of the potential energy stored during the stretch phase. To feel the impact of the SSC, stand up and see how high you can jump with a little flexion and then with moderate flexion at your hip, knee, and ankle joints. Then try a rebound jump from a small stool. This latter task is an example of a

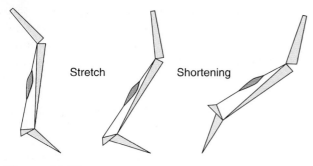

Stretch   Shortening

FIGURE 18.12

Stretch-Shortening Cycle

Source: P. V. Komi. Physiological and biomechanical correlates of muscle function: Effects of muscle structure and stretch-shortening cycle of force and speed. In R. Terjung (ed.), *Exercise and Sport Sciences Reviews* (Vol. 12). Lexington, MA: Collamore Press, 81–122 (1984). Reprinted by permission of Williams & Wilkins.

plyometric exercise. Plyometrics will be discussed more completely in the neural flexibility chapter (Chapter 20), since more than just elasticity is involved in the physiological basis for their execution. As a result of additional power generation with increasing stretch-proceeding contraction, you should be able to jump successively higher in the three examples.

Not only does the stretch-shortening cycle lead to more powerful muscle contractions, but it also has an impact on mechanical efficiency. Efficiency is discussed at length in the unit on metabolism (Chapter 11). Here you simply need to be aware that efficiency is the relationship between external work performed and the energy cost of doing that work. Prestretching is positively and rectilinearly related to mechanical efficiency in positive work.[24] That is, more work can be done with less energy expenditure following a prestretch.

Architectural Design. The maximal force that can be developed within a muscle fiber is related to its cross-sectional area. Also, the force that can be developed by a whole muscle is related to its cross-sectional area. However, this relationship is not as strong as the one within a single muscle fiber, largely owing to different arrangements of the muscle fiber within a muscle. Muscles that are designed for a high–force generation rate (pennate, bipennate, and multipennate muscles) are arranged so as

to maximize cross-sectional area. Muscles that are designed for a high velocity of shortening have parallel fibers and are arranged in a fusiform manner.[18]

Muscular Fatigue and Soreness

Despite all the benefits and enjoyment of exercise, there are also some unpleasant outcomes that can occur as a result of unaccustomed muscular activity. This section will deal with two of those consequences: muscular fatigue and muscular soreness.

Muscular Fatigue   Anyone who has participated in vigorous activity is familiar with muscular fatigue. Although exercise physiologists have studied fatigue for a long time, it is still to be precisely defined, and many questions remain regarding the basic causes of fatigue. Here is how one exercise physiologist summarizes the issue:

> Fatigue, generally defined as transient loss of work capacity resulting from preceding work, is one of the most fundamental problems both for research and for practical application. Fatigue limits performance in normal conditions and even more so in disease. It produces a general feeling of discomfort and frustration and interferes with well-being.[36]

Fatigue results in the cessation of muscular work or the inability to maintain a given intensity of work. Figure 18.13 depicts graphically the force that

FIGURE 18.13

Hypothetical Fatigue Curve for Handgrip

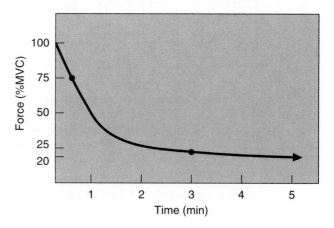

a muscle can produce isometrically as a function of time. This figure suggests that if an individual is asked to sustain an isometric contraction (in this case, a handgrip exercise) at less than 20% MVC, the load can be maintained indefinitely. However, as the % MVC increases, the time that the contraction can be maintained decreases rapidly. A force equal to 50% MVC can only be maintained for approximately 1 min for a handgrip exercise. The precise shape of the fatigue curve varies among muscle groups, reflecting the differences in fiber type distribution and architectural design. In addition to causing a decrease in force-generating capabilities, fatigue results in a decreased velocity and an increase in time to relax.

That force will decrease over time is probably obvious, but what causes muscle fatigue? Muscle fatigue is a complex phenomenon that includes failure at one or more of the sites along the chain of events that leads to muscular contraction. As diagramed in Figure 18.14, fatigue can be classified as central and peripheral on the basis of the location of the site of fatigue.

Possible causes for central fatigue include a malfunction of the nerve cells or inhibition of voluntary effort in the central nervous system. Other factors that may influence central fatigue include psychological factors and motivation that influence how much effort an individual will give, particularly if pain is associated with continuing an activity.

Peripheral fatigue refers to fatigue at a site beyond the central nervous system; this may include sites within the peripheral nervous system or within the skeletal muscle. Peripheral fatigue can occur at several sites: the neuromuscular junction, the sarcolemma–T tubules–sarcoplasmic reticulum system, and the myofilaments. Failure of neuromuscular transmission is a possible cause of fatigue. This failure could include (1) inhibition of the axon terminal, (2) depletion of the neurotransmitter, and/or (3) problems with the binding of the neurotransmitter to the receptors on the motor end plate. Fatigue can also result from a failure of the electrical excitation along the sarcolemma and T tubules and an inability of the sarcoplasmic reticulum to release sufficient calcium. Likewise, fatigue could result from any alteration in the ability of calcium to bind to troponin and thereby remove tropomyosin from its blocking position on actin.

FIGURE 18.14

Possible Sites of Muscle Fatigue

It is also possible that fatigue results from biochemical and metabolic changes within the contractile elements (myofilaments of the muscle cell). Notice in Figure 18.14 the categorizations of *electrophysiological considerations* and *metabolic and biochemical considerations* that relate to muscle fatigue. Electrophysiological considerations are concerned with steps within the central nervous system, the peripheral nervous system, or the muscle fiber leading up to the binding of the actin and myosin filaments. Metabolic and biochemical considerations involve the ability of actin and myosin to continue their cross-bridge attachment-detachment cycles, thus producing force and are therefore confined to the skeletal muscle fiber.

There are two primary hypotheses for the metabolic and biochemical causes of fatigue within muscle: the depletion (or exhaustion) hypothesis and the accumulation hypothesis.[29] The depletion hypothesis suggests that fatigue results from depletion of certain metabolites, specifically, ATP, CP, and glycogen. Hence, the muscle fibers are no longer able to produce force. The accumulation hypothesis suggests that fatigue is caused by the accumulation of certain metabolites that have been shown to impair force generation within muscles, specifically, hydrogen ions, ammonia, and phosphate.

Muscular Soreness   Muscle soreness is a familiar consequence of overexertion. There are two generally recognized types of muscle soreness. One type of muscular soreness is characterized by pain during and immediately after exercise, which may persist for several hours. The second type of muscular soreness is characterized by a local pain, which appears 24 to 48 hr after exercise and may persist for 7 days postexercise.[13] The former is thought to be caused by stimulation of the pain receptors by metabolic by-products of cellular respiration. It is generally relieved by discontinuing exercise, or it subsides shortly thereafter.

The second type of soreness is called **delayed-onset muscle soreness (DOMS)**. This soreness increases in intensity for the first 24 hr after activity, peaks from 24 to 48 hr, and then declines during the next 5 to 7 days.[14] Delayed-onset muscle soreness is generally considered to be an adult phenomena, but some children also exhibit DOMS.[39]

DOMS is of concern to exercise professionals because it affects athletic performance and exercise participation. Despite its importance and considerable research attention, the causative factors and cellular mechanisms of DOMS remain elusive. There are, however, several theories that have attempted to integrate the findings of research on this topic. Two of the primary theories of DOMS are presented here: the mechanical trauma theory and the local ischemic theory. These theories are not mutually exclusive; on the contrary, they share many of the same elements.

Etiology and Mechanisms.   The mechanical trauma model has been proposed by Armstrong[2] to describe the mechanisms responsible for DOMS. As the name implies, this model suggests that the mechanical forces in the contractile or elastic tissue result in structural damage to the muscle fibers. Damage to the sarcolemma of the cell leads to disruption in calcium homeostasis, which results in necrosis (death of tissue). The presence of cellular debris and immune cells (macrophages) leads to swelling and inflammation, which is responsible for the sensation of DOMS.

The local ischemic model has been proposed by DeVries & Housh.[13] This model suggests that exercise—even moderate, atraumatic activities—causes swelling in the muscle tissue, which increases tissue pressure. This increase in tissue pressure is thought to result in local ischemia (reduced blood flow), which causes pain and leads to tonic muscle constriction (spasm). This spasm causes additional swelling and perpetuates a cycle of swelling and ischemia that results in the painful sensation known as DOMS. DeVries also suggests that local ischemia can result in structural damage that leads to inflammation and swelling and, thus, exacerbates the cycle.

Figure 18.15 summarizes both the mechanical trauma and spasm models of DOMS. Note the considerable overlap in mechanisms that are proposed by the two models, which accounts for the considerable research evidence that supports each model. The major distinction between the models is the

Delayed-Onset Muscle Soreness (DOMS) Muscle soreness that increases in intensity for the first 24 hr after activity, peaks from 24 to 28 hr, and then declines during the next 5 to 7 days.

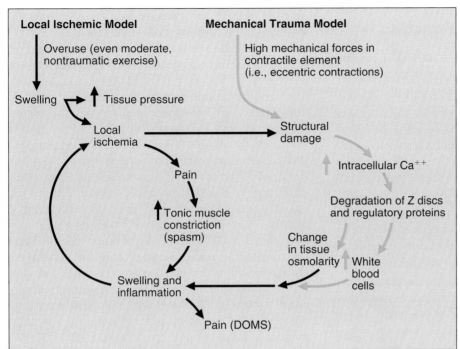

FIGURE 18.15

An Integrated Model to Explain DOMS

event that initiates the cycle. It is possible that both models are viable. DeVries points out that overexertion involving long-duration and moderate-intensity activities leads to DOMS. On the other hand, Armstrong concentrates on the manifestation of DOMS after activities that place considerable mechanical force on the muscle, specifically, eccentric contractions that are known to cause DOMS. Much of the research that supports the mechanical trauma model has used eccentric exercise as a means of eliciting DOMS.

One of the popular concepts (or rather misconceptions) regarding DOMS is that it is caused by the accumulation of lactic acid. Although this theory was originally proposed by researchers,[4,14] its popularity now rests in the lay public. There is now considerable research evidence to argue against this theory, including the fact that individuals who have McArdles's syndrome and do not produce lactic acid also suffer from DOMS. Additional evidence against lactic acid as the cause of muscle soreness is that the type of activity that produces the greatest degree of soreness, namely eccentric contractions, produces lower lactic acid levels than concentric contractions of the same power output.[3,6,11] Perhaps the most compelling evidence is that lactic acid has a half-life of 15–25 min and is

fully cleared from muscle within an hour (see Chapter 10). Since lactic acid is not present (at least not at elevated levels) it cannot cause soreness 24–48 hr later.

Treatment for Relief and Prevention.   The primary means of providing relief from muscular soreness appears to be static stretching of the sore muscle, acute exercise, and anti-inflammatory drugs. Muscular stretch is thought to initiate the inverse myotatic reflex (by stimulation of the golgi tendon organ, GTO), which results in a relaxation of the stretched muscle[13] (reflexes will be discussed in detail in Chapter 20). Although some research has demonstrated a reduction in soreness as a result of stretching,[13] more recent research has failed to demonstrate the same reduction in pain following static stretching.[31]

Acute exercise also diminishes DOMS.[3] Researchers suggest that this relief is due to an increased release of endorphins as a result of exercise.[23] The use of anti-inflammatory drugs has been suggested, too, since inflammation is clearly part of the DOMS cycle. Although the use of aspirin and ibuprofen do help relieve DOMS, these drugs appear to be most effective if taken prior to exercise.[21]

Assessing Muscular Function

Accurate assessment of the strength, endurance, and power a muscle is capable of generating is important for five reasons.

1. Assessment is an aid in *screening* to determine the extent of muscle weaknesses and/or imbalances. Both weakness and imbalance have been implicated as making an individual more prone to injury. Assessment also establishes baseline values for an individual.

2. Assessment can be used as a guide to *rehabilitation*. Assessment of the loss of function after an injury or accident is needed to determine rehabilitation workloads and to monitor progress.

3. Assessment is necessary for *exercise prescription*. Both athletes and fitness participants need realistic programs based on their own performance capabilities.

4. Assessment is an aid in *selection* of the best exercises for working on specific problems.

5. Assessment is a tool in *research* to study which types of training programs produce the greatest changes in muscle function.

Strength refers to the ability of a muscle or muscle group to exert force against a resistance. It is usually measured as one maximal effort and is sometimes referred to as maximal voluntary contraction (MVC). *Torque* is the more correct term if movement is made through a range of motion, but *strength* is the more commonly used term. **Muscular endurance** is the ability of a muscle or muscle group to repeatedly exert force against a resistance. That is, the activity is typically performed at a given percentage of maximal voluntary contraction (% MVC). The amount of work done per unit of time is **power,** and it is the

product of force and velocity ($P = F \times V$). Thus, it is the expression of strength exerted quickly.

Strength and muscular endurance can be expressed either as absolute values or as relative values. *Absolute values* represent the actual external load and are commonly measured in pounds (lb), kilograms (kg), newtons (N), or newton-meters ($N \cdot m$). *Relative values* are expressed in relation to body weight. Both values are useful. For example, if two individuals are doing a two-arm curl and individual A can lift 70 kg and individual B can only lift 60 kg, you would probably conclude that individual A is stronger. However, if individual A weighs 55 kg and individual B weighs 47 kg, they both are lifting 1.27 kg per kg of body weight. Thus, on a relative basis, neither can be considered stronger. So if a comparison is to be made between individuals, a relative expression of strength is generally preferred. On the other hand, absolute values are preferred for comparisons made on the same person.

In terms of endurance, if the two individuals (A and B) were asked to hold a 40-kg weight, you would assume that individual A could do so for a longer period of time, since that load represents 57% MVC for individual A and 67% MVC for individual B. Thus, an absolute load puts the individual who can lift less at a disadvantage. However, if both were asked to hold a load that represented a 50% MVC, and if they were equally motivated, you would expect that both individuals could hold that load for the same amount of time. To check that you understand the influence of body weight on the expression of strength, complete Box 18.1.

Laboratory Methods

In order to quantify the various aspects of muscular function just discussed, exercise physiologists use various laboratory and field methods. Laboratory methods are generally more accurate and precise than field methods in measuring different aspects of muscular function, but they have the disadvantage of being expensive and inaccessible to many people.

Electromyography Electromyography **(EMG)** is the measurement of the neural or electrical activity, known as muscle action potentials, that brings about muscle contraction. Motor unit activity can be recorded by the use of needle electrodes, or

---

Strength The ability of a muscle or muscle group to exert maximal force against a resistance in a single repetition.

Muscular Endurance The ability of a muscle or muscle group to repeatedly exert force against a resistance.

Power The amount of work done per unit of time; the product of force and velocity; the ability to exert force quickly.

Box 18.1   A Question of Understanding

Listed below are the body weight (BW) and MVC for a handgrip task.

Name	Gender	BW (kg)	Absolute Strength MVC (kg)	Relative Strength kg · kg⁻¹	50% MVC
Jody	F	60.0	40.0		
Jill	F	68.0	60.0		
Pat	F	70.0	36.0		
Scott	M	63.0	50.0		
Tom	M	82.0	72.0		
Mike	M	70.0	71.0		

1. Calculate the relative strength for each individual (strength ÷ BW).
2. Calculate the load that would need to be held for each of the subjects to be working at 50% MVC (absolute strength × 0.5).
3. Who is the strongest person on an absolute basis? on a relative basis?
4. For whom would 50% MVC represent the most absolute force?

---

whole-muscle activity can be recorded by the use of surface electrodes. The EMG voltage is proportional to the force of an isometric contraction, proportional to the tension developed in constant-velocity contractions,[28] and proportional to velocity in isotonic contractions.[5] Therefore, one can obtain a reasonably valid estimation of tension development in a muscle by EMG.

EMG does not give an absolute value of force or torque; instead, it provides a direct functional indication of muscle activity. If it is plotted against incremental loads or values resulting from a submaximal hold, it can be used to predict strength or endurance, respectively. Such submaximal testing using EMG is particularly important in situations where an individual either cannot or is not motivated to perform maximally. In addition, since weak individuals produce a greater EMG signal than strong individuals for any absolute load,[17] EMG activity can be used to monitor rehabilitation or training progress.

Perhaps the most valuable contribution of EMG to muscle function assessment, however, is its ability to show which muscles are primarily responsible for specific actions. For example, when training or testing individuals for abdominal strength, one should select an exercise that maximizes the involvement of the abdominal muscles (the rectus abdominous and the external obliques) and that minimizes the involvement of the hip flexors and

thigh muscles (rectus femoris). EMG helps in this selection.

Box 18.2 provides an example of the EMG activity of the muscles just mentioned during a sit-up with the feet supported and unsupported and the knees at various angles.[19,20] Work through the questions in the box to check on your understanding.

Isokinetic Machines   Isokinetic machines, such as a Cybex or MERAC (Figure 18.16), allow the velocity of limb movement to be kept constant throughout a contraction. These devices provide accurate and reliable measurements of muscular strength, muscular endurance, and power while the speed of the limb is kept constant at a predetermined velocity. Any increase in muscular force results in increased resistance rather than increased acceleration of the limb.[22] Measurements obtained on isokinetic machines serve as a reference against which other methods of assessment can be compared. These devices can be configured to test the limbs of the upper or the lower body.

Electromyography (EMG) The measurement of the neural or electrical activity that brings about muscle contraction.

Box 18.2 **A Question of Understanding**

Study the EMG data for each of the muscle groups with the feet supported (●) and with the feet unsupported (●), and answer the following questions.

● Feet supported   ● Feet unsupported

1. Does bending the knees eliminate the involvement of thigh muscles (rectis femoris) if the feet are held down? Which muscles are more active if the feet are held, the abdominal or thigh muscles?

2. Which muscle group does the angle of knee bend affect most?

3. Should the feet be held or not held to maximize the involvement of the abdominal muscles?

4. On the basis of your answers in 1–3, which sit-up form (feet held or not held) and which knee angle would you recommend?

Force Transducers   Force transducers measure static strength and endurance. The displacement of the transducer sends an electrical signal to a computer, which displays the force output in digital form. By having the subject exert as much force

FIGURE 18.16

Isokinetic Exercise Equipment
The measurement of isokinetic strength of quadriceps is recorded throughout normal range of motion.

as possible in a single maximal trial, these devices can be used to measure maximal strength during a maximal voluntary contraction. They can also be used to measure static muscular endurance by having the subject hold a given percentage of the predetermined maximal value (% MVC). Static muscular endurance is then calculated by determining either how long an individual can maintain the predetermined value or how long it takes the subject to drop to a specified percentage of his or her maximal contraction.

Laboratory and Field Methods

There are several other methods of assessing muscle function that require relatively simple testing devices. They may be encountered in a laboratory or in a field-testing environment.

Dynamometers   Dynamometers measure static strength and static muscular endurance. Two dynamometers are commercially available: the handgrip dynamometer and the back and leg dynamometer (Figure 18.17). Like the force transducer, these devices can be used to measure maximal strength by having the subject exert as much force as possible in a single maximal trial. Because of its availability and ease of administration, the handgrip dynamometer has been extensively used to measure grip strength.

FIGURE 18.17

Back and Leg Dynamometer

A back and leg dynamometer is used here to test leg strength.

Dynamometers use a spring device; as force is applied to the dynamometer, the spring is compressed and moves the needle to indicate force produced. Dynamometers can also be used to measure static muscular endurance by having the subject perform at a given percentage of the predetermined maximal value. Muscular endurance is then calculated by determining either how long an individual can maintain the predetermined (submaximal) value or how long it takes the subject to drop to his or her specified percentage of maximal contraction.

Constant-Resistance Equipment   The most common method of measuring dynamic strength is to determine the maximal amount an individual can lift in a single repetition using the constant resistance offered by free weight or weight machines. This is known as a one repetition max (1RM) and is a trial-and-error method of determining how much an individual can lift. If the selected weight is too heavy to be lifted, then a lower weight is used. If the weight is successfully lifted, then additional weight is added. Care must be taken in the use of this method, how-

ever, because too many trials will cause fatigue, thereby decreasing the true maximal strength value.

Constant-resistance equipment can also be used to measure dynamic muscular endurance by determining how many times an individual can lift a submaximal load. The submaximal load is usually a predetermined load (such as the 80-lb bench press test for males or the 35-lb test for females used in the YMCA assessment battery); or it may be expressed as a percentage of body weight or as a percentage of 1 RM.

Field Tests

There are several easily administered tests commonly used in the field to assess muscle function. Common field tests include calisthenic and jumping activities.

Calisthenic Activities   Calisthenic activities are often used in field settings to assess muscular endurance and, to a lesser extent, muscular strength. The most commonly administered tests include some version of sit-ups or curl-ups, push-ups, and pull-ups or flexed-arm hang. Although it is often reported that these tests measure strength, they are in fact usually endurance tests. That is, they measure the maximum number of times an individual can perform a given test (often within a specified time period, such as the number of curl-ups per minute). If the participant is able to complete more than one repetition of the task, the result represents muscular endurance. If the subject is able to complete one repetition (or sometimes no repetitions), the result represents strength (or lack thereof). Note that these tests indicate relative strength or endurance, because the amount of resistance is determined by individual body size.

Vertical Jump/Standing Broad Jump   The jump tests are used to measure the explosive muscular power of the legs. Although they are easy to administer, they are also influenced by the weight of the individual. Furthermore, there may be a strong neural component and there is a definite alactic anaerobic metabolic component to these tests (see Chapter 10).

Although all of these calisthenic (performance) tests are commonly used, they have not been definitively validated as tests of strength, muscular endurance, and/or power. Therefore, it may be best just to call them what they are—that is, a push-up test, for example—rather than trying to say they are a substitute for a certain laboratory assessment.

*A*ge, Sex, and Muscle Function

Strength development in humans is evident from infancy through maturity. Figure 18.18 shows a common pattern of development. Strength increases rectilinearly from early childhood (3–7 yr) through early adolescence (13–14 yr) for both sexes. Then a marked increase in strength occurs during the rest of adolescence and into early adulthood (15–20 yr) for boys. Girls, however, do not show an accelerated increase in strength in late adolescence. They either maintain a slow rectilinear rise, as shown for grip strength (Figure 18.18b), or decline after age 16, as shown for both elbow flexion and knee extension (Figures 18.18c and d).[30] The in-

crease in strength during childhood and adolescence, even without training, is more than can be accounted for just from growth in size.

During early childhood there is virtually no difference in strength measurements between boys and girls. As puberty begins and progresses, though, the gap progressively widens. On the average, at 11–12 yr of age girls achieve approximately 90% of boys' strength; at 13–14 yr, this percentage has been reduced to 80%, and at 15–16 yr, to 75%. These percentages vary not only with age but also with the muscle group being measured.

Adult females average only about 56% of the static strength values of adult males in upper-body locations, about 64% in trunk strength, and about 72% in lower-body locations.[27] As shown in Figure 18.19, the variation between upper- and lower-body strength has also been shown for the bench press and the leg press.[41] Note that there is considerable overlap in the distribution of leg strength even in untrained males and females (Figure 18.19a),

FIGURE 18.18

Strength Development in Boys and Girls

(a) Grip strength in young children. (b) Grip strength in children 6–18 years old. (c) Biceps strength. (d) Quadriceps strength.

Source: From *Growth, Maturation and Physical Activity* (pp. 189, 191) by Robert M. Malina and Claude Bouchard. Champaign, IL: Human Kinetics Publishers. Copyright 1991 by Robert M. Malina and Claude Bouchard. Reprinted by permission.

FIGURE 18.19

Frequency Distribution for Leg Press and Bench Press Values for Men and Women Before and After a Training Program

Source: Reprinted with permission from Wells & Plowman.[40]

FIGURE 18.20

Performance on Field Tests of Muscular Function in Children

(a) Flexed-arm hang (muscular endurance).
(b) Standing long jump (muscular power).

Source: From *Growth, Maturation and Physical Activity* (pp. 192, 193) by Robert M. Malina and Claude Bouchard. Champaign, IL: Human Kinetics Publishers. Copyright 1991 by Robert M. Malina and Claude Bouchard. Reprinted by permission.

whereas virtually no overlap exists for the arm strength (bench press) distributions (Figure 18.19b).

Although field tests are not pure tests of muscle function, differences in these tests parallel those seen in strength with growth and maturation and between boys and girls. Figure 18.20 illustrates these relationships for the flexed-arm hang and the standing long jump. Adult performances also appear to parallel adolescent male-female strength differences. Part of what can be interpreted from Figure 18.21 is that throughout the adult age span men perform more push-ups than women, even if the men are inactive. For leg lift exercise, however, the performance gap is smaller, with considerable overlap between inactive men and active women.

Why do these differences occur? Strength and other muscle functions increase as children grow because muscle mass increases parallel increases in body mass. The pubertal hormonal changes—

particularly in the level of testosterone, which is involved with the anabolic process of muscle growth—favor the males. While the young males are adding muscle mass under the influence of testosterone, the young females are adding fat under the influence of estrogen (Figure 18.22).[30] The

FIGURE 18.21

Performance on Field Tests of Muscular Function in Adults

(a) Push-up (muscular endurance). (b) Leg lifts.

Source: From "Age-Related Changes in Strength and Special Groups" by Siegfried Israel. In *Strength and Power in Sport* (p. 323) by P. V. Komi (ed.). Champaign, Il: Human Kinetics Publishers. Copyright 1992 by International Olympic Committee. Reprinted by permission.

FIGURE 18.22

Growth Curves for Mass and Percent Fat in Children

Source: From *Growth, Maturation and Physical Activity* (p. 97) by Robert M. Malina and Claude Bouchard. Champaign, IL: Human Kinetics Publishers. Copyright 1991 by Robert M. Malina and Claude Bouchard. Reprinted by permission.

similarities among the graphic representations of fat-free mass (Figure 18.22), strength (Figure 18.18), and muscle performance (Figure 18.20) are striking, leading to the conclusion that the quantity of muscle mass is what accounts for the difference in the expression of strength.

Another way to emphasize that it is the quantity of muscle and not the quality of muscle that is responsible for the male-female inequities is to calculate relative strength values.[40, 42] In one study the percentage of handgrip strength exhibited by the females in relation to the males increased from 57%, when expressed in absolute strength terms, to 73% and to 83% when expressed on a relative basis (absolute strength divided by total body weight and absolute strength divided by lean body mass, respectively).[42] For the bench press the corresponding figures were 37%, 46%, and 53%; and for the leg press they were 73%, 92%, and 106%. Thus, in leg strength relative to lean body mass female performance actually exceeded that of males!

In addition, studies relating strength to cross-sectional area of muscle show no inequities between the sexes. From all these studies it must therefore be concluded that it is the larger size of males in general, their greater muscle mass, and their larger fiber size (FT) that are physiologically responsible for their greater strength, rather than any inherent difference in the potential or function of the muscle fibers per se.

Another factor that cannot be ignored is cultural expectations. Many adolescent girls become less active as they grow up, detraining to some extent. Some detraining may be anatomically selective. That is, both males and females of all ages experience gravity equally in walking, climbing stairs, sitting down, and standing up. Yet individuals can selectively avoid upper-body activities, such as lifting heavy loads, opening jars, hammering, and weight lifting. Thus part of the reason for differences in upper-body versus lower-body activities in males and females may be cultural. Future studies may note a change in these relationships as more girls have the opportunity to enter sports at an early age and continue to be active into middle age and old age.

It is well documented that significant declines occur in muscular strength in both males and females from middle age to old age, but the rate of loss varies substantially among muscle groups.[34] Figure 18.23 represents a generalized change in strength (grip strength) over the normal lifespan for males and females. From the establishment of peak values in late adolescence or early adulthood, described previously, there is a maintenance of strength until approximately 45–50 years of age and then a fairly gradual decline into and beyond the 70s. The decline in muscle strength, in general, amounts to about 15% in the sixth and seventh decades of life and 30% per decade after that.[34] Relative static endurance (at approximately 40–50% MVC) is similar between older and younger individuals. Figures 18.21 and 18.23 show parallel declines in performance and illustrate the fact that different muscle groups decline at different rates, even between the sexes.

What causes the age related decline in strength? Three possibilities exist: (1) a loss of muscle mass, (2) a loss of mechanical or contractile properties

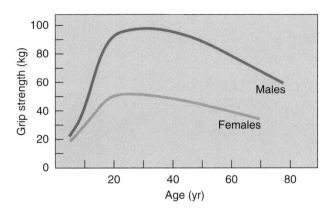

FIGURE 18.23

Maximal Handgrip Strength
Source: Komi

(namely, fiber type changes, fiber size changes, fiber number changes), and (3) reduced activation of motor units or denervation.

There is no doubt that muscle mass is lost with age. Between the ages of 30 and 70 yr almost 25% of muscle mass is lost in both males and females.[34] This loss leads to a reduction in force production. There is, however, some evidence to support the contention that the decline in strength with aging is greater than can be accounted for just by the loss of muscle mass. The capacity to exert force per unit of cross-sectional area also declines.[34]

Early studies using traditional biopsy techniques seemed to show a preferential loss of FT and, especially, FG fibers. Since these fibers are the high-force fibers, this result was intuitively logical. More recent studies utilizing whole-muscle cross-sectional techniques have shown that both ST and FT fibers are lost equally with aging.

As shown in Figure 18.24, the loss of muscle fibers begins at about age 25, and by age 80 a reduction of between 25 and 40% has occurred in females and males.[34] The genetically predetermined percentages of ST and FT fibers remain constant.

The SO fibers appear to maintain their size longer than do FT fibers. Thus, although FT fibers are not lost at a faster rate than SO fibers, they do atrophy faster; and FG fibers atrophy faster than FOG fibers. Since FT fibers are generally the larger fibers, the preferential loss in size of these fibers accounts in large part for the overall decrease in muscle size and strength with aging.

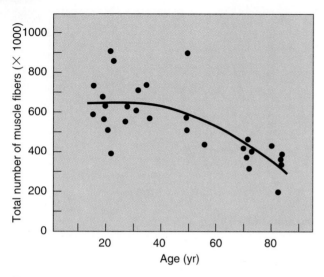

FIGURE 18.24

Loss of Muscle Fibers with Age

Source: M. A. Rogers & W. J. Evans. Changes in skeletal muscle with aging: Effects of exercise training. In J. O. Holloszy (ed.), *Exercise and Sport Science Reviews* (Vol. 21). Baltimore: Williams & Wilkins, 65–107 (1993). Reprinted by permission.

Of great concern is the practical meaning of these changes. Weakened respiratory muscles restrict aerobic activity. Weakened muscles around joints lead to instability, difficulty in restoring balance, and, potentially, falls.[1] Insufficient strength to get in and out of chairs, carry groceries, or take caps off medicine or food jars can lead to a loss of independent living. The most effective way to prevent these difficulties is by systematic exercise training. Aging of muscles cannot be prevented, but it can be delayed. Thus, maintaining and/or increasing muscular strength, endurance, and power is important for different reasons throughout the life span. However, muscles respond to exercise training in basically the same fashion at all ages; that is, trained muscles produce greater force.

*H*eritability of Muscular Function

Many characteristics of an individual, including fitness measures, are partially determined by genetics. The precise extent to which measures of muscle fitness are determined by biological heritability is difficult to determine because of sampling and population variation, methodological differences, and variations in subjects' levels of physical activity.[30] However, most studies suggest that genetics are an important determinant of muscle function, with heritability estimates of 20–40% being reported for muscular strength and endurance.[9, 30, 32]

The expression of muscular function is determined largely by the fiber type distribution and metabolic properties of muscle fibers. Both fiber type distribution and muscle content of enzymes that control metabolism have a significant genetic effect.[30]

It also appears that genetic variation accounts for a substantial fraction of the individual differences in responses to exercise training.[7, 8, 9] Individual differences in sensitivity to exercise training are largely inherited, with some individuals being high responders and others being low responders.[7, 8] These differences are the basis for the individualization principle of training, which states in part that even when individuals engage in the same training program, different results should be expected.

SUMMARY

1. The force developed when a contracting muscle acts on an object is called muscle tension, whereas the force exerted on the muscle by the object is called the load. In order for a muscle to move a load, the force of muscle tension must exceed the force of the load.

2. In isotonic contractions of muscle fibers force production is constant as the muscle fiber contracts. In the intact human system such a contraction is practically impossible. Instead, the load is constant but the force produced to move it through the range of motion is not. Thus, the term *dynamic* more accurately describes contraction within the intact human.

3. If movement results from a contraction in which muscle shortening occurs, it is a concentric dynamic contraction. If movement results from a contraction in which muscle lengthening occurs, the contraction is referred to as an eccentric dynamic contraction.

4. In isokinetic contractions of muscle fibers the velocity of contraction is constant. In the intact human the velocity of movement varies with joint angle. Specialized equipment can be used to hold the rate of limb displacement constant, resulting in isokinematic contraction.

5. A muscle fiber contraction that does not result in a meaningful length change in the muscle fiber is termed isometric. An intact fiber has an elastic element, and so some fiber shortening actually occurs even though no limb displacement takes place. Thus, the term *static* is preferable to isometric to describe this type of contraction in humans.

6. The amount of force produced by muscles is affected by neural and mechanical factors. Important mechanical factors include length-tension-angle relationships, force-velocity relationships, elasticity-force relationships, and architectural design.

7. Muscular fatigue results in a loss of muscle function and may be caused by a variety of factors, which can be described as central or peripheral, or as electrophysiological or biochemical in nature.

8. Muscular soreness may result from local ischema, mechanical trauma, or some combination of these factors.

9. Differences in strength between the sexes are largely due to the greater muscle mass of males. The magnitude of the difference in strength between males and females is influenced by the units used to express strength, the region of the body where strength is measured, and the training status of the individuals.

REVIEW QUESTIONS

1. Define isotonic, isokinetic, and isometric contractions. Discuss how they relate to dynamic and static contractions.

2. Diagram the force-length relationship in a muscle fiber. Diagram a strength curve for biceps flexion, knee flexion, and knee extension. Discuss the relationship between the force-length relationship in the muscle fiber and in the whole muscle.

3. Graph the force-velocity relationship in (a) a muscle fiber and in (b) a whole muscle. Identify the eccentric contraction on graph (a) and identify a static contraction on graph (b).

4. Provide a schematic representation of the possible sites of muscular fatigue.

5. Compare and contrast the two models proposed to explain delayed-onset muscle soreness. Is it possible that both models are correct? Why or why not?

6. What are the primary laboratory methods of assessing muscular function? What are the primary field tests to assess muscular function? What are the limitations of the various methods? What determines which is the appropriate test to administer?

7. Compare male and female strength development during childhood and adolescence.

8. Discuss differences in strength between adult males and females. How is the difference in strength affected by the units used to express strength (that is, absolute or relative values)? How does it vary among different regions of the body? What are the most likely causes of sex-related differences in muscular function?

9. What factors account for the age-related decline in muscular strength? Can this loss be minimized or slowed? If so, how?

10. What is the role of genetics in determining an individuals' strength or an individuals' response to a training program?

Box 18.1 **Answers**

Name	Absolute Strength MVC (kg)	Relative Strength kg · kg^{-1}	50% MVC
Jody	40.0	0.66	20.0
Jill	60.0	0.88	30.0
Pat	36.0	0.51	18.0
Scott	50.0	0.79	25.0
Tom	72.0	0.88	36.0
Mike	71.0	1.01	35.5

3. Tom; Mike

4. Tom

Box 18.2 **Answers**

1. No, bending the knees (changing knee angle) does not eliminate the involvement of the thigh muscles. If the feet are supported (held down), the thigh muscles are more active than the rectus abdominis.

2. External obliques

3. Not held

4. From the available choices you should have selected feet unsupported and knees bent at a 105° position in order to maximize the use of the abdominal muscles. These results indicate the best form of the sit-up from the standpoint of hip angle and foot support, but they do not take into account arm position. Also, they do not permit comparison with a curl-up or crunch (in which the head, shoulders, and trunk are lifted off the floor only about 30°). Other research has actually shown that the abdominal muscles are responsible for only the first 30–45° of the sit-up motion, and it is easier on the spinal discs if only a partial sit-up and not a full sit-up is performed. Combining this information, it must be concluded that on the basis of currently available information, a curl-up test with knees bent and feet unsupported is the exercise of choice for the abdominal muscles for most individuals.

REFERENCES

1. Aoyug, Y., & R. J. Shepard: Aging and muscle function. *Sports Medicine.* 14(6):376–396 (1992).

2. Armstrong, R. B.: Mechanisms of exercise-induced delayed onset muscular soreness: A brief review. *Medicine and Science in Sports and Exercise.* 16(6):529–538 (1984).

3. Armstrong, R. B., M. H. Laughlin, L. Rome, & C. R. Taylor: Metabolism of rats running up and down an incline. *Journal of Applied Physiology.* 55:518–521 (1983).

4. Asmussen, E.: Observations on experimental muscular soreness. *Acta Rheumatologica Scandinavia.* 2:109–116 (1956).

5. Bigland, B., & O. C. J. Lippold: The relation between force, velocity, and integrated electrical activity in human muscles. *Journal of Physiology.* 123:214–224 (1954).

6. Bonde-Petersen, F., H. G. Knuttgen, & J. Henriksson: Muscle metabolism during exercise with concentric and eccentric contractions. *Journal of Applied Physiology.* 33:792–795 (1972).

7. Bouchard, C., F. T. Dionne, J. A. Simoneau, & M. R. Boulay: Genetics of aerobic and anaerobic performances. *Exercise and Sport Science Reviews.* 20:27–58 (1992).

8. Bouchard, C., M. Chagnon, M. Thibault, M. Boulay, M. Marcotte, C. Cote, & J. Simoneau: Muscle genetic variants and relationship with performance and trainability. *Medicine and Science in Sports and Exercise.* 21(1):71–77 (1989).

9. Bouchard, C., & L. Pérusse: Heredity, activity level, fitness, and health. In C. Bouchard, R. J. Shephard, & T. Stephens (eds.), *Physical Activity, Fitness, and Health: International Proceedings and Consensus Statement.* Champaign, IL: Human Kinetics Publishers, 106–118 (1994).

10. Coyle, E. F., D. L. Costill, & G. R. Lesmes: Leg extension power and muscle fiber composition. *Medicine and Science in Sports.* 11(1):12–15 (1976).

11. Davies, C. T. M., & C. Barnes: Negative (eccentric) work. II. Physiological responses to walking uphill and downhill on motor-driven treadmill. *Ergonomics.* 15:121–131 (1972).

12. DeLorme, T. L., & A. L. Watkins: Techniques of progressive resistance exercise. *Archives of Physical Medicine.* 29:263–273 (1948).

13. DeVries, H. A., & T. J. Housh: *Physiology of Exercise: For Physical Education, Athletics and Exercise Science.* Madison, WI: Brown & Benchmark (1994).

14. Edington, D. W., & V. R. Edgerton: *The Biology of Physical Activity.* Boston: Houghton Mifflin, 282 (1976).

15. Edman, K. A. P.: Contractile performance of skeletal muscle fibers. In P. V. Komi (ed.), *Strength and Power in Sport.* Boston: Blackwell Scientific, 96–114 (1992).

16. Enoka, R. M.: *Neuromechanical Basis of Kinesiology.* Champaign, IL: Human Kinetics Publishers, 31–64 (1988).

17. Fischer, A., & Merhautova: Electromyographic manifestations of individual stages of adapted sports technique. In *Health and Fitness in the Modern World.* Chicago: Athletic Institute, 134–147 (1961).

18. Goldspink, G.: Cellular and molecular aspects of adaptation in skeletal muscles. In P. V. Komi (ed.), *Strength and Power in Sport.* Boston, MA: Blackwell Scientific, 211–229 (1992).

19. Hall, S. J., J. Lee, & T. M. Wood: Evaluation of selected sit-up variations for the individual with low back pain. *Journal of Applied Sport Science Research.* 4(2):42–46 (1990).

20. Halpern, A. A., & E. E. Bleck: Sit-up exercises: an electromyographic study. *Clinical Orthopaedics and Related Research.* 145:172–178 (1979).

21. Hasson, S. M., J. C. Daniels, J. G. Divine, B. R. Niebuhr, S. Richmond, P. G. Stein, & J. Williams: Effect of ibuprofen use on muscle soreness, damage, and performance: A preliminary investigation. *Medicine and Science in Sports and Exercise.* 25(1):9–17 (1990).

22. Heyward, V. H.: *Advanced Fitness Assessment and Exercise Prescription.* Champaign, IL: Human Kinetics Publishers (1991).

23. Kelly, D. D.: The role of endorphins in stress-induced analgesia. *Annals of the New York Academy of Sciences.* 398:260–270 (1982).

24. Komi, P. V.: Stretch-shortening cycle. In P. Komi (ed), *Strength and Power in Sport.* London: Blackwell Scientific, 169–180 (1992).

25. Komi, P. V.: Physiological and biomechanical correlates of muscle function: Effects of muscle structure and stretch-shortening cycle of force and speed. In R. Terjung (ed.), *Exercise and Sport Sciences Reviews* (Vol. 12). Lexington, MA: Collamore Press, 81–122 (1984).

26. Kulig, K., J. G. Andrews, & J. G. Hay: Human strength curves. In R. Terjung (ed.), *Exercise and Sport Sciences Reviews* (vol. 12). Lexington, MA: Collamore Press, 417–466 (1984).

27. Lauback, L. L.: Comparative muscle strength of men and women: A review of the literature. *Aviation, Space and Environmental Medicine.* 47:534–542 (1976).

28. Lippold, D. C. J.: The relation between integrated action potentials in a human muscle and its isometric tension. *Journal of Physiology.* 117:492–499 (1952).

29. MacLaren, D. P., H. Gibson, M. Parry-Billings, & R. H. T. Edwards: A review of metabolic and physiological factors in fatigue. *Exercise and Sport Sciences Reviews.* 17:29–66 (1989).

30. Malina, R. M., & C. Bouchard: *Growth, Maturation, and Physical Activity.* Champaign, IL: Human Kinetics Publishers (1991).

31. McGlynn, G. H., N. T. Laughlin, & V. Rowe: Effect of electromyographic feedback and static stretching on artificially induced muscle soreness. *American Journal of Physical Medicine.* 58:139–148 (1979).

32. Pérusse, L., G. Lortie, A. LeBlanc, A. Tremblay, G. Thériault, & C. Bouchard: Genetic and environmental sources of variation in physical fitness. *Annals of Human Biology.* 14:425–434 (198).

33. Powers, S. K., & E. T. Howley: *Exercise Physiology: Theory and Application to Fitness and Performance.* Dubuque, IA: Brown (1990).

34. Rogers, M. A., & W. J. Evans: Changes in skeletal muscle with aging: Effects of exercise training. In J. O. Holloszy (ed.), *Exercise and Sport Sciences Reviews* (Vol. 21). Baltimore: Williams & Wilkins, 65–102 (1993).

35. Roy, R. R., & V. R. Edgerton: Skeletal muscle architecture and performance. In P. V. Komi (ed.), *Strength and Power in Sport.* Boston: Blackwell Scientific, 115–129 (1992).

36. Simonson, E.: *Physiology of Work Capacity and Fatigue.* Springfield, IL: Thomas (1971).

37. Stauber, W. T.: Eccentric action of muscles: Physiology, injury, and adaptation. *Exercise and Sport Sciences Reviews.* 17:157–186 (1989).

38. Thomas, C. L. (ed.), *Taber's Cyclopedia Medical Dictionary.* Philadelphia: Davis (1989).

39. Webber, L. M., W. C. Pyrnes, T. W. Rowland & V. L. Foster: Serum creatine kinase activity and delayed onset muscle soreness in pre-pubescent children: A preliminary study. *Pediatric Exercise Science.* 1:351–359 (1989).

40. Wells, C. L., & S. A. Plowman: Sexual differences in athletic performance: Biological or behavioral? *The Physician and Sports Medicine.* 11(8):52–63 (1983).

41. Williams, J. H.: Normal musculoskeletal and neuromuscular anatomy, physiology and responses to training. In S. M. Hasson (ed.), *Clinical Exercise Physiology.* St. Louis: Mosby (1994).

42. Wilmore, J. H.: Alterations in strength, body composition, and anthropometric measurements consequent to a 10-week weight training program. *Medicine and Science in Sports.* 6:133–138 (1974).

19

Muscular Training Principles and Adaptations

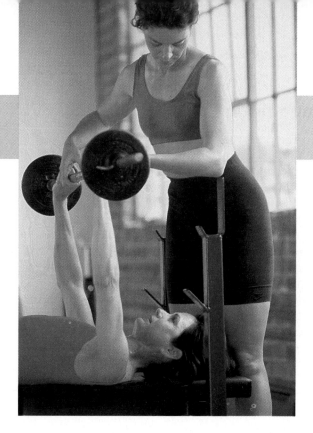

After studying the chapter, you should be able to:

- Apply each of the training principles to the development of a resistance training program.

- Describe muscular adaptations to dynamic resistance training and dynamic aerobic endurance training programs.

- Discuss the relationship between muscle function and lower-back pain.

- List the effects of anabolic steroid use, and summarize the position of the American College of Sports Medicine on the use of anabolic steroids in athletic competition.

Introduction

The previous chapters have provided a basis for an understanding of how isolated muscle fibers contract and how intact muscles contract to produce coordinated movements. This chapter will discuss the specific applications of the training principles for the development of muscular fitness and the training adaptations that occur as a result of an exercise training program. The final section addresses the applications of this information to the problems of lower-back pain and the use of anabolic steroids.

Although it is possible to develop a training program using static contractions, in reality such programs are rare. Therefore, this section will be limited to dynamic resistance and isokinetic training programs. The term *resistance training program* will be used as an inclusive term encompassing dynamic resistance and isokinetic training unless otherwise specified.

Overview of Resistance Training

Resistance training is a systematic program of exercises involving the exertion of force against a load used to develop strength, endurance, and/or hypertrophy of the muscular system;[8] it is commonly referred to as weight training. Resistance training is used by a wide range of individuals, including those seeking to improve overall health, improve athletic performance, rehabilitate an injury, change their physical appearance, or compete in power lifting or bodybuilding contests.

Resistance training—if done under skilled adult supervision with proper instruction in form, breathing, body mechanics, and prescription of loads—can be enjoyed by all individuals and carries relatively low risk of harm for prepubescent children (approximately 7–13 yr of age). Participation, however, should take into account the desire of the child and should be only one of a variety of activities and sports that the child participates in. Note that chil-

> **Resistance Training** A systematic program of exercises involving the exertion of force against a load used to develop strength, endurance, and/or hypertrophy of the muscular system.

dren should not participate in competitive weight lifting, power lifting, and bodybuilding. It is also important that expectations be realistic. For example, resistance training programs of less than 20 weeks duration have shown no significant positive influences on body composition, sports performance, injury rate, or recovery from injury in this age group. On the other hand, no detrimental effects have been shown on growth or injury rate.[3]

Application of the Training Principles

The training principles that govern a safe and effective resistance training program are the same principles that guide other types of exercise programs.

Specificity

As in any training program, a plan for muscular fitness must be specific to the goals of the individual. These goals may include the development of muscular strength, muscular endurance, power, muscle hypertrophy, or any combination of the above.

Muscles respond specifically to the type of contraction being performed and to the load imposed. Many sports, including basketball, utilize dynamic resistance programs to increase muscle strength and mass. Other sports, including swimming, are more likely to utilize isokinetic training programs in an attempt to develop strength through a specified range of motion.

Resistance training is also specific to the muscle groups being trained. Therefore, a resistance training program should include at least one exercise for all the major muscle groups of the body.[13] To avoid fatigue, it is often recommended that exercises be arranged in a specific order, alternating lower-body exercises with exercises of the upper body. This tactic allows the muscles to recover between exercises or exercise sessions. Generally, large muscle groups should be exercised first, followed by smaller muscle groups. For example, if an exerciser is interested in working the latissimus dorsi (lats) and the biceps, the lats should be worked first (pull-downs), because they involve a larger muscle group. This schedule helps to ensure the fatigue of the smaller muscle group (the biceps), but does not limit the work that can be performed by the larger muscle group (the lats).

The amount of stress applied to the muscle will determine, to a large extent, the response of the muscle. A muscle that is exposed to near-maximal stress will develop greater strength than a muscle that is required to repeat many submaximal trials. On the other hand, the muscle that performs in many submaximal trials will develop relatively more muscular endurance than one exposed to a small number of near-maximal trials.

Specificity also appears to apply to the velocity of contraction for isokinetic exercises.[19] Exercise performed at slow velocities tends to produce increases in torque specific to the training velocity. Training at high velocities tends to increase strength at and below the exercise velocity and, thus, is not as specific as slow-velocity training. Furthermore, it is a misconception that the velocity of isokinetic exercise should be specific to athletic events.[19] In reality the angular velocities of joint movements found in many athletic events (such as throwing) far exceed what can be performed during isokinetic exercise.

Overload

The successful application of the overload principle, as it applies to resistance training, necessitates the manipulation of intensity (load), frequency, and duration (number of repetitions, sets, and rest periods). Of these variables, intensity appears to have the greatest effect on the outcome of the program.

Historically, the development of programs based on these variables began in 1948 when De-Lorme and Watkins[9] introduced *progressive resistance exercise.* The DeLorme and Watkins program uses 30 repetitions per training session for each muscle group exercised. The 30 repetitions are broken down into 3 sets of 10 repetitions (reps) each, as follows:

set 1 = 10 repetitions at 50% of 10-RM
set 2 = 10 repetitions at 75% of 10-RM
set 3 = 10 repetitions at 100% of 10-RM

Since the 1950s, considerable research has been done to determine the optimal number of repetitions and sets, the workload, and the frequency necessary to develop muscular strength, endurance, and power. This research has resulted in the development of many training systems.

Apparently, there is no single combination of repetitions and sets that produces the best results; rather, the ideal number of sets is determined by individual goals and differences. In general, if your primary goal is the development of muscular strength, it's more advantageous to perform a smaller number of repetitions at a higher load. Research indicates that 3–6 repetitions per set for 3–5 sets is probably best for developing muscular strength.[13] If the primary goal is muscular endurance, an increased number of repetitions should be performed with a lesser load. Keep in mind that the muscle must still be "overloaded" in order to achieve a positive adaptation. If strength gains are sought, exercise intensity must be at least 60% of maximum. Gains in endurance can be achieved with an intensity of 30% of maximum if the muscle group is exercised until fatigued.[7] Figure 19.1 depicts a theoretical continuum for the development of muscular strength and power and muscular endurance.[13]

For isokinetic exercise, however, the duration of a single exercise bout appears more important than the total amount of work performed or the number of repetitions completed. Thus, isokinetic exercises are generally based on duration of exercise rather than the number of repetitions.

The length of rest periods between exercise sets is also related to the overload placed on the muscles. If the goal is maximal strength gains, relatively long (several minutes) rest periods should be used between sets. If endurance is the primary goal, shorter (less than 1 minute) rest periods should be used between sets.[13]

The frequency of resistance training varies with the goals of the individual. Obviously, a competitive bodybuilder will train more frequently than an adult fitness participant hoping to derive the health-related benefits of resistance training. The American College of Sports Medicine (ACSM) currently recommends that strengthening exercises should be done two to three times a week to achieve the health-related benefits of such exercises.[1] Training between two and four days a week appears to be most popular with weight lifters. Twice a week is considered the minimum requirement necessary to improve muscular strength; training less than twice a week may predispose the individual to muscle soreness and injury. It is common for athletes who train four days a week to follow a program that

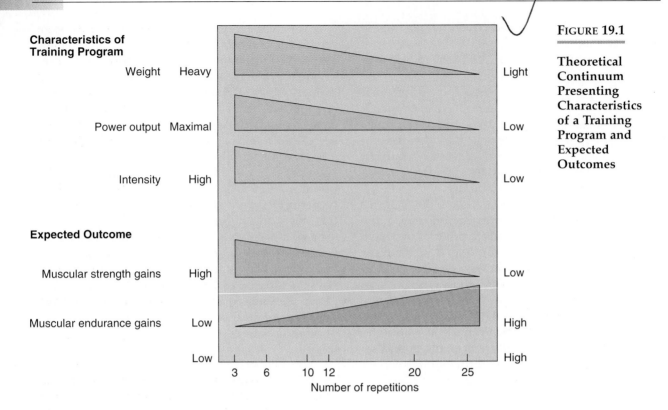

Characteristics of Training Program

Weight   Heavy — Light

Power output   Maximal — Low

Intensity   High — Low

Expected Outcome

Muscular strength gains   High — Low

Muscular endurance gains   Low — High

Low — High

Number of repetitions: 3 6 10 12 20 25

FIGURE 19.1

Theoretical Continuum Presenting Characteristics of a Training Program and Expected Outcomes

alternates an upper-body workout day with a lower-body workout day, so that two days a week are devoted to the upper body and two days a week to the lower body.

Competitive resistance-trained athletes often follow a training program whereby they train three to four days consecutively and then take a day off. When utilizing this type of program, they follow a split routine: Each muscle group is only exercised twice a week. A split routine emphasizes a single muscle group in a workout. This muscle group is then rested for 48–72 hr. A variation of this program is the double-split routine in which two exercise sessions are performed on each workout day.

The duration—the amount of time spent in the weight room—will largely be determined by the number of repetitions, the sets, and the number of different exercises performed. The average duration is 20–30 min per session, although many people will spend more time than that. The volume of training for a given training session is defined as the number of sets multiplied by the number of repetitions multiplied by the load.[22] Larger volumes of training are important not only to individuals seeking greater strength gains but also to those seeking a decrease in percentage of body fat. Novice lifters, however, should avoid excessive volume in order to prevent injury, particularly early in the program. It is prudent to begin a program at a low intensity and a low volume and to increase the amount of training after the body has had time to adapt to the training stress.

Overloading for prepubescent children should involve the same factors as outlined for adults, with some modification. A beginning program should stress learning proper form, techniques, and safety considerations, such as spotting. The equipment chosen should fit the child, which may mean that some exercise machines (designed primarily for adult males) should not be used. Exercises should include major muscle groups and work both agonist and antagonist muscles at each joint. Isolated eccentric training should be avoided.[3] Children should be started on a program consisting of a single set for the first several (2–6) weeks while skill development is being emphasized. Rest periods should be between 2 and 3 min. Low-intensity work of 12–15 RM is best as a starting point. Maximal lifts should be avoided. A frequency of two to three times per week is recommended.[16] Virtually no information is available on a preferred order of the exercises for children.

Adaptation

Muscles adapt to the stress placed upon them. For example, at some point during the program individuals will realize that their initial 10-repetition maximum can now be lifted more than 10 times. This result indicates that adaptation has occurred. The rate of adaptation depends on several factors, including rest periods and adequate diet, and it may not be the same for all muscle groups trained. The importance of rest (recovery) between exercise sessions to allow for the positive adaptations of exercise training cannot be overstressed. At least one day of rest should follow a day of training for a particular muscle group. Adequate rest periods and alternating heavy and light days are important to allow the training adaptations to occur and to prevent injury and soreness. As mentioned earlier, many competitive athletes who lift high volumes will allow 72-hr rest periods before training the same muscle group again.

Adaptation occurs in children as it does in adults. Careful monitoring of recovery between sessions is probably even more important for children to make sure that adequate rest (at least 48 hr) occurs.

Progression

Once the body has adapted to the current training level, exercise stress should be increased as dictated by the overload principle if further increases in strength are desired. This principle is the basis of progressive resistance exercise.

When indicated, progression should be done gradually. Progression can be accomplished by increasing the load, the repetitions, the number of sets, or the frequency of the workout, or by decreasing the rest period between sets. The variables that are most often manipulated are the load and the number of repetitions. Again, the choice will depend largely upon the individual's goals. If strength is the primary goal, then a heavier weight should be used. If endurance is the goal, then the same weight should be lifted more times. It is not uncommon for a combination of these two variables to be used. For instance, many people will begin with a weight they can lift for 6 repetitions. As they adapt to this stress, they will progress to 7 repetitions, then 8 repetitions, and so on. Once they can perform 8–10 repetitions, they will increase the weight to something they can again only lift for 6 repetitions. As recommended earlier, a novice lifter should begin by doing more repetitions with a lighter load. Once the body has adapted, the individual can lift heavier weights.

Progression in prepubescent children should be done slowly, especially in terms of intensity. Moderate loads of 10–12 RM are recommended for the first two to six months of a program; after that, heavier intensities of 8–10 RM can be introduced. Loads heavier than 6 RM are never recommended for children, and the 8–10-RM load gives a safety zone. Shorter rest periods can be introduced, but frequency should be maintained at three times per week.[16]

Individualization

The first step in individualizing a resistance training program is to determine the individual goals of the participant. Once the individual's goals are established, the next step is to evaluate his or her current strength level. This assessment is usually done by determining the individual's one repetition maximum (1 RM). A 1 RM should be established for each muscle group exercised; it is then used to determine the work intensity. For example, a program may call for an individual to do 6 repetitions per set at 80% of the 1 RM.

The final step is determining the training cycle to be used. This technique is often referred to as the periodization of training (see Chapter 1), and it is a common step among athletes who use resistance training to supplement their training programs for athletic competition. For instance, a player who is using resistance training as part of conditioning for basketball would follow a different weight training program during the active rest phase, off-season phase, and preseason phase than during basketball season. Periodization is also important to individuals who use weight training to maintain health-related muscular fitness; it prevents boredom by changing the training program on a regular basis. Competitive resistance-trained athletes also use periodization techniques to vary their training and to prepare for a peak season. Table 19.1

TABLE 19.1 ▪ **Developing a Resistance Training Program**

STEP	SPECIAL CONSIDERATIONS	APPLICABLE TRAINING PRINCIPLES
1. Goal identification	Desired outcome Component of muscular fitness to be stressed Mode of contraction most appropriate Muscle groups to be stressed	Specificity Individualization
2. Evaluation of initial strength or muscular endurance levels	Each muscle group to be used Proper lifting techniques	Specificity
3. Determination of the training system (design of a single session)	Exercises to be included Load Number of sets Rest periods Order in which exercises are to be done Warm-up and cool-down	Specificity Overload Individualization Warm-up and cool-down
4. Determination of the training cycle (periodization)	Prevention of boredom	Adaptation Progression Plateau/Retrogression Individualization

provides an outline for developing a training program based on the individualization of the training principles.

Even if the same program is followed by different individuals, training effects should be expected to occur at different rates. The principle of individualization states that responses to exercise vary among individuals because of factors unique to the individual. In terms of resistance training, these factors include age, body size and type, initial strength, and, perhaps most importantly, genetic makeup (including fiber type distribution).

A coach or exercise leader must be sensitive to the differences in the rate of individual adaptation because it directly affects the progression of training. Unfortunately, it is a common mistake for a coach to design a program for the entire team and expect adaptations to occur at the same rate. The result is often frustration on the part of the coach and the athletes and sometimes even overtraining and/or injuries.

Individually prescribing a resistance training program is probably more important for the prepubescent child than for the adult. Children are growing both physiologically and psychologically, and the rate of growth varies greatly among children. Periodization can be used with children as well as

adults.[22] Competition between individuals should be discouraged for children.

Maintenance

Once a desired level of muscular strength and endurance is achieved, it can be maintained by reduced amounts of work provided the intensity (workload) is maintained. That is, as long as the individual continues to lift the same weight, he or she can maintain strength with only one session per week. A reasonable program would allow individuals to train at a similar workload but with fewer days per week or at a lesser volume to maintain muscular strength and endurance.

Little information is available on maintenance in prepubescent children.[3] One study that is available showed that one day of high-intensity training for 8 weeks was not sufficient to maintain gains achieved in a 20-week program.

Retrogression/Plateau/Reversibility

Despite the best laid plans of coaches, training improvements do not occur in a linear fashion. Even with progressively increasing workloads, there will be times when performance stays at the same level (plateau) or shows a decrease (retrogression). The causes may be overtraining or individual differences. If overtraining is suspected, it is wise to include more rest days or include light days in the training regimen. Additionally, it may be beneficial to consider altering the training program by using the periodization technique discussed earlier.

Detraining (reversibility) occurs when an individual ceases to train. The rate of detraining depends upon the level of strength and endurance the individual has attained. Muscular strength is maintained to a greater degree during detraining than is muscular endurance. Although much of the individual's strength remains after discontinuation of a resistance program, detraining is evidenced on a cellular level. This evidence suggests that there are changes in the size and metabolic properties of the muscle fibers following detraining.

The impact of detraining in children is confounded by the concomitant effects of growth-related strength increases. The actual gains above this growth level do appear to be lost once training ceases.[3]

Warm-Up and Cool-Down

A proper warm-up raises the body temperature and is often recommended to prevent injury and muscle soreness. Although it has not been conclusively proven that a warm-up will decrease the incidence of injury, there is evidence that is consistent with this theory. An increase in temperature decreases the viscosity of the joint capsule. Increased temperatures also increase the speed of muscle contraction and relaxation and enzymatic reactions.[10]

Warm-ups for resistance training may be considered either general or specific and are recommended for weight lifting and isokinetic exercises.[19] A general warm-up involves the major muscles of the body; it is similar to the warm-up used for aerobic activities and includes such activities as jumping rope or jogging. Specific warm-up activities for weight training involve performing the same lifts that are part of the normal program but at a weight well below the training level. The duration and the intensity of the warm-up need to be suited to the individual and to the task to be performed. A proper warm-up should cause a rise in core body temperature of 1–2°F but should not be so strenuous that it causes fatigue. Generally, a warm-up is considered adequate when the individual begins to sweat.

A cool-down period, followed by stretching, is recommended after a training session. Cool-down may prevent muscle soreness and lead to an increase in flexibility, an aspect of muscular fitness that is often overlooked in resistance training programs. Cooling down is important in preventing venous pooling of blood in the lower extremities.

Warm-up and cool-down are just as important for children as for adults. The same pattern of activities should be followed to increase body temperature and to stretch the muscles.

Specific Application of Training Principles to Bodybuilding

The sport of competitive bodybuilding has gained great popularity in the past two decades. Furthermore, many individuals who initiate resistance training programs do so to enhance their physique. For many athletes weight lifting is not only about gaining strength but also about "sculpting" the body.

The goals of bodybuilding are to develop superior muscularity and mass, to develop symmetry and harmony between different body parts, and to enhance muscle density and visual separation of muscles.[22] The effect of such programs is shown in Figure 19.2. In order to achieve their goals, body-

FIGURE 19.2

Bodybuilder
A goal of bodybuilding is to "sculpt" the body.

builders follow specific training strategies and a strict diet.

The training strategies of bodybuilders are designed to increase muscle hypertrophy. Muscle strength is not the primary goal, although strength undoubtedly increases as a result of training. Bodybuilders typically use loads that can be lifted 6–12 times, whereas power lifters lift heavier loads but complete fewer repetitions. Bodybuilders commonly end each set with muscular fatigue or failure. That is, the lifter performs the exercise until the muscles are no longer capable of lifting the weight. Bodybuilders typically use short rest periods (1–2 min) between sets and perform as many as 15–20 sets per muscle group per session for smaller muscle groups. As many as 6 repetitions may be performed with larger muscle groups. Therefore, bodybuilders use a very high volume of training.

The frequency of training for bodybuilders varies; however, split routines or double splits are most common among competitive bodybuilders. These programs typically allow for training on three or four consecutive days, followed by a day of rest. This schedule allows for more than 48 hr of recovery for each muscle group. Although this program is common, there is little scientific evidence to suggest it is the best training schedule. Furthermore, the overall cycle of training (periodization) is important to bodybuilders. Bodybuilders commonly do more strength training in the off-season in order to build muscle mass. As the season approaches, the load is reduced and more repetitions are performed in an attempt to gain muscle symmetry.

Diet is perhaps as important to the success of bodybuilders as is an appropriate training program. In order to enhance muscle definition and promote visual separation of the various muscle groups, bodybuilders maintain a low percentage of body fat. Low body fat is accomplished through a combination of training and diet. Bodybuilders follow a strict low-fat diet, despite the large number of calories they consume. The practice of **cutting** *and ripping* refers to the bodybuilder's attempt to decrease

body fat and body water to very low levels prior to competition in order to increase muscle definition.

*M*uscular Adaptations to Exercise Training

This section will address how skeletal muscles adapt as a result of resistance training and dynamic endurance training. Emphasis will be placed on the changes that occur within muscle tissue.

Neuromuscular Adaptations to Resistance Training Programs

The initiation of a resistance training program typically results in strength gains within the first few weeks despite little or no change in muscle mass, suggesting that neural factors are largely responsible for early strength gains. Figure 19.3 provides a schematic representation of the relative roles of neural and muscular adaptations that contribute to strength gains. Neural adaptation is related to increased neural drive to the muscle, as indicated

FIGURE 19.3

Contribution of Neural and Muscular Adaptations to Strength Gains

Source: D. G. Sale. Neural adaptation to resistance training. *Medicine and Science in Sports and Exercise.* 20(suppl.):S135–S145. Reprinted with permission of William & Wilkins.

Cutting Decreasing body fat and body water content to very low levels in order to increase muscle definition.

by EMG studies; increased synchronization of the motor units; and an inhibition of the protective mechanism of the Golgi tendon organs.[13]

Participation in resistance training programs typically results in increased strength and increased cross-sectional area of muscle. There is also an increase in the fiber area of both ST and FT muscle fibers; however, FT fiber area appears to be increased to a greater extent.

The magnitude of the changes seen in muscles is specific to the muscle group being tested and depends upon the training program followed. The muscle hypertrophy that occurs is due to an increase in the total contractile protein, an increase in the size and number of the myofibrils per fiber, and an increase in the amount of connective tissue surrounding the muscle fibers.[20] Interestingly, there is some evidence that strength gains that occur as a result of isokinetic training can occur in the absence of muscle hypertrophy.[19] This may be due to the absence of an eccentric mode of contraction during these training protocols.

Although men are typically stronger than women, both sexes respond to resistance training in a similar fashion.[7,22,23] Figure 19.4 shows the percentage change in muscle strength for men and women for the elbow flexors, elbow extensors, knee flexor, and knee extensors after 16 weeks of participation in a weight training program.[7] In addition to having similar patterns of strength gains, the men

and women in this study both showed similar changes in muscle cross-sectional area (as determined from CAT scans). The cross-sectional area of the upper arm muscles for the men and women increased 15 and 23%, respectively, after the 16-week training program. Although the men had a greater cross-sectional area than the women, both before and after training, both sexes increased the muscle strength and the muscle cross-sectional area of the upper arm following training.

Until recently, exercise physiologists generally believed that resistance training programs would not increase strength in prepubescent children owing to their lack of testosterone. Results from early studies seemed to confirm this belief. Newer studies that used higher-intensity loads, volumes, and duration, though, have shown that children can increase strength, isometrically and isokinetically. When strength gains are expressed in absolute terms, preadolescents appear somewhat less trainable than either adolescents or adults. However, if the gains are expressed in relative percentages, preadolescents appear to be equally as trainable as adolescents and adults.[3]

In one research study fourteen 8–12-yr-old boys and girls trained twice a week for 8 weeks using 3 sets of 10–15 repetitions on 5 exercises with intensities varying between 50 and 100% of their 10-RM.[11] Following the training period these subjects increased their strength by 74.3%, while a control group increased their strength by 13%. The increase in strength reported in the control group was probably related to growth and maturation of the subjects.

Although the improvement in strength in this study is consistent with improvements documented in adults, the underlying physiological adaptations that account for increased strength appear to be somewhat different. It does not appear that resistance training induces muscle fiber hypertrophy in preadolescents. Changes do occur in the ability of the nervous system to activate motor units, as shown by increased EMG activity with training. Improved motor coordination is also thought to be a contributing neural factor. Thus, neurological factors rather than muscular factors are believed to be responsible for the strength changes in this age group.[3]

Resistance training is also effective in increasing muscular strength and cross-sectional area in

FIGURE 19.4

Improvement in Muscular Strength

Source: Cureton et al.[7]

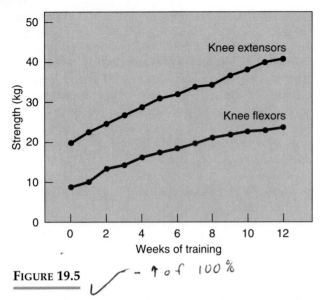

FIGURE 19.5 — ↑ of 100%

Effects of Dynamic Resistance Exercise on Muscular Strength in Older Men

Source: M. A. Rogers & W. J. Evans. Changes in skeletal muscle with aging: Effects of exercise training. In J. O. Holloszy (ed.), *Exercise and Sport Science Reviews* (Vol. 21). Baltimore: Williams & Wilkins, 65–102 (1993). Reprinted by permission.

elderly individuals.[4,5,14,17] In fact, older men and women show similar or even greater strength gains than young individuals after resistance training.[13] Figure 19.5 shows the improvements in dynamic strength of the knee extensors (quadriceps) and the knee flexors (hamstrings) following the 12 weeks of training in older men.[14] By the end of the training period both muscle groups had increased by over 100%. Additionally, these men demonstrated an 11% increase in muscle cross-sectional area, which was accompanied by a 34% increase in ST fiber area and a 28% increase in FT fiber area. A similar response to resistance training has been shown in older women.[23] For example, following a resistance training program of 12 weeks elderly women had improved their strength from 28 to 115%, depending upon the muscle group tested.[5]

In addition to being beneficial to healthy older individuals, resistance training is also beneficial for frail, institutionalized men and women.[12] When a group of 90–100-yr-old men and women engaged in a resistance training program for eight weeks, they increased their strength by 174% (from an average initial value of 8 kg to 21 kg). Additionally, these subjects increased the muscle cross-sectional area by 15%. These improvements demonstrate rather re-

markably the capacity of the muscular system to adapt to progressive resistance exercise as long as a person is willing to participate in a program that utilizes an appropriate intensity of stimulus.

Figure 19.6 summarizes the changes in muscle strength (a) and cross-sectional area (b) that occurs in the quadriceps for males and females of various ages following a resistance training program. These values indicate a percentage change from initial values; thus, they imply neither that females are stronger than males as adults nor that the elderly are stronger than the younger subjects. In fact, those who are weakest initially may be in the best position

FIGURE 19.6

Percentage of Strength Increases in Quadriceps Following Program of Resistance Training

Sources: Faigenbaum;[11] Cureton et al.;[7] Frontere et al.;[14] Charette;[5] Fiatarone.[12]

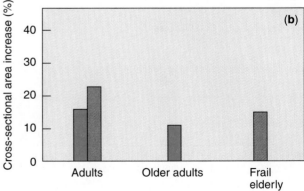

> ## Box 19.1 **A Question of Understanding**
>
> The table gives data for initial strength and final strength in the biceps following a 16-week strength training program for older adults.
>
> | Name | Initial Strength (kg) | Final Strength (kg) |
> |------|----------------------|---------------------|
> | Mary | 45 | 54 |
> | Dick | 47 | 50 |
> | Jim | 68 | 80 |
> | Ben | 62 | 68 |
> | Ralph | 84 | 88 |
> | Debbie | 40 | 55 |
>
> 1. Calculate strength gain for each of the individuals (final – initial).
>
> 2. Calculate percentage improvement [(final – initial)/(initial) × 100].

to show a percentage improvement. To make sure that you understand how to calculate and interpret strength gains, complete Box 19.1.

Muscular Adaptations to Dynamic Aerobic Endurance Training Programs

Dynamic endurance training results in an increase in ST fiber size in adult males and no change in FT fiber size.[15] There is also evidence to suggest that dynamic endurance training can result in the transformation of FG muscle fibers to FOG muscle fibers.[13] Dynamic endurance training in older men and women also results in an increase in the cross-sectional area of the ST fibers (averaging 12%) and an increase in the percentage of FOG fibers.[6]

Special Applications

Muscular Strength and Endurance and Lower-Back Pain

At some point in their lives, 60–80% of all individuals experience lower-back pain (LBP). The condition is disabling to 1–5% of the population. Most cases of LBP occur between the ages of 25 and 60 yr, but 12–26% of children and adolescents are LBP sufferers. Males and females are affected equally.

Neither exact causes nor established risk factors for LBP have been identified. However, there has been and still is great interest in the link between muscular fitness and the absence or occurrence of LBP. The interest is high enough that some tests of health-related physical fitness have included sit-and-reach, sit-ups or curl-ups, and trunk extension tests as means of testing lower-back function. The theoretical link between physical fitness and LBP is largely based on functional anatomy (Table 19.2), and at this time the anatomical logic is stronger than the research evidence.

In order to have a healthy, well-functioning back, an individual must have flexible lower-back (lumbar) muscles, hamstrings, and hip flexors and strong, fatigue-resistant abdominal and back extensor muscles. The goal is to keep the vertebrae aligned properly without excessive disk pressure, allowing a full range of motion in all directions. In addition, the pelvis must freely rotate both posteriorly and anteriorly without strain on the muscle or fascia.

Research evidence shows that individuals suffering from LBP exhibit lower levels of strength in both abdominal and back extensors. EMG activity is also increased in the back muscles of individuals with LBP. These differences, however, are more likely to be the result of LBP rather than the cause. Studies that have attempted to predict who might get LBP, either for a first time or in recurrent episodes, from strength and muscular endurance measures have identified back extension endurance as the critical variable. That is, individuals with low levels of back extension endurance are more likely to develop LBP at a later date than individuals with high levels of back extensor endurance. Although high levels of back extensor strength and abdominal flexion strength or endurance have not proven to offer this same predictive value, they have never been shown to be detrimental. Thus, a total body workout for strength and muscular endurance should include exercises for the back and abdominals. This program does not mean that individuals who follow it will be protected absolutely from LBP.

Anabolic Steroids

Despite warnings about the adverse effects of anabolic steroids, the use of these androgens appears to be widespread among athletes, particularly those involved in resistance training.[24] In fact, anabolic

TABLE 19.2 ■ Theoretical Relationship Between Physical Fitness Components and Healthy or Unhealthy Lower-Back or Spinal Function

PHYSICAL FITNESS COMPONENT (NEUROMUSCULAR)	NORMAL ANATOMICAL FUNCTION IN LOWER BACK: HEALTHY	DYSFUNCTION	RESULTS OF DYSFUNCTION: UNHEALTHY
Lumbar flexibility	Allows the lumbar curve to almost be reversed in forward flexion	Inflexible	Disrupts forward and lateral movement; places excessive stretch on hamstrings, leading to lower-back and hamstring pain
Hamstring flexibility	Allows anterior rotation (tilt) of the pelvis in forward flexion and posterior rotation in the sitting position	Inflexible	Restricts anterior pelvic rotation and exaggerates posterior tilt; both cause increased disk compression; excessive stretching causes strain and pain
Hip flexor flexibility	Allows achievement of neutral pelvic position	Inflexible	Exaggerates anterior pelvic tilt if not counteracted by strong abdominal muscles, thereby increasing disk compression
Abdominal strength or endurance	Maintains pelvic position; reinforces back extensor fascia and pulls it laterally on forward flexion, providing support	Weak, easily fatigued	Allows abnormal pelvic tilt; increases strain on back extensor muscles
Back extensor strength or endurance	Provides stability for the spine; maintains erect posture; controls forward flexion	Weak, easily fatigued	Increases loading on the spine; causes increased disk compression

steroids have been used by professional athletes for decades in their attempt to become stronger, leaner, and more aggressive. Furthermore, the use of steroids extends to high school athletes and individuals wishing to enhance their physique.

Anabolic steroids are synthetic androgens that mimic the effects of the male hormone testosterone. Although anabolic steroids are derived from testosterone, they have been altered to enhance their anabolic effect.

Although steroids build muscle mass, their use is dangerous, illegal, and unethical. After reviewing the available literature concerning anabolic steroids, the American College of Sports Medicine (ACSM) issued a position statement concerning the use of anabolic-androgenic steroids in sport.[2] This paper addresses the following adverse effects of steroid use:

- ■ *Effects on the liver.* Anabolic steroids are associated with impaired excretory function (resulting in jaundice), blood filled cysts (peliosis hepatis), and liver tumors.

- ■ *Effects on the cardiovascular system.* The use of anabolic steroids results in hyperinsulinism and altered glucose tolerance, decreased levels of high-density lipoprotein, and elevated blood pressure.

- ■ *Effects on the male reproductive system.* Anabolic steroid use has the effect of decreasing the number of sperm, decreasing testicular size, and reducing the levels of testosterone.

- ■ *Effects on the female reproductive system.* The effects of anabolic steroids include a reduction in circulating levels of luteinizing hormone,

Anabolic Steroids Synthetic androgens that mimic the effects of the male hormone testosterone.

follicle-stimulating hormone, estrogens and progesterone; inhibition of folliculogenesis and ovulation; and menstrual cycle changes.

- *Effects on psychological status.* The use of anabolic steroids decreases libido and causes mood swings and aggressive behavior.

- *Other effects.* Other side effects associated with anabolic steroids include premature closure of epiphysial plates, acne, and hair loss.

Clearly, the use of anabolic steroids can have serious short-term and long-term effects. Exercise scientists thus have a responsibility to be involved in the ongoing educational efforts regarding the effects of steroid use.

SUMMARY

1. Resistance training is used to improve overall health, improve athletic performance, rehabilitate an injury, and change physical appearance. It is also the primary activity of the sports of power lifting and bodybuilding.

2. A plan for muscular fitness is specific to the goals of the individual, which may include the development of muscular strength, muscular endurance, power, muscle hypertrophy, or any combination of these properties.

3. Overload of the muscular system is achieved by manipulating the intensity (load), frequency, and duration of training. The duration is determined by the number of repetitions and sets performed and the recovery period between lifts.

4. If the same training program is followed by different individuals, adaptation will occur at different rates owing to individual differences in age, body size and type, initial strength, and genetic makeup.

5. A coach or exercise leader must be sensitive to the differences in the rate of individual adaptation because it directly affects the progression of training. A common mistake is for coaches to design a program for the entire team and expect adaptations to occur at the same rate.

6. Adaptation to resistance training in children and the elderly is very similar to adaptations that occur in adults.

REVIEW QUESTIONS

1. Give several reasons why an individual may engage in a resistance training program, and specify the different goals of a program.

2. Discuss how each of the training principles is applied in the development of a resistance training program. How do these applications vary if the exerciser is a child?

3. Is there an ideal number of repetitions and sets that should be performed by everyone? Defend your answer.

4. Discuss the importance of adequate recovery time in training adaptations to a resistance training program.

5. Do all individuals respond to a training program with the same adaptation (or magnitude of adaptation)? Why or why not?

6. What is the importance of a warm-up period prior to resistance training?

7. Compare and contrast the training adaptations that occur in skeletal muscle as a result of resistance training and endurance training.

8. What is the relationship between muscle function and lower-back pain?

9. Why are anabolic steroids dangerous?

Box 19.1 Answers

$$\text{strength gain} = \text{final strength} - \text{initial strength}$$

$$\text{for Mary:} \quad 9\,\text{kg} = 54\,\text{kg} - 45\,\text{kg}$$

$$\% \text{ improvement} = [(\text{final strength} - \text{initial strength}) \div \text{initial strength}] \times 100$$

$$\text{for Mary:} \quad \frac{9\,\text{kg}}{45\,\text{kg}} \times 100 = 20\%$$

	Strength Gain	*% Improvement*
Mary	9	20
Dick	3	6
Jim	12	18
Ben	6	10
Ralph	4	5
Debbie	15	38

REFERENCES

1. American College of Sports Medicine: *Guidelines for Exercise Testing and Prescription.* Philadelphia: Lea & Febiger (1991).

2. American College of Sports Medicine: Position paper: The use of anabolic-steroids in sports. *Medicine and Science in Sports and Exercise.* 19(6):534–539 (1987).

3. Blimkie, C. J. R.: Resistance training during preadolescence: Issues and controversies. *Sports Medicine.* 15(6):389–407 (1988).

4. Brown, C. H., & J. H. Wilmore: The effects of maximal resistance training on the strength and body composition of women athletes. *Medicine and Science in Sports and Exercise.* 6:174–177 (1974).

5. Charette, S. L., L. McEvovy, G. Pyka, C. Snow-Harter, D. Guido, R. A. Wiswell, & R. Marcus: Muscle hypertrophy response to resistance training in older women. *Journal of Applied Physiology.* 70:1912–1916 (1991).

6. Coggan, A. R., R. J. Pina, D. S. King, M. A. Rogers, M. Brown, P. M. Nemeth, & J. O. Holloszy: Skeletal muscle adaptations to endurance training in 60- to 70-year-old men and women. *Journal of Applied Physiology.* 68:1896–1901 (1990).

7. Cureton, K. J., M. A. Collins, D. W. Hill, & F. M. Mcelhannon: Muscle hypertrophy in men and women. *Medicine and Science in Sports and Exercise.* 20(4):338–344 (1988).

8. Davies, C. T. M., & C. Barnes: Negative (eccentric) work. II. Physiological responses to walking uphill and downhill on motor-driven treadmill. *Ergonomics.* 15:121–131 (1972).

9. DeLorme, T. L., & A. L. Watkins: Techniques of progressive resistance exercise. *Archives of Physical Medicine.* 29:263–273 (1948).

10. Enoka, R. M.: *Neuromechanical Basis of Kinesiology.* Champaign, IL: Human Kinetics Publishers, 31–64 (1988).

11. Faigenbaum, A. D., L. D. Zaichkowsky, W. L. Westcott, L. J. Micheli, & A. F. Fehlandt: The effects of a twice-a-week strength training program on children. *Pediatric Exercise Science.* 5:339–346 (1993).

12. Fiatarone, M. A., E. C. Marks, N. D. Ryan, C. N. Meedith, L. A. Lipsitz, & W. J. Evans: High intensity strength training in nonagenarians. Effects on skeletal muscle. *Journal of the American Medical Association.* 263:3029–3034 (1990).

13. Fleck, S. J., & W. J. Kramer: *Designing Resistance Training Programs.* Champaign, IL: Human Kinetics Publishers (1987).

14. Frontera, W. R., V. A. Hughs, K. J. Lutz, & W. J. Evans: A cross-sectional study of muscle strength and mass in 45- to 78-yr-old men and women. *Journal of Applied Physiology.* 71:644–650 (1991).

15. Gollnick, P. D., R. B Armstrong, C. W. Saubert IV, K. Piehl, & B. Saltin: Enzyme activity and fiber composition in skeletal muscle of untrained and trained men. *Journal of Applied Physiology.* 33(3):312–319 (1972).

16. Kramer, W. J., A. D. Fry, P. N. Frykman, & B. Conroy: Resistance training and youth. *Pediatric Exercise Science.* 1:336–350 (1989).

17. Larsson, L.: Physical training effects on muscle morphology in sedentary males at different ages. *Medicine and Science in Sports and Exercise.* 14:203–206 (1982).

18. McGlynn, G. H., N. T. Laughlin, & V. Rowe: Effect of electromyographic feedback and static stretching on artificially induced muscle soreness. *American Journal of Physical Medicine.* 58:139–148 (1979).

19. Perrin, D. H.: *Isokinetic Exercise and Assessment.* Champaign, IL: Human Kinetics Publishers (1993).

20. Rogers, M. A., & W. J. Evans: Changes in skeletal muscle with aging: Effects of exercise training. In J. O. Holloszy (ed.), *Exercise and Sport Sciences Reviews* (Vol. 21). Baltimore: Williams & Wilkins, 65–102 (1993).

21. Sale, D. G.: Neural adaptation to resistance training. *Medicine and Science in Sports and Exercise.* 20(suppl.):S135–S145 (1988).

22. Tesch, P. A.: Training for body building. In P. V. Komi (ed.), *Strength and Power in Sport.* London: Blackwell Scientific, 357–369 (1992).

23. Wilmore, J. H.: Alterations in strength, body composition, and anthropometric measurements consequent to a 10 week weight training program. *Medicine and Science in Sports.* 6:133–138 (1974).

24. Yesalis, C. E., S. P. Courson, & J. Wright: History of anabolic steroid use in sport and exercise. In C. E. Yesalis (ed.), *Anabolic Steroids in Sport and Exercise.* Champaign, IL: Human Kinetics Publishers (1993).

20

Neuromuscular Aspects of Movement

After studying the chapter, you should be able to:

- Describe the nerve supply to muscle.

- Describe the sequence of events at the neuromuscular junction.

- Identify the components of a reflex arc.

- Describe the structure and innervation of the muscle spindle, and explain how the muscle spindle functions in the myotatic reflex.

- Describe the structure and innervation of the Golgi tendon organ, and explain how it functions in the inverse myotatic reflex.

- Provide research and clinical evidence that individual motor units can be volitionally controlled.

- Diagram the sequence of events involved in volitional control of movement.

- Differentiate between dynamic and static flexibility.

- Identify the anatomical factors that influence flexibility.

- Describe the basic methods of assessing flexibility.

- Discuss the relationship between flexibility and low-back pain.

- Differentiate among the different types of flexibility training.

- Apply the training principles to the development of a flexibility program.

Introduction

As spectators watching the Olympic games, we marvel at the grace and skill of figure skaters and stare in amazement at the incredible feats of gymnasts. As adults, we look on with wonder as a child learns a new task: rolling over, walking, tying a shoe. As coaches or fitness leaders, we experience the satisfaction of seeing individuals incorporate our suggestions to improve their skill. To understand the awe-inspiring accomplishments of athletes and the simple movements that are often taken for granted requires a knowledge of the nervous system.

The nervous system is made up of the brain, spinal cord, and nerves. It is the primary control and communication center for the entire body. As discussed in Chapter 1, the nervous system functions with the endocrine system to control and regulate the internal environment of the body; that is, it maintains homeostasis. All human movement depends on the nervous system; skeletal muscles will not contract unless they receive a signal from the nervous system.

This chapter will introduce some basic neuroanatomy and examine the role of the nervous system in controlling human movement. It will also discuss the influence of the nervous system on flexibility and flexibility training.

Neural Control of Muscle Contraction

Nerve Supply

All skeletal muscles require nervous stimulation to produce the electrical excitation in the muscle cells that leads to contraction. The neurons that carry information from the central nervous system to the muscle are called *efferent neurons.* Efferent neurons that innervate skeletal muscle are referred to as *motor neurons;* motor neurons may be classified as alpha motor neurons or gamma motor neurons. The *alpha* (α) *motor neurons* are relatively large motor neurons that innervate (connect to) skeletal muscle fibers and result in contraction of muscles. You should recall from Chapter 17 that α_1 motor neurons innervate FT muscle fibers, whereas α_2 motor neu-

rons innervate ST muscle fibers. *Gamma* (γ) *motor neurons* innervate proprioceptors.

As a nerve enters the connective tissue of the muscle, it divides into branches, with each branch ending near the surface of a muscle fiber (cell). Because the axon of the motor neuron branches, each neuron is connected to several muscle fibers. As defined in Chapter 17 a motor neuron and the muscle fibers it innervates is called a *motor unit* (Figure 20.1). The motor unit is the basic unit of contraction. Because each muscle fiber in a motor unit is connected to the same neuron, the electrical activity in that neuron controls the contractile activity of all the muscle fibers in that motor unit. The number of muscle fibers controlled by a single neuron (that is, the number of muscle cells in a motor unit) varies tremendously, depending on the size and function of the muscle involved. Although a single neuron may innervate many muscle fibers, each muscle fiber is only innervated by a single motor neuron.

Figure 20.2 illustrates the relationship between the motor neuron (originating in the central nervous system) and the muscle fibers. The cell body of the motor neuron is located within the gray matter of the spinal cord [(2) in Figure 20.2], and the axon

FIGURE 20.1

Motor Units

Two motor units are depicted. Notice that the muscle fibers of the two motor units are intermingled.

Dorsal root
(sensory)
Cell body
Posterior
Upper motor
neuron
Fascicle
Ventral root
(motor)
Anterior
Alpha motor neuron
(lower motor neuron)
Myelin sheath
Blood vessels
Muscle fibers

FIGURE 20.2

Functional Relationship Between Motor (Efferent) Neurons and Muscle Cells

A motor neuron and the muscle cells it innervates is called a motor unit. (1) Schematic of central nervous system, (2) cross-sectional view of the spinal cord, (3) cross-sectional view of peripheral nerve emphasizing axon of motor neuron, and (4) the motor neuron branching near its terminal end where it forms the neuromuscular junction with the muscle fibers.

extends out through the ventral root of the spinal nerve [(3) in Figure 20.2] to carry the electrical signal to the muscle fiber [(4) in Figure 20.2]. Each branch of the motor neuron terminates in a slight bulge called the axon terminal, which lies very close to but does not touch the underlying muscle fiber [(4) in Figure 20.2].

The space between the membrane of the neuron at the motor end plate and the muscle cell membrane is called the neuromuscular (or synaptic) cleft. The entire region is referred to as the *neuromuscular junction*. The neuromuscular junction is important because it is here that the electrical signal from the motor neuron is transmitted to the surface of the muscle cell which is to contract.

Muscle cells are also supplied with afferent (sensory) nerve endings, which are sensitive to mechanical and chemical changes in the muscle tissue and which relay this information back to the central nervous system. The information carried by afferent neurons is used by the central nervous system to make adjustments in muscular contractions.

The Neuromuscular Junction

The neuromuscular junction is a specialized synapse formed between a terminal end of a motor neuron and a muscle fiber. Figure 20.3 summarizes the events that occur at the neuromuscular junction. When an action potential reaches the axon terminal, the membrane of the neuron increases its permeability to calcium, and calcium is taken up into the cell (Figure 20.3a). The increased levels of calcium cause the synaptic vesicles to migrate to the cell membrane (by the process of exocytosis) and release neurotransmitter (acetylcholine, ACh) into the synaptic cleft (Figure 20.3b). The ACh then diffuses across the synaptic cleft and binds to the sarcolemma, causing changes in the ionic permeability and leading to the depolarization of the sarcolemma (Figure 20.3c). This change in permeability and subsequent depolarization leads to the generation of an action potential in the sarcolemma of the muscle fiber. The action potential spreads in all directions from the neuromuscular junction, depolarizing the entire sarcolemma. The action potential is then

(a)

(b)

(c)

(d)

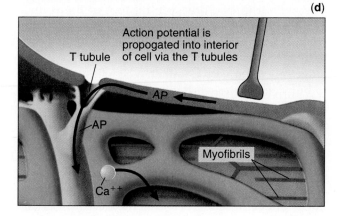

FIGURE 20.3

Events at the Neuromuscular Junction

(a) An action potential (AP) in the axon terminal causes the uptake of Ca^{++} into the axon terminal and the subsequent release of the neurotransmitter. (b) The neurotransmitter (ACh) is released from the synaptic vesicles and diffuses across the synaptic cleft. (c) Generation of action potential: The binding of ACh to the sarcolemma causes a change in membrane permeability, causing an AP to be initiated in the sarcolemma. (d) The AP is propagated into the interior of the cells via the T tubules.

spread into the interior of the cell through the T tubules (Figure 20.3d).

Although the neuromuscular junction functions much like other synapses, there are three important differences.

1. At a neuromuscular junction, a single presynaptic action potential leads to a postsynaptic action potential.

2. The synapse can only be excitatory.

3. A muscle fiber only receives synaptic input from one motor neuron.

Note the two distinct roles that calcium plays in controlling muscular contraction. The first role is to facilitate the release of ACh from the synaptic vesicles in the motor neuron terminal. The second (and most often discussed) role of calcium is to control the position of the regulatory proteins troponin and tropomyosin on actin.

Reflex Control of Movement

Reflexes play an important role in maintaining an upright posture and in responding to movement in a coordinated fashion. A **reflex** is a rapid, involuntary response to a stimuli in which a specific stimulus results in a specific motor response. Reflexes can be classified into two types: *Autonomic reflexes,* which activate cardiac and smooth muscle and glands, and *somatic reflexes,* which result in skeletal muscle contraction. This section will focus on somatic reflexes, which play an important role in movement.

Many spinal reflexes do not require the participation of higher brain centers to initiate a response. The higher brain centers, however, are often notified of the resultant movement by neurons that synapse with the afferent neuron.

Spinal Cord

The spinal cord is involved in both involuntary and voluntary movements. It performs two essential functions: It connects the peripheral nervous system with the brain, and it serves as the site of reflex integration.

Figure 20.4 displays a cross-sectional view of the spinal cord; notice the spinal nerves extending from each side of the cord. Each spinal nerve con-

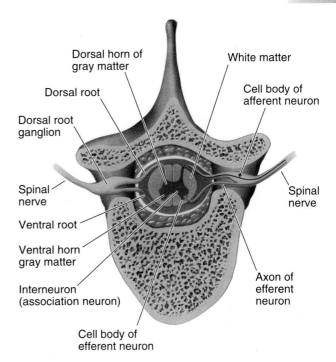

Dorsal horn of gray matter

White matter

Dorsal root

Cell body of afferent neuron

Dorsal root ganglion

Spinal nerve

Spinal nerve

Ventral root

Ventral horn gray matter

Interneuron (association neuron)

Axon of efferent neuron

Cell body of efferent neuron

FIGURE 20.4

Cross-Sectional View of the Spinal Cord Showing the Relationships Between the Spinal Cord and Vertebra

tains afferent (sensory) fibers and efferent (motor) fibers. The cell bodies of the afferent neurons are located in the dorsal root ganglion of the spinal nerve, which is part of the peripheral nervous system. The cell bodies of the efferent neurons, however, are located within the central nervous system, and the axon exits through the ventral root of the spinal nerve. The most familiar efferent neurons are the alpha motor neurons that innervate skeletal muscles. The dorsal root and ventral roots refer to the area of the spinal nerve that carries only afferent and efferent fibers, respectively. Once the two roots come together, it is referred to as a spinal nerve. Therefore, even though individual neurons have only sensory or motor functions, a nerve typically contains both afferent and efferent neurons, and hence has both sensory and motor functions.

Reflex Rapid, involuntary response to a stimuli in which a specific stimulus results in a specific motor response.

Information is carried up and down the spinal cord by a series of tracts. A *tract* is a bundle of fibers in the central nervous system. The tracts that carry sensory (afferent) information are called ascending tracts. The tracts that carry motor (efferent) information are called descending tracts. There are specific tracts that are responsible for carrying different types of sensory information (such as pressure and temperature) and motor information (such as fine distal movement).

The descending pathways of the spinal cord can be divided into the pyramidal and extrapyramidal pathways, each of which includes several descending tracts that carry specific information. Voluntary motor impulses are transmitted from the motor area of the brain to somatic efferent neurons leading to skeletal muscles via the *pyramidal pathways.*[33]

Pyramidal System   The pyramidal (corticospinal) system is composed of neurons with cell bodies that originate in the cerebral cortex and axons that travel through the spinal cord. The neurons that extend from the brain down through the descending tract are called the upper motor neurons (see Figure 20.2). These neurons synapse with the lower motor neurons, also known as the alpha (α) motor neurons, in the anterior gray matter of the spinal cord. The lower motor neurons then carry the message to the skeletal muscles that specifically control precise, discrete movement.[33]

Both the lateral and anterior corticospinal (pyramidal) tracts decussate, or cross over, as they descend from the brain. Therefore, the motor cortex of the right side of the brain controls the muscles on the left side of the body, and vice versa. Thus, a patient who has had a cerebral vascular accident on the right side of the brain will lose the motor function of the left side of the body.

Extrapyramidal System   The extrapyramidal system consists of all descending tracts not included in the pyramidal system. Typically, the neurons found in these tracts have cell bodies located in the basal nuclei or reticular formation of the brain. The extrapyramidal system not only carries information that dictates muscle tone and posture but also controls head movements in response to visual stimuli and changes in equilibrium.

Components of a Reflex Arc

Many of the movements that individuals make daily depend upon spinal reflexes. The neural pathway over which a reflex occurs is called a *reflex arc.* The basic components of a reflex arc are described in the following list and are shown in Figure 20.5.

1. The *receptor* is the organ that responds to the stimulus by converting it into a neural (electrical) signal.

2. The *afferent* (sensory) *neuron* carries the signal to the central nervous system.

3. The *integration center* is located in the central nervous system. Here, the incoming neural signal is processed through the connection of the afferent neuron with *association neurons* (also called interneurons) and efferent neurons. The incoming afferent neuron may synapse directly with the efferent neuron or with association neurons, depending upon the complexity of the reflex.

4. The *efferent* (motor) *neuron* carries the impulse from the central nervous system to the organ

FIGURE 20.5

Components of a Reflex Arc

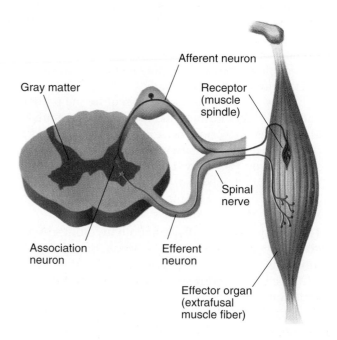

Afferent neuron

Receptor (muscle spindle)

Gray matter

Spinal nerve

Association neuron

Efferent neuron

Effector organ (extrafusal muscle fiber)

of the body that is to respond to the original stimulus.

5. The *effector organ* is the organ of the body that responds to the original stimulus. The effector organ may be a muscle or a gland.

Proprioceptors and Related Reflexes

Proprioceptive sensations provide an awareness of the activities of the muscles, tendons, and joints and provide a sense of equilibrium. Although all of the senses are important, this section emphasizes the role of the proprioceptive senses in order to explain the somatosensory system. Although the proprioceptive receptors will be emphasized, the other senses and receptors should not be forgotten; they too play a major role in human movement. For example, we use our visual senses to provide important information regarding the speed and direction of a tennis ball during a tennis match. And we may listen to the sound created by the impact of the ball on the opponent's racket in order to judge the return. So keep in mind that human movement is not only extremely complex but also affected by a host of factors, including sensory receptors of all types.

Stimulation of the proprioceptors gives rise to kinesthetic perceptions. Historically, *kinesthesis* was defined as a person's perception of his or her own motion, specifically, the motion of the limbs with respect to one another and to the body as a whole. *Proprioception* was defined as the perception of movement of the body plus its orientation in space. Over the years these terms have become practically synonymous.[29]

Vestibular Apparatus
Specialized equilibrium receptors in the inner ear, called the vestibular apparatus, provide important proprioceptive sensations. The primary function of the vestibular apparatus is to maintain equilibrium and to preserve a constant plane of head position by modifying muscle tone.[28] Receptors of the vestibular apparatus can be divided into two categories: those located in the vestibule and those located in the semicircular canals.

The vestibule is comprised of two fluid-filled, saclike structures called the utricle and saccule. The receptors in these structures, the maculae, sense information about the position of the head when the body is not moving and as a result of linear acceleration. The semicircular canals are oriented in three planes of space; that is, each of the semicircular canals is positioned at right angles to the other. This arrangement allows the equilibrium receptors in the semicircular canals, the crista ampullaris, to detect angular movement of the head in any plane. The receptors in the semicircular canals are sensitive to changes in the velocity of head movements—that is, to angular acceleration.[20, 28]

Information from the vestibular apparatus is transmitted to the brain via the vestibulochoclear nerve. This information is carried to the vestibular nuclear complex and the cerebellum. Here, it is processed along with information from visual receptors and the somatic receptors of the muscles, tendons, and joints. Although the vestibular receptors are very important, they can be overruled by information from other receptors. For example, the spotting technique (keeping the eyes focused on one spot) used by figure skaters allows them to perform spins without becoming dizzy.

Muscle Spindles and the Myotatic Reflex
Muscle spindles (sometimes called neuromuscular spindles, NMS) are located in skeletal muscle; they lie parallel to and are imbedded in the muscle fibers. These receptors are stimulated by stretch, and they provide information to the central nervous system regarding the length and rate of length change in skeletal muscles. Stimulation of the muscle spindles results in reflex contraction of the stretched muscle via a myotatic reflex also known as a stretch reflex.[3] Thus, the muscle spindle performs both a sensory and a motor function.

Figure 20.6 represents a muscle spindle and its nerve supply. The muscle spindle consists of a fluid-filled capsule composed of connective tissue; it is long and cylindrical with tapered ends. The typical spindle is 4–7 mm long and approximately $\frac{1}{5}$ the diameter of a muscle fiber (extrafusal fiber).[28] The capsule contains specialized muscle fibers called *intrafusal muscle fibers*. Note that in contrast to intrafusal fibers, the muscle fibers that produce muscular movement are sometimes called *extrafusal fibers*. Each end of the spindle is attached to extrafusal muscle fibers.

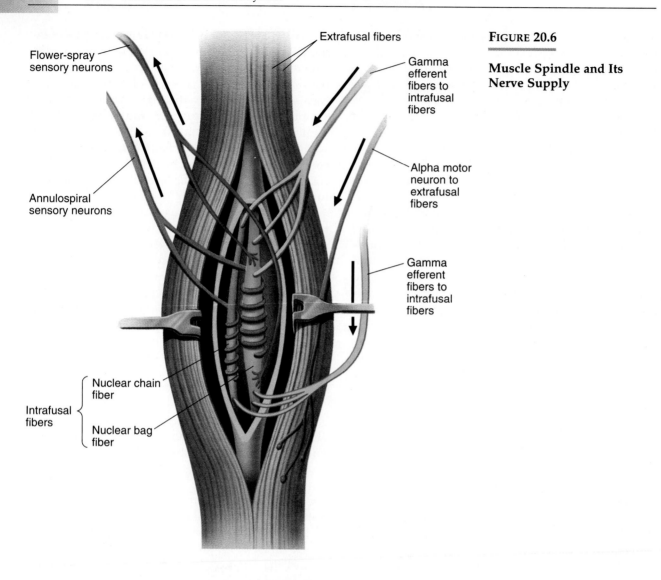

FIGURE 20.6

Muscle Spindle and Its Nerve Supply

There are two types of intrafusal fibers located within the muscle spindle: nuclear bag fibers and nuclear chain fibers. *Nuclear bag fibers* are thicker and contain many nuclei that are centrally located. These fibers extend beyond the spindle capsule and attach to the connective tissue of the extrafusal fibers. *Nuclear chain fibers* are shorter and thinner and have fewer nuclei in the central area of the fiber. Both types of intrafusal fibers contain contractile elements at their distal poles. The central region of the fibers do not contain contractile elements; this represents the sensory receptor area of the spindle.

A typical muscle spindle contains two nuclear bag fibers and approximately five nuclear chain fibers.[3] The intrafusal fibers of the spindle are innervated by sensory nerves called annulospiral and flower-spray neurons. The branches of the *annulospiral neurons* wrap around the center of both types of intrafusal fibers. These annulospiral fibers are large, myelinated fibers.[3]

The branches of the *flower-spray neurons* are located on either side of the annulospiral[33] and wrap around only the nuclear chain fibers. The flower-spray fibers are smaller than and conduct impulses slower than the annulospiral fibers. Both types of afferent fibers are stimulated when the central portion of the spindle is stretched. Since the intrafusal fibers are arranged in parallel with the extrafusal fibers, they are stretched or shortened with the whole muscle. The flower-spray nerve endings have a higher threshold of excitation than the annulospiral nerve endings. The flower-spray nerve endings provide information about relative muscle length; the annulospiral nerve endings are concerned primarily with the rate of length change.

The contractile intrafusal fibers also receive motor innervation from the central nervous system. The efferent fibers that terminate on the intrafusal fibers are called gamma efferents (γ motor neurons) or fusimotor neurons. The axons of the gamma motor neurons travel in the spinal nerve and terminate on the distal ends of the intrafusal fibers. Stimulation of the gamma motor neurons produces contraction of the intrafusal fiber, which causes the central region of the spindle to be stretched. Gamma motor neurons are important enough to comprise almost a third of all motor neurons in the body.

Myotatic Reflex.   The myotatic or stretch reflex is comprised of two separate components: a dynamic reaction and a static reaction. The dynamic reaction occurs in response to a sudden change in length of the muscle. When a muscle is quickly stretched, the annulospiral nerve endings (but not the flower-spray endings) transmit an impulse to the spinal cord, which results in an immediate strong reflex contraction of the same muscle from which the signal originated.[10] This is what happens in the knee jerk response, diagrammed in Figure 20.7, or in the head jerk response when you fall asleep sitting up reading a book not nearly as interesting as this one.

Stretching of the skeletal muscle results in the stimulation of the muscle spindle fibers, which monitor changes in muscle length. In this example the stretch is initiated by a tapping on the patellar tendon, thereby causing a deformation that will

FIGURE 20.7

Myotatic (Stretch) Reflex

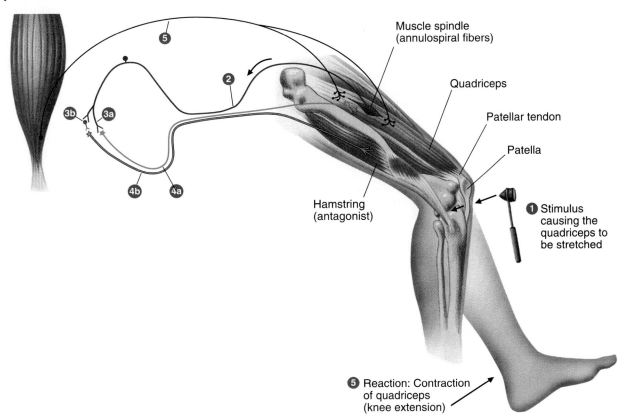

Muscle spindle (annulospiral fibers)

Quadriceps

Patellar tendon

Patella

Hamstring (antagonist)

❶ Stimulus causing the quadriceps to be stretched

❺ Reaction: Contraction of quadriceps (knee extension)

cause the quadriceps muscle group to be stretched [(1) in Figure 20.7]. Sudden stretching of the muscle spindle causes an impulse to be sent to the spinal cord by way of the annulospiral nerve fibers [(2) in Figure 20.7]. In the gray matter of the spinal cord this sensory fiber bifurcates, with one branch synapsing with an alpha motor neuron [(3a) in Figure 20.7]. The other branch synapses with an association neuron [(3b) in Figure 20.7]. The alpha motor neuron exits the spinal cord and synapses with the skeletal muscle, which was originally stretched, resulting in a contraction that is roughly equal in force and distance to the original stretch [(4a) in Figure 20.7]. The inhibitory association neuron synapses with another efferent neuron, which innervates the antagonist muscle (hamstring group in this example), where it causes inhibition; this reflex relaxation of the antagonist muscle in response to the contraction of the agonist is called **reciprocal inhibition.** This response facilitates contraction of the agonist muscle that was stimulated; the inhibited antagonist cannot resist the contraction of the agonist [(4b) in Figure 20.7]. The muscle spindle is also supplied with a gamma efferent neuron; for clarity, this neuron is shown on the opposite side of the spinal cord [(5) in Figure 20.7].

As soon as the lengthening of the muscle has ceased to increase, the rate of impulse discharge returns to its original level, except for a small static response that is maintained as long as the muscle is longer than its normal length. The static response is elicited by both the annulospiral and flower-spray nerve endings. The resultant low-level muscle contractions oppose the force that is causing the excess length, with the ultimate goal of returning to the resting length. A static response is also invoked if the sensory receptor portion of the neuromuscular spindle is stretched slowly.

Normally, the muscle spindles emit low-level sensory nerve signals that assist in the maintenance of muscle tonus and postural adjustments. **Muscle tonus** is a state of low-level muscle contraction at rest. Muscle spindles also respond to stretch by an antagonistic muscle, to gravity, or to a load being applied to the muscle. The head jerk is an example of the response to gravity, but other muscles such as the back extensors and quadriceps function the same way for unconscious postural adjustments. As an example of the load stimulus, think about what happens if you stand with your elbows at 90°, palms up, and someone places a 10-lb weight in your hands. Before you can consciously adjust to this weight, and because the weight stretches your biceps, the muscle spindles will have caused a reflex contraction to stop your hands from dropping too far.

In addition to providing maintenance of muscle tone and adjustments for posture and load, the neuromuscular spindle serves as a damping mechanism that facilitates smooth muscle contractions. This is accomplished by a gamma loop.

In a gamma loop the stretch reflex is activated by the gamma motor neurons [(5) in Figure 20.7]. Recall that the gamma motor neurons originate in the spinal cord and innervate the distal contractile portions of the intrafusal fibers. Pick up a rubber band and hold it at its maximal, unstretched length with your fingers. Now pull against both ends. What happens to the rubber band in the middle? Obviously, it is stretched. This is precisely what happens when the gamma motor neurons stimulate contractions at both ends of the intrafusal fibers. The central, noncontractile portion of the fibers is stretched, deforming the sensory nerve endings and eliciting the myotatic stretch response. The questions then are: What stimulates the gamma motor neurons, and why are they stimulated?

When signals are transmitted to the alpha motor neurons from the motor cortex or other areas of the brain, the gamma motor neurons are almost always simultaneously stimulated. This action is called *coactivation,* and it serves several purposes. First, it provides damping, as mentioned earlier. Sometimes, the alpha and gamma neural signals to contract arrive asynchronously. But since the response to the gamma motor neuron stimulation is contraction anyway, the gaps can be filled in by reflex contractions—hence smoothing out the force of contraction. Second, coactivation maintains proper load responsiveness regardless of the muscle length.

Reciprocal Inhibition The reflex relaxation of the antagonist muscle in response to the contraction of the agonist.

Muscle Tonus A state of low-level muscle contraction at rest.

If, for example, the extrafusal fibers contract less than the intrafusal fibers owing to a heavy external load, the mismatch would elicit the stretch reflex and the additional extrafusal fiber excitation would cause more shortening.[10] Similarly, because the intrafusal and extrafusal lengths are adjusted to each other, the neuromuscular spindle may be able to help compensate for fatigue by recruiting additional extrafusal fibers by reflex action. Finally, sensory information from the neuromuscular spindles is always carried to the higher brain centers, where it is unconsciously integrated with other sensory information. If the muscle spindles were not adjusted to the length of the extrafusal fibers during contraction, information on muscle length and the rate of change of that length could not be transmitted.[20] Since the gamma fibers do adjust the muscle spindle fibers, the gamma loop can assist voluntary motor activity, but it does not actually control voluntary motor activity.

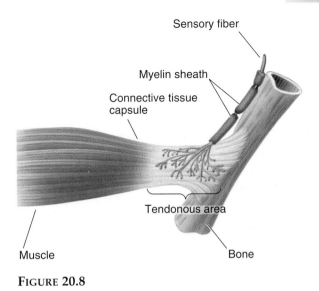

FIGURE 20.8

Golgi Tendon Organ

Plyometrics. Plyometrics, also known as depth jumping or rebound training, is a training exercise that involves eccentric-concentric sequences of muscle activity. It involves such activities as jumping off a box with both feet together and then immediately performing a maximal jump back into the box. While the training has proven effective in increasing jumping performance, the mechanisms responsible for the improved performance have not been fully elucidated, although the stretch-shortening cycle, which relies on the elastic properties of the muscle, is thought to be involved (see Chapter 18). It is also thought that the myotatic reflex plays a role. During the eccentric phase (lengthening) muscle spindles are believed to be activated, thus enhancing the contraction of the muscle during the concentric phase.[33]

Golgi Tendon Organ   Golgi tendon organs (GTOs) are receptors that are activated by stretch or active contraction of a muscle and that transmit information about muscle tension. Activation of these receptors results in a reflex inhibition of the muscle via the inverse myotatic reflex.[3] GTOs are located in the tendons, close to the point of muscular attachment. As shown in Figure 20.8, each Golgi tendon organ consists of a thin capsule of connective tissue that encloses collagenous fibers. The collagenous fibers within the capsule are penetrated by fibers of

sensory neuron whose terminal branches intertwine with the collagenous fibers. This afferent neuron relays information about muscle tension to the spinal cord. The information is then transmitted to muscle efferents and/or to higher brain centers, particularly the cerebellum.

The Golgi tendon organ is in series with the muscle. Thus, the Golgi tendon organ can be stimulated by either stretch or contraction of the muscle. Because of elongation properties of the muscle during stretch, however, active contraction of a muscle is more effective in initiating action potentials within the Golgi tendon organ.

As with the myotatic reflex, the inverse myotatic reflex has both a static and dynamic component. When tension increases abruptly and intensely, the dynamic response is invoked. Within milliseconds this dynamic response becomes a lower-level static response within the GTO that is proportional to the muscle tension. The sequence of events in the inverse myotatic reflex is diagramed in Figure 20.9.

Contraction of a skeletal muscle (or stretching) results in tension that stimulates the Golgi tendon organs in the tendon attached to the skeletal muscle [(1) in Figure 20.9]. Stimulation of the Golgi tendon organ results in the transmission of impulses to the spinal cord by afferent neurons [(2) in Figure 20.9]. In the spinal cord the afferent neuron synapses with

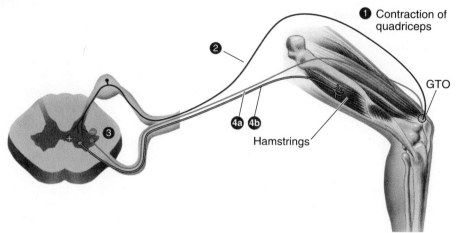

1 Contraction of quadriceps

GTO

Hamstrings

FIGURE 20.9

Inverse Myotatic Reflex

an inhibitory association neuron and an excitatory motor neuron [(3) in Figure 20.9]. In turn, the inhibitory association neuron synapses with a motor neuron that innervates the muscle attached to the tendon; the inhibitory impulses lead to the relaxation of the contracted muscle [(4a) in Figure 20.9]. The excitatory association neuron synapses with a motor neuron that innervates the antagonist muscle [(4b) in Figure 20.9].

Note that as the muscle group originally exhibiting the tension (the agonist) is relaxed, the opposing muscle group (or antagonists) is reciprocally activated. The relaxing action of the Golgi tendon organ serves several important functions.[10] First, excessive tension that might cause muscles and tendons to be torn or pulled away from their attachments is avoided. For example, a weight lifter who manages to get a heavier barbell off the ground than he or she can really handle may suddenly find that his or her muscle gives out. The Golgi tendon organs are responsible for the muscles giving out. It is speculated that increases in the amount of weight that can be lifted following resistance training are in part due to an inhibition of the Golgi tendon organ, allowing for a more forceful muscle contraction.[10]

The second important advantage of Golgi tendon organ–mediated relaxation is that muscle fibers that are relaxed can be stretched further without damage. This response is useful in the development of flexibility. Third, the sensory information regarding tension, which is provided to the cerebellum, allows for muscle adjustment so that only the amount

of tension needed to complete the movement is produced. This feature ensures both a smooth beginning and a smooth ending to a movement and is particularly important in movements such as running that involve a rapid cycling between flexion and extension.[4]

Volitional Control of Movement

Although reflexes are important in controlling human movement, the volitional control of movement is more important in skilled movement. This section discusses the volitional control of motor units and of whole muscles.

Volitional Control of Individual Motor Units

Healthy people often take the ability to move for granted; they assume that if the proper signal is sent from their brain, the desired action will simply occur. An appreciation that it is not quite that simple occurs when one attempts to learn a new sport or when one has an illness or injury. Conscious control of single motor units is not something we normally think about. Most people think of reflex action as the most basic, albeit unconscious, form of muscle action. But even reflexes involve more than one motor unit and result in muscle activity that can be felt by the individual. In reality, motor unit control is really the most basic level of volitional control of movement that can be achieved.

Basmajian[2] and his colleagues performed a series of experiments using intramuscular electrodes attached to a tape recorder and audio-amplifier for sound and an oscilloscope and camera for visual feedback. Initially, when subjects were asked to activate a motor unit, say, in the little finger, they moved the finger and got a typical EMG tracing such as the one shown in Figure 20.10d. Gradually, when movement was decreased to virtually nothing but neural signals continued to be sent, a single motor unit (identifiable by a characteristic sound and spike pattern) (Figure 20.10a) was isolated. Once one motor unit had been isolated, the frequency of its recruitment could be varied. Additionally, other motor units could be isolated (Figures 20.10b and 20.10c), and firings could be varied between the motor units. Thus, it has been shown that motor units truly can be controlled. Precisely *how* this control is achieved is unclear both to the sub-

jects doing it and the scientists observing it, although some type of proprioceptive feedback is suspected.

Such delicate, discrete control has obvious implications for the refinement of motor skills. Perhaps its greatest benefit, however, is in the area of therapeutic rehabilitation. For example, bioengineers have been able to utilize trained motor units to control myoelectric protheses and orthoses. Individuals disabled with conditions such as cerebral palsy can learn better motor control. And some individuals whose spinal cords have been injured but not totally destroyed can learn through such biofeedback to control first one motor unit and then another until muscle movement is regained.

Volitional Control of Muscle Movement

Figure 20.11 provides an overview of volitional movement. The brain initiates movement; [(1) in Figure 20.11]; that is, the plan for a desired movement, whether it be to lift a book or perform the high jump, originates in the brain. This information is then transmitted down the appropriate descending tract [(2) in Figure 20.11]. The neurons of the descending tract synapse with the motor neurons in the gray matter of the spinal cord. The efferent motor neuron then carries the impulse to the muscle, the effector organ [(3) in Figure 20.11].

Upon receiving the signal from the nervous system, the muscle contracts and produces movement [(4) in Figure 20.11]. Changes in muscle length, tension, and position stimulate receptors in the muscles and joints of surrounding muscles [(5) in Figure 20.11]. This information is transmitted to the central nervous system through afferent sensory neurons [(6) in Figure 20.11]. The afferent neurons synapse with various association neurons in the gray matter of the spinal cord. In some instances the neurons synapse with association neurons, which synapse with efferent motor neurons to reflexively control movement [(7a) in Figure 20.11]. In other cases, the association neurons synapse with neurons of the ascending tract, which will carry the information to the brain [(7b) in Figure 20.11].

The signals from the ascending pathway are transmitted to the brain, where the information is perceived, compared, evaluated, and integrated in light of past experience, desired outcome, and

FIGURE 20.10

Volitional Control of a Single Motor Unit

Source: J. V. Basmajian. Control of individual motor units. *American Journal of Physical Medicine.* (48)1: 480–486 (1967). Reprinted by permission of Williams & Wilkins.

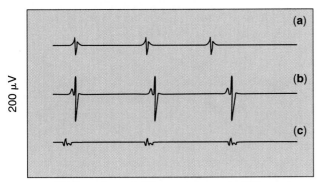

EMG tracings of different motor units (25 msec)

EMG tracing of muscle contraction in little finger
(many motor units firing) (25 msec)

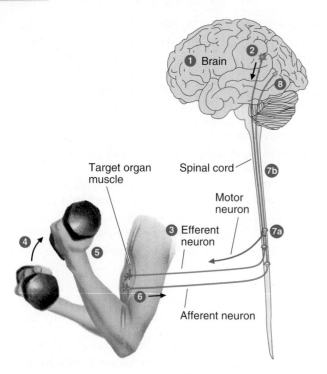

FIGURE 20.11

Overview of Volitional Movement

additional sensory information [(8) in Figure 20.11]. The brain then makes adjustments to its original message, which is again sent to the muscles via the descending pathway and the motor neuron.

This cycle continues throughout the duration of a given activity. The speed at which the information is transmitted is as remarkable as the degree of integration that occurs. What seems to be an instantaneous response on, say, a racquetball court (such as reaction to a powerful serve) actually requires a vast amount of communication within the neuromuscular system.

As already stated, many movements rely on both involuntary reflex action and volitional control of movement. An example is flexibility exercise. Although we decide to initiate stretches, the responses to them depend largely on reflexes.

> **Flexibility** The range of motion in a joint or series of joints that reflects the ability of the musculotendon structures to elongate within the physical limits of the joint.

Flexibility

Flexibility is defined as the range of motion (ROM) in a joint or series of joints that reflects the ability of the musculotendon structures to elongate within the physical limitations of the joint.[13] There are two basic types of flexibility: static and dynamic. *Static flexibility* refers to the range of motion about a joint with no consideration of how easily or quickly the range of motion is achieved. *Dynamic flexibility* refers to the resistance to motion in a joint that will affect how easily and quickly a joint can move through the range of motion. Despite the fact that dynamic flexibility is undoubtedly the more important of the two when one considers athletic performances (especially speed events) and the health or diseased condition of the joints (such as arthritis), no standardized measurement technique exists that can be used in practical settings for evaluating dynamic flexibility.[26] Thus, there is very little information available on dynamic flexibility.[30] Therefore, unless specifically stated otherwise, the discussion that follows is limited to static flexibility.

Several anatomical factors affect the range of motion in any given joint. The first is the actual structural arrangement of the joint—that is, the way the bones articulate. Each joint has a specific bony configuration that, in general, cannot and should not be altered. The soft tissue surrounding the joint, including the skin, ligaments, fascia, muscles, and tendons, also affects joint range of motion. The skin has very little influence on the range of motion under normal circumstances. The ligaments provide joint stability, and whatever restriction to the range of motion they provide is generally considered to be both necessary and beneficial. Thus, the muscles and their connective tissues are the critical factors that determine flexibility and that are altered by flexibility training.

Muscles actively resist elongation through contraction and passively resist elongation owing to the noncontractile elements of elasticity and plasticity. The difference between elastic and plastic properties can best be exemplified by thinking about a rubber band versus a balloon. If the rubber band is stretched and then let go, it should rebound to its original length—at least it should when it is new and has not been frequently stretched. That is elasticity. Blowing up a balloon also stretches it. However, if the air is let out of the previously fully in-flated balloon, the balloon does not return to its original size. That is plasticity. What one is attempt-ing to do in flexibility training is to influence the plastic deformation so that a degree of elongation remains when the force causing the stretch is re-moved.[26] Neuromuscular disorders characterized by spasticity and rigidity, any injuries resulting in scar tissue, or adaptive muscle shortening from casting will impact flexibility.

Flexibility and stretching are important for everyday living (putting on shoes, reaching the top shelf), for muscle relaxation and proper posture, and for relief of muscle soreness (discussed in Chap-ter 18). In relation to exercise it is advocated for two primary reasons: (1) as preparation for activity, which will enhance the performance of that activity, and (2) as a means of decreasing the likelihood of in-jury during physical activity.

There can be no doubt that flexibility is impor-tant to sport performance. The degree of importance differs, of course, with the sport. Table 20.1 gives a partial listing of popular sport and fitness activities according to the degree of flexibility required. The three degrees of flexibility listed are a normal range of motion, a slightly above average range of motion in one or more joints, and an extreme range of mo-tion in specific joints.

It is obvious that the gymnast needs to be more flexible than long-distance runners and cyclists. However, there are no scientific studies that directly link selected flexibility values with performance if the athletes can move through the required range of motion.[26] For example, a bicyclist with normal range of motion in the ankle, knee, hip, and trunk will not become a better cyclist just by increasing her flexibility in those joints. But what about pre-venting injury?

Muscles, tendons, and ligaments are the tissues injured most frequently in work and in fitness and sport participation. Presently, however, there is no conclusive evidence that high levels of flexibility or improvements in flexibility either protect against in-jury or reduce the severity of injury,[26,30] including low-back pain. Indeed, there is some indication that hypermobility, or loose ligamentous structure, may predispose some individuals to injury or low-back pain.[26]

Nevertheless individuals with poor flexibility for the task they are expected to perform probably have an increased risk of exceeding the extensibility limits of the musculotendon unit. Such individuals should work on improving their flexibility. Like-wise, individuals whose sports may cause maladap-tive shortening in certain muscles should perform stretching exercises to counteract this tendency.

TABLE 20.1 ▪ Flexibility in Sport and Fitness Activities

SKILLS REQUIRING EXTREME RANGE OF MOTION IN SPECIFIC JOINTS	SKILLS REQUIRING GREATER-THAN-NORMAL RANGE OF MOTION IN ONE OR MORE JOINTS	SKILLS REQUIRING ONLY NORMAL RANGE OF MOTION IN INVOLVED JOINTS	
Figure skating	Jumping	Boxing	Bicycling
Gymnastics	Swimming	Long distance jogging or running	Stair stepping
Diving	Wrestling		Skating (in-line, roller)
Hurdles	Sprinting	Archery	
Pitching	Racquet sports	Shooting	Horseback riding
Dancing (ballet, modern)	Most team sports	Curling	Resistance training
Karate		Basketball	
Yoga		Cross-country skiing	

Source: Modified from Hubley-Kozey.[13]

Note: Because the skills involved with a particular sport do not require greater-than-normal-flexibility does not mean that stretching exercises should not be included in the exercise program.

Individuals who are shown to be hypermobile need to concentrate on strengthening the musculature around those joints.

Assessing Flexibility

The measurement of flexibility is not an exact, standardized procedure with a well-established criterion test. Direct measurement in the laboratory usually measures angular displacement (in degrees) between adjacent segments or from a reference point. Such measurements are usually obtained by a goniometer or flexometer (Figure 20.12). A goniometer resembles a protractor with two arms, one of which is movable. The center of the goniometer is placed over the joint about which movement will occur, and the arms are aligned with the body segments about the joint. Thus, for a measurement of the range of motion at the elbow joint, the center of the goniometer would coincide with the elbow, the stationary arm would be aligned with the upper arm, and the movable arm would be aligned with the forearm. The angle would be measured at the extreme range of motion for extension and flexion—that is, with the arm completely extended and completely flexed. The range of motion for this joint is the difference between the angles measured.

Flexibility measures can also be obtained by a flexometer. This instrument has a weighted 360° dial and pointer. Range of motion is measured relative to gravity. The instrument is attached to the body segment that is going to be moved, and the dial is locked at 0° at one extreme of the range of motion. The individual then performs the movement and the pointer is locked at the other extreme range of motion. Thus, the range of motion can be read from the dial.

Flexibility measurements can be made passively, in which case an external force causes the movement through the range of motion. Or they can be made actively, in which case the individual being tested uses muscle action to produce the movement. One must indicate which technique is used since passive measurements generally give a higher value than active ones.[26]

The field methods of assessing flexibility typically involve linear measurements of distances between segments or from an external object. Some variation of the stand or sit-and-reach test is the most popular field test of flexibility. The sit-and-reach test is performed by having the individual being tested assume a sitting position with one (now recommended) or both (previously used) stocking feet flat against a testing box. The hands are

FIGURE 20.12

Range of Motion Measurements

The range of motion of the hip joint is measured by a goniometer (left), by a flexometer (right).

positioned fully extended from the shoulders onto a scale on top of the testing box. The individual flexes as far forward as possible in a controlled fashion, sliding the fingertips along the scale. The point of maximum reach is recorded.

From the mid 1940s until the mid 1980s the stand or sit-and-reach test was described as a test of low-back (lumbar) and hip (hamstring) flexibility, mobility, or extensibility. In the mid to late 1980s several studies were published showing clearly that although the stand or sit-and-reach test is a valid test of hamstring flexibility, it is *not* a valid test of low-back flexibility.[4,15,16,17,24]

Because of its widespread use as the only flexibility test in physical fitness test batteries, the sit-and-reach test was often interpreted, although incorrectly, as a measure of total body flexibility. That is, if an individual was shown to have good flexibility using this test, equally good flexibility was assumed in other joint-muscle units. Although this idea is appealing in terms of simplicity and ease of testing, it is *not* accurate.[5,31] Joint flexibility is highly specific to individual locations; it is not a general trait common to all joints. Thus, if the goal of testing is to determine whether an individual is flexible, a profile of major joints must be compiled; one representative test does not indicate total body flexibility. Joint specificity for flexibility is true throughout the age span of childhood to old age.

The Influence of Age and Sex on Flexibility

The specificity of flexibility to each joint makes generalizations regarding sex differences difficult. But as shown in one study, across the entire age spectrum from 10 to 75 yr, males exhibited greater anterior trunk flexion (also called lumbar mobility or low-back flexibility) than did females (Figure 20.13a). Conversely, across most of the same age span, females exhibited greater right lateral trunk flexibility than males (Figure 20.13b). Although not shown in the figure, females had greater left lateral flexibility than males, at least in the adults.

The differences graphed in Figure 20.13a and b did not reach statistical significance at all ages and/or were not always tested for significance, so another interpretation can be that there really aren't any differences in flexibility between the sexes. Either way, these observations are vastly different from the usual assumption that females are more flexible than males. Other data have shown that adult men are more flexible than adult women in trunk extension[23] and rotation (both left and right)[9] but are not significantly different in trunk flexion, trunk extension, and lateral trunk flexion (both left and right),[9] head rotation (both left and right), external shoulder rotation, and ankle flexion (both plantar and dorsi) but are less flexible than adult women in internal shoulder rotation and hip flexion.[32]

The often-stated, but apparently insupportable, assumption that females are more flexible than males is probably attributable to results from the sit-and-reach test. Since studies have shown that females have greater hip flexibility,[31] it is expected that females would score better than males on the sit-and-reach test. Figure 20.14 clearly shows that from 5 to 18 yr girls do have a higher sit-and-reach score than boys.

Despite the sit-and-reach results, it must be concluded from the results of many other studies that there is no consistent generalized pattern of sex differences in flexibility. Depending on which specific joint is being measured, females may have a larger, equal, or smaller range of motion than males.

The impact of age on flexibility is only slightly less confusing. Again Figures 20.13a and 20.13b can be used to illustrate specificity through the pubertal growth years. The general trend is for lumbar flexibility to decrease between 10 and 15 yr of age, while lateral flexion generally increases during the same period. The sit-and-reach data (Figure 20.14) show an interaction of age and sex.[19] Basically, the girls show a consistent improvement from age 5 to 18, while the boys show a U-shaped response—that is, a gradual decline from age 5 to 13 yr and then an improvement from 13 to 18 yr—so that they are more flexible in the hip and posterior thigh by adulthood. Thus, whether and how the range of motion changes through the growing years is joint specific.

Although Figure 20.13 shows a pattern of declining flexibility as people progress from young adulthood through middle age and into old age, other studies investigating different joints suggest that flexibility does not change.[9,31] What has not been shown is an increase, without training, in range of motion with age through the adult years. Therefore, it can be concluded that through the adult years flexibility either declines or stays the same. This is probably joint-specific both in terms of direction and

FIGURE 20.13

Flexibility in Males and Females

(a) Anterior trunk flexion (lumbar mobility). (b) Lateral trunk flexibility (right).

Source: Plotted from data of Morau et al., Moll & Wright.[23]

magnitude. Changes in flexibility with aging may also be confounded by the decreasing activity that often accompanies aging. Most of the information on flexibility is from cross-sectional rather than longitudinal studies, and this information has not been analyzed taking activity level into account.

All ages appear to be trainable in terms of flexibility.[5,27] This adaptation may be especially important to the elderly, where healthy, independent living is at stake.

Flexibility and Low-Back Pain

The theoretical link between muscle function and low-back pain (LBP) was described in Chapter 19

(Table 19.2), with particular emphasis at that time being placed on muscle strength and endurance. In this chapter emphasis will be given to the flexibility needs for a healthy, well-functioning back. Flexibility of the low back and hip area and strong and balanced lumbar, hamstrings, and hip flexor muscles are crucial for controlled pelvic movement. Controlled pelvic movement means having neither an exaggerated anterior tilt (lordotic curve) nor a restricted anterior tilt (no low-back curvature). Either an exaggerated or a restricted pelvic tilt can increase vertebral disc compression and cause pain and strain in the lower-back area.

Research evidence shows that individuals suffering from LBP exhibit lower values for range of

FIGURE 20.14

Flexibility as Measured by the Sit-and-Reach Test

Source: From *Growth, Maturation and Physical Activity* (p. 196) by Robert M. Malina & Claude Bouchard. Champaign, IL: Human Kinetics Publishers. Copyright 1991 by Robert M. Malina and Claude Bouchard. Reprinted by permission.

motion, particularly in the lower-back and hamstring areas. As with the reduced strength and endurance values, however, these differences are more likely the result of LBP than a cause of it.

One study found that first-time low-back pain could be predicted from lumbar flexibility.[15] However, in this study high lumbar flexibility predicted LBP, not low flexibility, as might be expected; and it was only predictive in men. On the other hand, recurrent LBP has been found to be predictable from both low-lumbar extension (not flexion) range of motion and low-hamstring flexibility.[4]

Exactly what value constitutes too low or too high a range of motion is unknown. From the research that has been conducted, though, it can be recommended that flexibility of the hip, low back, and hamstrings be part of a general overall fitness program. Flexibility should be developed specifically for athletes as needed. However, flexibility should not be taken to extremes, nor should one expect that flexibility will mean absolute protection from LBP.

Flexibility Training

The biggest decision in setting up a flexibility training program is determining which stretching technique to employ. There are three techniques used to increase flexibility: ballistic stretching, static stretching, and proprioceptive neuromuscular facilitation (PNF). **Ballistic stretching,** characterized by an action-reaction bouncing motion, is a form of stretch-

ing in which the joints involved are placed into an extreme range of motion limits by fast, active contractions of agonistic muscle groups. As a result, the antagonistic muscles are stretched quickly and forced to elongate. This quick stretch distorts the intrafusal fibers of the neuromuscular spindle and activates the annulospiral nerve endings, which transmit an impulse to the spinal cord, resulting in an immediate strong reflex contraction (the myotatic reflex) of the muscles that had been stretched.[7] This rebound bounce is proportional in force and distance to the original move. Although ballistic action is frequently seen in sport performance—for example, punting a football or a high kick in dance—and although ballistic stretching has been shown to be effective in increasing flexibility, this type of stretching is generally not recommended. Ballistic stretching may cause muscle soreness; and even though there is virtually no research or clinical evidence to support it, the fear is that the forces generated by the series of pulls will exceed the extensibility limits of the tissues involved and result in injury.[30] Fortunately, there are alternative means of increasing flexibility that do not invoke this (real or imagined) fear of injury.

Static stretching is a form of stretching in which the muscle to be stretched (the antagonist) is slowly put into a position of controlled maximal or near-maximal stretch. The position is then held for 30–60 sec. Because the rate of change in muscle length is slow as the individual gets into position and then is nonexistent as the position is held, the annulospiral nerve endings of the neuromuscular spindle (NMS) are not stimulated to fire and a strong reflex contraction does not occur. That is, the dynamic phase of the NMS response is bypassed. Instead, if the stretch continues for at least 6 sec, the Golgi tendon organs (GTOs) respond, leading to the inverse myo-

---

Ballistic Stretching A form of stretching, characterized by an action-reaction bouncing motion, in which the joints involved are placed into an extreme range of motion limits by fast, active contractions of agonistic muscle groups.

Static Stretching A form of stretching in which the muscle to be stretched is slowly put into a position of controlled maximal or near-maximal stretch by contraction of the opposing muscle group and held for 30–60 sec.

tatic reflex and causing relaxation in the stretched muscle group. This response is called *autogenic inhibition*.[7] This relaxation is easily felt by the exerciser, and it allows the muscle to be elongated even further. The impulses from the GTO are able to override the weaker static response impulses coming from the NMS to allow this reflex relaxation and a continuous sustained stretch. Ultimately, the muscle being stretched will reach a point of **myoclonus**—twitching or spasm in the muscle group—indicating the endpoint of an effective stretch.

Because no uncontrolled sudden forces are involved, injury is unlikely with this type of stretch.[30] Indeed, static stretch has been touted as a means not only of avoiding injury but also of relieving muscle soreness. Static stretch done prior to dynamic activity involving eccentric muscle contractions does not prevent muscle soreness, however.[12]

Proprioceptive neuromuscular facilitation (PNF) is a stretching technique in which the muscle to be stretched is first contracted maximally. The muscle is then relaxed and is either actively stretched by contraction of the opposing muscle or is passively stretched. There are a number of different proprioceptive neuromuscular techniques currently being used for stretching, but the two most popular are the contract-relax (CR) and contract-relax-agonist-contract (CRAC) techniques. In both the CR and CRAC techniques the muscle to be stretched (the antagonist) is first placed in a position of maximal stretch by action of the agonist and then is contracted maximally, using either a dynamic concentric or static contraction. Both techniques also require the assistance of a partner or an implement that can provide resistance and elongation.

The contraction phase, which originates from the position of maximal stretch, typically lasts for at least 6 sec. Because of the slow rate of change of the muscle length as the individual gets to the maximal

---

Myoclonus A twitching or spasm in the muscle group that is maximally stretched.

Proprioceptive Neuromuscular Facilitation (PNF) A stretching technique in which the muscle to be stretched is first contracted maximally. The muscle is then relaxed and is either actively stretched by contraction of the opposing muscle or is passively stretched.

---

stretch position, the annulospiral nerve endings of the NMS are not stimulated to fire, and no reflex contraction occurs. As with a static stretch, the dynamic phase of the NMS response is bypassed. The exerciser then contracts the antagonists against the resistance provided by a partner. As tension is created in the muscle by the maximal contraction, the Golgi tendon organs respond and the inverse myotatic reflex is initiated, causing a relaxation in the stretched muscle group.[7] At this point in the CR technique the partner who has been resisting the contraction moves the relaxed limb into a greater stretch. That is, the antagonist is further elongated passively until resistance to the stretch is again felt.

In the CRAC technique the exerciser actively contracts the agonist to assist the stretching of the antagonist. By reciprocal inhibition, the contraction of the agonist is thought to aid in the relaxation of the antagonist, allowing it to be stretched further. There is some danger of injury in PNF stretching if the partner attempts to push the relaxed limb too far. However, if the partner stops at the point of myoclonus, which can be easily felt with proper hand placement, injury is avoided.

The role of the Golgi tendon organ in bringing about an inhibitory relaxation of stretched muscle has generally been supported by research studies.[7,8,14] When needle electrodes were implanted in the stretched muscles, very little EMG activity was recorded, indicating relaxation.

Table 20.2 summarizes the three stretching techniques. Although you have undoubtedly stretched using all three techniques before, try them again now using the stretches given next. Be very conscious of what you are feeling and why.

1. Stand up with your feet shoulder's width apart, legs straight, and quickly attempt to place your palms (or if that is easy, your elbows) on the floor. You should have bounced back up, but you probably didn't go down forcefully because you didn't want to pull your hamstring. Review the action of the NMS in your mind.

2. Stand up with your feet shoulder's width apart, legs straight, and bend over at the waist with your head and arms dangling down. Hold that position until you feel your hamstring muscles relax and allow you to bend even further. Repeat until your hamstring starts to quiver (myoclonus) or you

Table 20.2 ■ Summary of Stretching Techniques

	BALLISTIC	STATIC	PNF: CR	PNF: CRAC
Action	Antagonist stretched by dynamic contraction of agonist	Antagonist moved slowly to limit of ROM and held	Antagonist moved slowly to limit of ROM by action of agonist, where it contracts maximally for about 6–10 sec	Antagonist moved slowly to limit of ROM by action of agonist, where it contracts maximally for about 6–10 sec
Reaction	Bounce back proportional to force of original contraction	Relaxation and further elongation, usually gravity-assisted	Relaxation and further passive elongation by partner or implement, such as towel or jump rope	Relaxation and further passive elongation by active dynamic concentric contraction of agonist
Mechanism	Neuromuscular spindle (myotatic reflex)	Golgi tendon organ, autogenetic inhibition (inverse myotatic reflex)	Golgi tendon organ, autogenetic inhibition (inverse myotatic reflex)	Golgi tendon organ, autogenetic inhibition (inverse myotatic reflex) plus reciprocal inhibition
Advantages	Improves flexibility; may mimic action in sport performance	Improves flexibility and is safest; may provide relief from delayed-onset muscle soreness	Improves flexibility and is safe	Improves flexibility and is safe
Disadvantages	Muscle soreness or injury may result		Requires partner or implement, such as towel, jump rope, or sweats	Requires partner or implement

Note: ROM = range of motion.

can't go any further. If you can easily touch the floor initially, stand on a stable box that allows you to go beyond your feet. Think about the interaction of the GTO and NMS.

3. Lie supine on the floor and place a towel around the heel of one foot so that you can pull on it. Elevate that leg straight until resistance is felt. Statically, contract the hamstrings against the resistance being provided by your towel for 6 sec. Then pull on the towel with your arms to further stretch the hamstrings. This is the CR PNF technique. From the new position, repeat the isometric contraction for another 10 sec. This time, stretch the hamstrings by actively contracting the quadriceps of that leg. This is the CRAC PNF technique. Think about the interaction of the NMS, GTO, and reciprocal inhibition needed to perform these actions.

Work through the problems provided in Box 20.1 to ensure that you understand these concepts.

Application of the Training Principles

The application of the training principles to flexibility development has not received a great deal of attention in the research literature. Some guidelines, however, can be suggested and are given in the following sections.

Specificity

Flexibility is joint-specific.[21,31] Hence, flexibility is also task- or sport-specific. Thus, the first step in developing a flexibility program is to analyze the task or sport to determine both the specific joint(s) involved and the plane of action involved. For example, hurdling requires flexion and extension at both the hip and the knee joints and also hip adduction, abduction, and rotation. Swimming requires the same hip flexibility as hurdling; but instead of knee flexion and extension, swimming requires ankle flexion and extension plus inversion, eversion, and shoulder flexion and extension, adduction, abduction, and rotation.[13] A general fitness participant should emphasize a total body workout of the major joints and muscle groups.

Specificity need not refer to the type of action the individual is planning on doing. How muscle and connective tissue are elongated does not matter as long as the elongation occurs. Because a movement will be done ballistically does not mean that ballistic flexibility work should be done.[7, 11]

Overload

Overload in flexibility training is achieved by placing the muscle and connective tissue at or near the normal limits of extensibility and manipulating the NMS and GTO by holding the position or contracting the muscle to achieve an elongation. The duration of the static stretch hold should be between 30 and 60 sec, although an individual may need to start with a shorter hold and work up to this time. PNF stretches with 6–10 sec of contraction followed by 6–10 sec of relaxation and elongation are repeated to myoclonus or extensibility limits.

Usually, two or three relaxation periods can be achieved in one repetition of static stretch. A high number of repetitions is not necessary. Two to six

are frequently recommended for both the static and PNF flexibility techniques.

The intensity of the stretching exercises should be monitored both by myoclonus and pain. Stretched muscles that begin to twitch or spasm (myoclonus) are stretched too far and are fighting that stretch by reflexly trying to contract. Such a muscle should be shortened to the point where the myoclonus ceases before proceeding. Pain also means the stretch is too intense and should not be tolerated.

The frequency of the workout should be at least three days per week in the development phase. Reasonable daily stretching, however, should have no detrimental effects.

Adaptation and Progression

Short-term improvements in flexibility have been shown to occur after as little as one week of daily sessions.[11] On the other hand, anecdotal evidence indicates that some people do not seem to improve at all. At any rate, since the individual begins both static and PNF stretching exercises at the limit of extensibility, progression will naturally follow whatever adaptation does occur. What is most important is that, except in the case of specific athletic requirements, progression not continue to extreme flexibility.

Individualization

As stated previously, the most important consideration in flexibility training is that the goals and technique preferences of the individual be considered. In a school situation the maturity of the individuals might also need to be considered. For example, if a PNF technique with a partner is going to be used, the partner has to be able to detect the onset of myoclonus and not try to just push as far as possible. Otherwise, individualization is inherent in the flexibility exercises themselves. Each individual stretches to his or her own limits at his or her own rate. Joint looseness is an individual characteristic.[21]

Maintenance

Once the appropriate or desired level of flexibility has been attained, it can be maintained by just one day per week of training at the same intensity level.[34]

Retrogression/Plateau/Reversibility

Little is known about when or even if a plateau is achieved in a flexibility training program, although there will be a point, probably set by genetics, when further improvement ceases.[7] Improvements in flexibility have been shown to continue for a least eight weeks after the cessation of exercise.[5]

Warm-Up and Cool-Down

Considerable confusion exists about the relationship between warming up and stretching prior to an activity and flexibility training. A *flexibility training program* is a planned, deliberate, and regular program of exercises that can permanently and progressively increase the usable range of motion of a joint or set of joints over time.[1] A w*arm-up and cooldown stretching program* is a planned, deliberate, and regular program of exercises that are done immediately before and after an activity to improve performance and reduce the risk of injury.[1]

Stretching does not cause an elevation in body temperature and therefore it is not a warm-up. In fact, a cardiovascular warm-up to elevate body temperature should precede flexibility exercises regardless of the reason for stretching. The cardiovascular warm-up will increase the body temperature and therefore make the muscles and joints more viscous and receptive to stretch.

Despite the fact that an increase in body temperature should make stretching more effective, studies have not shown that flexibility gains after 3–4 min of warm-up are any different from flexibility gains after 3–4 min of warm-up plus 20–30 min of aerobic work.[6]

*A*daptation to Flexibility Training

Flexibility exercises and flexibility training improve range of motion, whether the technique used is ballistic, static, or one of the PNF techniques.[7,14,30] Which technique brings about the greatest improvement has been the subject of a great number of studies. Results from these studies have occasionally shown that one type of athlete, or males as opposed to females, responds better to one stretching technique than another.[7,25] But no consistent pattern

has emerged. Thus, we can only conclude at this point that the question of which stretching method is most effective has not been definitively answered. Indeed, the exact position in which the stretching exercises are done may be more important than the method of stretching.[32]

There is little scientific or empirical evidence to suggest that resistance training will decrease flexibility. In fact, studies have shown that heavy resistance training results in either an improvement or no change in flexibility.[22] Furthermore, competitive weight lifters have average or above-average flexibility in most joints.[18] So that flexibility is not lost, those engaged in resistance training should stress the full range of motion of both the agonists and the antagonists.

SUMMARY

1. The spinal cord performs the essential functions of connecting the peripheral nervous system with the brain and serving as a site of reflex integration.

2. Voluntary motor impulses are transmitted from the motor area of the brain to somatic efferent neurons leading to skeletal muscles via the pyramidal pathways.

3. Reflexes play an important role in maintaining an upright posture and responding to movement in a coordinated fashion. Reflexes are defined as rapid, automatic responses to stimuli in which a specific stimulus results in a specific motor response.

4. The myotatic reflex is initiated in response to a sudden change in length of the muscle. When a muscle is quickly stretched, the annulospiral nerve endings in the NMS transmit an impulse to the spinal cord, which results in an immediate strong reflex contraction of the same muscle from which the signal originated.

5. The inverse myotatic reflex is initiated when tension increases abruptly and intensely and stimulates Golgi tendon organs; it results in inhibition of the tensed muscle group, causing relaxation.

6. Volitional control of movement can be evidenced at the level of the motor unit as well as at the whole muscle level.

7. Flexibility is joint-specific, and the degree or flexibility is specific to the individual. Static stretching or proprioceptive neuromuscular facilitation techniques are recommended to enhance flexibility.

8. There is little scientific evidence to suggest that resistance training will decrease flexibility. In fact, studies

have shown that heavy resistance training results in either an improvement or no change in flexibility.

Box 20.1   Answers

1. A ballistic technique is to stand on a step and bounce on your toes so that your heel goes below step height and then above it. This exercise will not work on a level surface.

2. A static technique is the wall stretch. Extend one leg straight back and stretch it, with the other bent at the knee and forward. Hold the position.

3. A CR PNF technique is to assume the long sitting position, a jump rope (or a towel or sweats) around your foot in a neutral position. Resist a maximal isometric contraction of foot, attempting to plantarflex. Relax and pull your foot into dorsiflexion with the implement. Repeat.

4. A CRAC PNF technique is the same as the CR technique, except that you actively contract the shin muscles (dorsiflex). Repeat.

REVIEW QUESTIONS

1. Describe the anatomical relationship between nerves and muscles. What is the functional significance of this relationship?

2. Diagram the sequence of events that occur at the neuromuscular junction.

3. Diagram the components of a generalized reflex arc.

4. Diagram the components of the myotatic reflex. Pay careful attention to the afferent and efferent neurons involved.

5. Diagram the components of the inverse myotatic reflex.

6. Outline the sequence of events involved in volitional control of movement.

7. Provide a rationale for incorporating a flexibility training program into an overall fitness program.

8. Critique the appropriateness of the sit-and-reach test to predict low-back pain.

9. What are the anatomical requirements of a healthy low back?

10. Describe static stretching, and explain the involvement of reflexes in providing for muscle elongation during this type of stretching.

11. Describe the proprioceptive neuromuscular facilitation technique, and explain the involvement of reflexes in providing for muscle elongation during this type of stretching.

12. Discuss the application of the individual training principles to the development of a flexibility program.

REFERENCES

1. Alter, M. J.: *The Science of Stretching.* Champaign, IL: Human Kinetics Publishers (1988).

2. Basmajian, J. V.: Control of individual motor units. *American Journal of Physical Medicine.* 48(1):480–486 (1967).

3. Berne, R. M., & M. N. Levy: *Physiology.* St. Louis: Mosby (1988).

4. Biering-Sorenseu, F.: Physical measurements as risk indicators for low-back trouble over a one year period. *Spine.* 9(2):106–119 (1984).

5. Clarke, H. H.: Joint and body range of motion. In *Physical Fitness Research Digest* (series 5, no 4). Washington, DC: President's Council on Physical Fitness and Sports (1975).

6. Cornelius, W. L., R. W. Hagemann, & A. W. Jackson: A study on placement of stretching within a workout. *Journal of Sports Medicine and Physical Fitness.* 28:234–236 (1988).

7. Ethyre, B. R., & E. J. Lee: Dialogue: Comments on proprioceptive neuromuscular facilitation stretching techniques. *Research Quarterly for Exercise and Sport.* 58:184–188 (1987).

8. Etnyre, B. R., & L. D. Abraham: Antagonist muscle activity during stretching: A paradox reassessed. *Medicine and Science in Sports and Exercise.* 20:285–289 (1988).

9. Gomez, T. G., G. Beach, C. Cooke, W. Hrudey, & P. Goyert: Normative database for trunk range of motion, strength, velocity, and endurance with the isostation B-200 lumbar dynamometer. *Spine.* 16:15–21 (1991).

10. Guyton, A. C.: *Textbook of Medical Physiology.* Philadelphia: Saunders (1986).

11. Hardy, L., & D. Jones: Dynamic flexibility and proprioceptive neuromuscular facilitation. *Research Quarterly for Exercise and Sport.* 57:150–153 (1986).

12. High, D. M., E. T. Howley, & B. D. Franks: The effects of static stretching and warm-up on prevention of delayed-onset muscle soreness. *Research Quarterly for Exercise and Sport.* 60:356–361 (1989).

13. Hubley-Kozey, C. L.: Testing flexibility. In J. D. MacDougall, H. A. Weuger, & H. J. Green (eds.), *Physiological Testing of the High-Performance Athlete.* Champaign, IL: Human Kinetics Publishers (1991).

14. Hutton, R. S.: Neuromuscular basis of stretching exercises. In P. V. Komi (ed.), *Strength and Power in Sport.* London: Blackwell Scientific (1992).

15. Jackson, A. W., & A. A. Baker: The relationship of the sit and reach test to criterion measures of hamstring and back flexibility in young females. *Research Quarterly for Exercise and Sport.* 57:183–186 (1986).

16. Jackson, A. W., & N. J. Langford: The criterion-related validity of the sit and reach test: Replication and exten-

sion of previous findings. *Research Quarterly for Exercise and Sport.* 60:384–387 (1989).

17. Kippers, V., & A. W. Parker: Toe-touch test: A measure of its validity. *Physical Therapy.* 67:1680–1684 (1987).

18. Leighton, J.: Flexibility characteristics of three specialized skill groups of champion athletes. *Archives of Physical Medicine and Rehabilitation.* 36:580–583 (1957).

19. Malina, R. M., & C. Bouchard: *Growth, Maturation, and Physical Activity.* Champaign, IL: Human Kinetics Publishers (1991).

20. Marieb, E. N.: *Human Anatomy and Physiology.* New York: Benjamin-Cummings (1992).

21. Marshall, J. L., N. Johnson, T. L. Wickiewicz, H. M. Tischler, B. L. Koslin, S. Zeno & A. Meyers: Joint looseness: a function of the person and joint. *Medicine and Science in Sports.* 12(3):189–194 (1980).

22. Massey, B. H., & N. L. Chaudet: Effects of heavy resistance exercise on range of joint movement in young male adults. *Research Quarterly.* 27:41–51 (1956).

23. Moll, J. M. H., & V. Wright: Normal range of spinal mobility: An objective clinical study. *Annals of Rheumatic Diseases.* 30:381–386 (1971).

24. Nicolaisen, T., & K. Jorgensen: Trunk strength, back muscle endurance and low-back trouble. *Scandinavian Journal of Rehabilitation Medicine.* 17:121–127 (1985).

25. Osternig, L. R., R. N. Robertson, R. K. Troxel, & P. Hansen: Differential response to proprioceptive neuromuscular facilitation (PNF) stretch techniques. *Medicine and Science in Sports and Exercise.* 22:106–111 (1990).

26. Plowman, S. A.: Physical activity, physical fitness and low back pain. In J. O. Holloszy (ed.), *Exercise and Sport Science Reviews.* 20:221–242 (1992).

27. Rider, R. A., & J. Daly: Effects of flexibility training on enhancing spinal mobility in older women. *Journal of Sports Medicine and Physical Fitness.* 31:213–217 (1991).

28. Sage, G.: *Introduction to Motor Behavior: A Neurophysiological Approach.* Reading, MA: Addison-Wesley (1971).

29. Schmidt, R. A.: *Motor Control and Learning: A Behavioral Emphasis.* Champaign, IL; Human Kinetics Publishers (1988).

30. Shellock, F. G., & W. E. Prentice: Warming-up and stretching for improved physical performance and prevention of sports-related injuries. *Sports Medicine.* 2(4):267–278 (1985).

31. Shephard, R. J., M. Berridge, & W. Montelpare: On the generality of the "sit and reach" test: An analysis of flexibility data for an aging population. *Research Quarterly for Exercise and Sport.* 61:326–330 (1990).

32. Sullivan, M. K., J. J. DeJulia, & T. W. Worrell: Effect of pelvic position and stretching method on hamstring muscle flexibility. *Medicine and Science in Sports and Exercise.* 24:1383–1389 (1992).

33. Tortora, G. J., & N. P. Anagnostakos: *Principles of Anatomy and Physiology* (5th edition). New York: Harper & Row, 280–305 (1987).

34. Wallin, D., B. Ekblom, R. Grahn, & T. Nordenborg: Improvement of muscle flexibility: A comparison between two techniques. *American Journal of Sports Medicine.* 13:263–268 (1985).

A

Appendix: Units of Measure, the Metric System, and Conversions Between the English and Metric Systems of Measurement

TABLE A.1 ▪ SI Units (*Systeme International*) (Metric)

PHYSICAL QUANTITY	UNIT	SYMBOL
Mass	kilogram	kg
Distance	meter	m
Volume (liquid or gas)	liter	L
Time	second	sec
Force	newton	N
Work	joule	J
Power	watt	W
Angle	radian	rad
Linear velocity	meters per second	$m \cdot sec^{-1}$
Angular velocity	radians per second	$rad \cdot sec^{-1}$
Temperature	degrees	°
Velocity	meters per sec	$m \cdot sec^{-1}$
Torque	newton-meter	N-m
Acceleration	meters per second	$m \cdot sec^{-1}$
Amount of substance	mole	mol

TABLE A.2 ▪ **SI Prefixes (*Systeme International*) (Metric)**

PREFIX*	MEANING	SCIENTIFIC NOTATION	SYMBOL
Makes smaller			
deci-	one tenth of (0.1)	10^{-1}	d
centi-	one hundredth of (0.01)	10^{-2}	c
milli-	one thousandth of (0.001)	10^{-3}	m
micro-	one millionth of (0.000001)	10^{-6}	μm
Makes larger			
kilo-	a thousand times (1000)	10^{3}	K

*Most commonly used in this text.

TABLE A.3 ▪ **Conversions Between the English and Metric Systems of Measurement**

MEASUREMENT	UNIT AND ABBREVIATION	METRIC EQUIVALENT	ENGLISH-TO-METRIC CONVERSION FACTOR	METRIC-TO-ENGLISH CONVERSION FACTOR
Length	1 kilometer (km)	= 1000 meters	1 mile = 1.61 km	1 km = 0.62 mile
	1 meter (m)	= 100 centimeters	1 yard = 0.914 m	1 m = 1.09 yards
		= 1000 millimeters	1 foot = 0.305 m	1 m = 3.28 feet
			1 foot = 30.5 cm	1 m = 39.37 inches
	1 centimeter (cm)	= 0.01 meter	1 inch = 2.54 cm	1 cm = 0.394 inch
	1 millimeter (mm)	= 0.001 meter		
	1 micrometer (μm)	= 0.000001 meter		
Mass	1 kilogram (kg)	= 1000 grams	1 pound = 0.454 kg	1 kg = 2.205 pounds
	1 gram (g)	= 1000 milligrams	1 ounce = 28.35 g	1 g = 0.035 ounce
	1 milligram (mg)	= 0.001 gram		
Volume (liquids and gases)	1 liter (L)	= 1000 milliliters	1 quart = 0.946 L	1 L = 0.264 gallon
			1 quart = 946 ml	1 L = 1.057 quarts
			1 gallon = 3.785 L	
	1 milliliter (mL}	= 0.001 liter		1 ml = 0.034 fluid ounce
		= 1 cubic centimeter	1 pint = 473 ml	
			1 fluid ounce = 29.57 ml	
	1 microliter (μL)	= 0.000001 liter		
Area	1 square meter (m²)	= 1000 square centimeters	1 square yard = 0.836 m²	1 m² = 1.196 square yards
	1 square centimeter (cm²)	= 100 square millimeters	1 square inch = 6.452 cm²	1 cm² = 0.155 square inch
Temperature	Degrees Celsius (°C)		$°C = \frac{5}{9}(°F - 32)$	$°F = (\frac{9}{5}°C) + 32$

TABLE A.3 ▪ *(continued)*

Measurement	Unit and Abbreviation	Metric Equivalent	English-to-Metric Conversion Factor	Metric-to-English Conversion Factor
Force	1 Newton (N)	= 0.1019 kilopond	1 ft-lb · sec^1 = 0.138 N	
Linear velocity	1 (m · sec^{-1})		1 mi · hr^{-1} = 26.8 m · min^{-1}	
Angular velocity	1 radian per second (rad · s^{-1})			1 radian^{-1} = 57.3° · s^{-1}
Work & energy	1 Joule (J)	= 1 N-m		1 J = 0.784 ft · lb
	1 Kcal	= 426.85 kgm = 4.18 KJ		1 J = 0.239 cal
	1 kgm	= 1 kpm = 0.00234 Kcal		
Power	1 watt (W)	1 W = 1 joule per sec (J · sec^{-1}) 1 W = 6.12 kgm · min^{-1}	1 hp = 745.7 W	1 W = 0.0013 hp
Pressure	1 Newton per square meter (N · m^2)		1 mmHg = 133.32 N · m^2 1 atmosphere = 760 mmHg	760 mmHg = 29.02 inches

Appendix: Metabolic Calculations

This appendix will explain the calculations for oxygen consumption ($\dot{V}O_2$cons) in three sets of circumstances. The first series of equations will be direct calculations using data obtained from open-circuit spirometry. This technique also allows for the calculation of carbon dioxide produced ($\dot{V}CO_2$prod), which the other two, because they are indirect techniques, do not. The second series of equations will calculate submaximal oxygen consumption values for selected activities (walking, running, cycle ergometer riding, and bench stepping) using known rates of work. The third set of calculations will determine an estimation of maximal oxygen consumption ($\dot{V}O_2$max) from selected field tests (the PACER or 20-meter shuttle test and the Rockport Fitness Walking Test).

The Calculation of Oxygen Consumed and Carbon Dioxide Produced from Data Obtained by Open-Circuit Spirometry

Basic Formulas

Theoretically, the amount of oxygen consumed is simply equal to the amount of oxygen in inspired air minus the amount of oxygen in the expired air. All values are expressed in $mL \cdot min^{-1}$ or $L \cdot min^{-1}$.

(B.1) oxygen consumption ($L \cdot min^{-1}$) = amount of oxygen inspired ($L \cdot min^{-1}$) – amount of oxygen expired ($L \cdot min^{-1}$)

or
$$\dot{V}O_2\text{cons} = \dot{V}_IO_2 - \dot{V}_EO_2$$

In practice, there is no way to obtain $\dot{V}_IO_2$ or $\dot{V}_EO_2$ directly, so a working formula is used. The working formula is based on the fact that the amount of a gas depends on the fraction (F) of that gas and the volume of air containing that gas.

(B.2) oxygen consumption ($L \cdot min^{-1}$) = [fraction of oxygen in inspired air × volume of inspired air ($L \cdot min^{-1}$)] – [fraction of oxygen in expired air × volume of expired air ($L \cdot min^{-1}$)]

or
$$\dot{V}O_2\text{cons} = (F_IO_2 \times \dot{V}_I) - (F_EO_2 \times \dot{V}_2)$$

Although the term *fraction* and the symbol F are always used in this equation, these values really represent the percentages of oxygen in inspired or expired air and are expressed mathematically as decimals. Thus, F_IO_2 is a constant 20.93%, or 0.2093. The inspired ventilation values can either be directly measured by a spirometer or pneumoscan as described in Chapters 2 and 11 or they can be calculated. The F_EO_2 is measured by an oxygen analyzer, as described in Chapter 11. As with inspired ventilation, expired ventilation can be either directly measured by a spirometer or pneumoscan or calculated. Either $\dot{V}_I$ or $\dot{V}_E$ must be directly measured. When the value from one of them is known, the other can be calculated.

Ventilation Conversions

You will recall from Chapter 2 (respiration) that the volume of air (either inspired or expired) is collected under conditions known as ambient temperature and pressure saturated, or ATPS. To do metabolic calculations, air volumes must first be converted to standard temperature and pressure (STPD) values. This conversion is necessary so that the number of gas molecules in any given volume is equal. The equations vary slightly depending on whether the measured volume is inspired or expired.

The Conversion of $\dot{V}_E$ from ATPS to STPD   The formula for converting $\dot{V}_E$ ATPS to $\dot{V}_E$ STPD accounts for changes in temperature (T) and pressure (P) as follows:
In this equation the 273 represents the standard tem-

> **(B.3)** minute ventilation (L · min^{-1}) STPD = minute ventilation (L · min^{-1}) ATPS × temperature correction (°Kelvin) × pressure correction (mmHg)
>
> or $\dot{V}_E$ STPD = $\dot{V}_E$ ATPS $\left(\dfrac{273}{273 + T°C}\right)\left(\dfrac{P_B - PH_2O}{760}\right)$

perature of 0°C, which equals 273°Kelvin. The T°C represents the ambient temperature in degrees Celsius. Since Charles's law (Chapter 2) states that the volume of a gas is related directly to the temperature of the gas, the relationship would be

$$\frac{V_1 (\dot{V}_E \text{ ATPS})}{V_2 (\dot{V}_E \text{ STPD})} = \frac{T_1 (T \text{ ATPS})}{T_2 (T \text{ STPD})}$$

Rearranging, we get

$$\dot{V}_E \text{ STPD} \times \text{T ATPS} = \dot{V}_E \text{ ATPS} \times \text{T STPD}$$
$$(V_2) \times (T_1) = (V_1) \times (T_2)$$

Finally, the relationship becomes

$$V_2 = \frac{V_1 \times T_2}{T_1} \quad \text{or} \quad \dot{V}_E \text{ STPD} = \frac{\dot{V}_E \text{ ATPS} \times \text{T STPD}}{\text{T ATPS}}$$

This is the volume and temperature factor in Eq. C.3:

$$\dot{V}_E \text{ ATPS} \left(\frac{273}{273 + T°C}\right)$$

The pressure conversion portion of Eq. B.3 follows Boyle's law (Chapter 2), which states that the volume of a gas is inversely related to the pressure as follows:

$$\frac{V_1 (\dot{V}_E \text{ ATPS})}{V_2 (\dot{V}_E \text{ STPD})} = \frac{P_2 (P \text{ STPD})}{P_1 (P \text{ ATPS})}$$

or

$$\dot{V}_E \text{ STPD} \times \text{P STPD} = \dot{V}_E \text{ ATPS} \times \text{P ATPS}$$
$$(V_2) \times (P_2) = (V_1) \times (P_1)$$

Finally, the relationship is rearranged to give us

$$V_2 = \frac{V_1 \times P_1}{P_2} \quad \text{or} \quad \dot{V}_E \text{ STPD} = \frac{\dot{V}_E \text{ ATPS} \times \text{P ATPS}}{\text{P STPD}}$$

The volume portion of this conversion is already accounted for. The pressure relationship is the last element in Eq. B.3, $(P_B - P_{H_2O})/760$. The standard pressure (P STPD) in this equation is very straightforward, since standard pressure is always 760 mmHg. The ambient pressure (P_B, read from a barometer in the laboratory where the test is being done) must be adjusted for the water vapor at body temperature, so that this conversion also goes from saturated or wet air to unsaturated or dry air. A normal body temperature of 37°C is usually assumed. Water vapor pressure (PH_2O) at 37°C is 47 mmHg.

Thus, given the following information, we can correct $\dot{V}_E$ from ATPS to STPD conditions.

$\dot{V}_E$ ATPS = 12 L · min^{-1}

T ATPS = 22°C

P_B = 745 mmHg

$\dot{V}_E$ STPD = 12 L · min^{-1} ×
$$\left(\frac{273°}{273° + 22°C}\right)\left(\frac{745 \text{ mmHg} - 47 \text{ mmHg}}{760 \text{ mmHg}}\right)$$

$\dot{V}_E$ STPD = 10.2 L · min^{-1}

The Conversion of $\dot{V}_I$ from ATPS to STPD   The conversion of $\dot{V}_I$ ATPS to $\dot{V}_I$ STPD follows the same gas laws and general logic as described for the conversion of $\dot{V}_E$ ATPS to $\dot{V}_E$ STPD with one small addition. Specifically, in most laboratory settings the inspired air is not totally saturated. That is, the relative humidity is not 100%. For this reason the equation must be modified to adjust for the measured relative humidity (RH) expressed as a decimal fraction at the ambient temperature. Thus, the conversion equation becomes:

$$(\text{B.4}) \quad \dot{V}_I \text{ STPD} = \dot{V}_I \text{ ATPS} \times$$
$$\left(\frac{273}{273 + T°C}\right)\left(\frac{P_B - [RH \times PH_2O]}{760}\right)$$

Table B.1 presents the water vapor pressures (PH_2O) at temperatures generally encountered in a laboratory (20–25°C or 68–77°F). Thus, under the conditions given in the previous example, but with a RH of 46%, the calculations become

$$\dot{V}_I \text{ STPD} = 12 \text{ L} \cdot \text{min}^{-1} \times$$
$$\left(\frac{273°}{273° + 22°}\right)\left(\frac{745 \text{ mmHg} - [0.46 \times 19.8 \text{ mmHg}]}{760 \text{ mmHg}}\right)$$

$$\dot{V}_I \text{ STPD} = 10.8 \text{ L} \cdot \text{min}^{-1}$$

Calculation of the Unknown Ventilation Value

The Calculation of $\dot{V}_E$ from $\dot{V}_I$ Open-circuit metabolic systems measure either inspired or expired air, not both. The volume of expired air does not equal the volume of inspired air. This is because, except when an individual is burning pure carbohydrate and has an RER of exactly 1.0, the number of oxygen molecules used from the inspired air is not replaced by the same number of carbon dioxide

molecules. If the RER value is greater than 1.0, $\dot{V}_E$ will be larger than $\dot{V}_I$. If the RER value is less than 1.0, $\dot{V}_E$ will be smaller than $\dot{V}_I$.

To solve Eq. B.2 we must have values for both $\dot{V}_E$ and $\dot{V}_I$. Fortunately, there is a way to mathematically convert $\dot{V}_E$ to $\dot{V}_I$ or $\dot{V}_I$ to $\dot{V}_E$. This conversion is called the *Haldane transformation* and is based upon the fact that nitrogen (N_2) is an inert gas that does not participate in human metabolism. That is, the number of particles of nitrogen does not change although the concentration or fraction of the nitrogen will change because the fractions of oxygen and carbon dioxide are changing. The following equation is used for the Haldane transformation:

$$(\text{B.5}) \quad \text{expired minute ventilation (L} \cdot \text{min}^{-1}) \text{ STPD}$$
$$= \text{inspired minute ventilation (L} \cdot \text{min}^{-1}) \text{ STPD}$$
$$\times [(\text{the ratio of the fraction of inspired nitrogen})$$
$$\div (\text{the fraction of expired nitrogen})]$$

or $\quad \dot{V}_E = \dot{V}_I\left(\dfrac{F_I N_2}{F_E N_2}\right)$

As usual in these formulas, the measurements are percentages but are expressed as decimal fractions. The fraction of nitrogen in a subject breathing room air ($F_I N_2$) is the constant 0.7904. $F_E N_2$ is determined by subtracting the measured values of oxygen and carbon dioxide obtained from the gas analyzers from 1.0.

$$(\text{B.6}) \quad F_E N_2 = (1 - [F_E O_2 + F_E CO_2])$$

For example, if

$$\dot{V}_I \text{ STPD} = 10.8 \text{ L} \cdot \text{min}^{-1}$$
$$O_2\% = 16.38$$
$$CO_2\% = 4.03$$

the computation becomes

$$\dot{V}_E \text{ STPD L} \cdot \text{min}^{-1} = 10.8 \text{ L} \cdot \text{min}^{-1} \times$$
$$\left(\frac{0.7904}{1 - [0.1638 + 0.0403]}\right) = 10.73 \text{ L} \cdot \text{min}^{-1}$$

The Calculation of $\dot{V}_I$ from $\dot{V}_E$ The calculation of inspired air volume when expired air volume is known is based upon the same reasoning as the calculation of expired air volume when the inspired air volume is known. The formula now becomes

TABLE B.1 ■ Water Vapor Pressure (PH_2O) at Selected Ambient Temperatures

AMBIENT (°C)	TEMPERATURE (°F)	PH$_2$O (mmHg)
20	68	17.5
21	70	18.7
22	72	19.8
23	73	21.1
24	75	22.4
25	77	23.8

$$\dot{V}_I = \dot{V}_E \left(\frac{F_E N_2}{F_I N_2} \right)$$

or, using the fraction of oxygen and carbon dioxide as in Eq. B.6,

(B.7)

$$\dot{V}_I = \dot{V}_E \left(\frac{1 - [F_E O_2 + F_E CO_2]}{0.7904} \right)$$

Using the same O_2% and CO_2% from the previous example, but with $\dot{V}_E$ STPD = 10.2 L · min^{-1}, the computation becomes

$\dot{V}_I$ STPD L · min^{-1} =

$$10.2 \text{ L} \cdot \text{min}^{-1} \left(\frac{1 - [0.1638 + 0.0403]}{0.7904} \right)$$

$$= 10.3 \text{ L} \cdot \text{min}^{-1}$$

The Calculation of Oxygen Consumed

Now we are finally ready to solve Eq. B.2.

$$\dot{V}O_2 \text{ L} \cdot \text{min}^{-1} = (F_I O_2 \times \dot{V}_I) - (F_E O_2 \times \dot{V}_E)$$

The following information is available:

$F_I O_2$	= 0.2093 (assumed constant)
$\dot{V}_I$ STPD	= 10.8 L · min^{-1} (measured as $\dot{V}_I$ ATPS by pneumoscan and converted by Eq. B.4)
$F_E O_2$	= 0.1638 (measured by oxygen analyzer)
$\dot{V}_E$ STPD	= 10.73 L · min^{-1} (calculated by Haldane transformation)
$\dot{V}O_2$ L · min^{-1}	= (0.2093 × 10.8 L · min^{-1}) − (0.1638 × 10.73 L · min^{-1})
	= 0.5 L · min^{-1} or 500 mL · min^{-1}

The Calculation of Carbon Dioxide Produced

The calculation of the amount of carbon dioxide produced is very similar to the calculation of oxygen consumed.

(B.8)   carbon dioxide produced (L · min^{-1}) = [fraction of carbon dioxide in expired air × volume of expired air (L · min^{-1})] − [fraction of inspired carbon dioxide × volume of inspired air (L · min^{-1})]

or $\dot{V}CO_2$ (L · min^{-1}) = $(F_E CO_2 \times \dot{V}_E) - (F_I CO_2 \times \dot{V}_I)$

The $F_I CO_2$ is a constant 0.0003 since the percentage of carbon dioxide in room air is assumed to be 0.03%. Because this number is so small and would have no meaningful effect on the calculation in Eq. B.8, it is generally considered to be 0.0. As a result, only the expired portion of the equation needs to be computed. $F_E CO_2$ is measured by a carbon dioxide analyzer as described in Chapter 11. $\dot{V}_E$ is either directly measured by a spirometer or pneumoscan or calculated as previously described.

Using the values for CO_2% and $\dot{V}_E$ given previously, the calculation example becomes

$$\dot{V}CO_2 \text{ (L} \cdot \text{min}^{-1}) = (0.0403 \times 10.2 \text{ L} \cdot \text{min}^{-1})$$
$$= 0.41 \text{ L} \cdot \text{min}^{-1} \text{ or } 410 \text{ mL} \cdot \text{min}^{-1}$$

Note that as mentioned (in the calculation of $\dot{V}_E$ from $\dot{V}_I$), the oxygen consumed (500 mL · min^{-1}) is not equaled by the amount of carbon dioxide produced (410 mL · min^{-1}).

The Calculation of Oxygen Consumed Using Mechanical Work or Speed of Movement

In exercise situations where an accurate assessment of mechanical work or speed of movement is possible, but the actual measurement of oxygen consumed and carbon dioxide produced is not, the oxygen consumed can be estimated. These situations include walking, running, cycling on an ergometer, and bench stepping. Specific formulas recommended by the American College of Sports Medicine[1] are available for each activity. The resultant oxygen consumption values will not be as accurate as the direct measurement of oxygen consumed which was described in the last section. However, these estimated oxygen consumptions are much less difficult and much less expensive to obtain. They can be very useful in the practical field settings of health clubs, hospitals, and/or school gymnasia as the initial step in determining exercise prescriptions by MET level or determining the caloric cost of any activity. Because of differences in economy (Chapter 11), none of these equations should be used for children. Since no systematic differences in economy have been found between males and females, all of these equations can be used for both sexes.

The following computations will show how to determine the oxygen consumption values of the four activities specified earlier. Recall from Chapter 11 that converting to METs requires dividing the O_2 mL · kg^{-1} · min^{-1} value by 3.5 mL · kg^{-1} · min^{-1}. Caloric cost (also discussed in Chapter 11) can be estimated by multiplying the O_2 (L^{-1} · min^{-1}) value by 5 kcal · L^{-1} · min^{-1}, since 5 kcal · L^{-1} · min^{-1} is the estimated caloric equivalent if the RER is unknown.

The Oxygen Consumed During Horizontal (Level) and Vertical (Graded) Walking

Level Walking   To determine the oxygen consumed while walking on level ground or on a treadmill at zero percent elevation, it is necessary to determine the walking speed (in meters per minute). It is known that, for speeds between 1.9 and 3.7 mi · hr^{-1} (or 50–100 m · min^{-1}; 26.8 m · min^{-1} = 1 mi · hr^{-1}), the net oxygen cost of level walking is 0.1 mL · kg^{-1} · min^{-1}. Because this oxygen consumption constant is a net value, the oxygen consumed during rest (1 MET or 3.5 mL · kg^{-1} · min^{-1}) is added to obtain the total amount of oxygen consumed. Therefore, the equation can be stated as follows.

(B.9)   oxygen consumed during horizontal walking (mL · kg^{-1} · min^{-1}) = horizontal component (mL · kg^{-1} · min^{-1}) + resting component (mL · kg^{-1} · min^{-1})

or $\dot{V}O_2$cons (mL · kg^{-1} · min^{-1}) = speed (m · min^{-1})

$$\times \frac{0.1 \text{ mL} \cdot \text{kg}^{-1} \cdot \text{min}^{-1}}{\text{m} \cdot \text{min}^{-1}} + 3.5 \text{ mL} \cdot \text{kg}^{-1} \cdot \text{min}^{-1}$$

For example, if an individual were walking on a treadmill at 0% grade and 3 mi · hr^{-1}, it would first be necessary to convert the speed to meters per minute (3 mi · hr^{-1} × 26.8 m · min^{-1}/mi · hr^{-1} = 80.4 m · min^{-1}). Then, substituting this value into Eq. B.9, we get

$$\dot{V}O_2\text{cons (mL} \cdot \text{kg}^{-1} \cdot \text{min}^{-1}) = 80.4 \text{ m} \cdot \text{min}^{-1}$$
$$\times \frac{0.1 \text{ mL} \cdot \text{kg}^{-1} \cdot \text{min}^{-1}}{\text{m} \cdot \text{min}^{-1}} + 3.5 \text{ mL} \cdot \text{kg}^{-1} \cdot \text{min}^{-1}$$
$$= 11.54 \text{ mL} \cdot \text{kg}^{-1} \cdot \text{min}^{-1}$$

Graded Walking   To determine the oxygen consumed during uphill walking or walking on a treadmill at a grade, a vertical component is added to Eq. B.9. The vertical component is determined by the percent grade expressed as a decimal. Each m · min^{-1} of vertical rise consumes an additional 1.8 mL · kg^{-1} · min^{-1} for each m · min^{-1} of speed. The following formula incorporates the vertical component in Eq. B.9.

(B.10)   oxygen consumed during vertical walking (mL · kg^{-1} · min^{-1}) = horizontal component (mL · kg^{-1} · min^{-1}) + resting component (mL · kg^{-1} · min^{-1}) + vertical component (mL · kg^{-1} · min^{-1})

or $\dot{V}O_2$cons (mL · kg^{-1} · min^{-1}) = [speed (m · min^{-1})

$$\times \frac{0.1 \text{ mL} \cdot \text{kg}^{-1} \cdot \text{min}^{-1}}{\text{m} \cdot \text{min}^{-1}} + 3.5 \text{ mL} \cdot \text{kg}^{-1} \cdot \text{min}^{-1}$$
$$+ \text{ decimal grade}] \times [\text{speed (m} \cdot \text{min}^{-1})$$
$$\times \frac{1.8 \text{ mL} \cdot \text{kg}^{-1} \cdot \text{min}^{-1}}{\text{m} \cdot \text{min}^{-1}}]$$

If we change the percent grade in the previous example from 0 to 5%, we now have only to calculate the vertical component.

$$\text{Vertical component} = 0.05 \times 80.4 \text{ m} \cdot \text{min}^{-1}$$
$$\times \frac{1.8 \text{ mL} \cdot \text{kg}^{-1} \cdot \text{min}^{-1}}{\text{m} \cdot \text{min}^{-1}} = 7.24 \text{ mL} \cdot \text{kg}^{-1} \cdot \text{min}^{-1}$$

The vertical component is then added to the horizontal and resting components to get the total amount of oxygen consumed while walking at a speed of 3 mi · hr^{-1} with a 5% grade on a treadmill.

Horizontal component =	8.04 mL · kg^{-1} · min^{-1}
Resting component =	3.50 mL · kg^{-1} · min^{-1}
Vertical component =	7.24 mL · kg^{-1} · min^{-1}
Total $\dot{V}O_2$cons =	18.78 mL · kg^{-1} · min^{-1}

The Oxygen Consumed During Horizontal (level) and Vertical (graded) Running

The formulas for estimating the amount of oxygen consumed during running differ from those for walking only in two factors. The first is that the net oxygen cost of level running is 0.2 mL · kg^{-1} · min^{-1}, or double the same cost for walking. Conversely, the additional cost for the vertical component is only half as much as for walking due to differences in the biomechanics of the two gaits, especially the greater forefoot pushoff in running. This difference necessitates multiplying the vertical component by 0.5.

Running is defined as speeds greater than 5 mi · hr^{-1} (134 m · min^{-1}). This leaves a gap between the top walking speed (3.7 mi · hr^{-1} or 100 m · min^{-1}) and the lowest running speed. The best formula for these intermediate speeds depends on whether the individual is actually running or walking.

To determine the oxygen consumed while running on level ground or a treadmill, the formula is

$$\text{(B.11)} \quad \dot{V}O_2\text{cons (mL · kg}^{-1} \cdot \text{min}^{-1}) = \text{speed (m · min}^{-1})$$
$$\times \frac{0.2 \text{ mL · kg}^{-1} \cdot \text{min}^{-1}}{\text{m · min}^{-1}} + 3.5 \text{ mL · kg}^{-1} \cdot \text{min}^{-1}$$

Graded running adds a vertical component to Eq. B.11:

$$\text{(B.12)} \quad \dot{V}O_2\text{cons (mL · kg}^{-1} \cdot \text{min}^{-1}) = \text{speed m · min}^{-1}$$
$$\times \frac{0.2 \text{ mL · kg}^{-1} \cdot \text{min}^{-1}}{\text{m · min}^{-1}} + 3.5 \text{ mL · kg}^{-1} \cdot \text{min}^{-1}$$
$$+ \text{ decimal grade} \times \text{speed (m · min}^{-1}) \times$$
$$\frac{1.8 \text{ mL · kg}^{-1} \cdot \text{min}^{-1}}{\text{m · min}^{-1}} \times 0.5$$

This added vertical component is not accurate for over ground uphill running; therefore the use of Eq. B.12 should be restricted to treadmill running.

If the individual in the previous example switches from walking at 3 mi · hr^{-1} up a 5% grade to running the same grade at 7 mi · hr^{-1} (188 m · min^{-1}), this example works out as follows:

$$\dot{V}O_2\text{cons (mL · kg}^{-1} \cdot \text{min}^{-1}) = 188 \text{ m · min}^{-1}$$
$$\times \frac{0.2 \text{ mL · kg}^{-1} \cdot \text{min}^{-1}}{\text{m · min}^{-1}} + 3.5 \text{ mL · kg}^{-1} \cdot \text{min}^{-1}$$
$$+ 0.05 \times 188 \text{ m · min}^{-1} \times \frac{1.8 \text{ mL · kg}^{-1} \cdot \text{min}^{-1}}{\text{m · min}^{-1}} \times 0.5$$

Horizontal component =	37.60 mL · kg^{-1} · min^{-1}
Resting component =	3.50 mL · kg^{-1} · min^{-1}
Vertical component =	8.46 mL · kg^{-1} · min^{-1}
Total $\dot{V}O_2$cons =	49.56 mL · kg^{-1} · min^{-1}

The Oxygen Consumed During Cycling Using Either the Legs or the Arms

The formulas for calculating the amount of oxygen consumed during cycling are intended only for cycling on an ergometer, which permits the actual measurement of the workload. The mechanical work completed (as described in Chapter 11) is determined by multiplying the force exerted, in the form of the load or resistance overcome, in kilograms, by the distance traveled (m · min^{-1}) using the following equation.

$$\text{(B.13)} \quad \text{work (kgm · min}^{-1}) = \text{kg of resistance}$$
$$\times \text{ m · rev}^{-1} \times \text{rev · min}^{-1}$$

The distance traveled per revolution is the circumference of the flywheel. On many ergometers, including the often-used Monark friction ergometers, this distance is 6 m. The pedaling rate, or revolutions per minute value, is typically displayed on the console of the ergometer and can vary from 30 to 110 rev · min^{-1} with 50 or 60 rev · min^{-1} being the most common.

Because cycling is assumed to be independent of body weight (that is, the body weight is supported by the seat and handle bars of the ergometer), oxygen consumption is determined in liters or milliliters per minute, not milliliters per kilogram of body weight per minute. Each kilogram-meter of work is known to require 2 milliliters of oxygen for leg work.

Leg Cycling   Oxygen consumed during leg cycling can be estimated using the following equation. This formula is most accurate when the workload is between 300 and 1200 kgm · min^{-1}, but it may be used up to loads of 4200 kgm · min^{-1}.

$$\text{(B.14)} \quad \text{oxygen consumed during leg cycling}$$
(mL · min^{-1}) = oxygen consumed during the resistance component (mL · min^{-1}) + oxygen consumed during the resting component (mL · min^{-1})

or $\dot{V}O_2$cons (mL · min^{-1}) = kgm · min^{-1} × 2 mL · kgm^{-1} + 3.5 mL · kg^{-1} · min^{-1} × kg WT

For example, if a 50-kg individual pedals a Monark bike at 60 rev · min^{-1} at a load of 2 kg (denoted as 2 kp on the ergometer itself; 1 kg = 1 kp), she consumes 1615 mL · min⁻¹, which is calculated as follows:

$$\dot{V}O_2\text{cons (mL · min}^{-1}) = 2 \text{ kg} \times 6 \text{ m · rev}^{-1} \times 60$$
$$\text{rev · min}^{-1} \times 2 \text{ mL · kgm}^{-1} + 3.5 \text{ mL · kg}^{-1} \cdot \text{min}^{-1} \times 50 \text{ kg}$$

Resistance component	= 1440 mL · min⁻¹
Resting component	= 175 mL · min⁻¹
Total $\dot{V}O_2$cons	= 1615 mL · min⁻¹ or 1.615 L · min⁻¹

Arm Cranking Cycling with the arms is more properly referred to as arm cranking. The formula for arm cranking differs from leg cycling only in the constant for oxygen use per kilogram of resistance. Although the arm musculature used in cranking is smaller than the leg musculature used in cycling, additional muscles in the shoulders, back, and chest are recruited to stabilize the arms, hence elevating the oxygen cost. Thus, instead of a constant 2 mL · kgm⁻¹ the value is 3 mL · kgm⁻¹.

(B.15)
$$\dot{V}O_2\text{cons (mL · min}^{-1}) = \text{kgm · min}^{-1} \times$$
$$3 \text{ mL · kgm}^{-1} + 3.5 \text{ mL · kg}^{-1} \cdot \text{min}^{-1} \times \text{kg WT}$$

If the individual in the previous example switches from leg cycling to arm cranking, she now consumes 2335 mL · min⁻¹ of oxygen, calculated as follows:

$$\dot{V}O_2\text{cons (mL · min}^{-1}) = 2 \text{ kg} \times 6 \text{ m · rev}^{-1} \times 60$$
$$\text{rev · min}^{-1} \times 3 \text{ mL · kgm}^{-1} + 3.5 \text{ mL · kg}^{-1} \cdot \text{min}^{-1} \times 50 \text{ kg}$$

Resistance component	= 2160 mL · min⁻¹
Resting component	= 175 mL · min⁻¹
Total $\dot{V}O_2$cons	= 2335 mL · min⁻¹

The Oxygen Consumed During Bench Stepping

Like cycling, bench stepping allows for the exact computation of the work being done if the height of the step, the rate of stepping, and the body weight of the stepper are known. Like walking and running, the body weight must be carried and so the unit of measurement is milliliters (or liters) per kilogram of body weight per minute. Unlike all of the other exercise modalities (walking, running, leg cycling, and arm cranking), the resting component is not separate but is inherent in the horizontal and vertical components. Thus, they are gross, not net, values.

(B.16) oxygen consumption during bench stepping (mL · kg⁻¹ · min⁻¹) = oxygen consumed during the horizontal component (mL · kg⁻¹ · min⁻¹) + oxygen consumed during the vertical component (mL · kg⁻¹ · min⁻¹)

or $\dot{V}O_2$cons (mL · kg⁻¹ · min⁻¹) = [step rate

$$(\text{steps · min}^{-1}) \times \frac{0.35 \text{ mL · kg}^{-1} \cdot \text{min}^{-1}}{\text{steps · min}^{-1}}] + [\text{step}$$

height (m · step⁻¹) × step rate (steps · min⁻¹)

$$\times \frac{1.8 \text{ mL · kg}^{-1} \cdot \text{min}^{-1}}{\text{m · min}^{-1}} \times 1.33]$$

In the first component 0.35 mL · kg⁻¹ · min⁻¹ is the oxygen cost of stepping back and forth along the horizontal plane. In the second component, as with walking or running, each m · min⁻¹ of vertical rise requires 1.8 mL · kg⁻¹ · min⁻¹ of oxygen. The 0.33 in the constant 1.33 at the end accounts for the fact that bench stepping has both a positive (up) and a negative (down) action. Negative work in this situation requires one-third as much oxygen as positive work.

An example for an individual stepping up and down on a 10-inch (0.254-m) bench at 24 steps · min⁻¹ is calculated as follows:

$$\dot{V}O_2\text{cons (mL · kg}^{-1} \cdot \text{min}^{-1}) = [24 \text{ steps · min}^{-1}$$

$$\times \frac{0.35 \text{ mL · kg}^{-1} \cdot \text{min}^{-1}}{\text{steps · min}^{-1}}] + [0.254 \text{ m · step}^{-1} \times$$

$$24 \text{ steps · min}^{-1} \times \frac{1.8 \text{mL · kg}^{-1} \cdot \text{min}^{-1}}{\text{m · min}^{-1}} \times 1.33]$$

Horizontal component	= 8.4 mL · kg⁻¹ · min⁻¹
Vertical component	= 14.6 mL · kg⁻¹ · min⁻¹
Total $\dot{V}O_2$cons	= 23.0 mL · kg⁻¹ · min⁻¹

*T*he Calculation of Maximal Oxygen Consumption from Cardiovascular Endurance Field Tests

The direct measurement of maximal oxygen consumption ($\dot{V}O_2$max) is the best indicator of cardiovascular respiratory fitness. However, the direct measurement of $\dot{V}O_2$max requires expensive equipment, trained technicians, and considerable time, rendering it unsuitable for mass testing. Therefore, as indicated in Chapter 4, field tests are often used to estimate $\dot{V}O_2$max. The calculation of $\dot{V}O_2$max from the one-mile run/walk was explained in Chapter 4. This section will detail the calculation of $\dot{V}O_2$max from the PACER and from the Rockport Fitness Walking Test (RFWT).

PACER $\dot{V}O_2$max

Several formulas are available to determine $\dot{V}O_2$max from the results of the PACER test. The two included here cover as wide an age span as possible. The first equation should be used for both male and female children and adolescents.[4] It requires knowing only the final speed at which the individual ran and the age of the individual.

(B.17) $\dot{V}O_2$max = 31.025 + 3.238 (final speed in km · hr^{-1}) − 3.248 (age in yr) + 0.1536 (final speed × age).

For example, if a 9-yr-old boy had a final speed of 11 km · hr^{-1}, we would substitute into the equation as follows.

$$\dot{V}O_2 \text{ max} = 31.025 + 3.238(11) - 3.248(9)$$
$$+ 0.1536(11 \times 9) = 52.62 \text{ mL} \cdot \text{kg}^{-1} \cdot \text{min}^{-1}$$

The second equation should be used for young adult males and females.[5] It requires knowing only the total number of minutes the individual completed.

(B.18) $\dot{V}O_2$max = 14.4 + 3.48(minutes completed)

Thus if a 20-yr-old college student ran for 10 min, the calculation would be

$$\dot{V}O_2\text{max} = 14.4 + 3.48(10) = 49.2 \text{ mL} \cdot \text{kg}^{-1} \cdot \text{min}^{-1}$$

RFWT $\dot{V}O_2$max

The RFWT can be used to estimate $\dot{V}O_2$max in male and female adults from approximately age 30 to 70 yr.[3] Individuals younger than 30 will not obtain sufficiently accurate results from this formula to warrant doing this test.

Five variables are needed to estimate $\dot{V}O_2$max: body weight in pounds, age in years, sex (females are coded as 0 and males are coded as 1), time for completion of the mile walk (in minutes including a decimal), and heart rate in beats per minute (recorded by a heart rate monitor during the final quarter-mile or in the 15 sec immediately postexercise).

(B.19) $\dot{V}O_2$max = 132.853 − 0.0769(body weight) − 0.3877(age) + 6.3150(sex) − 3.2649(walk time) − 0.1565(heart rate)

For example, if a 64-yr-old, 195-lb male completed the mile walk in 19.01 min with a last quarter heart rate of 113 b · min^{-1}, the calculation would be as follows:

$$\dot{V}O_2\text{max} = 132.853 - 0.0769(195) - 0.3877(64)$$
$$+ 6.3150(1) - 3.2649(19.01) - 0.1565(113)$$
$$= 19.61 \text{ mL} \cdot \text{kg}^{-1} \cdot \text{min}^{-1}$$

Standard Error of the Estimate

Since all these formulas are estimates, knowing the accuracy of the estimate is helpful. Accuracy is determined during the development of the equations when the estimated values are compared to the actual values statistically and a standard error of the estimate (SEE) is obtained. The PACER equation for children and adolescents (B.17) has a SEE of 5.9 mL · kg^{-1} · min^{-1}. The PACER equation for young adults (B.18) has a SEE of 3.5 mL · kg^{-1} · min^{-1}. The RFWT equation (B.19) has a SEE of 5.0 mL · kg^{-1} · min^{-1}. Each SEE means that the calculated $\dot{V}O_2$max could differ from an actual measured value by one or two times the amount of the SEE. Most scores (68%) should vary only plus or minus one SEE from the calculated estimated value.

Thus, the $\dot{V}O_2$max of 49.2 mL · kg^{-1} · min^{-1} calculated for the college student from Eq. B.18 could actually be anywhere from 45.7 to 52.7 mL · kg^{-1} · min^{-1}. Obviously, the smaller the SEE, the better, since this means greater accuracy.[2] All three of these estimation equations are deemed to have acceptable accuracy.

*P*ractice Problems

Use the data in Table B.2 to work the problems that follow. Answers are provided at the end of all of the problems.

TABLE B.2 ▪ Practice Problem Data

VARIABLES	Subjects			
	No. 1	No. 2	No. 3	No. 4
Descriptive Information				
Sex	Female	Female	Male	Male
Age (yr)	15	24	32	58
Weight (lb)	108	132	175	201
Maximal Treadmill Data				
$\dot{V}_E$ ATPS (L · min^{-1})	45		130	
P_B (mmHg)	740	742	738	739
T (°C)	20	23	21	24
F_EO_2 (%)	16.08	16.2	16.04	16.75
F_ECO_2 (%)	4.94	5.01	5.12	4.73
$\dot{V}_I$ ATPS (L · min^{-1})		70		75
RH (%)		50		25
Submaximal Exercise Data				
Speed (m · min^{-1})	90	161		
Grade	11	0		
Ergometer load (kp)			4	3
Pedaling rate (rev · min^{-1})			80	50
Flywheel circumference (m)			6	3
Step height (m)		.305		
Step rate (steps · min^{-1})		30		
Field Test Data				
PACER speed (km · hr^{-1})	10			
Pacer time (min)		9	16	
1 mi walk time (min)				17.6
HR (b · min^{-1})				108

Note that not all data are available for each of the four subjects. In some problems you will first have to decide what information you need and select the appropriate subject. In other problems more than one subject can be used for additional practice.

1. Correct the expired minute ventilations from ATPS to STPD.

2. Correct the inspired minute ventilations from ATPS to STPD.

3. Calculate the inspired minute ventilations from the expired minute ventilations using the Haldane transformation.

4. Calculate the expired minute ventilations from the inspired minute ventilations using the Haldane transformation.

5. Calculate $\dot{V}O_2$cons substituting the information given and computed from the maximal treadmill results in Eq. B.2. Present your answer in both relative (mL · kg · min^{-1}) and absolute (L · min^{-1}) oxygen units.

6. Calculate the $\dot{V}CO_2$ produced using the information given and computed from the maximal treadmill results in L · min^{-1}.

7. Calculate the oxygen consumed during submaximal walking.

8. Calculate the oxygen consumed during submaximal running.

9. Calculate the oxygen consumed during submaximal cycling, assuming that subject 3 is doing leg work and subject 4 is doing arm cranking.

10. Calculate the oxygen consumed during bench stepping.

11. Calculate the estimated $\dot{V}O_2max$ for each subject using the appropriate formula for the information presented.

Solutions and Answers

1. Subject No. 1

$$\dot{V}_E \text{ STPD} = 45 \text{ L} \cdot \text{min}^{-1}\left(\frac{273°}{273° + 20°}\right)\left(\frac{740 - 47 \text{ mmHg}}{760}\right)$$

$$= 38.23 \text{ L} \cdot \text{min}^{-1}$$

Subject No. 3

$$\dot{V}_E \text{ STPD} =$$

$$130 \text{ L} \cdot \text{min}^{-1}\left(\frac{273°}{273° + 21°}\right)\left(\frac{738 - 47 \text{ mmHg}}{760}\right)$$

$$= 109.76 \text{ L} \cdot \text{min}^{-1}$$

2. Subject No. 2

$$\dot{V}_I \text{ STPD} =$$

$$70 \text{ L} \cdot \text{min}^{-1}\left(\frac{273°}{273° + 23°}\right)\left(\frac{742 - [0.5 \times 21.1] \text{ mmHg}}{760 \text{ mmHg}}\right)$$

$$= 60.14 \text{ L} \cdot \text{min}^{-1}$$

Subject No. 4

$$\dot{V}_I \text{ STPD} =$$

$$75 \text{ L} \cdot \text{min}^{-1}\left(\frac{273°}{273° + 22°}\right)\left(\frac{739 - [0.25 \times 22.4] \text{ mmHg}}{760}\right)$$

$$= 66.98 \text{ L} \cdot \text{min}^{-1}$$

3. Subject No. 1

$$\dot{V}_I \text{ STPD} = 38.23 \text{ L} \cdot \text{min}^{-1}\left(\frac{1 - [0.1608 + 0.0494]}{0.7904}\right)$$

$$= 38.20 \text{ L} \cdot \text{min}^{-1}$$

Subject No. 3

$$\dot{V}_I \text{ STPD} = 109.76 \text{ L} \cdot \text{min}^{-1}\left(\frac{1 - [0.1604 + 0.0512]}{0.7904}\right)$$

$$= 109.48 \text{ L} \cdot \text{min}^{-1}$$

4. Subject No. 2

$$\dot{V}_E \text{ STPD} = 60.14 \text{ L} \cdot \text{min}^{-1}\left(\frac{0.7904}{1 - [0.1620 + 0.0501]}\right)$$

$$= 60.33 \text{ L} \cdot \text{min}^{-1}$$

Subject No. 4

$$\dot{V}_E \text{ STPD} = 66.98 \text{ L} \cdot \text{min}^{-1}\left(\frac{0.7904}{1 - [0.1675 + 0.0473]}\right)$$

$$= 60.33 \text{ L} \cdot \text{min}^{-1}$$

5. Subject No. 1

$$\dot{V}O_2cons = (0.2093 \times 38.20 \text{ L} \cdot \text{min}^{-1})$$
$$- (0.1608 \times 38.23 \text{ L} \cdot \text{min}^{-1}) = 1.85 \text{ L} \cdot \text{min}^{-1}$$
$$= 1850 \text{ mL} \cdot \text{min}^{-1} \div 49.1 \text{ kg}$$
$$= 37.68 \text{ mL} \cdot \text{kg}^{-1} \cdot \text{min}^{-1}$$

Subject No. 2

$$\dot{V}O_2cons = (0.2093 \times 60.14 \text{ L} \cdot \text{min}^{-1})$$
$$- (0.1620 \times 60.33 \text{ L} \cdot \text{min}^{-1}) = 2.81 \text{ L} \cdot \text{min}^{-1}$$
$$= 2810 \text{ mL} \cdot \text{min}^{-1} \div 60 \text{ kg}$$
$$= 46.83 \text{ mL} \cdot \text{kg}^{-1} \cdot \text{min}^{-1}$$

Subject No. 3

$$\dot{V}O_2cons = (0.2093 \times 109.48 \text{ L} \cdot \text{min}^{-1})$$
$$- (0.1604 \times 109.76 \text{ L} \cdot \text{min}^{-1}) = 5.31 \text{ L} \cdot \text{min}^{-1}$$
$$= 5310 \text{ mL} \cdot \text{min}^{-1} \div 79.55 \text{ kg}$$
$$= 66.75 \text{ mL} \cdot \text{kg}^{-1} \cdot \text{min}^{-1}$$

Subject No. 4

$$\dot{V}O_2cons = (0.2093 \times 66.98 \text{ L} \cdot \text{min}^{-1})$$
$$- (0.1675 \times 67.42 \text{ L} \cdot \text{min}^{-1}) = 2.73 \text{ L} \cdot \text{min}^{-1}$$
$$= 2730 \text{ mL} \cdot \text{min}^{-1} \div 91.36 \text{ kg}$$
$$= 29.88 \text{ mL} \cdot \text{kg}^{-1} \cdot \text{min}^{-1}$$

6. Subject No. 1

$\dot{V}CO_2 \text{ prod} = (0.0494 \times 38.23 \text{ L} \cdot \text{min}^{-1}) = 1.89 \text{ L} \cdot \text{min}^{-1}$
$\dot{V}CO_2 \text{ prod} = (0.0501 \times 60.33 \text{ L} \cdot \text{min}^{-1}) = 3.02 \text{ L} \cdot \text{min}^{-1}$
$\dot{V}CO_2 \text{ prod} = (0.0512 \times 109.76 \text{ L} \cdot \text{min}^{-1}) = 5.62 \text{ L} \cdot \text{min}^{-1}$
$\dot{V}CO_2 \text{ prod} = (0.0473 \times 67.42 \text{ L} \cdot \text{min}^{-1}) = 3.19 \text{ L} \cdot \text{min}^{-1}$

7. Subject No. 1

$$\dot{V}O_2cons = 90 \text{ m} \cdot \text{min}^{-1} \times \frac{0.1 \text{ mL} \cdot \text{kg}^{-1} \cdot \text{min}^{-1}}{\text{m} \cdot \text{min}^{-1}}$$
$$+ 3.5 \text{ mL} \cdot \text{kg}^{-1} \cdot \text{min}^{-1} + 0.11 \times 90 \text{ m} \cdot \text{min}^{-1}$$
$$\times \frac{1.8 \text{mL} \cdot \text{kg}^{-1} \cdot \text{min}^{-1}}{\text{m} \cdot \text{min}^{-1}} = 30.32 \text{ mL} \cdot \text{kg}^{-1} \cdot \text{min}^{-1}$$

8. Subject No. 2

$$\dot{V}O_2cons = 161 \text{ m} \cdot \text{min}^{-1} \times \frac{0.2 \text{ mL} \cdot \text{kg}^{-1} \cdot \text{min}^{-1}}{\text{m} \cdot \text{min}^{-1}}$$
$$+ 3.5 \text{ mL} \cdot \text{kg}^{-1} \cdot \text{min}^{-1} = 35.7 \times \text{mL} \cdot \text{kg}^{-1} \cdot \text{min}^{-1}$$

9. Subject No. 3

$$\dot{V}O_2cons = (4 \text{ kg} \times 6 \text{ m} \cdot \text{rev}^{-1}$$
$$\times 80 \text{ rev} \cdot \text{min}^{-1}) \times 2 \text{ mL} \cdot \text{kg}^{-1} \cdot \text{min}^{-1}$$
$$+ 3.5 \text{ mL} \cdot \text{kg}^{-1} \cdot \text{min}^{-1} \times 79.55 \text{ kg}$$
$$= 4118.43 \text{ mL} \cdot \text{min}^{-1} = 4.12 \text{ L} \cdot \text{min}^{-1}$$

Subject No. 4

$$\dot{V}O_2cons = (3 \text{ kg} \times 3 \text{ m} \cdot \text{rev}^{-1} \times 50 \text{ rev} \cdot \text{min}^{-1})$$
$$\times 3 \text{ mL} \cdot \text{kg}^{-1} \cdot \text{min}^{-1}$$
$$+ 3.5 \text{ mL} \cdot \text{kg}^{-1} \cdot \text{min}^{-1} \times 91.4 \text{ kg}$$
$$= 1669.8 \text{ mL} \cdot \text{min}^{-1} = 1.67 \text{ L} \cdot \text{min}^{-1}$$

10. Subject No. 2

$$\dot{V}O_2cons = 30 \text{ steps} \cdot \text{min}^{-1} \times \frac{0.35 \text{ mL} \cdot \text{kg}^{-1} \cdot \text{min}^{-1}}{\text{steps} \cdot \text{min}^{-1}}$$
$$+ 0.305 \text{ m} \cdot \text{step}^{-1} \times 30 \text{ steps} \cdot \text{min}^{-1}$$
$$\times \frac{1.8 \text{ mL} \cdot \text{kg}^{-1} \cdot \text{min}^{-1}}{\text{m} \cdot \text{min}^{-1}} \times 1.33$$
$$= 32.41 \text{ mL} \cdot \text{kg}^{-1} \cdot \text{min}^{-1}$$

11. Subject No. 1 PACER $\dot{V}O_2$max (Eq. B.17)

$$\dot{V}O_2max = 31.025 + 3.238 \ (10) - 3.248 \ (15)$$
$$+ 0.1536 \ (10 \times 15) = 37.73 \text{ mL} \cdot \text{kg}^{-1} \cdot \text{min}^{-1}$$

Subject No. 2 PACER $\dot{V}O_2$max (Eq. B.18)

$$\dot{V}O_2max = 14.4 - 3.48 \ (9) = 48.72 \text{ mL} \cdot \text{kg}^{-1} \cdot \text{min}^{-1}$$

Subject No. 3 PACER $\dot{V}O_2$max (Eq. B.18)

$$\dot{V}O_2max = 14.4 + 3.48 \ (16) = 70.08 \text{ mL} \cdot \text{kg}^{-1} \cdot \text{min}^{-1}$$

Subject No. 4 (RWFT)

$$\dot{V}O_2max = 132.853 - 0.0769(201) - 0.3877(58) + 6.3150(1)$$
$$- 3.2649 \ (17.6) - 0.1565 \ (108) = 26.86 \text{ mL} \cdot \text{kg}^{-1} \cdot \text{min}^{-1}$$

REFERENCES

1. American College of Sports Medicine: *Guidelines for Exercise Testing and Prescription* (5th edition). Baltimore: Williams & Williams (1995).

2. Jackson, A. S.: Application of regression analysis to exercise science. In M. J. Safrit & T. M. Wood (eds.), *Measurement Concepts in Physical Education and Exercise Science.* Champaign, IL: Human Kinetics Books (1989).

3. Kline, G. M., J. P. Porcari, R. Huntermeister, P. S. Freedson, A. Ward, R. F. McCarron, J. Ross, & J. M. Rippe: Estimation of VO₂max from a one mile track walk, gender, age, and body weight. *Medicine and Science in Sports and Exercise.* 19:253–259 (1987).

4. Leger, L. A., D. Mercier, C. Gadoury, & J. Lambert: The multistage 20 metre shuttle run test for aerobic fitness. *Journal of Sport Sciences.* 6:93–101 (1988).

5. Ramsbottom, R., J. Brewer, & C. Williams: A progressive shuttle run test to estimate maximal oxygen uptake. *British Journal of Sports Medicine.* 22(4): 141–144 (1988).

Glossary

Absolute Submaximal Workload A set exercise load performed at any intensity from just above resting to just below maximum.

Acclimatization The adaptive changes that occur when an individual undergoes prolonged or repeated exposure to a stressful environment; these changes reduce the physiological strain produced by such an environment.

Adenosine Triphosphate (ATP) Stored chemical energy that links the energy-yielding and energy-requiring functions within all cells.

Aerobic In the presence of, requiring, or utilizing oxygen.

Afterload Resistance presented to the contracting ventricle.

All-or-None Principle When a motor neuron is stimulated, all of the muscle fibers in that motor unit contract to their fullest extent or they do not contract at all.

Alveolar Ventilation ($\dot{V}_A$) The volume of air available for gas exchange; calculated as tidal volume minus dead space volume times frequency.

Amenorrhea The absence of menses.

Anabolic Steroids Synthetic androgens that mimic the effects of the male hormone testosterone.

Anaerobic In the absence of, not requiring, nor utilizing oxygen.

Anorexia Athletica An eating disorder occurring primarily in young, female athletes that is characterized by a food intake less than that required to support the training regimen and by body weight no more than 95% of normal.

Anorexia Nervosa An eating disorder characterized by marked self-induced weight loss accompanied by an intense fear of fatness and reproductive hormonal changes.

Apolipoprotein The protein portion of lipoproteins.

Archimedes' Principle The principle that a partially or fully submerged object will experience an upward buoyant force equal to the weight or the volume of fluid displaced by the object.

Arteriosclerosis The natural aging changes that occur in blood vessels—namely thickening of the walls, loss of elastic connective tissue, and hardening of the vessel wall.

Arteriovenous Oxygen Difference (a-vO_2 diff) The difference between the amount of oxygen returned in venous blood and the amount originally carried in arterial blood.

Atherosclerosis A pathological process that results in the buildup of plaque inside the blood vessels.

Ballistic Stretching A form of stretching, characterized by an action-reaction bouncing motion, in which the joints involved are placed into an extreme range of motion limits by fast, active contractions of agonistic muscle groups.

Basal Metabolic Rate (BMR) The level of energy required to sustain the body's vital functions in the waking state, when the individual is in a fasted condition, at normal body and room temperature, and without psychological stress.

Beta Oxidation A cyclic series of steps that breaks off successive pairs of carbon atoms from FFA, which are then used to form acetyl CoA.

Blood Pressure (BP) The force exerted on the wall of the blood vessel by the blood as a result of contraction of the heart (systole) or relaxation of the heart (diastole).

Body Composition The partitioning of body mass into fat-free mass (weight or percentage) and fat mass (weight or percentage).

Bone Modeling The process of altering the shape of bone by bone resorption and bone deposition.

Bone Remodeling The continual process of bone breakdown (resorption) and formation (deposition of new bone).

Bradycardia A heart rate less than $60 \text{ b} \cdot \text{min}^{-1}$.

Bulimia Nervosa An eating disorder marked by an unrealistic appraisal of body weight and/or shape that is manifested by alternating bingeing and purging behavior.

Caloric Balance Equation The mathematical summation of the caloric intake (+) and energy expenditure (−) from all sources.

Caloric Cost Energy expenditure of an activity performed for a specified period of time. It may be expressed as total calories (kcal), calories or kjoules per minute ($\text{kcal} \cdot \text{min}^{-1}$ or $\text{kJ} \cdot \text{min}^{-1}$) or relative to body weight ($\text{kcal} \cdot \text{kg}^{-1} \cdot \text{min}^{-1}$ or $\text{kJ} \cdot \text{kg}^{-1} \cdot \text{min}^{-1}$).

Caloric Equivalent The number of kilocalories produced per liter of oxygen consumed.

Calorimetry The measurement of heat energy liberated or absorbed in metabolic processes.

Capacitance Vessels Another name for veins, owing to their distensibility, which enables them to pool large volumes of blood and become reservoirs for blood.

Carbohydrate Loading (Glycogen Supercompensation) A process of nutritional modification that results in an additional storage of glycogen in muscle fiber that can be approximately three to four times the normal levels.

Carbon Dioxide Produced ($\dot{V}CO_2$) The amount of carbon dioxide generated during metabolism.

Cardiac Cycle One complete sequence of contraction and relaxation of the heart.

Cardiac Output The amount of blood pumped per unit of time, in liters per minute.

Cardiorespiratory Fitness The ability to deliver and use oxygen under the demands of intensive, prolonged exercise or work.

Cardiovascular Drift The changes in observed cardiovascular variables that occur during prolonged, heavy submaximal exercise without a change in workload.

Cellular Respiration The process by which cells transfer energy from food to ATP in a stepwise series of reactions; relies heavily upon the use of oxygen.

Central Cardiovascular Adaptations Adaptations that occur in the heart and contribute to an increased ability to deliver oxygen.

Cholesterol A derived fat that is essential for the body but may be detrimental in excessive amounts.

Coenzyme A A nonprotein substance derived from a vitamin that activates an enzyme.

Concentric Contraction A dynamic muscle contraction that produces tension during shortening.

Contractility The force of contraction of the heart. Also the ability of a muscle to respond to a stimuli by shortening.

Coupled Reactions Linked chemical processes in which a change in one substance is accompanied by a change in another.

Criterion Test The standard against which other tests are judged.

Cross-Bridging Cycle The sequence of events that are necessary for the generation of force or tension exerted by the myosin heads during muscle contraction.

Cross Training The development or maintenance of cardiovascular fitness by alternating between or concurrently training in two or more modalities.

Cutting Decreasing body fat and body water content to very low levels in order to increase muscle definition.

Delayed-Onset Muscle Soreness (DOMS) Muscle soreness that increases in intensity for the first 24 hr after activity, peaks from 24 to 28 hr, and then declines during the next 5 to 7 days.

Densitometry The measurement of mass per unit volume.

Diet (a) The food regularly consumed during the course of normal living; (b) a restriction of caloric intake.

Diffusion The tendency of gaseous, liquid, or solid molecules to move from areas of high concentration to areas of low concentration by constant random action.

Doppler Echocardiography A technique that calculates stroke volume from measurements of aortic cross-sectional area and time-velocity integrals in the ascending aorta.

Dynamic Contraction A muscle contraction in which the force exerted varies as the muscle shortens to accommodate change in muscle length and/or joint angle throughout the range of motion while moving a constant external load.

Eccentric Contraction A dynamic muscle contraction that produces tension (force) while lengthening.

Economy The oxygen cost of walking or running at varying speeds.

Ejection Fraction (EF) The percentage of LVEDV that is ejected from the heart.

Elasticity The ability of a muscle to return to resting length after being stretched.

Electromyography (EMG) The measurement of the neural or electrical activity that brings about muscle contraction.

Electron Transport System (ETS) The final metabolic pathway; it proceeds as a series of chemical reactions in the mitochondria that transfer electrons from the hydrogen atom carriers NAD and FAD to oxygen; water is formed as a by-product; the electrochemical energy released by the hydrogen ions is coupled to the formation of ATP from ADP and P_i.

Energy System Capacity The total amount of energy that can be produced by an energy system.

Energy System Power The maximal amount of energy that can be produced per unit of time.

Entrainment The synchronization of limb movement and breathing frequency that accompanies rhythmical exercise.

Enzyme A protein that accelerates the speed of a chemical reaction without itself being changed by the reaction.

Eupnea Normal respiration rate and rhythm.

Excess Postexercise Oxygen Consumption (EPOC) Oxygen consumption during recovery that is above normal resting values.

Excitation-Contraction Coupling The sequence of events by which an action potential in the sarco-lemma initiates the sliding of the myofilaments, resulting in contraction.

Exercise A single acute bout of bodily exertion or muscular activity that requires an expenditure of energy above resting level and that in most, but not all, cases results in voluntary movement.

Exercise-Induced Hypoxemia (EIH) A condition found in elite male endurance athletes in which the amount of oxygen carried in arterial blood is severely reduced.

Exercise Modality or Mode The type of activity or sport; usually classified by energy demand or type of muscle action.

Exercise Physiology A basic and an applied science that describes, explains, and uses the body's response to exercise and adaptation to exercise training to maximize human physical potential.

Extensibility The ability of a muscle to be stretched or lengthened.

External Respiration The exchange of gases between the lungs and the blood.

Fartlek Workout A type of training session, named from the Swedish word meaning "speed play," that combines the aerobic demands of a continuous run with the anaerobic demands of sporadic speed intervals.

Fast Glycolytic (FG) Fibers Fast-twitch muscle fibers that perform primarily under glycolytic conditions.

Fast Oxidative Glycolytic (FOG) Fibers Fast-twitch muscle fibers that have the ability to work under oxidative and glycolytic conditions.

Fat-Free Weight The weight of body tissue excluding extractable fat.

Fatigue Index (FI) Percentage of peak power drop-off during high-intensity, short-duration work.

Fick Equation An equation used to calculate cardiac output from oxygen consumption and arterio-venous oxygen difference (a-vO_2 diff).

Field Test A test that can be conducted anywhere; is performance-based and estimates the values measured by the criterion test.

First Law of Thermodynamics or the Law of Conservation of Energy Energy can neither be created nor destroyed but only changed in form.

Flavin Adenine Dinucleotide (FAD) A hydrogen carrier in cellular respiration.

Flexibility The range of motion in a joint or series of joints that reflects the ability of the musculotendon structures to elongate within the physical limits of the joint.

Food Efficiency An index of the amount of calories an individual needs to ingest in order to maintain a given weight or percent body fat.

Gluconeogenesis The creation of glucose in the liver from noncarbohydrate sources, particularly glycerol, lactate or pyruvate, and alanine.

Glycemic Index A measure that compares the elevation in blood glucose caused by the ingestion of 50 g of any carbohydrate food with the elevation caused by the ingestion of 50 g of white bread.

Glycogen Stored form of carbohydrate composed of chains of glucose molecules chemically linked together.

Glycogenolysis The process by which stored glycogen is broken down (hydrolyzed) to provide glucose.

Glycolysis The energy pathway responsible for the initial catabolism of glucose in a 10- or 11-step process that begins with glucose or glycogen and ends with the production of pyruvate (aerobic glycolysis) or lactate (anaerobic glycolysis).

Health-Related Physical Fitness That portion of physical fitness directed toward the prevention of or rehabilitation from disease as well as the development of a high level of functional capacity for the necessary and discretionary tasks of life.

Heart Rate (HR) The number of cardiac cycles per minute, expressed as beats per min ($b \cdot min^{-1}$).

Heat Illness A spectrum of disorders that range in intensity and severity from mild cardiovascular and central nervous system disruptions to severe cell damage, including the brain, kidney, and liver.

Heat Stress Index A scale used to determine the risk of heat stress from measures of ambient temperature and relative humidity.

Hematocrit The ratio of blood cells to total blood volume, expressed as a percentage.

Hemoglobin (Hb) The protein portion of the red blood cell that binds with oxygen, consisting of four iron-containing pigments called hemes and a protein called globin.

High-Density Lipoprotein (HDL) A lipoprotein in blood plasma composed primarily of protein and a minimum of cholesterol or triglyceride whose purpose is to transport cholesterol from the tissues to the liver.

Hydrolysis A chemical process in which a substance is split into simpler compounds by the addition of water.

Hydrostatic Weighing Criterion measure for determining body composition through the calculation of body density.

Hydroxyapatite Calcium and phosphate salts that are responsible for the hardness of the bone matrix.

Hyperplasia Growth in a tissue or organ through an increase in the number of cells.

Hyperpnea Increased pulmonary ventilation that matches an increased metabolic demand, as in an exercise situation.

Hypertension High blood pressure, defined as values equal to or greater than 140/90 mmHg.

Hyperventilation Increased pulmonary ventilation, especially ventilation that exceeds metabolic requirements; carbon dioxide is blown off, leading to a decrease in its partial pressure in arterial blood.

Hypokinetic Diseases Diseases caused by and/or associated with lack of physical activity.

Immune System A precisely ordered system of cells, hormones, and chemicals that regulate susceptibility to, severity of, and recovery from infection and illness.

Intercalated Discs The junction between cardiac muscle cells that forms the mechanical and electrical connection between the two cells.

Internal Respiration The exchange of gases at the cellular level.

Interval Training An aerobic and/or anaerobic workout that consists of three elements: a selected work interval (usually a distance), a target time for that distance, and a predetermined recovery period before the next repetition of the work interval.

Irritability The ability of a muscle to receive and respond to stimuli.

Isokinematic Contraction A muscle contraction in which the rate of limb displacement or joint rotation is held constant with the use of specialized equipment.

Isokinetic Contraction A muscle fiber contraction in which the velocity of the contraction is kept constant.

Isometric Contraction A muscle fiber contraction that does not result in a length change in muscle fiber.

Isotonic Contraction A muscle fiber contraction in which the tension generated by the muscle is constant through the range of motion.

Kilocalorie The amount of heat needed to raise the temperature of 1 kg of water 1°C.

Krebs Cycle A series of eight chemical reactions that begins and ends with the same substance; energy is liberated for direct substrate phosphorylation of ATP from ADP and P_i; carbon dioxide is formed and hydrogen atoms removed and carried by NAD and FAD to the electron transport system; does not directly utilize oxygen but requires its presence.

Laboratory Test Precise, direct measurement of physiological functions for the assessment of exercise responses or training adaptations; usually involves monitoring, collection, and analysis of expired air, blood, or electrical signals.

Lactate Thresholds Points on the linear-curvilinear continuum of lactate accumulation that appear to indicate sharp rises, often labeled as the first (LT1) and second (LT2) lactate threshold.

Left Ventricular End–Diastolic Volume (LVEDV) The volume of blood in the left ventricle at the end of diastole.

Left Ventricular End–Systolic Volume (LVESV) The volume of blood in the left ventricle at the end of systole.

Lipoprotein Water-soluble compound composed of apolipoprotein and lipid components that transport fat in the bloodstream.

Long Slow Distance (LSD) Workout A continuous aerobic training session performed at a steady-state pace for an extended period of time or distance.

Low-Density Lipoprotein (LDL) A lipoprotein in blood plasma composed of protein, a small portion of triglyceride, and a large portion of cholesterol whose purpose is to transport cholesterol to the cells.

Maximal Exercise The highest intensity, greatest load, or longest duration exercise of which an individual is capable.

Maximal Oxygen Consumption ($\dot{V}O_2$max) The highest amount of oxygen an individual can take in and utilize to produce ATP aerobically while breathing air during heavy exercise.

Maximal Voluntary Contraction The maximal force (100%) that a muscle can exert.

Mean Power (MP) The average power (force times distance divided by time) exerted during short- (typically 30 sec) duration work.

Mechanical Efficiency The percentage of energy input that appears as useful external work.

MET A unit that represents the metabolic equivalent in multiples of the resting rate of oxygen consumption of any given activity.

Metabolic Pathway A sequence of enzyme-mediated chemical reactions resulting in a specified product.

Metabolism The total of all energy transformations that occur in the body.

Minerals Elements not of animal or plant origin which are essential constituents of all cells and of many functions in the body.

Minute Ventilation (Minute Volume) ($\dot{V}_I$ or $\dot{V}_E$) The amount of air inspired or expired each minute; the pulmonary ventilation rate per minute; calculated as tidal volume times frequency of breathing.

Mitochondria Cell organelles in which the Krebs cycle, electron transport, and oxidative phosphorylation take place.

Motor Unit A motor neuron and the muscle fibers it innervates.

Muscle Tonus A state of low-level muscle contraction at rest.

Muscular Endurance The ability of a muscle or muscle group to repeatedly exert force against a resistance.

Myoclonus A twitching or spasm in the muscle group that is maximally stretched.

Myofibril Contractile structures composed of myofilaments.

Myofilaments Contractile (thick and thin) proteins that are responsible for muscle contraction.

Nicotinamide Adenine Dinucleotide (NAD) A hydrogen carrier in cellular respiration.

Non-Weight-Bearing Exercise A movement performed in which the body weight is supported or suspended and thereby not working against the pull of gravity.

Osteoblasts Bone cells that cause the deposition of bone tissue (bone-forming cells).

Osteoclasts Bone cells that cause the resorption of bone tissue (bone-destroying cells).

Osteocytes Mature osteoblasts surrounded by calcified bone that help regulate the process of bone remodeling.

Osteopenia A condition of decreased bone mineral density (BMD), diagnosed when BMD is greater than one standard deviation (SD) below (but not more than 2.5 SD below) values for young, normal adults.

Osteoporosis A condition of porosity and decreased bone mineral density that is defined as a BMD greater than 2.5 standard deviations (SD) below values for young, normal adults.

Overtraining A state of overstress or failure to adapt to an exercise training load.

Oxidation A gain of oxygen, a loss of hydrogen, or the direct loss or electrons by an atom or substance.

Oxidative Phosphorylation (OP) The process in which NADH   H   and FADH$_2$ are oxidized in the electron transport system and the energy released is used to synthesize ATP from ADP and P$_i$.

Oxygen Consumption ($\dot{V}O_2$) The amount of oxygen taken up, transported, and used at the cellular level.

Oxygen Deficit The difference between the oxygen required during exercise and the oxygen supplied and utilized. Occurs at the onset of all activity.

Oxygen Dissociation The separation or release of oxygen from the red blood cells to the tissues.

Oxygen Drift A situation that occurs in submaximal activity of long duration, or above 70% $\dot{V}O_2$max, or in hot and humid conditions where the oxygen consumption increases, despite the fact that the oxygen requirement of the activity has not changed.

Partial Pressure of a Gas (P$_G$) The pressure exerted by an individual gas in a mixture; determined by multiplying the fraction of the gas by the total barometric pressure.

Peak Power (PP) The maximum power (force times distance divided by time) exerted during very short (5 sec or less) duration work.

Percent Saturation of Hemoglobin (SbO$_2$%) The ratio of the amount of oxygen combined with hemoglobin to the total oxygen capacity for combining with hemoglobin, expressed as a percentage; indicated generally as SbO$_2$% or specifically as SaO$_2$% for arterial blood or as SvO$_2$% for venous blood.

Perfusion of the Lung Pulmonary circulation, especially capillary blood flow.

Periodization Plans for training based on a manipulation of the fitness components with the intent of peaking the athlete for the competitive season or varying health-related fitness training in cycles of harder or easier training.

Peripheral Cardiovascular Adaptations Adaptations that occur in the vasculature or the muscles that contribute to an increased ability to extract oxygen.

Physical Fitness A physiological state of well-being that provides the foundation for the tasks of daily living, a degree of protection against hypokinetic disease, and a basis for participation in sport.

Power The amount of work done per unit of time; the product of force and velocity; the ability to exert force quickly.

Preload Volume of blood returned to the heart.

Pressor Response The rapid increase in both systolic pressure and diastolic pressure during static exercise.

Proprioceptive Neuromuscular Facilitation (PNF) A stretching technique in which the muscle to be stretched is first contracted maximally. The muscle is then relaxed and is either actively stretched by contraction of the opposing muscle or is passively stretched.

Pulmonary Ventilation   The process by which air is moved into the lungs.

Reciprocal Inhibition   The reflex relaxation of the antagonist muscle in response to the contraction of the agonist.

Reduction   A loss of oxygen, a gain of electrons, or a gain of hydrogen by an atom or substance.

Reflex   Rapid, involuntary response to a stimuli in which a specific stimulus results in a specific motor response.

Relative Humidity   The moisture in the air relative to how much moisture, or water vapor, can be held by the air at any given ambient temperature.

Relative Submaximal Workload   A workload above resting but below maximum that is prorated to each individual; typically set as some percentage of maximum.

Residual Volume (RV)   The amount of air left in the lungs following a maximal exhalation.

Resistance Training   A systematic program of exercises involving the exertion of force against a load used to develop strength, endurance, and/or hypertrophy of the muscular system.

Resistance Vessels   Another name for arterioles due to their ability to vasodilate and vasoconstrict; changing diameter allows them to control the flow of blood.

Resistance   The factors that oppose blood flow.

Respiratory Cycle   Inspiration and expiration.

Respiratory Exchange Ratio (RER)   The ratio of the volume of CO_2 produced divided by the volume of O_2 consumed.

Respiratory Quotient (RQ)   The ratio of the amount of carbon dioxide produced divided by the amount of oxygen consumed at the cellular level.

Resting Metabolic Rate (RMR)   The energy expended while an individual is resting quietly in a supine position.

Risk Factor   An aspect of personal behavior or lifestyle, an environmental exposure, or an inher-

ited characteristic that has been shown by epidemiological evidence to predispose an individual to the development of a specific disease.

Sarcomere   The functional unit (contractile unit) of muscle fibers.

Sarcoplasmic Reticulum (SR)   The specialized muscle cell organelle that stores calcium.

Skinfolds   The double thickness of skin plus the adipose tissue between the parallel layers of skin.

Sliding Filament Theory of Muscle Contraction   The theory that explains muscle contraction as the result of the myofilaments sliding over one another.

Slow Oxidative (SO) Fibers   Slow-twitch muscle fibers that rely primarily on oxidative metabolism to produce energy.

Spirometry   An indirect calorimetry method for estimating heat production or calorimetry in which expired air is measured and analyzed for the amount of oxygen consumed and carbon dioxide produced.

Sport-Specific Physical Fitness   That portion of physical fitness which is directed toward optimizing athletic performance.

Sports Anemia   A transient decrease in red blood cells and hemoglobin levels (grams per deciliter of blood).

Static Contraction   A muscle contraction that produces an increase in muscle tension but does not cause meaningful limb displacement or joint displacement and therefore does not result in movement of the skeleton.

Static Stretching   A form of stretching in which the muscle to be stretched is slowly put into a position of controlled maximal or near-maximal stretch by contraction of the opposing muscle group and held for 30–60 sec.

Steady State   A condition in which the energy expenditure provided during exercise is balanced with the energy required to perform that exercise and factors responsible for the provision of this energy reach elevated levels of equilibrium.

Strength   The ability of a muscle or muscle group to exert maximal force against a resistance in a single repetition.

Stress The state manifested by the specific syndrome that consists of all the nonspecifically induced changes within a biological system; a disruption in body homeostasis and all attempts by the body to regain homeostasis.

Stress Fracture A fine hairline break in bone that occurs in the absence of acute trauma, is clinically symptomatic, and is detectable by X rays or bone scans.

Stress Reactions Maladaptive areas of bone hyperactivity where the balance between resorption and deposition is progressively lost such that resorption exceeds deposition.

Stroke Volume (SV) Amount of blood ejected from the ventricles with each beat of the heart.

Substrate A substance acted upon by an enzyme.

Substrate-Level Phosphorylation The transfer of P_i directly from a phosphorylated intermediate or substrates to ADP without any oxidation occurring.

Syncytium The individual cells of the myocardium that function collectively as a unit during depolarization.

Thermic Effect of a Meal (TEM) The increased heat production as a result of food ingestion.

Thermogenesis The production of heat.

Tidal Volume (V_T) The amount of air that is inspired or expired in a normal breath.

Torque The capability of a force to produce rotation.

Total Lung Capacity (TLC) The greatest amount of air that the lungs can contain.

Tracking A phenomenon in which a characteristic is maintained, in terms of relative rank, over a long time span or even a lifetime.

Training A consistent or chronic progression of exercise sessions designed to improve physiological function for better health or sport performance.

Training Adaptations Physiological changes or adjustments resulting from an exercise training program that promote optimal functioning.

Training Principles Fundamental guidelines that form the basis for the development of an exercise training program.

Training Taper A reduction in training prior to important competitions that is intended to allow the athlete to recover from previous hard training, maintain physiological conditioning, and improve performance.

Training Volume The total amount of work done, usually expressed as mileage or load.

Transamination The transfer of the NH_2 amino group from an amino acid to a keto acid.

Transverse Tubules (T tubules) Organelles that carry the electrical signal from the sarcolemma into the interior of the cell.

Type A Behavior Pattern (TABP) Behavior that is characterized by hard-driving competitiveness; time urgency, haste, and impatience; a workaholic lifestyle; and hostility.

Type B Behavior Pattern (TBBP) Behavior associated with characteristics of relaxation without guilt and no sense of time urgency.

Valsalva Maneuver Breath-holding that involves closing of the glottis and contraction of the diaphragm and abdominal musculature.

Velocity at $\dot{V}O_2$max The speed at which an individual can run when working at his or her maximal oxygen consumption; based both on submaximal running economy and $\dot{V}O_2$max.

Ventilatory Thresholds Points where the rectilinear rise in minute ventilation breaks from linearity during an incremental exercise to maximum.

Vital Capacity (VC) The greatest amount of air that can be exhaled following a maximal inhalation.

Vitamins Organic substances of plant or animal origin which are essential for normal growth, development, metabolic processes, and energy transformations.

Voluntary Dehydration Exercise-induced dehydration that develops despite an individual's access to unlimited water.

Weight Cycling Repeated bouts of weight loss and regain.

Weight-Bearing Exercise A movement performed in which the body weight is supported by muscles and bones.

Index

PHOTO CREDITS

P. 1: Will Hart; p. 18: David Madison/Tony Stone Images; p. 20: Robert Harbison; p. 29: Courtesy of Northern Illinois University Media Services; p. 40: CNRI/SPL/Photo Researchers; p. 47: Tony Neste; p. 79: Brian Smith; p. 111: Dugald Bremner/Tony Stone Images; p. 142: Robert Harbison; p. 210: Will Hart; p. 221: K. R. Porter/Photo Researchers; p. 229: Professor P. Motta/Department of Anatomy, University "La Spienza" Rome/Science Photo Library/Photo Researchers; p. 243: Mike Powell/Tony Stone Images; p. 247: Will Hart (left), Courtesy of Northern Illinois University Media Services (right); p. 249: Courtesy of Northern Illinois University Media Services; p. 264: Will Faller; p. 267: Robert Daemmrich/Tony Stone Images; p. 274: Amwell/Tony Stone Images; p. 277: Courtesy of Northern Illinois University Media Services; p. 294: Will Hart; p. 309: Will Hart; p. 351: Brian Smith; p. 355: Yoav Levy/Phototake NY; p. 359: Tony Neste; p. 361: Courtesy of Northern Illinois University Media Services; p. 375: Will Hart; p. 395: Brian Smith; p. 400: Will Hart; p. 415: Custom Medical Stock; p. 423: Tony Neste; p. 425: Lewis Portney/The Stock Market; p. 430: Biology Media/Science Source/Photo Researchers; p. 437: Biology Media/Science Source/Photo Researchers; p. 445: Sohm/Chromosohn/Stock Market; p. 462: Courtesy of Northern Illinois University Media Services; p. 463: Will Hart; p. 471: David Madison/Tony Stone Images; p. 477: Bill Aron/Tony Stone Images; p. 485: Warren Bolster/Tony Stone Images; p. 500: Courtesy of Northern Illinois University Media Services.